Pediatric Ophthalmology and Strabismus

Section 6

2004–2005

(Last major revision 2002–2003)

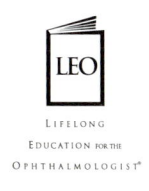

BASIC AND CLINICAL SCIENCE COURSE

AMERICAN ACADEMY
OF OPHTHALMOLOGY
The Eye M.D. Association

LEO
LIFELONG
EDUCATION FOR THE
OPHTHALMOLOGIST

The Basic and Clinical Science Course is one component of the Lifelong Education for the Ophthalmologist (LEO) framework, which assists members in planning their continuing medical education. LEO includes an array of clinical education products that members may select to form individualized, self-directed learning plans for updating their clinical knowledge. Active members or fellows who use LEO components may accumulate sufficient CME credits to earn the LEO Award. Contact the Academy's Clinical Education Division for further information on LEO.

> The American Academy of Ophthalmology is accredited by the Accreditation Council for Continuing Medical Education to provide continuing medical education for physicians.
>
> The American Academy of Ophthalmology designates this educational activity for a maximum of 40 category 1 credits toward the AMA Physician's Recognition Award. Each physician should claim only those hours of credit that he/she actually spent in the activity.
>
> The American Medical Association has determined that non-US licensed physicians who participate in this CME activity are elegible for AMA PRA category 1 credit.

The Academy provides this material for educational purposes only. It is not intended to represent the only or best method or procedure in every case, nor to replace a physician's own judgment or give specific advice for case management. Including all indications, contraindications, side effects, and alternative agents for each drug or treatment is beyond the scope of this material. All information and recommendations should be verified, prior to use, with current information included in the manufacturers' package inserts or other independent sources, and considered in light of the patient's condition and history. Reference to certain drugs, instruments, and other products in this publication is made for illustrative purposes only and is not intended to constitute an endorsement of such. Some material may include information on applications that are not considered community standard, that reflect indications not included in approved FDA labeling, or that are approved for use only in restricted research settings. The FDA has stated that it is the responsibility of the physician to determine the FDA status of each drug or device he or she wishes to use, and to use them with appropriate patient consent in compliance with applicable law. The Academy specifically disclaims any and all liability for injury or other damages of any kind, from negligence or otherwise, for any and all claims that may arise from the use of any recommendations or other information contained herein.

Copyright © 2004
American Academy of Ophthalmology
All rights reserved
Printed in the United States of America

Basic and Clinical Science Course

Thomas J. Liesegang, MD, Jacksonville, Florida, *Senior Secretary for Clinical Education*
Gregory L. Skuta, MD, Oklahoma City, Oklahoma, *Secretary for Ophthalmic Knowledge*
Louis B. Cantor, MD, Indianapolis, Indiana, *BCSC Course Chair*

Section 6

Faculty Responsible for This Edition

John W. Simon, MD, *Chair*, Albany, New York
Edward G. Buckley, MD, Durham, North Carolina
Arlene V. Drack, MD, Atlanta, Georgia
Amy K. Hutchinson, MD, Charleston, South Carolina
David A. Plager, MD, Indianapolis, Indiana
Edward L. Raab, MD, New York, New York
Mark S. Ruttum, MD, Milwaukee, Wisconsin
Aazy A. Aaby, MD, Portland, Oregon
   Practicing Ophthalmologists Advisory Committee for Education

Each author states that he or she has no significant financial interest or other relationship with the manufacturer of any commercial product discussed in the chapters that he or she contributed to this publication or with the manufacturer of any competing commercial product.

Recent Past Faculty

Carol G. Blackwell, MD
Joseph H. Calhoun, MD
Monte A. Del Monte, MD
Allan M. Eisenbaum, MD
David S. Friendly, MD
J. Allen Gammon, MD
Mark J. Greenwald, MD
Jane D. Kivlin, MD
Elbert H. Magoon, MD
Marilyn B. Mets, MD

Marilyn T. Miller, MD
R. Hugh Minor, MD
Ronald L. Price, MD
James M. Richard, MD
Paul E. Romano, MD
William E. Scott, MD
Wilson K. Wallace, MD
M. Edward Wilson, MD
Kenneth W. Wright, MD

In addition, the Academy gratefully acknowledges the contributions of numerous past faculty and advisory committee members who have played an important role in the development of previous editions of the Basic and Clinical Science Course.

American Academy of Ophthalmology Staff

Richard A. Zorab, *Vice President, Ophthalmic Knowledge*
Hal Straus, *Director, Publications Department*
Carol L. Dondrea, *Publications Editor*
Christine Arturo, *Acquisitions Editor*
Maxine Garrett, *Administrative Coordinator*

Cover design: Paula Shuhert Design
Cover photograph: Choroidal folds, by Patrick J. Saine, MEd, CRA, Dartmouth-Hitchcock Medical Center

AMERICAN ACADEMY OF OPHTHALMOLOGY
The Eye M.D. Association

655 Beach Street
Box 7424
San Francisco, CA 94120-7424

Contents

General Introduction xvii

Objectives 1
Introduction: Rapport With Children: Tips for a Productive Examination 3
Preparation 3
The Examination 3
Eye Drops 5
Use of Anesthesia for Foreign Body Removal 5

PART I   Strabismus 7

1   Introduction to Strabismus 9
Terminology 9
   Prefixes 9
   Suffixes 10
   Usage 10
Classification 10
   Fusional Status 10
   Variation of the Deviation With Gaze Position or Fixating Eye 10
   Fixation 11
   Age of Onset 11
   Type of Deviation 11
   Abbreviated Designations for Types of Strabismus 11

2   Anatomy of the Extraocular Muscles and Their Fascia 13
Origin, Course, Insertion, Innervation, and Action of the Extraocular Muscles 13
   Horizontal Rectus Muscles 13
   Vertical Rectus Muscles 14
   Oblique Muscles 14
   Levator Palpebrae Superioris Muscle 16
   Insertion Relationships of the Rectus Muscles 17
Blood Supply of the Extraocular Muscles 17
   Arterial System 17
   Venous System 18
Fine Structure of the Extraocular Muscles 18
   Fiber Types 19
Orbital and Fascial Relationships 22
   Tenon's Capsule (the Fascia Bulbi) 22

Muscle Cone 24
Muscle Capsule 24
Intermuscular Septum (Membrane) 25
Lockwood's Ligament 25
Adipose Tissue 25
Anatomical Implications 25

3 Motor Physiology 29
Basic Principles and Terms 29
Axes of Fick, Center of Rotation, Listing's Plane,
and Median Plane 29
Positions of Gaze 30
Arc of Contact 30
Primary, Secondary, and Tertiary Action 30
Field of Action 30
Changing Muscle Action With Different Gaze Positions 31
Physiology of Muscle 32
Eye Movements 33
Monocular Eye Movements (Ductions) 33
Binocular Eye Movements (Versions and Vergences) 33
Supranuclear Control Systems for Eye Movement 36

4 Sensory Physiology and Pathology 39
Physiology of Normal Binocular Vision 39
Correspondence 39
Fusion 40
Selected Aspects of the Neurophysiology of Vision ...42
Retino-Geniculo-Cortical Pathway 42
Visual Development 44
Effects of Abnormal Visual Experience on the
Retino-Geniculo-Cortical Pathway 46
Abnormalities of Binocular Vision 49
Confusion 49
Diplopia 49
Sensory Adaptations in Strabismus 50
Suppression 50
Anomalous Retinal Correspondence 51
Monofixation Syndrome 53
Subjective Testing for Suppression and Anomalous Retinal
Correspondence 54

5 Amblyopia 63
Classification 64
Strabismic Amblyopia 64
Anisometropic Amblyopia 65
Amblyopia Due to Bilateral High Refractive Errors (Isometropia) ...65
Deprivation Amblyopia 65
Diagnosis 66

Treatment 67
    Cataract Removal 67
    Refractive Correction 67
    Occlusion and Optical Degradation 67
    Complications of Therapy 69

6 Diagnostic Techniques for Strabismus and Amblyopia 71

History and Characteristics of the Presenting Complaint 71
Assessment of Visual Acuity 72
    Distance Visual Acuity 72
    Near Visual Acuity 74
Assessment of Eye Movements 74
    Tests of Ocular Alignment 74
    Confounding Factors in Ocular Alignment Assessment 80
    Positions of Gaze 80
    Convergence 81
    Fusional Vergence 82
    Tests of Binocular Sensory Cooperation 83
    Special Motor Tests 84
    Three-Step Test 85
    Cycloplegic Refraction 87
    Prism Adaptation Test 88

7 Esodeviations 91

Pseudoesotropia 91
Infantile (Congenital) Esotropia 91
    Classic Congenital (Essential Infantile) Esotropia 91
    Nystagmus and Esotropia 94
Accommodative Esotropia 95
    Refractive Accommodative Esotropia 96
    Nonrefractive Accommodative Esotropia 96
    Partially Accommodative Esotropia 98
Nonaccommodative Acquired Esotropia 99
    Basic (Acquired) Esotropia 99
    Acute Esotropia 99
    Cyclic Esotropia 100
    Sensory Deprivation Esodeviation 100
    Divergence Insufficiency 100
    Spasm of the Near Synkinetic Reflex 101
    Surgical (Consecutive) Esodeviation 101
Incomitant Esodeviation 101
    Sixth Nerve (Abducens) Paralysis 101
    Other Forms of Incomitant Esodeviation 103

8 Exodeviations 105

Pseudoexotropia 105
Exophoria 105

Intermittent Exotropia 105
    Clinical Characteristics 106
    Clinical Evaluation 107
    Nonsurgical Management 108
    Surgical Treatment 109
Constant Exotropia 111
    Congenital Exotropia 111
    Sensory Exotropia 112
    Consecutive Exotropia 112
    Exotropic Duane (Retraction) Syndrome 112
    Neuromuscular Abnormalities 112
    Dissociated Horizontal Deviation 112
Convergence Insufficiency 113
Convergence Paralysis 114

9 Vertical Deviations 115

Inferior Oblique Muscle Overaction 115
    Clinical Features 115
    Management 116
Superior Oblique Muscle Overaction 116
    Clinical Features 117
    Management 117
Dissociated Vertical Deviation 118
    Clinical Features 118
    Management 119
Superior Oblique Muscle Palsy (or Paresis) 119
    Clinical Features 120
    Management 120
Brown Syndrome 123
    Clinical Features 123
    Management 124
Inferior Oblique Muscle Palsy 125
    Clinical Features 125
    Management 125
Monocular Elevation Deficiency (Double Elevator Palsy) 125
    Clinical Features 126
    Management 126
Orbital Floor Fractures 127
    Clinical Features 128
    Management 129

10 A and V Patterns 131

Clinical Features 131
Management 132
Sample Treatment Plans for the Various Patterns 135
    V-Pattern Esotropia 135
    V-Pattern Exotropia 136
    A-Pattern Esotropia 136
    A-Pattern Exotropia 136

11 Special Forms of Strabismus ... **137**
- Duane Syndrome ... 137
  - Clinical Features ... 138
  - Management ... 139
- Third Cranial Nerve (Oculomotor) Palsy ... 140
  - Clinical Features ... 140
  - Management ... 140
- Graves Eye Disease (Thyroid Ophthalmopathy) ... 141
  - Clinical Features ... 141
  - Management ... 142
- Chronic Progressive External Ophthalmoplegia ... 143
  - Clinical Features ... 143
  - Management ... 143
- Myasthenia Gravis ... 143
  - Clinical Features ... 144
  - Management ... 144
- Congenital Fibrosis Syndrome ... 145
  - Clinical Features ... 146
  - Management ... 146
- Möbius Syndrome (Sequence) ... 147
  - Clinical Features ... 147
  - Management ... 147
- Internuclear Ophthalmoplegia ... 147
  - Clinical Features ... 147
  - Management ... 148
  - Congenital Ocular Motor Apraxia ... 148
  - Clinical Features ... 148
- Special Settings for Strabismus ... 148

12 Childhood Nystagmus ... **151**
- Nomenclature ... 151
- Evaluation ... 152
  - History ... 152
  - Ocular Examination ... 152
- Childhood Nystagmus Types ... 155
  - Congenital Nystagmus ... 155
  - Acquired Nystagmus ... 158
  - Differential Diagnosis ... 160
- Treatment ... 160
  - Prisms ... 160
  - Nystagmus Surgery ... 162

13 Surgery of the Extraocular Muscles ... **165**
- Indications for Surgery ... 165
- Surgical Techniques for the Muscles and Tendons ... 166
  - Weakening Procedures ... 166
  - Strengthening Procedures ... 166
  - Adjustable Suture Techniques ... 167

x • Contents

       Transposition Procedures 168
    Considerations in Planning Surgery for Strabismus 169
       Incomitance 169
       Prior Surgery 169
       Cyclovertical Strabismus 170
       Visual Acuity 170
    Guidelines for Strabismus Surgery 170
       Esodeviation 170
       Exodeviation 171
       Oblique Muscle-Weakening Procedures 172
       Vertical Rectus Muscle Surgery for Hypotropia and Hypertropia . . 173
       Other Rectus Muscle Surgery 174
    Anesthesia for Extraocular Muscle Surgery 175
    Conjunctival Incisions 175
       Fornix Incision 175
       Limbal or Peritomy Incision 176
    Complications of Strabismus Surgery 176
       Unsatisfactory Alignment 176
       Refractive Changes 176
       Diplopia 176
       Perforation of the Sclera 177
       Postoperative Infections 178
       Foreign Body Granuloma and Allergic Reaction 178
       Conjunctival Inclusion Cyst 179
       Conjunctival Scarring 179
       Adherence Syndrome 180
       Dellen 180
       Anterior Segment Ischemia 180
       Change in Eyelid Position 181
       Lost Muscle 182
       Slipped Muscle 182
       Postoperative Nausea and Vomiting 183
       Oculocardiac Reflex 183
       Malignant Hyperthermia 183

14 Chemodenervation Treatment of Strabismus and Blepharospasm Using Botulinum Toxin 187

Pharmacology and Mechanism of Action 187
Indications, Techniques, and Results 187
    Strabismus Correction 187
Complications 188

PART II Pediatric Ophthalmology 189

Introduction to Part II: Growth and Development of the Child's Eye 191

Evaluation of the Child With Congenital or Juvenile Ocular
    Anomalies 192

15 Congenital Anomalies ... **195**
Glossary ... 196

16 Eyelid Disorders ... **197**
Cryptophthalmos ... 197
Congenital Coloboma of the Eyelid ... 197
Ankyloblepharon ... 197
Congenital Ectropion ... 197
Congenital Entropion ... 198
Epiblepharon ... 198
Congenital Tarsal Kink ... 198
Distichiasis ... 199
Euryblepharon ... 199
Epicanthus ... 199
Telecanthus ... 200
Palpebral Fissure Slants ... 200
Blepharophimosis, Epicanthus Inversus, Telecanthus, and Ptosis (Kohn-Ramono Syndrome) ... 201
Ptosis (Blepharoptosis) ... 201
Marcus Gunn Jaw Winking ... 202

17 Infectious and Allergic Ocular Diseases ... **203**
Intrauterine and Perinatal Infections of the Eye ... 203
   Toxoplasmosis ... 203
   Rubella (German Measles) ... 205
   Cytomegalovirus (Cytomegalic Inclusion Disease) ... 206
   Herpes Simplex ... 207
   Syphilis ... 208
Ophthalmia Neonatorum ... 209
   Etiology ... 209
   Most Important Agents ... 209
   Prophylaxis for Ophthalmia Neonatorum ... 211
Conjunctivitis ... 211
   Bacterial Conjunctivitis ... 211
   Viral Conjunctivitis ... 212
   Other Types of Conjunctivitis ... 216
Orbital and Adnexal Infections ... 217
   Preseptal Cellulitis ... 217
   Orbital Cellulitis ... 218
Ocular Allergy ... 220
   Seasonal Allergic Conjunctivitis ... 220
   Vernal Keratoconjunctivitis ... 221
   Atopic Keratoconjunctivitis ... 222
Stevens-Johnson Syndrome (Erythema Multiforme) ... 223
   Treatment ... 224
Kawasaki Syndrome ... 224

18 The Lacrimal Drainage System 227
- Developmental Anomalies 227
  - Atresia of the Lacrimal Puncta 227
  - Supernumerary Puncta 228
  - Congenital Lacrimal Fistula 228
- Dacryocele 228
  - Clinical Features 228
  - Management 229
- Nasolacrimal Duct Obstruction 229
  - Clinical Features 229
  - Nonsurgical Management 230
  - Surgical Management 231

19 Diseases of the Cornea and Anterior Segment 237
- Embryology of the Cornea and Anterior Segment 237
- Congenital Corneal Anomalies 238
  - Abnormalities of Corneal Size and Shape 238
  - Anterior Segment Dysgenesis: Peripheral Developmental Abnormalities 239
  - Anterior Segment Dysgenesis: Central Developmental Abnormalities 241
- Infantile Corneal Opacities 242
  - Treatment 245
- Systemic Diseases With Corneal Manifestations in Childhood . . . 246

20 Iris Abnormalities 249
- Aniridia 249
- Coloboma of the Iris 250
- Iris Nodules 251
  - Lisch Nodules 251
  - Juvenile Xanthogranuloma 252
- Primary Iris Cysts 252
  - Cysts of Iris Pigment Epithelium 252
  - Central (Pupillary) Cysts 253
  - Cysts of Iris Stroma 253
- Secondary Iris Cysts 253
- Brushfield Spots (Wofflin Nodules) 254
- Heterochromia Iridis 254
- Persistent Pupillary Membranes 255
- Abnormalities in the Size, Shape, or Location of the Pupil 255
  - Congenital Miosis 255
  - Congenital Mydriasis 256
  - Dyscoria 256
  - Corectopia 256
  - Polycoria and Pseudopolycoria 256
- Congenital Iris Ectropion 257
- Iris Transillumination 257
- Posterior Synechiae 258

21 Pediatric Glaucomas 259
Primary Congenital Glaucoma 259
Genetics 259
Pathophysiology 260
Clinical Manifestations and Diagnosis 260
Natural History 264
Other Primary Developmental and Secondary Pediatric Glaucomas . . 265
Primary Developmental Glaucomas 265
Secondary Glaucoma 266
Treatment 266
Surgical Therapy 267
Medical Therapy 267
Prognosis and Follow-Up 269

22 Childhood Cataracts and Other Pediatric Lens Disorders 271
Structural or Positional Lens Abnormalities 271
Dislocated Lenses in Children 273
Treatment 276
Pediatric Cataracts 277
Onset 278
Location 278
Morphologic Types of Cataracts 279
Evaluation 282
History 283
Visual Function 283
Anterior Segment Evaluation 283
Funduscopic Examination 284
Workup 284
Surgery 284
Lensectomy (No Intraocular Lens) 284
Intraocular Lens Implant 286
Postoperative Care 288
Visual Outcome After Cataract Extraction . . . 288

23 Uveitis in the Pediatric Age Group 291
Classification 291
Clinical Features 291
Anterior Uveitis 292
Juvenile Rheumatoid Arthritis 293
Trauma 295
Sarcoidosis 295
Diseases Related to HLA-B27 296
Herpetic Iridocyclitis 297
Sympathetic Ophthalmia 297
Syphilis 297
Other Causes 297
Intermediate Uveitis (Pars Planitis) 297

Posterior Uveitis 299
    Toxoplasmosis 299
    Ocular Histoplasmosis 300
    Toxocariasis 300
    Other Causes 301
Masquerade Syndromes 301
Treatment of Uveitis in Children 301
    Medical Treatment 301
    Surgical Treatment 303

24 Vitreous and Retinal Diseases and Disorders 305

Leukocoria 305
    Persistent Hyperplastic Primary Vitreous 306
    Retinopathy of Prematurity 307
    Coats Disease 314
Hereditary Retinal Disease 315
    Leber Congenital Amaurosis 316
    Achromatopsia 317
    Blue-Cone Monochromatism 318
    Congenital Stationary Night Blindness 318
    Foveal Hypoplasia 319
    Aicardi Syndrome 319
Hereditary Macular Dystrophies 320
    Stargardt Disease 320
    Best Vitelliform Dystrophy 321
    Familial Drusen 322
Hereditary Vitreoretinopathies 322
    Juvenile Retinoschisis 322
    Stickler Syndrome 322
    Familial Exudative Vitreoretinopathy 323
    Norrie Disease 324
    Goldmann-Favre Vitreoretinal Dystrophy 324
Systemic Diseases and Disorders With Retinal Manifestations 324
    Diabetes Mellitus 324
    Leukemia 325
    Albinism 327
    Familial Oculorenal Syndromes 330
    Cherry-Red Spot 331
    Gangliosidoses 332

SCREENING EXAMINATION OF PREMATURE INFANTS FOR RETINOPATHY
    OF PREMATURITY 333

25 Optic Disc Abnormalities 339

Developmental Anomalies 339
Optic Atrophy 343
    Hereditary Optic Atrophy 344
Optic Neuritis 345
Papilledema 346

Pseudotumor Cerebri 346
Pseudopapilledema 346
Drusen 347

26 Ocular Tumors in Childhood 349
Differential Diagnosis 349
Orbital Tumors 351
    Primary Malignant Neoplasms 351
    Metastatic Tumors 352
    Benign Tumors 355
    Ectopic Tissue Masses 358
    Childhood Orbital Inflammations 362
Eyelid and Epibulbar Tumors 363
    Inflammatory Conditions 365
Intraocular Tumors 366
    Iris and Ciliary Body Lesions 366
    Choroidal and Retinal Pigment Epithelial Lesions . . . 367
    Retinoblastoma 368

27 Phakomatoses 375
Neurofibromatosis 375
    Melanocytic Lesions 377
    Glial Cell Lesions 378
    Other Manifestations 381
Tuberous Sclerosis (Bourneville Disease) 383
von Hippel–Lindau Disease (Retinal Angiomatosis) 386
Sturge-Weber Syndrome (Encephalofacial Angiomatosis) . . 387
    Ocular Involvement 389
    Management 390
Ataxia-Telangiectasia (Louis-Bar Syndrome) 390
Incontinentia Pigmenti (Bloch-Sulzberger Syndrome) . . . 391
Wyburn-Mason Syndrome (Racemose Angioma) 393

28 Craniofacial Malformations 395
Approach to the Child With Craniofacial and Ocular Malformations . . 395
    Intrinsic Ocular Pathology 395
    Secondary Ocular Complications 395
Selected Craniofacial Syndromes 396
    Craniosynostosis 396
    Other Craniofacial Anomalies 399
    Fetal Alcohol Syndrome 401
    Fetal Hydantoin Syndrome 403

29 Ocular Findings in Inborn Errors of Metabolism . . . 405
Treatment 408

30 Ocular Trauma in Childhood 409
Child Abuse 410
    Shaking Injury 410

Superficial Injury 413
Penetrating Injury 414
Blunt Injury 414
    Hyphema 414
    Orbital Fractures 417

31 Decreased Vision in Infants and Children 419

Normal Visual Development 419
Approach to the Infant With Decreased Vision 420
Anterior Segment Anomalies, Glaucoma, Cataract 421
Optic Nerve Hypoplasia 421
Optic Atrophy 422
Leber Congenital Amaurosis 423
Achromatopsia (Rod Monochromatism) 423
Congenital Infection Syndrome/TORCH Syndrome 424
Cortical Visual Impairment 424
Delay in Visual Maturation 424
Acquired Vision Loss Later in Childhood 425

Basic Texts 429
Related Academy Materials 431
Credit Reporting Form 433
Study Questions 437
Answers 446
Index 453

General Introduction

The Basic and Clinical Science Course (BCSC) is designed to meet the needs of residents and practitioners for a comprehensive yet concise curriculum of the field of ophthalmology. The BCSC has developed from its original brief outline format, which relied heavily on outside readings, to a more convenient and educationally useful self-contained text. The Academy regularly updates and revises the course, with the goals of integrating the basic science and clinical practice of ophthalmology and of keeping ophthalmologists current with new developments in the various subspecialties.

The BCSC incorporates the effort and expertise of more than 80 ophthalmologists, organized into 14 section faculties, working with Academy editorial staff. In addition, the course continues to benefit from many lasting contributions made by the faculties of previous editions. Members of the Academy's Practicing Ophthalmologists Advisory Committee for Education serve on each faculty and, as a group, review every volume before and after major revisions.

Organization of the Course

The Basic and Clinical Science Course comprises 14 volumes, incorporating fundamental ophthalmic knowledge, subspecialty areas, and special topics:

1. Update on General Medicine
2. Fundamentals and Principles of Ophthalmology
3. Optics, Refraction, and Contact Lenses
4. Ophthalmic Pathology and Intraocular Tumors
5. Neuro-Ophthalmology
6. Pediatric Ophthalmology and Strabismus
7. Orbit, Eyelids, and Lacrimal System
8. External Disease and Cornea
9. Intraocular Inflammation and Uveitis
10. Glaucoma
11. Lens and Cataract
12. Retina and Vitreous
13. International Ophthalmology
14. Refractive Surgery

In addition, a comprehensive Master Index allows the reader to easily locate subjects throughout the entire series.

References

Readers who wish to explore specific topics in greater detail may consult the journal references cited within each chapter and the Basic Texts listed at the back of the book.

These references are intended to be selective rather than exhaustive, chosen by the BCSC faculty as being important, current, and readily available to residents and practitioners.

Related Academy educational materials are also listed in the appropriate sections. They include books, audiovisual materials, self-assessment programs, clinical modules, and interactive programs.

Study Questions and CME Credit

Each volume of the BCSC is designed as an independent study activity for ophthalmology residents and practitioners. The learning objectives for this volume are given on page 1. The text, illustrations, and references provide the information necessary to achieve the objectives; the study questions allow readers to test their understanding of the material and their mastery of the objectives. Physicians who wish to claim CME credit for this educational activity may do so by mail, by fax, or online. The necessary forms and instructions are given at the end of the book.

Conclusion

The Basic and Clinical Science Course has expanded greatly over the years, with the addition of much new text and numerous illustrations. Recent editions have sought to place a greater emphasis on clinical applicability, while maintaining a solid foundation in basic science. As with any educational program, it reflects the experience of its authors. As its faculties change and as medicine progresses, new viewpoints are always emerging on controversial subjects and techniques. Not all alternate approaches can be included in this series; as with any educational endeavor, the learner should seek additional sources, including such carefully balanced opinions as the Academy's Preferred Practice Patterns.

The BCSC faculty and staff are continuously striving to improve the educational usefulness of the course; you, the reader, can contribute to this ongoing process. If you have any suggestions or questions about the series, please do not hesitate to contact the faculty or the editors.

The authors, editors, and reviewers hope that your study of the BCSC will be of lasting value and that each section will serve as a practical resource for quality patient care.

Objectives

Upon completion of BCSC Section 6, *Pediatric Ophthalmology and Strabismus*, the reader should be able to:

- Describe evaluation techniques for young children that provide the maximum gain of information with the least trauma and frustration

- Outline the anatomy and physiology of the extraocular muscles and their fascia

- Explain the classification, diagnosis, and treatment options for amblyopia

- Describe the commonly used diagnostic and measurement tests for strabismus

- Classify the various esodeviations and exodeviations and describe the management of each type

- Identify vertical strabismus and special forms of strabismus and formulate a treatment plan for each type

- List the possible complications of strabismus surgery and describe guidelines to minimize them

- Differentiate among various causes of congenital and acquired ocular infections in children and formulate a logical plan for the diagnosis and management of each type

- List the most common diseases and malformations of the cornea, lacrimal drainage system, anterior segment, and iris seen in children

- Describe the diagnostic findings and treatment options for childhood glaucoma

- Identify common types of childhood cataracts and other lens disorders

- Outline a diagnostic and management plan for childhood cataracts

- Identify appropriate diagnostic tests for pediatric uveitis

- Differentiate among various vitreoretinal diseases and disorders found in children

- List the characteristics of ocular tumors and phakomatoses seen in children

- Describe the characteristic findings of accidental and nonaccidental childhood trauma
- Outline the current joint policy statement regarding the role of vision in learning disabilities and dyslexia

INTRODUCTION

Rapport With Children: Tips for a Productive Examination

Children are not merely small adults. The most common ophthalmologic problems in children are different from the most common problems in adults. The varying developmental levels of children require different approaches to the ophthalmic examination. Proper preparation and attitude can make the ophthalmic examination of pediatric patients both enjoyable and rewarding.

Preparation

If at all possible, have a small room or corner of the waiting area designated for children. Both the parents and adult patients will be relieved by this separation. A small table and chairs, some books, and some toys are sufficient.

A dedicated long pediatric examination lane with different types of distance fixation targets is optimal. Following the *one toy, one look* rule, have several small toys readily available (Fig I-1). Light-colored plastic finger puppets become silent accommodative near targets that can also provide a corneal light reflex if placed over a muscle light or pen light.

Some children fear the white coat. You may choose to enter the room without yours.

The Examination

Examination of the pediatric patient begins with observing children at ease in the play area, in their parent's arms as you enter the room, and as they navigate their way to the lane. This may be the best look you get before children cry and bury their face in the parent's shoulder.

Observe the parents and siblings. Some ophthalmic conditions tend to run in families.

Some children are more comfortable sitting in the parent's lap.

Be relaxed, open, honest, and playfully engaging during the examination. Gaining the child's confidence makes for a faster and better examination, easier follow-up visits, and greater parental support.

Seat yourself at the child's eye level and introduce yourself to the child and the parent.

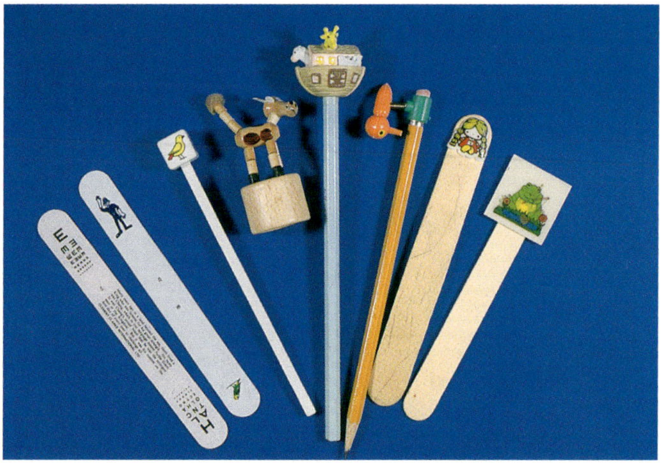

Figure I-1 Small toys, pictures, and reduced letter and E charts are used as near fixation targets. *(Reproduced with permission from Haldi BA, Mets MB. Nonsugical treatment of strabismus. In:* Focal Points: Clinical Modules for Ophthalmologists. *San Francisco: American Academy of Ophthalmology; 1997: vol 15, no 4. Photograph courtesy of Betty Anne Haldi, CO.)*

Establish and maintain eye contact with the child.

Initiate verbal contact by asking children easy questions with simple answers. For example, children enjoy being regarded as "big" and correcting adults when they are wrong. Tell them they look "so grown up"; grossly overestimate their age or grade level and then ask, "Is that right?" A simple joke can relax both child and parent.

To initiate physical contact with the child, you can ask them to "give me five" or admire an article of their clothing such as their shoes. Pushing the "magic button" on the nose of children as you surreptitiously activate the mechanical animals with your foot pedal allows you to work close to their face while they are distracted.

Go to where the action is—you may only have a few moments of cooperation, so check what you most need to see at the beginning of the examination.

If fusion is in doubt, check it first before disrupting it with other tests, including those for vision.

While checking vision, make the child feel successful by initially giving them objects they can readily discern, then say "that's too easy—let's try this one."

Develop a different vocabulary when working with children, such as "I want to show you something special" instead of "I want to examine you." Use *magic sunglasses* for the Polaroid stereo glasses, *special flashlight* for retinoscope, *funny hat* for the indirect ophthalmoscope, and *magnifying glass* for the indirect lens. Confrontation visual fields can be performed as a counting-fingers game or Simon Says. Talk children into a slit-lamp examination by saying that they can "drive the motorcycle" by having them grab the handles of the slit lamp. Use your imagination to "play" with children while rapidly proceeding with the examination. Children will be more cooperative if you are sharing an experience instead of doing something to them.

Save the most threatening or most unpleasant part of the examination for the end.

The least expensive test you can order is a return office visit. Children who become totally uncooperative can return later to finish the examination.

When dealing with a vision- or life-threatening problem, you must persist with the examination and even use sedation or anesthesia when necessary.

Eye Drops

Almost all children are apprehensive about eye drops. However, they do not have to *like* the drops; the important thing is to instill them. There are many approaches to giving eye drops. If possible, someone other than the examining physician should administer the drops. Some practitioners use a cycloplegic spray, some use a topical anesthetic drop first, and some simply use the cycloplegic drop. The drops can be described as being "like a splash of swimming pool water" that will "feel funny for about 30 seconds." Do not give children a long time to think about it. Dark irides are more difficult to dilate. In some cases, the parent can put the cycloplegic drops in at home or an atropine refraction can be performed. (See Table 21-2 in BCSC Section 2, *Fundamentals and Principles of Ophthalmology*, for a complete listing of mydriatics and cycloplegics.)

Use of Anesthesia for Foreign Body Removal

Procedures that provoke anxiety or are painful are best performed if children know that it is possible to numb the area. For example, the following process to remove foreign bodies can comfort the child:

1. Explain to the child that the eyes can be made numb.
2. Show the child that you have a drop that is cold but that most children say is also comfortable. You can call it a "magic drop." Drop it on the back of the child's hand first, before putting it in the eye. Tell the patient he or she might have felt that first drop but probably won't notice a second drop so much because the eye is already numb.
3. Demonstrate with a second drop that the eye has become numb. Show the child that a soft cotton-tipped applicator with drops on it can touch the eye without hurting or even being felt.
4. Instruments for foreign body removal can then be introduced similarly.

Day S. History, examination and further investigation. In: Taylor D, ed. *Pediatric Ophthalmology*. 2nd ed. Cambridge, MA: Blackwell; 1996.

McKeown CA. The pediatric eye examination. In: Albert DM, Jakobiec FA, eds. *Principles and Practice of Ophthalmology*. 2nd ed. Philadelphia: Saunders; 1991.

Preferred Practice Patterns Committee. Pediatric Ophthalmology Panel. *Pediatric Eye Evaluations*. San Francisco: American Academy of Ophthalmology; 1997.

PART I

Strabismus

CHAPTER 1

Introduction to Strabismus

Terminology

The term *strabismus* is derived from the Greek word *strabismos*, "to squint, to look obliquely or askance." Strabismus means ocular misalignment, whether caused by abnormalities in binocular vision or by anomalies of neuromuscular control of ocular motility. Many terms are employed in discussing strabismus, and unless they are used correctly and uniformly, confusion and misunderstanding can occur.

Orthophoria is the ideal condition of ocular balance. In reality, orthophoria is seldom encountered: a small heterophoria can be documented in most persons. Some ophthalmologists therefore prefer *orthotropia* to mean correct direction or position of the eyes even if a small heterophoria is present.

Heterophoria is an ocular deviation kept latent by the fusional mechanism *(latent strabismus)*. Heterotropia is a deviation that is manifest and not kept under control by the fusional mechanism *(manifest strabismus)*.

A detailed nomenclature has evolved to describe types of ocular deviations. This vocabulary uses many prefixes and suffixes based on the relative positions of the visual axes of both eyes to account for the multiple strabismic patterns encountered.

Prefixes

Eso- The eye is rotated so that the cornea is deviated nasally and the fovea is rotated temporally. Because the visual axes converge, this is also known as *convergent strabismus*.

Exo- The eye is rotated so that the cornea is deviated temporally and the fovea is rotated nasally. Because the visual axes diverge, this is also known as *divergent strabismus*.

Hyper- The eye is rotated so that the cornea is deviated superiorly and the fovea is rotated inferiorly. This is also known as *vertical strabismus*.

Hypo- The eye is rotated so that the cornea is deviated inferiorly and the fovea is rotated superiorly. This is also known as *vertical strabismus*.

Incyclo- The eye is rotated so that the superior portion of the vertical meridian is torted nasally and the inferior portion of the vertical meridian is torted temporally. This is also known as *intorsional strabismus*.

Excyclo- The eye is rotated so that the superior portion of the vertical meridian is torted temporally and the inferior portion of the vertical meridian is torted nasally. This is also known as *extorsional strabismus*.

Suffixes

-phoria A latent deviation (eg, esophoria, exophoria, right hyperphoria) that is controlled by the fusional mechanism so that the eyes remain aligned under normal binocular vision.

-tropia A manifest deviation (eg, esotropia, exotropia, right hypertropia, excyclotropia) that exceeds the control of the fusional mechanism so that the eyes are not aligned.

Usage

For all of the above deviations (eso-, exo-, hyper-, hypo-, incyclo-, and excyclo-), the deviating eye is assumed to be the nonfixating one because the fixating eye should be directed at the fixation target. Sometimes, it is important to identify the deviating eye, especially when seeking to call attention to the "offending" eye as causing the deviation. This usage is particularly helpful when dealing with vertical deviations, restrictive or paretic strabismus, or amblyopia in a preverbal child.

Classification

No classification is perfect or all-inclusive, and several methods of classifying eye alignment and motility disorders are used.

Fusional Status

Phoria A latent deviation in which fusional control is always present.

Intermittent tropia Fusional control is present part of the time.

Tropia A manifest deviation in which fusional control is not present.

Variation of the Deviation With Gaze Position or Fixating Eye

Comitant (concomitant) The deviation does not vary in size with direction of gaze or fixating eye.

Incomitant (noncomitant) The deviation varies in size with direction of gaze or fixating eye. Most incomitant strabismus is paralytic or restrictive. Especially if acquired, incomitant strabismus may indicate neurologic or orbital disease.

Fixation

Alternating Spontaneous alternation of fixation from one eye to the other

Monocular Definite preference for fixation with one eye

Age of Onset

Congenital A deviation documented in early infancy, presumably related to a defect present at birth; the term *infantile* might be more appropriate

Acquired A deviation with later onset, after a period of apparently normal visual development

Type of Deviation

Horizontal Esodeviation or exodeviation

Vertical Hyperdeviation or hypodeviation

Torsional Incyclodeviation or excyclodeviation

Combined Horizontal, vertical, torsional, or any combination thereof

Abbreviated Designations for Types of Strabismus

E, X, RH, LH Esophoria, exophoria, right hyperphoria, left hyperphoria at distance fixation, respectively. The addition of a prime (′) indicates near fixation (eg, E′, X′, RH′).

ET, XT, RHT, LHT Esotropia, exotropia, right hypertropia, left hypertropia at distance fixation, respectively. The addition of a prime (′) indicates near fixation (eg, ET′, XT′, RHT′).

E(T), X(T), RH(T), LH(T) Intermittent esotropia, intermittent exotropia, intermittent right hypertropia, intermittent left hypertropia at distance fixation, respectively. The addition of a prime (′) indicates near fixation (eg, E(T)′, X(T)′, RH(T)′).

RHoT, LHoT Right hypotropia, left hypotropia at distance fixation, respectively. The addition of a prime (′) indicates near fixation (eg, RHoT′, LHoT′).

CHAPTER 2

Anatomy of the Extraocular Muscles and Their Fascia

Origin, Course, Insertion, Innervation, and Action of the Extraocular Muscles

There are seven extraocular muscles: the four rectus muscles, the two oblique muscles, and the levator palpebrae superioris muscle. Cranial nerve VI (abducens) innervates the lateral rectus muscle; cranial nerve IV (trochlear) innervates the superior oblique muscle; and cranial nerve III (oculomotor) innervates the levator palpebrae, superior rectus, medial rectus, inferior rectus, and inferior oblique muscles. CN III has an upper and a lower division: the upper division supplies the levator palpebrae and superior rectus muscles; the lower division supplies the medial rectus, inferior rectus, and inferior oblique muscles. The parasympathetic innervation of the sphincter pupillae and ciliary muscle travels with the branch of the lower division of cranial nerve III that supplies the inferior oblique muscle. BCSC Section 5, *Neuro-Ophthalmology,* discusses the ocular motor nerves in more detail, and Section 2, *Fundamentals and Principles of Ophthalmology,* extensively illustrates the anatomical structures mentioned in this chapter.

When the eye is directed straight ahead and the head is also straight, the eye is said to be in *primary position.* The *primary action* of a muscle is its major effect on the position of the eye when the muscle contracts while the eye is in primary position. The secondary and tertiary actions of a muscle are the additional effects on the position of the eye in primary position. The globe usually can be moved about 50° in each direction from primary position. Under normal viewing circumstances, however, the eyes move only about 15°–20° from primary position before head movement occurs.

Horizontal Rectus Muscles

The horizontal rectus muscles are the medial and lateral rectus muscles. Both arise from the annulus of Zinn. The *medial rectus muscle* courses along the medial orbital wall and inserts 5.5 mm from the limbus; the *lateral rectus muscle* inserts 6.9 mm from the limbus after coursing along the lateral orbital wall. The medial and lateral rectus muscles have only horizontal action: the medial rectus is an adductor, and the lateral rectus is an abductor (Fig 2-1). The medial rectus muscle is the only rectus muscle that is not adjacent to an oblique muscle.

14 • Pediatric Ophthalmology and Strabismus

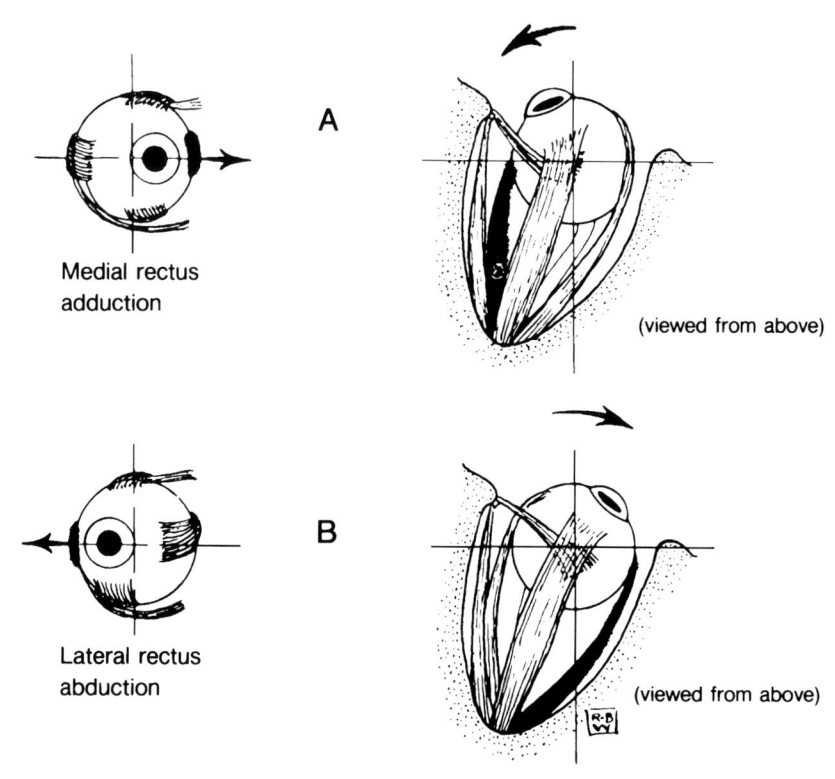

Figure 2-1 The right horizontal rectus muscles. **A,** Right medial rectus muscle. **B,** Right lateral rectus muscle. *(Reprinted from von Noorden GK.* Atlas of Strabismus. *4th ed. St Louis: Mosby; 1983:3.)*

Vertical Rectus Muscles

The vertical rectus muscles are the superior and inferior rectus muscles. The *superior rectus muscle* originates from the annulus of Zinn and courses anteriorly, upward over the eyeball, and laterally, forming an angle of 23° with the visual axis of the eye in primary position. The superior rectus muscle inserts 7.7 mm from the limbus. This muscle's primary action is elevation; secondary actions are adduction and intorsion (incycloduction) (Fig 2-2).

The *inferior rectus muscle* also arises from the annulus of Zinn, and it then courses anteriorly, downward, and laterally along the floor of the orbit, forming an angle of 23° with the visual axis of the eye in primary position. This muscle inserts 6.5 mm from the limbus. The inferior rectus muscle's primary action is depression; secondary actions are adduction and extorsion (excycloduction) (Fig 2-3).

Oblique Muscles

The *superior oblique muscle* originates from the orbital apex above the annulus of Zinn and passes anteriorly and upward along the superomedial wall of the orbit. The muscle becomes tendinous before passing through the *trochlea,* a cartilaginous saddle attached to the frontal bone in the superior nasal orbit. A bursa-like cleft separates the trochlea

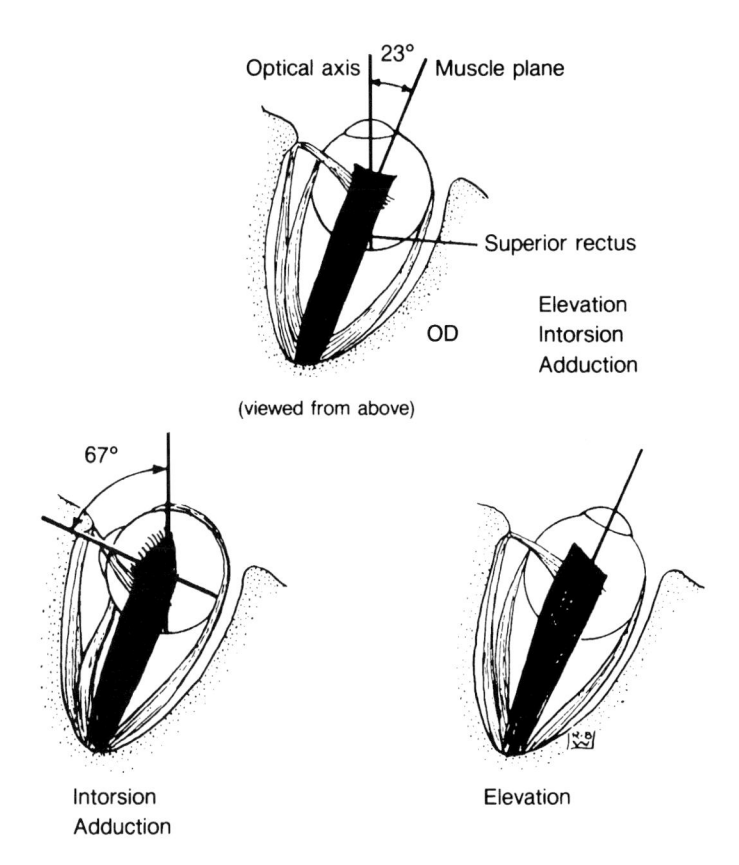

CHAPTER 2: Anatomy of the Extraocular Muscles and Their Fascia • 15

Figure 2-2 The right superior rectus muscle. *(Reprinted from von Noorden GK.* Atlas of Strabismus. *4th ed. St Louis: Mosby; 1983:3.)*

from the loose fibrovascular sheath surrounding the tendon. The discrete fibers of the tendon telescope as they move through the trochlea, the central fibers moving farther than the peripheral ones (Fig 2-4). The function of the trochlea is to redirect the tendon inferiorly, posteriorly, and laterally, forming an angle of 51° with the visual axis of the eye in primary position. The tendon penetrates Tenon's capsule 2 mm nasally and 5 mm posteriorly to the nasal insertion of the superior rectus muscle. The tendon inserts in the posterosuperior quadrant of the eyeball, almost or entirely lateral to the midvertical plane or center of rotation, passing under the superior rectus muscle. The primary action of the superior oblique muscle is intorsion (incycloduction); secondary actions are depression and abduction (Fig 2-5).

 Helveston EM. The influence of superior oblique anatomy on function and treatment. The 1998 Bielschowsky Lecture. *Binoc Vis Strabismus Q.* 1999;14:16–21.

The *inferior oblique muscle* originates from the periosteum of the maxillary bone, just posterior to the orbital rim and lateral to the orifice of the lacrimal fossa. It passes laterally, superiorly, and posteriorly, going inferior to the inferior rectus muscle and inserting under the lateral rectus muscle in the posterolateral portion of the globe, in the

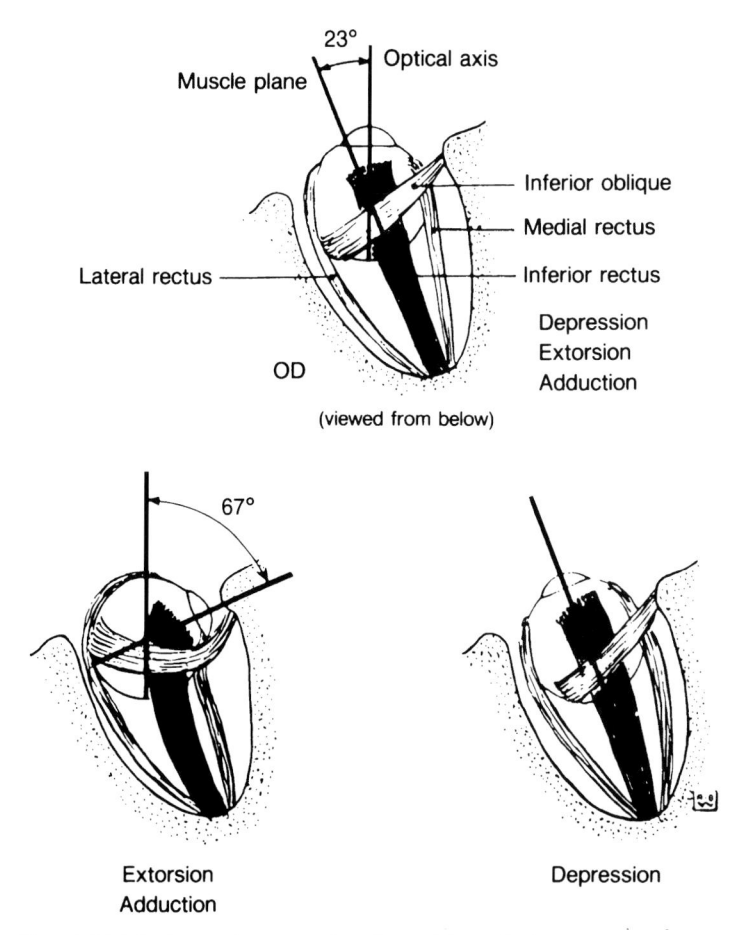

Figure 2-3 The right inferior rectus muscle, viewed from below. *(Reprinted from von Noorden GK. Atlas of Strabismus. 4th ed. St Louis: Mosby; 1983:5.)*

area of the macula. The inferior oblique muscle forms an angle of 51° with the visual axis of the eye in primary position. The muscle's primary action is extorsion (excycloduction); secondary actions are elevation and abduction (Fig 2-6).

Levator Palpebrae Superioris Muscle

The levator palpebrae superioris muscle arises at the apex of the orbit from the lesser wing of the sphenoid bone just superior to the annulus of Zinn. The origin of this muscle blends with the superior rectus muscle inferiorly and with the superior oblique muscle medially. The levator palpebrae superioris passes anteriorly, lying just above the superior rectus muscle; the fascial sheaths of these two muscles are connected. The levator palpebrae superioris muscle becomes an aponeurosis in the region of the superior fornix. This muscle has both a cutaneous and a tarsal insertion. BCSC Section 7, *Orbit, Eyelids, and Lacrimal System,* discusses this muscle in detail.

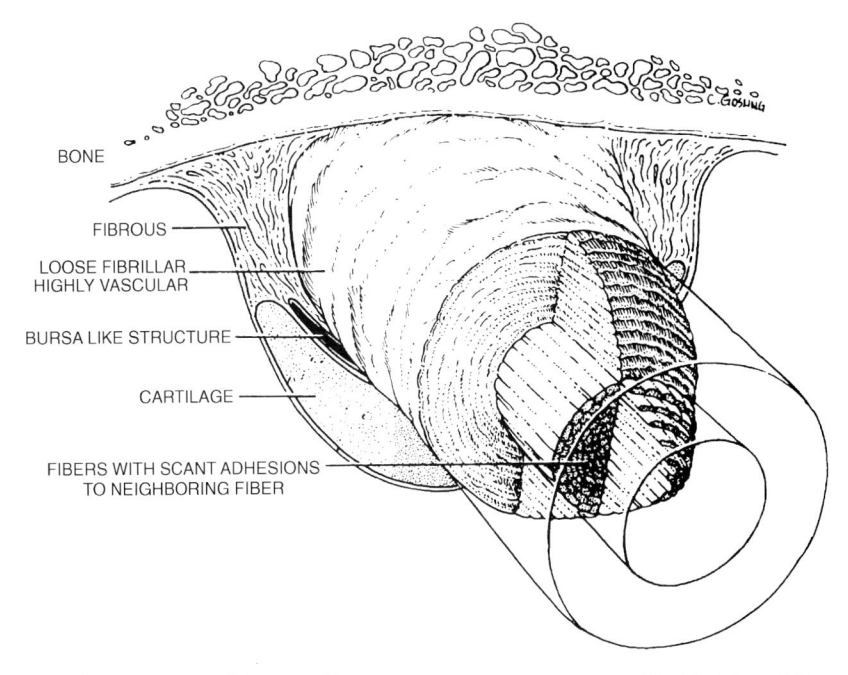

Figure 2-4 Components of the trochlea. *(From Helveston EM, Merriam WW, Ellis FD, et al. The trochlea: a study of the anatomy and physiology.* Ophthalmology. *1982;89:124–133.)*

Table 2-1 summarizes the characteristics of the extraocular muscles and reveals their relationship to one another (Fig 2-7).

Insertion Relationships of the Rectus Muscles

Starting at the medial rectus and proceeding to inferior rectus, lateral rectus, and superior rectus muscles, the rectus muscle tendons insert progressively farther from the limbus. A continuous curve drawn through these insertions yields a spiral, known as the *spiral of Tillaux* (Fig 2-8). The temporal side of the vertical rectus muscle insertion is farther from the limbus (ie, more posterior) than is the nasal side.

Blood Supply of the Extraocular Muscles

Arterial System

The muscular branches of the ophthalmic artery provide the most important blood supply for the extraocular muscles. The *lateral muscular branch* supplies the lateral rectus, superior rectus, superior oblique, and levator palpebrae superioris muscles; the *medial muscular branch*, the larger of the two, supplies the inferior rectus, medial rectus, and inferior oblique muscles.

The lateral rectus muscle is partially supplied by the *lacrimal artery;* the *infraorbital artery* partially supplies the inferior oblique and inferior rectus muscles. The muscular branches give rise to the *anterior ciliary arteries* accompanying the rectus muscles; each

18 • Pediatric Ophthalmology and Strabismus

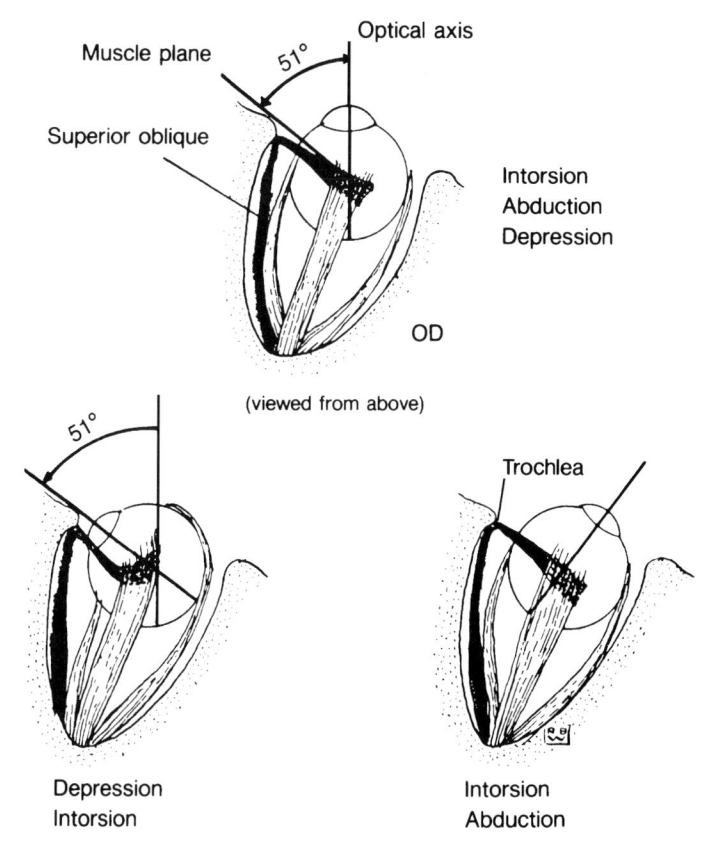

Figure 2-5 The right superior oblique muscle, viewed from above. *(Reprinted from von Noorden GK. Atlas of Strabismus. 4th ed. St Louis: Mosby; 1983:7.)*

rectus muscle has one to three anterior ciliary arteries. These pass to the episclera of the globe and then supply blood to the anterior segment. The superior and inferior rectus muscles carry the bulk of the blood supply.

Venous System

The venous system parallels the arterial system, emptying into the *superior* and *inferior orbital veins*. Generally, four *vortex veins* are located posterior to the equator; these are usually found near the nasal and temporal margins of the superior rectus and inferior rectus muscles.

Fine Structure of the Extraocular Muscles

The ratio of nerve fibers to eye muscle fibers in the extraocular muscles is high (1:3–1:5) compared with that found in other skeletal muscles (1:50–1:125), allowing for more accurate control. Extraocular muscle is a specialized form of skeletal muscle that incorporates several different fiber types, from a slow, tonic type resistant to fatigue and active

CHAPTER 2: Anatomy of the Extraocular Muscles and Their Fascia • 19

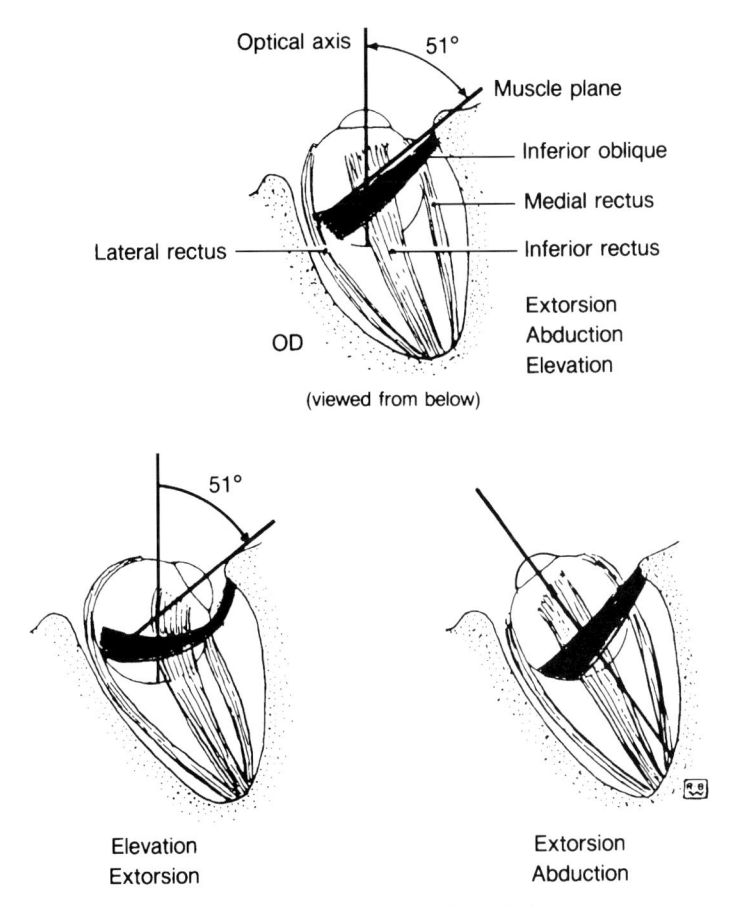

Figure 2-6 The right inferior oblique muscle, viewed from below. *(Reprinted from von Noorden GK. Atlas of Strabismus. 4th ed. St Louis: Mosby; 1983:9.)*

in holding gaze straight ahead to the type adapted for rapid (saccadic) eye movements. Intermediate fiber types also exist.

Fiber Types

Felderstruktur muscle fibers are unique to the extraocular muscles. These are slow, tonic, stamina-oriented muscle fibers that tend to be superficial in the muscle, near the orbital wall, and smaller. They usually have aerobic metabolism, many mitochondria, high capillary density, oxidative enzymes, innervation by multiple grapelike *(en grappe)* endings, and small nerve fibers. These fibers contract slowly, smoothly, and with a graded response, depending on repetitive stimuli, and participate in smooth pursuit.

Fibrillenstruktur muscle fibers, the usual type of fiber in skeletal muscle, correspond to striated muscles of the body. These fast, phasic fibers tend to be deeper in the center of the muscle and larger; they usually have platelike *(en plaque)* nerve endings, glycolytic enzymes, large nerve fibers that are myelinated, and fewer mitochondria. These muscle

Table 2-1 Extraocular Muscles

Muscle	Approx. Length of Active Muscle (mm)	Origin	Anatomic Insertion	Direction of Pull*	Tendon Length (mm)	Arc of Contact (mm)	Action From Primary Position	Innervation
Medial rectus (MR)	40	Annulus of Zinn	5.5 mm from medial limbus	90°	4.5	7	Adduction	Lower CN III
Lateral rectus (LR)	40	Annulus of Zinn	6.9 mm from lateral limbus	90°	7	12	Abduction	CN VI
Superior rectus (SR)	40	Annulus of Zinn	7.7 mm from superior limbus	23°	6	6.5	Elevation Intorsion Adduction	Upper CN III
Inferior rectus (IR)	40	Annulus of Zinn	6.5 mm from inferior limbus	23°	7	6.5	Depression Extorsion Adduction	Lower CN III
Superior oblique (SO)	32	Orbit apex above annulus of Zinn (functional origin at the trochlea)	Posterior to equator in superotemporal quadrant	51°	26	7–8	Intorsion Depression Abduction	CN IV
Inferior oblique (IO)	37	Behind lacrimal fossa	Macular area	51°	1	15	Extorsion Elevation Abduction	Lower CN III
Levator palpebrae superioris (LPS)	40	Orbit apex above annulus of Zinn	Septa of pretarsal orbicularis and anterior surface of tarsus	—	14–20	—	Eyelid elevation	Upper CN III

* relative to visual axis in primary position

CHAPTER 2: Anatomy of the Extraocular Muscles and Their Fascia • 21

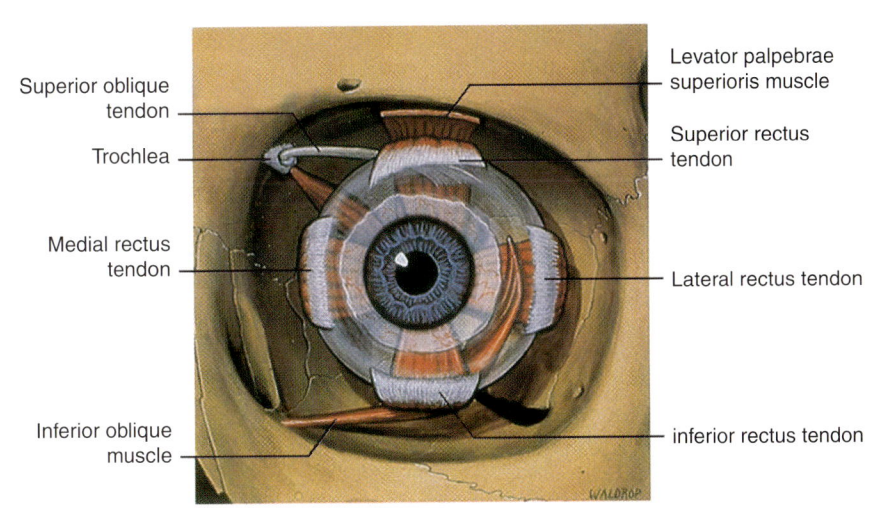

Figure 2-7 Extraocular muscles, frontal composite view, left eye. *(Reproduced with permission from Dutton JJ. Atlas of Clinical and Surgical Orbital Anatomy. Philadelphia: Saunders; 1994:23.)*

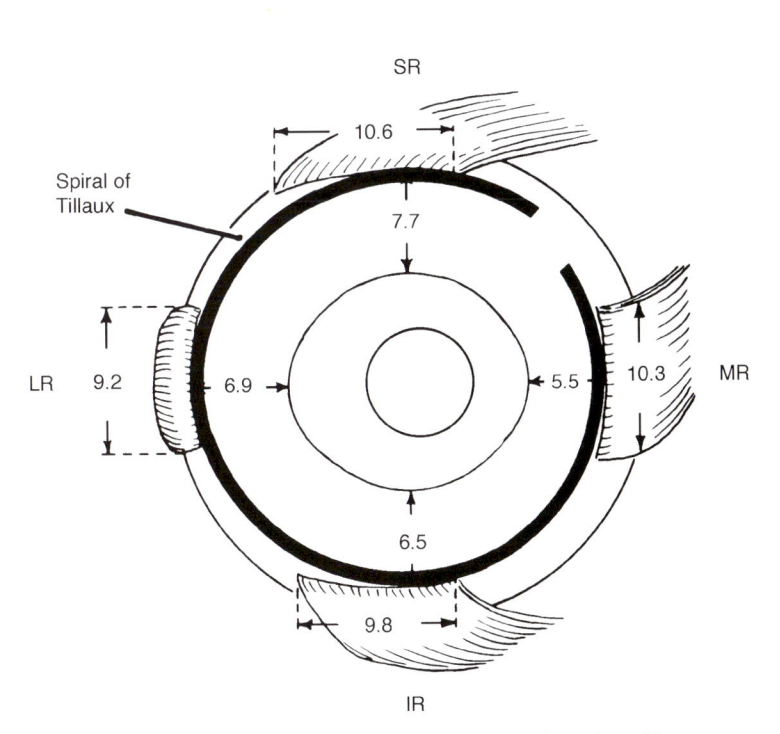

Figure 2-8 Spiral of Tillaux, right eye. *Note:* the distances given in millimeters are averages only and may vary greatly in individuals. IR, inferior rectus; LR, lateral rectus; MR, medial rectus; SR, superior rectus. *(Reprinted from von Noorden GK. Atlas of Strabismus. 4th ed. St Louis: Mosby; 1983:13.)*

22 • Pediatric Ophthalmology and Strabismus

fibers contract rapidly as a fast twitch in response to a single stimulus and function in saccadic movements of the eye.

Orbital and Fascial Relationships

Within the orbit, a complex musculofibroelastic structure suspends the globe, supports the extraocular muscles, and compartmentalizes the fat pads (Fig 2-9).

Tenon's Capsule (the Fascia Bulbi)

The bulk of the orbital fascial system is Tenon's capsule, which forms the cavity within which the eyeball moves (Fig 2-10). Tenon's capsule is an envelope of elastic connective tissue that fuses posteriorly with the optic nerve sheath and fuses anteriorly with the intermuscular septum at a position 3 mm from the limbus (Fig 2-11). The posterior portion of Tenon's capsule is thin and flexible, allowing for free movement of the optic

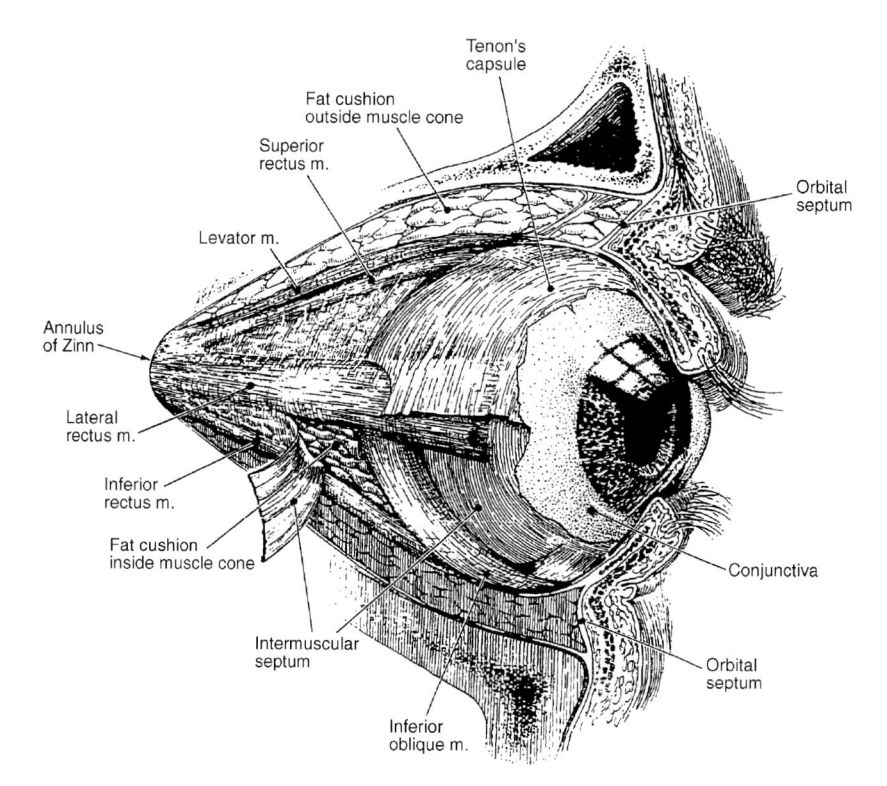

Figure 2-9 The muscle cone contains one fat cushion and is surrounded by another, and these two fat cushions are separated by the rectus muscles and intermuscular septa. Tenon's capsule anterior to the penetration of the rectus muscles and intermuscular septa is the inner surface of the compartment containing the fat cushion outside the muscle cone. Tenon's capsule posterior to the penetration of the rectus muscles and intermuscular septa is the anterior surface of the compartment containing the fat cushion inside the muscle cone. *(From Parks MM. Atlas of Strabismus Surgery. Philadelphia: Harper & Row; 1983:7.)*

CHAPTER 2: Anatomy of the Extraocular Muscles and Their Fascia • 23

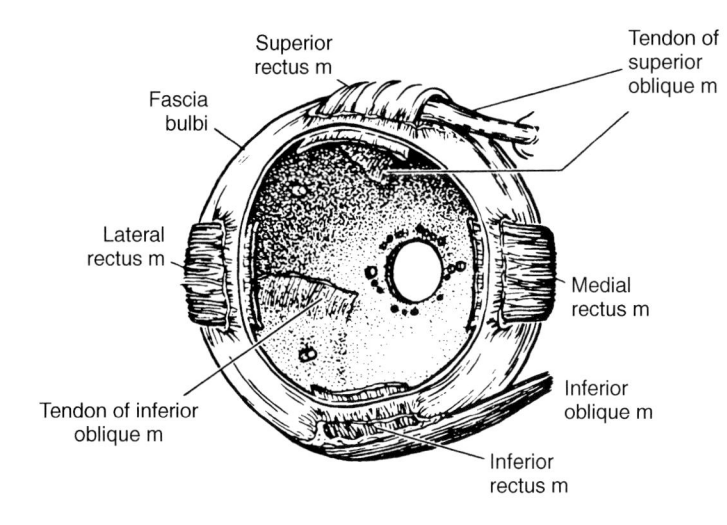

Figure 2-10 Anterior and posterior orifice of Tenon's capsule shown after enucleation of the globe. *(From von Noorden GK. Binocular Vision and Ocular Motility. 5th ed. St Louis: Mosby; 1996:47.)*

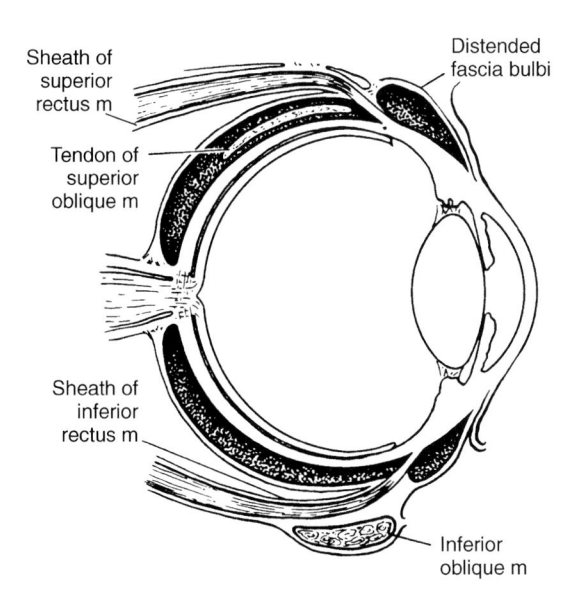

Figure 2-11 Tenon's space shown by injection with India ink. *(From von Noorden GK. Binocular Vision and Ocular Motility. 5th ed. St Louis: Mosby; 1996:46.)*

nerve, ciliary nerves, and ciliary vessels as the globe rotates while separating the orbital fat inside the muscle cone from the sclera. At and just posterior to the equator, Tenon's capsule is thick and tough and suspends the globe trampoline-like by means of connections to the periorbital tissues. The extraocular rectus muscles penetrate this thick musculofibroelastic tissue approximately 10 mm posterior to their insertions. This tissue complex forms a sleeve around the penetrating rectus muscles and creates a compliant pulley suspended from the periorbita, which acts as the functional origin of the muscle. The sleeves also extend anteriorly and posteriorly to form slings that stabilize the muscle path, preventing side-slipping or movement perpendicular to the muscle axis (Fig 2-12). Anterior to the equator, the oblique muscles penetrate Tenon's capsule. Tenon's capsule

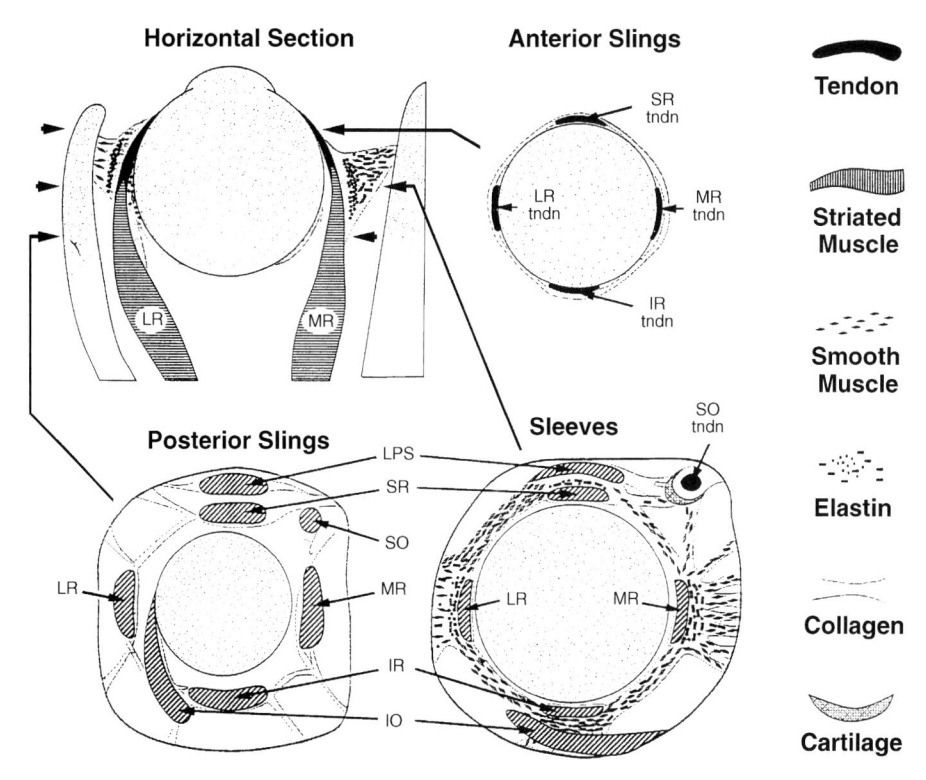

Figure 2-12 Structure of orbital connective tissues. IO, inferior oblique; IR, inferior rectus; LPS, levator palpebrae superioris; LR, lateral rectus; MR, medial rectus; SO, superior oblique; SR, superior rectus. The three coronal views are represented at the levels indicated by arrows in horizontal section. *(From Demer JL, Miller JM, Poukens V. Surgical implications of the rectus extraocular muscle pulleys.* J Pediatr Ophthalmol Strabismus. *1996;33:208–218.)*

continues forward over all six extraocular muscles and separates them from the orbital fat and structures lying outside the muscle cone.

Muscle Cone

The muscle cone lies posterior to the equator. It consists of the extraocular muscles, the extraocular muscle sheaths, and the intermuscular membrane. The muscle cone extends posteriorly to the annulus of Zinn in the orbital apex.

Muscle Capsule

Each rectus muscle has a surrounding fascial capsule that extends with the muscle from its origin to its insertion. These capsules are thin posteriorly, but near the equator they thicken as they pass through the Tenon's capsule sleeve, continuing anteriorly with the muscles to their insertions. Anterior to the equator between the undersurface of the muscle and the sclera there is almost no fascia, only connective tissue footplates that connect the muscle to the globe. The smooth avascular surface of the muscle capsule allows the muscles to slide smoothly over the globe.

Intermuscular Septum (Membrane)

The four rectus muscles are connected by a thin layer of tissue that underlies the conjunctiva. This is the intermuscular septum, which spans between rectus muscles and fuses with the conjunctiva 3 mm posterior to the limbus. Posterior to the globe, the intermuscular septum separates the intraconal fat pads from the extraconal ones. In addition, there are numerous extensions from all the extraocular muscle sheaths that attach them to the orbit and help support the globe.

Lockwood's Ligament

The muscle capsule of the inferior oblique muscle (but not the muscle itself) is bound to the inferior rectus muscle capsule. This fusion is called *Lockwood's ligament*, and it connects to the lower eyelid retractors.

Adipose Tissue

The eye is supported and cushioned in the orbit by a large amount of fatty tissue. External to the muscle cone, fatty tissue comes forward with the rectus muscles, stopping about 10 mm from the limbus. Fatty tissue is also present inside the muscle cone, kept away from the sclera by Tenon's capsule (see Fig 2-9).

Anatomical Implications

The nerves to the rectus muscles and the superior oblique muscle enter the muscles about one third of the distance from the origin to the insertion (or trochlea, in the case of the superior oblique muscle) (Fig 2-13). Damaging these nerves during anterior surgery is difficult but not impossible. An instrument thrust more than 26 mm posterior to the rectus muscle's insertion may cause injury to the nerve.

The nerve supplying the inferior oblique muscle enters the lateral portion of the muscle, where it crosses the inferior rectus muscle; the nerve can be damaged by surgery in this area. Because the parasympathetic innervation to the sphincter pupillae and ciliary muscle accompanies the nerve to the inferior oblique muscle, surgery in this area may also result in pupillary abnormalities.

Maintaining the integrity of the muscle capsules will decrease bleeding during surgery and will provide a smooth muscle surface with less risk of adhesion formation.

The intermuscular septum connections, especially between rectus muscles and oblique muscles, can help locate a lost muscle during surgery. Extensive intermuscular septum dissections are not necessary for rectus recession surgery. During resection surgery, the intermuscular septum connections should be severed to prevent, for example, the inferior oblique muscle from being advanced with the lateral rectus muscle.

The inferior rectus muscle is distinctly bound to the lower eyelid by the fascial extension from its sheath. *Recession*, or weakening, of the inferior rectus muscle tends to widen the palpebral fissure with an associated lower lid droop; *resection*, or strengthening, of the inferior rectus muscle tends to narrow the fissure by elevating the lower eyelid.

26 • Pediatric Ophthalmology and Strabismus

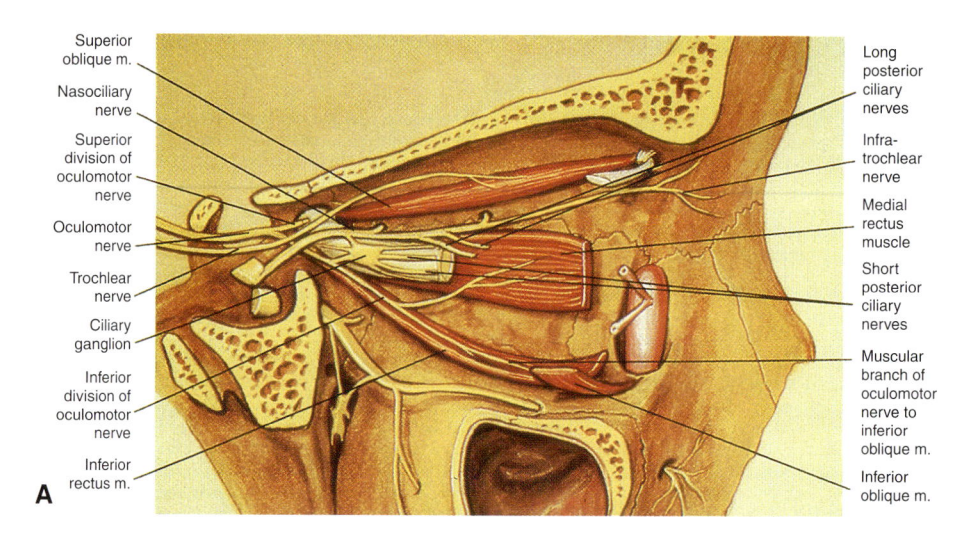

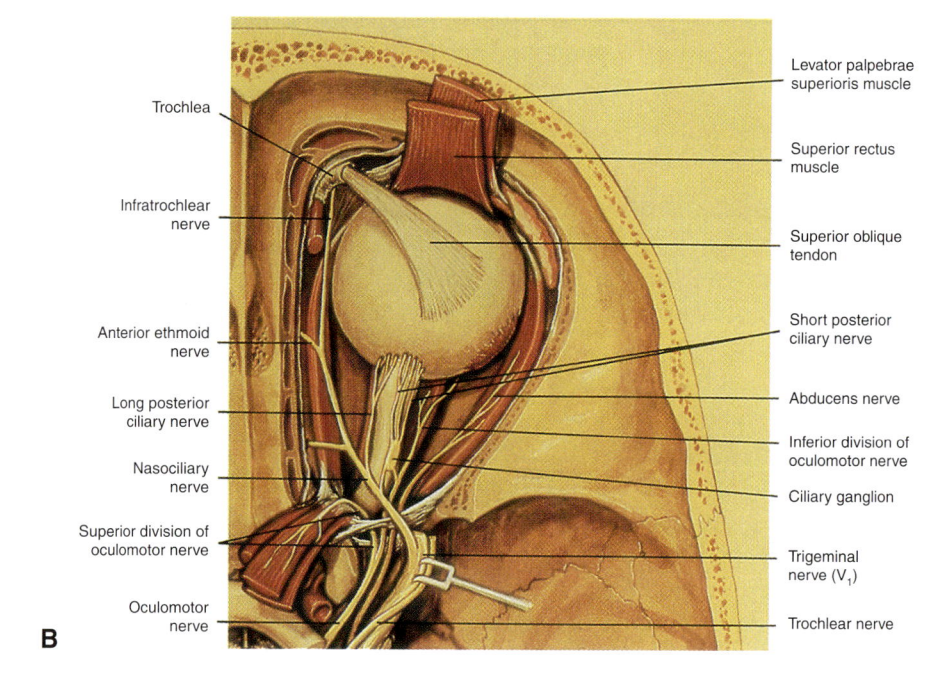

Figure 2-13 The extraocular muscles are innervated by cranial nerves III, IV, and VI. Cutaway views facing nasally **(A)** and down **(B)** show the course of these ocular motor nerves. CN III (oculomotor) divides into a superior and an inferior division in the cavernous sinus or at the superior orbital fissure. The superior division innervates the superior rectus and levator muscles. The inferior division sends branches to the medial rectus, inferior rectus, and inferior oblique muscles and the ciliary ganglion. CN IV (trochlear) enters the orbit through the superior orbital fissure, crosses over the superior rectus and levator muscle complex, and runs along the external surface of the superior oblique muscle, entering in the posterior third. CN VI (abducens) enters the orbit through the superior orbital fissure and annulus of Zinn to supply the lateral rectus muscle. *(Reproduced with permission from Buckley EG, Freedman S, Shields MB.* Atlas of Ophthalmic Surgery. Vol III: *Strabismus and Glaucoma. St Louis: Mosby; 1995:11.)*

CHAPTER 2: Anatomy of the Extraocular Muscles and Their Fascia • 27

Therefore, any alteration of the inferior rectus muscle may be associated with palpebral fissure change (Fig 2-14).

The superior rectus muscle is loosely bound to the levator palpebrae superioris muscle. The eyelid may be pulled forward following resection of the superior rectus muscle, thus narrowing the palpebral fissure, and pulled upward with a recession, widening the fissure. In hypotropia, a pseudoptosis may be present because the upper eyelid tends to follow the superior rectus.

The blood supply to the extraocular muscles provides almost all of the temporal half of the anterior segment circulation and the majority of the nasal half of the anterior segment circulation, which also receives some blood from the long posterior ciliary artery. Therefore, simultaneous surgery on three rectus muscles may induce anterior segment ischemia, particularly in older patients.

Whenever muscle surgery is performed, special care must be taken to avoid penetration of Tenon's capsule 10 mm or more posterior to the limbus. If the integrity of Tenon's capsule is violated posterior to this point, fatty tissue may prolapse through the capsule and form a restrictive adhesion to sclera, muscle, intermuscular membrane, or conjunctiva, limiting ocular motility.

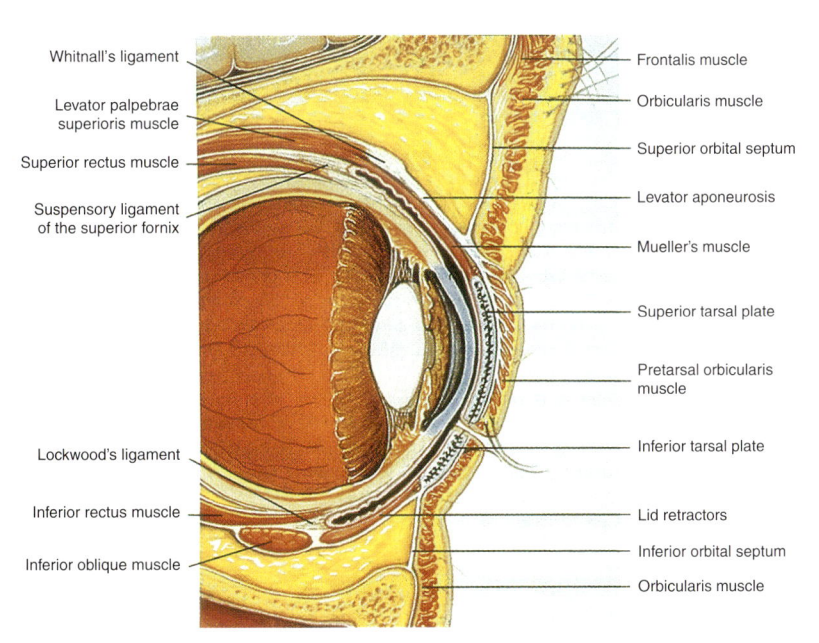

Figure 2-14 Attachments of the upper and lower eyelids to the vertical rectus muscles. Superiorly, the suspensory ligament acts to connect the superior rectus and levator, which facilitates movement of the eyelid on attempted upgaze. Large recessions of the superior rectus muscle can result in upper eyelid retraction, while resections can create a ptosis. Surgery on the inferior rectus can also cause changes in position of the lower eyelid because of the presence of Lockwood's ligament. A recession of the inferior rectus muscle can result in lower eyelid retraction, while a resection of the inferior rectus muscle can result in advancement of a lower eyelid and a narrowing of the palpebral fissure. *(Reproduced with permission from Buckley EG, Freedman S, Shields MB.* Atlas of Ophthalmic Surgery. Vol III: Strabismus and Glaucoma. *St Louis: Mosby; 1995:15.)*

When surgery is performed in the domain of the vortex veins, accidental severing of a vein is possible. The procedures that present the greatest risk for damaging a vortex vein are inferior rectus and superior rectus muscle recession or resection, inferior oblique muscle weakening procedures, and exposure of the superior oblique muscle tendon.

The sclera is thinnest just posterior to the four rectus muscle insertions. This area is the site for most muscle surgery, especially for recession procedures. Therefore, scleral perforation is always a risk during eye muscle surgery. This risk can be minimized by:

- Using spatulated needles with swedged sutures
- Working with a clean, dry, and blood-free surgical field
- Using loupe magnification or the operating microscope
- Employing a head-mounted fiberoptic light source in addition to the overhead operating lights

Chapter 13 discusses these procedures and complications in greater detail.

Bron AJ, Tripathi RC, Tripathi BJ, eds. *Wolff's Anatomy of the Eye and Orbit.* 8th ed. London: Chapman and Hall; 1997.

Buckley EG, Freedman S, Shields MB. *Atlas of Ophthalmic Surgery.* Vol III: *Strabismus and Glaucoma.* St Louis: Mosby; 1995.

Parks MM. Ocular motility and strabismus. In: *Duane's Clinical Ophthalmology.* Philadelphia: Lippincott; 1993; vol 1:1–20.

CHAPTER 3

Motor Physiology

Basic Principles and Terms

Axes of Fick, Center of Rotation, Listing's Plane, and Median Plane

The movement of the eye around a theoretical center of rotation is explained with specific terminology. Two helpful concepts are the axes of Fick and Listing's plane (Fig 3-1). The *axes of Fick* are designated as x, y, and z. The *x axis* is a transverse axis passing through the center of the eye at the equator; voluntary vertical rotations of the eye occur about this axis. The *y axis* is a sagittal axis passing through the pupil; involuntary torsional rotations occur about this axis. The *z axis* is a vertical axis; voluntary horizontal rotations occur about this axis. *Listing's equatorial plane* passes through the center of rotation and includes the x and z axes. The y axis is perpendicular to Listing's plane.

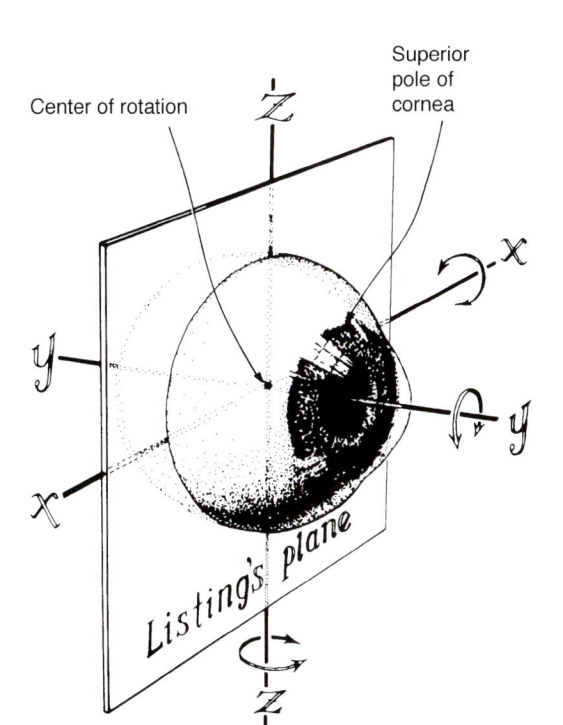

Figure 3-1 Axes of Fick, center of rotation, Listing's plane. *(Reprinted from Parks MM. Atlas of Strabismus. Philadelphia: Harper & Row; 1983.)*

Another helpful term for defining ocular movement is the median plane. The *median plane* is a sagittal plane that passes anteroposteriorly through the body, bisecting the head into symmetrical parts.

Positions of Gaze

Positions of gaze are also discussed in detail in Chapter 6. The following is basic terminology:

- *Primary position* is straight ahead
- *Secondary positions* are straight up, straight down, right gaze, left gaze
- *Tertiary positions* are the four oblique positions of gaze: up and right, up and left, down and right, down and left
- *Cardinal positions* are up and right, up and left, right, left, down and right, down and left

Arc of Contact

As the eye rotates, the extraocular muscle involved and the sclera act like a rope and pulley. The point of effective, or physiologic, insertion is the tangential point where the muscle first contacts the globe. The action of the eye muscle may be considered a vector of force that acts at this tangential point to rotate the eye. The length of muscle actually in contact with the globe constitutes the arc of contact.

Primary, Secondary, and Tertiary Action

With the eye in primary position, the horizontal rectus muscles are purely horizontal movers around the z (vertical) axis, and they have a primary action only. The vertical rectus muscles have a direction of pull that is mostly vertical as their primary action, but the angle of pull from origin to insertion is inclined 23° to the visual axis, giving rise also to *torsion,* which is defined as any rotation of the vertical corneal meridians. *Intorsion* (also called *incycloduction*) is the secondary action for the superior rectus; *extorsion* (also called *excycloduction*) is the secondary action for the inferior rectus; and *adduction* is the tertiary action for both muscles. Because the oblique muscles are inclined 51° to the visual axis, torsion is their primary action. Vertical rotation is their secondary and horizontal rotation their tertiary action (Table 3-1).

Field of Action

The term *field of action* is used in two ways to describe entirely separate and distinct concepts:

- To indicate the direction of rotation of the eye when a muscle contracts
- To refer to the gaze position in which the effect of the muscle is most readily observed

For the lateral rectus muscle, these two movements are both abduction; for the medial rectus, they are both adduction. However, the two movements are not the same for all muscles. For example, the inferior oblique muscle creates some vertical, torsional, and

Table 3-1 **Action of the Extraocular Muscles from Primary Position**

Muscle*	Primary	Secondary	Tertiary
Medial rectus	Adduction	—	—
Lateral rectus	Abduction	—	—
Inferior rectus	Depression	Extorsion	Adduction
Superior rectus	Elevation	Intorsion	Adduction
Inferior oblique	Extorsion	Elevation	Abduction
Superior oblique	Intorsion	Depression	Abduction

* The superior muscles are intortors; the inferior muscles are extortors. The vertical rectus muscles are adductors; the oblique muscles are abductors.

horizontal movement whenever it contracts. Furthermore, the amount of vertical, horizontal, and torsional change depends on the position of the eye. Only attempted elevation of the eye increases inferior oblique muscle activity, which is not increased with attempted abduction. Thus, a field of action is not a single unvarying movement for the inferior oblique muscle.

Field of activation would perhaps be a better term for this concept of what a muscle does. For example, the inferior oblique muscle is usually tested by its contribution to vertical eye movement in the adducted position because this is the muscle's field of greatest vertical action.

Thus, evaluation of fields of action must involve three separate aspects:

- Plane of the muscle action
- Gaze direction, which increases or decreases the innervation to the muscle
- Vector distribution of the muscle's force (vertical, horizontal, torsional) in various gaze positions

The importance of fields of action is that a deviation *(strabismus)* that increases with gaze in some directions may result from the weakness of the muscle normally pulling the eye in that direction. For example, esotropia increasing with gaze to the right may result from right lateral rectus muscle weakness.

Changing Muscle Action With Different Gaze Positions

The horizontal rectus muscles are the chief movers for horizontal gaze in all gaze positions. The vertical rectus muscles are the chief movers for vertical gaze in all gaze positions because of their greater size and power. When the eye abducts about 23°, it is codirectional with the line of pull of the vertical rectus muscles, and these muscles then primarily affect vertical rotation. In this position, the oblique muscles are now almost perpendicular to the y axis and function chiefly by cycloduction of the globe.

In adduction of 51°, the oblique muscles are nearly pure vertical rotators of the globe. The transverse x axis of the eye has been rotated to be almost perpendicular to their plane of muscle action; the vertical rectus muscles have become partial adductors and produce some increased torsional effect (Fig 3-2). (See also Chapter 2, Figs 2-5 and 2-6.)

Figure 3-2 The contribution of oblique muscles and vertical rectus muscles to vertical ductions is represented for the right eye. In abduction the rectus muscles contribute nearly the entire movement; in adduction both rectus and oblique muscles contribute. In abduction the superior rectus muscle is practically a pure elevator while the inferior oblique muscle is almost a pure tortor. IO, inferior oblique; IR, inferior rectus; SO, superior oblique; SR, superior rectus.

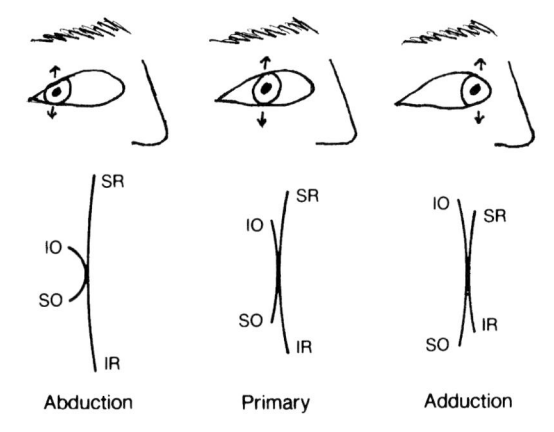

Physiology of Muscle

Position of rest

The position of each eye in the orbit without any innervation to the extraocular muscles is described as the position of rest. The position of each eye is slightly divergent in normal persons.

Motor units

An individual motor nerve fiber and its several muscle fibers is a motor unit. *Electromyography* records motor unit electrical activity. An electromyogram is useful in investigating normal and abnormal innervation and can be helpful in documenting paralysis, recovery from paralysis, and abnormalities of innervation in myasthenia gravis and muscle atrophy. However, this test is not helpful in ordinary comitant strabismus.

Recruitment during fixation or following movement

As the eye moves farther into abduction, for example, more and more lateral rectus motor units are activated and brought into play by the brain to help pull the eye. This process is called *recruitment*. In addition, as the eye fixates farther into abduction, the frequency of activity of each motor unit increases until it reaches a peak (for some motor units, several hundred contractions per second).

Saccades

Saccadic movements require a sudden, strong pulse of force from the extraocular muscles in order to move the eye rapidly against the viscosity produced by the fatty tissue and fascia in which the globe lies. For example, abducting the eye in a saccade requires a sudden great increase in lateral rectus muscle activity to get the eye moving and, at the same time, a total inhibition of the medial rectus muscle until the eye is again stabilized in the new gaze position. Velocity is nearly proportional to the size of the saccade and can be 10°–400°/sec. The velocity of the saccadic movement and the high forces that must be produced are affected by muscle paresis, and study of saccadic velocity is of practical value in determining paresis of muscles and abnormal innervation. BCSC Section 5, *Neuro-Ophthalmology*, discusses saccades in detail.

Scott AB. Ocular motility. In: Tasman W, Jaeger EA, eds. *Biomedical Foundations of Ophthalmology.* Vol 2. Philadelphia: Lippincott; 1997.

Eye Movements

Monocular Eye Movements (Ductions)

Ductions are monocular rotations of the eye. *Adduction* is movement of the eye nasally; *abduction* is movement of the eye temporally. *Elevation (supraduction* or *sursumduction)* is an upward rotation of the eye; *depression (infraduction* or *deorsumduction)* is a downward rotation of the eye. *Intorsion (incycloduction)* is defined as a nasal rotation of the superior portion of the vertical corneal meridian. *Extorsion (excycloduction)* is a temporal rotation of the superior portion of the vertical corneal meridian.

The following are also important terms relating to the muscles used in monocular eye movements:

- *Agonist:* the primary muscle moving the eye in a given direction
- *Synergist:* the muscle in the same eye as the agonist that acts with the agonist to produce a given movement (eg, the inferior oblique muscle is a synergist with the agonist superior rectus muscle for elevation of the eye)
- *Antagonist:* the muscle in the same eye as the agonist that acts in the direction opposite to that of the agonist; the medial rectus and lateral rectus muscles are antagonists

Sherrington's law of reciprocal innervation states that increased innervation and contraction of a given extraocular muscle are accompanied by a reciprocal decrease in innervation and contraction of its antagonist. For example, as the right eye abducts, the right lateral rectus muscle receives increased innervation while the right medial rectus receives decreased innervation.

Binocular Eye Movements (Versions and Vergences)

When binocular eye movements are conjugate and the eyes move in the same direction, such movements are called *versions.* When the eye movements are disconjugate and the eyes move in opposite directions, such movements are known as *vergences* (eg, convergence and divergence).

Versions: conjugate binocular eye movements

Right gaze (dextroversion) is movement of both eyes to the patient's right. *Left gaze (levoversion)* is movement of both eyes to the patient's left. *Elevation,* or *upgaze (sursumversion),* is an upward rotation of both eyes; *depression,* or *downgaze (deorsumversion),* is a downward rotation of both eyes. In *dextrocycloversion,* both eyes rotate so that the superior portion of the vertical corneal meridian moves to the patient's right. Similarly, *levocycloversion* is movement of both eyes so that the superior portion of the vertical corneal meridian rotates to the patient's left.

The term *yoke muscles* is used to describe two muscles (one in each eye) that are the prime movers of their respective eyes in a given position of gaze. For example, when the eyes move or attempt to move into right gaze, the right lateral rectus muscle and the left medial rectus muscle are simultaneously innervated and contracted. These muscles are said to be "yoked" together.

Each extraocular muscle in one eye has a yoke muscle in the other eye. Because the effect of a muscle is usually best seen in a given direction of gaze, the concept of yoke muscles is used to evaluate the contribution of each extraocular muscle to eye movement. The six positions of gaze in which one muscle of each eye is the prime mover are known as the *cardinal positions of gaze*. Figure 3-3 shows these six cardinal positions of gaze and the yoke muscles whose primary actions are in that field of gaze.

Hering's law of motor correspondence states that equal and simultaneous innervation flows to yoke muscles concerned with the desired direction of gaze. The most useful application of this law is in evaluating binocular eye movements and, in particular, the yoke muscles involved.

Hering's law has important clinical implications, especially when dealing with a paralytic or restrictive strabismus. Because the amount of innervation to both eyes is always determined by the fixating eye, the angle of deviation varies according to which eye is fixating. When the normal eye is fixating, the amount of misalignment is called the *primary deviation*. When the paretic or restrictive eye is fixating, the amount of misalignment is called the *secondary deviation*. The secondary deviation is larger than the primary deviation.

Hering's law is also necessary to explain the following example. If a patient has a right superior oblique muscle paresis and uses the right eye to fixate an object that is located up and to the patient's left, the innervation of the right inferior oblique muscle required to move the eye into this gaze position is reduced because the right inferior oblique does not have to overcome the normal antagonistic effect of the right superior oblique muscle. Therefore, according to Hering's law, less innervation is also received by the right inferior oblique muscle's yoke muscle, the left superior rectus muscle. This decreased innervation could lead to the incorrect impression that the left superior rectus muscle is paretic (Fig 3-4).

The above example is said to involve an inhibitional paresis of the *contralateral antagonist* when the paretic eye is fixating. However, the term *contralateral antagonist*, when used in conjunction with the concept of inhibitional paresis, is a contradiction. A more accurate description would be an inhibitional paresis of the antagonist (left superior rectus muscle) of the *yoke muscle* (left inferior rectus muscle) of the paretic muscle (right superior oblique muscle).

Vergences: disconjugate binocular eye movements

Convergence is movement of both eyes nasally relative to a given position; *divergence* is movement of both eyes temporally relative to a given position. *Incyclovergence* is a rotation of both eyes so that the superior portion of each vertical corneal meridian rotates toward the median plane; *excyclovergence* is a rotation of both eyes so that the superior portion of each vertical corneal meridian rotates away from the median plane. *Vertical vergence* movement, though less frequently encountered, can also occur: one eye moves upward and the other downward. Other important terms and concepts related to vergences include the following:

- *Tonic convergence* represents the constant innervational tone to the extraocular muscles when a person is awake and alert. Because of the anatomical shape of the bony orbits and the position of the rectus muscle origins, the alignment of the eyes under complete muscle paralysis is divergent. Therefore, convergence tone is necessary in the awake state to maintain straight eyes even in the absence of strabismus.
- *Accommodative convergence* of the visual axes occurs as part of the synkinetic near reflex. A fairly consistent increment of accommodative convergence (AC) occurs for each diopter of accommodation (A), giving the *accommodative convergence/accommodation (AC/A) ratio*.

Abnormalities of this ratio are common, and they are an important cause of strabismus. With an abnormally high AC/A ratio, the excess convergence tends to produce esotropia during accommodation on near targets. An abnormally low AC/A ratio tends to make the eyes exotropic when the person looks at near targets. For techniques of measuring this ratio, see the discussion of the AC/A ratio under Convergence in Chapter 6.

- *Voluntary convergence* is a conscious application of the near synkinesis.
- *Proximal (instrument) convergence* is an induced convergence movement caused by a psychological awareness of near; this movement is particularly apparent when a person looks through an instrument such as a binocular microscope.
- *Fusional convergence* is an optomotor reflex to converge and position the eyes so that similar retinal images project on corresponding retinal areas. Fusional convergence is accomplished without changing the refractive state of the eyes and is prompted by bitemporal retinal image disparity.
- *Fusional divergence* is the only clinically significant form of divergence. It is an optomotor reflex to diverge and align the eyes so that similar retinal images project on corresponding retinal areas. Fusional divergence is accomplished without changing the refractive state of the eyes and is prompted by binasal retinal image disparity.

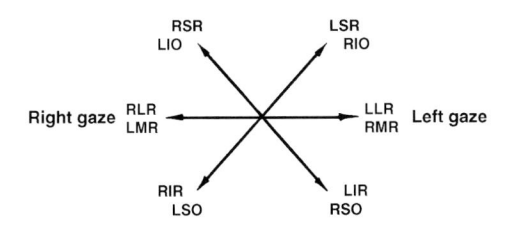

Figure 3-3 Cardinal positions and yoke muscles. RSR, right superior rectus; LIO, left inferior oblique; LSR, left superior rectus; RIO, right inferior oblique; RLR, right lateral rectus; LMR, left medial rectus; LLR, left lateral rectus; RMR, right medial rectus; RIR, right inferior rectus; LSO, left superior oblique; LIR, left inferior rectus; RSO, right superior oblique.

36 • Pediatric Ophthalmology and Strabismus

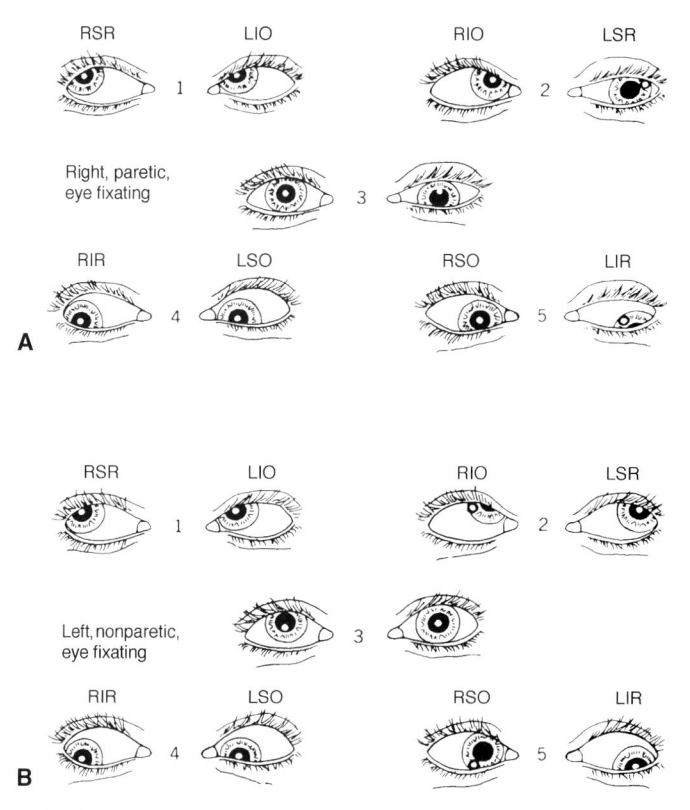

Figure 3-4 Paresis of right superior oblique muscle. **A,** With right paretic eye fixating, little or no vertical difference appears between the two eyes in the right (uninvolved) field of gaze *(1 and 4)*. In primary position *(3)*, a left hypotropia may be present because the right elevators require less innervation and thus the left elevators will receive less than normal innervation. When gaze is up and left *(2)*, the RIO needs less than normal innervation to elevate OD because its antagonist, the RSO, is paretic. Consequently, its yoke, the LSR, will be apparently underacting, and pseudoptosis with pseudoparesis of the LSR will be present. When gaze is toward the field of action of the paretic muscle *(5)*, maximal innervation is required to move OD down during adduction, and thus the LIR will be overacting. **B,** With left sound eye fixating, no vertical difference appears in the right field of gaze *(1 and 4)*. In primary position *(3)*, OD is elevated because of unbalanced elevators. When gaze is up and left *(2)*, the RIO shows marked overaction because its antagonist is paretic and there is contracture of the unopposed muscle. The action of the LSR is normal. When gaze is down and left *(5)*, normal innervation required by the fixating normal eye does not suffice to fully move the paretic eye. *(Reprinted from von Noorden GK. Atlas of Strabismus. 4th ed. St Louis: Mosby; 1983:24–25.)*

Supranuclear Control Systems for Eye Movement

There are five supranuclear eye movement systems:

- The *saccadic system* generates all fast (up to 400°–500°/sec) eye movements, or eye movements of refixation. This system functions to place the image of an object of interest on the fovea or to move the eyes from one object to another. Saccades are

initiated by burst cells within the paramedian pontine reticular formation. Activation of burst cells requires suppression of pause cell activity. Pause cells are inhibited by corticobulbar projections from the frontal lobe.
- The *smooth pursuit system* generates all following, or pursuit, eye movements. Pursuit latency is shorter than for saccades, but the maximum peak velocity of these slow pursuit movements is limited to 30°–60°/sec. The pathway starts with the striate cortex, which receives input from the lateral geniculate bodies. Extrastriate visual areas then receive input and project ipsilaterally to the dorsolateral pontine nuclei. Ultimately, the vestibular nuclei receive the input (probably through the cerebellar flocculus and dorsal vermis) and transmit it to ocular motor nuclei of cranial nerves III, IV, and VI.
- The *vergence system* controls disconjugate eye movement, as in convergence or divergence. Supranuclear control of vergence eye movements is not yet fully understood.
- The *position maintenance system* maintains a specific gaze position, allowing an object of interest to remain on the fovea. The site of this system is not known.
- The *nonoptic reflex systems* integrate eye movements and body movements. The most clinically important system is the labyrinthine reflex system involving the semicircular canals of the inner ears. Other, less important, systems involve the utricle and saccule of the inner ears. The cervical, or neck, receptors also provide input for this nonoptic reflex control.

These systems are discussed in depth in BCSC Section 5, *Neuro-Ophthalmology*.

CHAPTER 4

Sensory Physiology and Pathology

Objective visual space consists of actual visual objects in physical space outside of, and independent of, our visual system. *Subjective visual space* is our conscious awareness of these visual objects and their relationships to us as perceived and interpreted by the brain.

Physiology of Normal Binocular Vision

If an area of the retina is stimulated by any means—externally by light or internally by mechanical pressure or electrical processes—the resulting sensation is always one of *light*, and the light is subjectively localized as coming from a specific visual direction in space. This directional value of the retinal elements is an intrinsic physiologic property of the retina and the brain. Thus, the stimulation of any retinal area results in a visual sensation from a subjective visual direction relative to the visual direction of the fovea. The visual direction of the fovea is termed the *visual axis*, and normally, with central fixation, it is subjectively localized straight ahead. BCSC Section 12, *Retina and Vitreous*, illustrates and discusses in depth the anatomy and physiology of the retina.

Correspondence

If retinal areas in the two eyes share a common subjective visual direction—that is, if their simultaneous stimulation results in the subjective sensation that the stimulating target or targets come from the same direction in space—these retinal areas or points are said to be *corresponding*. If the simultaneous stimulation of retinal areas in the two eyes results in the sensation of two separate visual directions, or diplopia, these retinal areas or points are said to be *noncorresponding*, or *disparate*. If corresponding retinal areas in the two eyes bear identical relationships to the fovea in each eye (eg, both corresponding areas are located equidistantly to the right or left of and above or below the fovea), *normal retinal correspondence* (NRC) exists. Dissimilar relationships between two corresponding retinal areas and their respective foveas indicate *anomalous retinal correspondence* (ARC). (ARC is discussed at length later in the chapter.)

If the two eyes have NRC and each fovea fixates an identical point, this point is seen singly. Points to both sides of this fixation point likewise fall on corresponding retinal areas and also are seen singly, as long as these points lie on a horizontal construct known as the *Vieth-Müller circle*. This circle passes through the optical centers of each eye and the point of fixation. When attempts are made to duplicate the Vieth-Müller circle experimentally, the locus of all points seen singly falls not on the circle but on a curved surface called the *empirical horopter* (Fig 4-1). The horopter exists not only in two dimensions but is actually a three-dimensional space obtained by rotating the horizontal horopter around an axis connecting the centers of rotation of the two eyes. The geometric figure thus formed is a *torus*.

Each fixation point determines a specific horopter. By definition, all points lying on the horopter curve stimulate corresponding retinal elements and thus are seen singly. All points not lying on the horopter mathematically fall on disparate retinal elements and would therefore be expected to create double vision. However, double vision does not occur physiologically within a limited area surrounding the horopter curve because the visual system fuses the two disparate retinal images, resulting in single binocular vision with *stereopsis*. The slightly different images caused by the three-dimensional object stimulate stereoscopic perception.

The areas near the fovea allow very little overlap (small receptive fields) before diplopia is elicited, whereas more overlap (larger receptive fields) is tolerated farther toward the periphery of vision. Figure 4-1 shows objects in this space that fall mathematically on disparate retinal areas but are physiologically seen singly. This space is called *Panum's area of single binocular vision*. Objects outside of Panum's area fall on widely disparate retinal areas and are seen as coming from two different visual directions, causing diplopia.

A three-dimensional object is partly in front of and partly behind the empirical horopter and thus stimulates disparate retinal points and is seen stereoscopically. As long as the three-dimensional object falls entirely within Panum's area, it is seen singly. Objects that fall outside of Panum's area are seen double because the images are too disparate to be fused cortically into a single image. Stereopsis is a response to horizontally disparate retinal stimulation. The zone of stereopsis is actually wider than Panum's fusional area, creating a zone in front of and behind Panum's space in which double images can still be perceived as being farther away or closer than the object of regard (see Fig 4-1).

Fusion

Fusion is the cortical unification of visual objects into a single percept that is made possible by the simultaneous stimulation of corresponding retinal areas. For retinal images to be fused, they must be similar in size and shape. Fusion has been artificially divided into sensory fusion, motor fusion, and stereopsis.

Sensory fusion

Sensory fusion is based on the innate orderly topographic relationship between the retinas and the visual cortex whereby corresponding retinal points project to the same cortical locus, and corresponding adjacent retinal points have adjacent cortical representations.

Motor fusion

Motor fusion is a vergence movement that causes similar retinal images to fall and be maintained on corresponding retinal areas even though natural (eg, phorias) or artificial causes tend to induce disparities. For example, if progressive base-out prism is introduced before both eyes while a target is viewed, the retinal images move temporally over both retinas if the eyes remain in fixed position. However, fusional convergence movements maintain similar retinal images on corresponding retinal areas, and the eyes are observed to converge. This response is called *fusional convergence.* Motor fusion may be thought of as a diplopia avoidance mechanism. Fusional vergence amplitudes can be measured with rotary prisms, by major haploscopes, and by other devices. Representative normal values are given in Table 4-1. Fusional vergences are also discussed in Chapter 6.

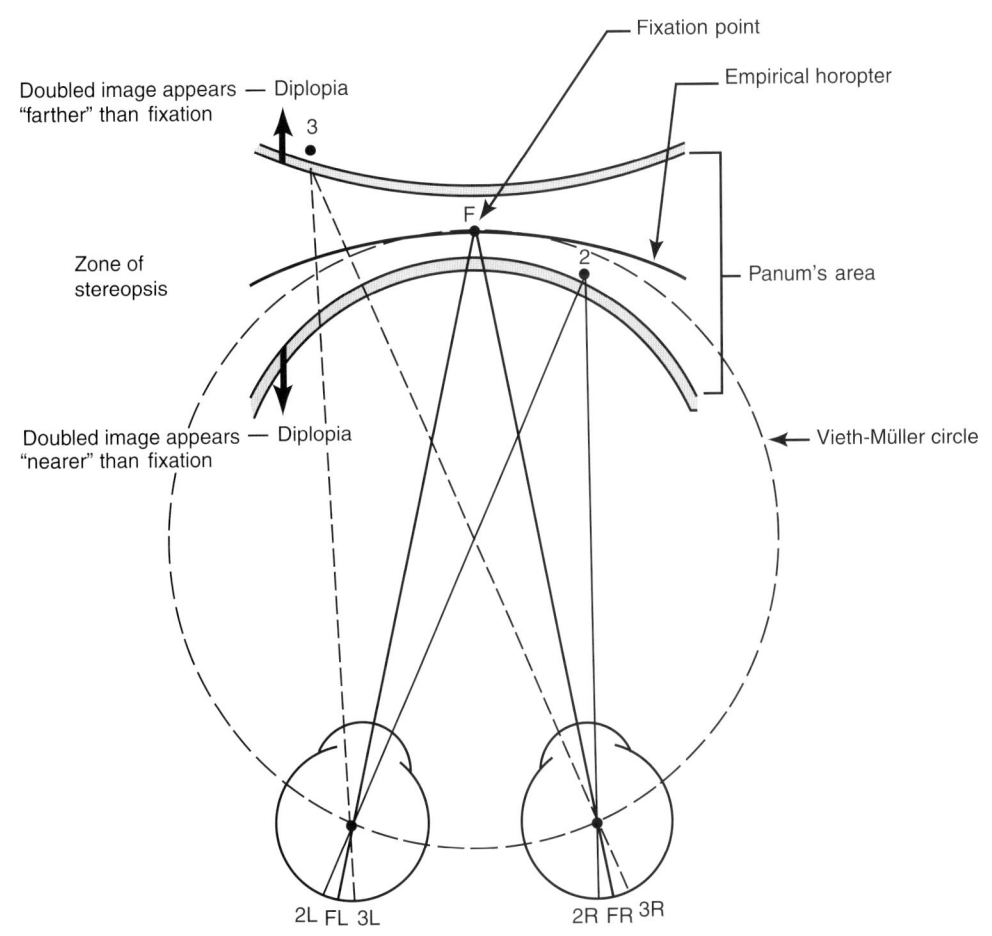

Figure 4-1 Empirical horopter. *F,* fixation point; *FL* and *FR,* left and right foveas, respectively. Point 2, falling within Panum's area, is seen singly and stereoscopically. Point 3 falls outside of Panum's area and is therefore seen double.

Table 4-1 Average Normal Fusional Amplitudes in Prism Diopters (Δ)

Testing Distance	Convergence Fusional Amplitudes	Divergence Fusional Amplitudes	Vertical Fusional Amplitudes
6 m	14Δ	6Δ	2.5Δ
25 cm	38Δ	16Δ	2.6Δ

Stereopsis

Stereopsis should not be thought of as a form of simple fusion. As discussed, stereopsis occurs when retinal disparity is too great to permit the simple superimposition or fusion of the two visual directions but is not great enough to elicit diplopia. Stereopsis, therefore, is a bridge between simple sensory and motor fusion and diplopia. Stereopsis is a relative or subjective ordering of visual objects in depth, or three dimensions.

Stereopsis and *depth perception* should not be considered synonymous. Monocular clues contribute to depth perception. These monocular clues include object overlap, relative object size, highlights and shadows, motion parallax, and perspective. Stereopsis is a binocular sensation of relative depth caused by horizontal retinal image disparity. Nasal disparity between two similar retinal images is interpreted by the brain as farther away from the fixation point, temporal disparity as nearer. At distances farther than 20 feet, we rely almost entirely on monocular clues for depth perception.

Selected Aspects of the Neurophysiology of Vision

Substantial research has recently focused on the neurophysiology of vision. For the purposes of this book, we will focus on the magno and parvo cells of the retinal ganglion cell layer; the lateral geniculate body (LGB), which consists of six purely monocular laminae (four dorsal parvocellular and two ventral magnocellular laminae); and the primary visual cortex, also called the *striate cortex, V1,* or *Brodmann's area 17*. This retino-geniculo-cortical pathway provides the neural substrate for visual perception (Fig 4-2).

The LGB is the principal thalamic visual nucleus linking the retina and the striate cortex. Of the approximately 1 million ganglion cells in the retina, approximately 90% of these terminate in the LGB. The LGB contains about 1.8 million neurons, which yields a ratio of ganglion cells to geniculate neurons of approximately 1:2. After a relatively direct transfer through the LGB, the signal activates a unit in the striate cortex containing approximately 1000 processing elements. According to the classic view, the striate cortex performs the basic analysis of geniculate input and then transmits its essence to higher peristriate cortical areas for further interpretation. These areas have been called *Brodmann's areas 18* and *19,* or *V2, V3, V3a, V4,* and *V5*.

Retino-Geniculo-Cortical Pathway

The magnocellular (M) system and the parvocellular (P) system are the main neural systems in the retino-geniculo-cortical pathway. The M pathway originates with the magnocellular retinal ganglion cells. These M retinal cells have large soma with large dendritic fields and large axons. These cells are rare in the foveal area and increase in number toward the near periphery. They synapse with the magnocellular neurons in the LGB. The M geniculate axons terminate in the striate cortex (V1) layer IV Cα. The neurons in this system have a fast response time, but these responses decay rapidly when the stimulus is maintained, making the M system especially sensitive to moving stimuli but not to stationary images. The M system is also relatively insensitive to color.

The P system originates in the P retinal ganglion cells, which have small soma and small dendritic fields; these cells are of relatively high density in the fovea and decrease

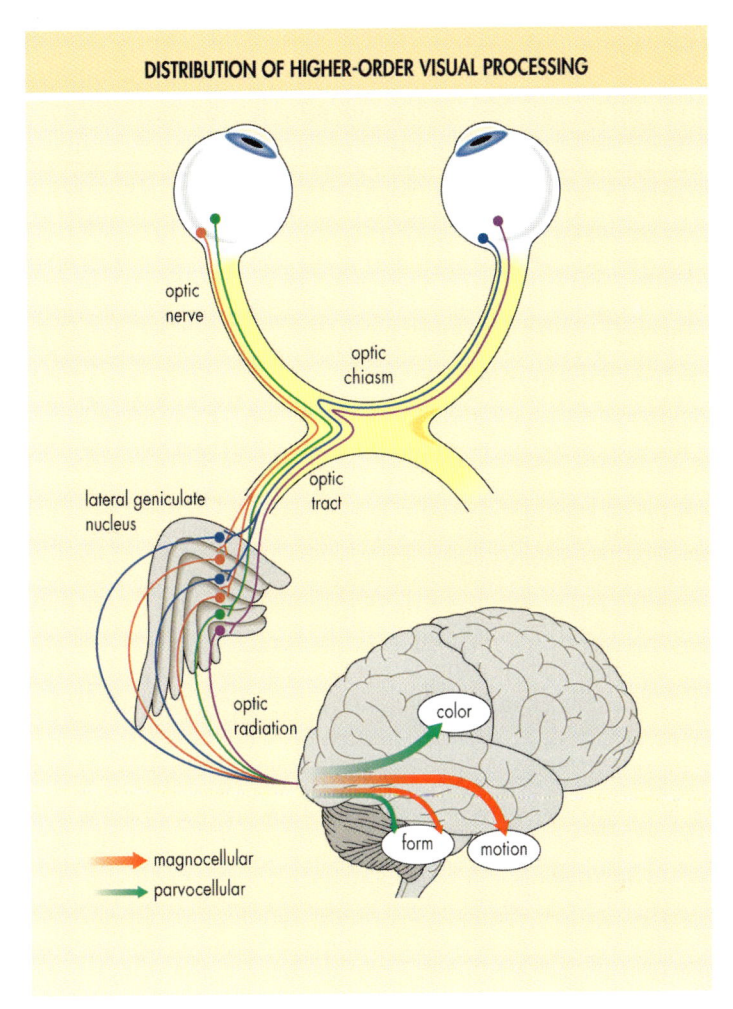

Figure 4-2 Distribution of higher-order visual processing among different cortical areas. The magnocellular system (inferior stream) is concerned generally with the location and motion of objects; the parvocellular system (superior stream) is concerned with the fine resolution (acuity), form, and color of objects. *(From Lawton A. The afferent visual system cortical representation of vision. In: Yanoff M, Duker J, eds.* Ophthalmology. *London: Mosby; 1999.)*

in number as retinal eccentricity increases. The P retinal ganglion cells synapse with the parvocellular LGB cells. The P geniculate axons terminate in layer IV Cβ of V1. The P system gives a slow tonic response to visual stimulation, carries high-resolution information about object borders and color contrast, and is important for shape perception and the ability to see standing objects in detail.

The fibers of the optic tract terminate in the LGB. Geniculate laminae 1 (parvo), 4 (parvo), and 6 (magno) receive axons from the contralateral nasal retina; laminae 2 (parvo), 3 (parvo), and 5 (magno) receive axons from the ipsilateral temporal retina. This monocular separation continues through the lateral geniculate laminae into the striate cortex (V1), where the geniculate axon terminals from the right and left eyes are segregated into a system of alternating parallel stripes called *ocular dominance columns* (Fig 4-3). In the P system, these strictly monocular geniculate axons terminate in layer IV Cβ. From there, the paired right and left monocular cells finally converge on the first binocular cells in layers II and III of V1. In the M system, after the monocular geniculate axons terminate in layer IV Cα, the paired right and left monocular cells converge on the first binocular cells in layer IV B of V1.

Visual Development

Data pertaining to the prenatal development of the central visual pathways in humans is limited by the practical difficulties in obtaining adequate fixed specimens and the fact that invasive experimental techniques suitable for animal studies cannot be used in human studies.

In the human retina, most of the ganglion cells are generated between the 8th and 15th weeks of gestation, reaching a plateau of 2.2–2.5 million by week 18. After week 30, the ganglion cell population falls dramatically during a period of rapid cell death that lasts 6–8 weeks. Thereafter, cell death continues at a low rate into the first few postnatal months. The retinal ganglion cell population is reduced to a final count of about 1 million. The loss of over 1 million optic axons may serve to refine topography and specificity of the retinogeniculate projection by eliminating inappropriate connections.

The neurons of the human LGB are probably formed between the 8th and 11th weeks of gestation. By week 10, the first retinal ganglion cells, those of the M system, invade the developing LGB. Segregation of the magno and parvo retinal ganglion cells occurs on a timetable that parallels the lamination in the LGB. Retinal afferents prune back their axon terminals so that the synaptic connections are preserved only within the appropriate geniculate laminae, which emerge between weeks 22 and 25. It is thought that ganglion cells die if their axons do not successfully synapse with the appropriate targets in the brain.

The cells that will become the striate cortex are probably formed between the 10th and 25th weeks of gestation. Initially, the geniculate afferents representing each eye overlap extensively in layer IV C (Fig 4-4). The maturation of the ocular dominance columns requires thousands of left and right eye geniculate afferents to gradually disentangle their overlapping axon terminals. This segregation transpires during the last few weeks of pregnancy and is almost complete at birth.

The continued development of visual function after birth is accompanied by major anatomical changes occurring simultaneously at all levels of the central visual pathways. The fovea is still covered by multiple cell layers and is sparsely packed with cones, which may account for the estimated visual acuity of 20/400 at birth. During the first years of life, the photoreceptors redistribute within the retina and peak foveal cone density increases fivefold to achieve the configuration found in the adult retina, with an improvement in visual acuity to the 20/20 level. In newborns, the white matter of the visual pathways is not fully myelinated. For the first 2 years after birth, myelin sheaths enlarge rapidly and then continue at a slower rate through the first decade of life. At birth, the neurons of the LGB are only 60% of their average size. Their volume gradually increases until age 2 years. Striate cortex refinement of synaptic connections continues for many

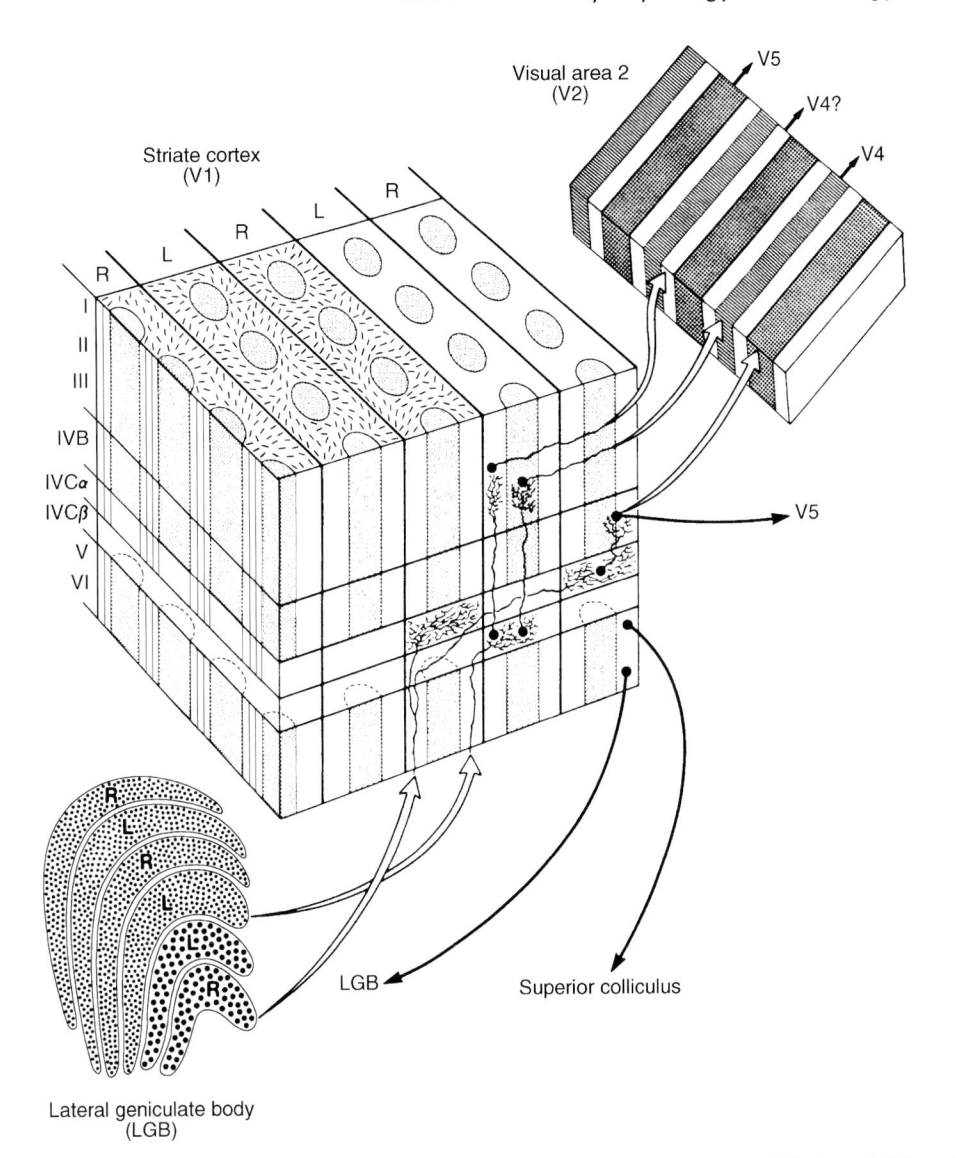

Figure 4-3 Magno and parvo pathways from the lateral geniculate body (LGB) through V1 and V2 to areas V4 and V5. Each module of striate cortex contains a few complete sets of ocular dominance columns (R + L). The magno stream courses through layer IV Cα, layer IV B, *thick stripes* in V2, and V5. The parvo stream projects through layer IV Cβ to layers II and III. In striate cortex, layers V and VI send projections to the superior colliculus and the lateral geniculate body, respectively. *(From Horton J. The central visual pathways. In: Hart WM, ed.* Adler's Physiology of the Eye: Clinical Applications. *9th ed. St Louis: Mosby; 1992:751.)*

years after birth. The density of synapses declines by 40% over several years to attain final adult levels at about age 10 years.

Surprisingly, physiologic activity in the fetus is vital to the development of normal anatomical connections in the visual system. In utero, mammalian retinal ganglion cells

46 • Pediatric Ophthalmology and Strabismus

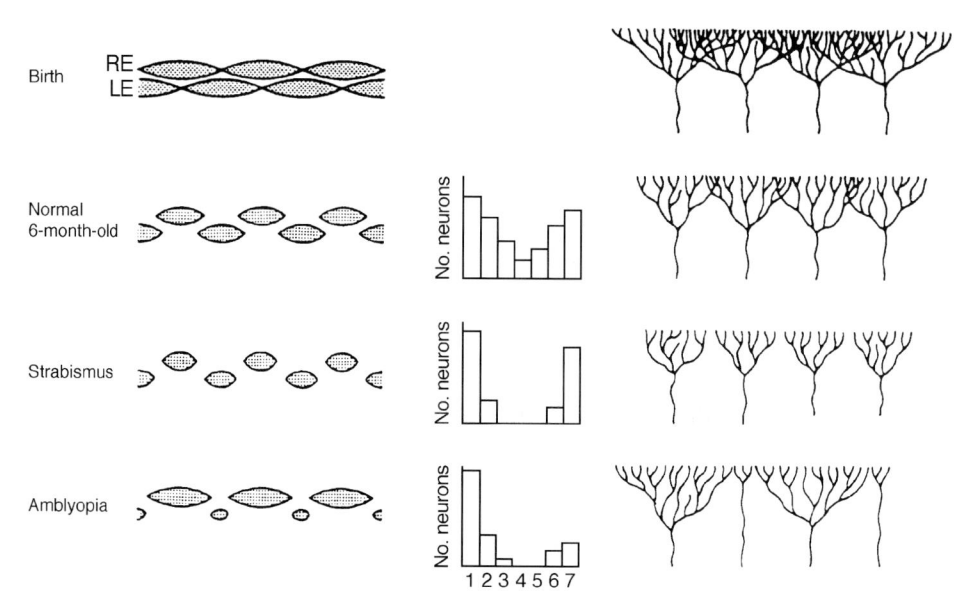

Figure 4-4 Anatomical and physiologic maturation of ocular dominance in lamina IV of left primary visual cortex in normal and deprived monkeys. *Birth:* Broad overlap of afferents from lateral geniculate nucleus to lamina 4, hence little dominance by right (RE) vs. left eye (LE). *Normal 6-month-old:* Regression of overlapping afferents from both eyes with distinct areas of monocular dominance. Bar graph shows the classic U-shaped distribution obtained by single-cell recordings from the visual cortex. About half the cells are driven predominantly by the contralateral right eye and the other half by the ipsilateral left eye. A small number are driven equally by the two eyes. 1 = driven only by contralateral eye; 7 = driven only by ipsilateral eye; 2–6 = driven binocularly. *Strabismus:* Effect of artificial eye misalignment in the neonatal period on ocular dominance. The monkey alternated fixation (no amblyopia) and lacked fusion. Lack of binocularity is evident as exaggerated segregation into dominance columns. Bar graph shows results of single-cell recordings obtained from this animal after age 1 year. Almost all neurons are driven exclusively by the right or left eye. *Amblyopia:* Effect of suturing the left eyelid shut shortly after birth. Dominance columns of the normal right eye are much wider than those of the amblyopic left eye. Bar graph shows markedly skewed ocular dominance. *(From Tychsen L. Binocular vision. In: Hart WM, ed. Adler's Physiology of the Eye: Clinical Applications. 9th ed. St Louis: Mosby; 1992:810.)*

discharge spontaneous action potentials in the absence of any visual stimulation. Abolishing these action potentials with tetrodoxin prevents the normal prenatal segregation of the retinogeniculate axons into appropriate geniculate laminae and blocks the formation of ocular dominance columns in the striate cortex. Thus, although the functional architecture of the visual system is ordained by genetics, the specificity and refinement are molded by physiologic vision-independent activity occurring in the fetus as well as by postnatal vision-dependent experience.

Effects of Abnormal Visual Experience on the Retino-Geniculo-Cortical Pathway

Abnormal visual experience can powerfully affect retino-geniculo-cortical development. Abnormal development produced by visual deprivation, anisometropia, or strabismus appears to result in changes in the primary visual cortex, which ceases to be a faithful relay of visual signals. The developing visual system's extreme sensitivity to unequal binocular competition and competitive inhibition is the price to be paid for the mechanisms that use patterns of activity to refine neural connections to a level of high precision.

If a newborn monkey is reared in the dark or with both eyes sutured closed, cells in the striate cortex eventually lose sharp orientation tuning and normal binocular responses. Some of the cells become unresponsive to visual stimulation and activate erratically and spontaneously. The remaining units give sluggish and unpredictable responses to visual stimulation. After a prolonged period of deprivation, if the monkey is introduced to a normal visual environment or the eyelids are reopened, the animal is left profoundly blind with minimal potential for recovery. Cells in the striate cortex do not recover their normal responses.

Following the postnatal critical period, the visual system becomes impervious to the effects of sensory deprivation. If an adult monkey is visually deprived by the suturing of both eyelids, the cells in the striate cortex remain unaffected.

Single eyelid suturing in baby macaque monkeys usually produced axial myopia but no other significant changes in the eye. There was minor shrinkage of both magno and parvo cells of the lateral geniculate laminae receiving input from that deprived eye, but these cells responded briskly to visual stimulation, implying that a defect in the LGB is not likely to account for amblyopia. In the striate cortex, monocular visual deprivation caused the ocular dominance columns of the closed eye to appear radically narrowed (see Fig 4-4). The most popular explanation is that the two eyes compete for synaptic contacts in the cortex. As a result, the deprived eye loses many of the connections already formed at birth with postsynaptic cortical targets. This leads to excessive pruning of the terminal arbors of geniculate cells driven by the deprived eye. In turn, the ocular dominance columns of the deprived eye begin to shrink, which leads to a reduction in the cell size of the LGB cells required to sustain a reduced arbor of axon terminals in layer IV C. The open eye profits by the sprouting of terminal arbors beyond their usual boundaries to occupy territory relinquished by the deprived eye. However, the benefit derived by invading the cortical territory of the deprived eye is unclear because visual acuity does not improve beyond normal. Positron emission testing has shown a reduction in the cortical blood flow and glucose metabolism during stimulation of the amblyopic eye compared with the normal eye, suggesting the visual cortex as the primary site of amblyopia. This monocular deprivation also devastates binocularity in that few cells can be driven by both eyes.

There is a critical period in which the eye of the macaque monkey is vulnerable to the effects of eyelid suturing. This critical period corresponds to when the wiring of the striate cortex is still vulnerable to the effects of visual deprivation. During the critical period, the deleterious effects of eyelid closure are correctable by reversal of the eyelid suture—that is, opening the sutured eye and closing the fellow eye. In this case, the ocular dominance columns of the initially closed eye appeared practically normal, indicating that anatomical recovery of the initially shrunken columns was induced by opening the right eye and penalizing the left eye. However, when the right eye was sewn closed beyond the critical period, then reopened and the fellow eye closed, the deprived eye columns did not reexpand.

Eyelid suturing in the baby macaque monkey is a good model for visual-deprivation amblyopia. In children, this condition can be caused by any dense opacity of the ocular media or occlusion by the eyelid. Amblyopia in children also has other causes. Optical defocus caused by anisometropia causes the cortical neurons driven by the defocused eye to be less sensitive (particularly to higher spatial frequencies because they are most affected by blur) and to send out a weaker signal. This results in a binocular neural imbalance, resulting in a less drastic narrowing of the ocular dominance columns and cell shrinkage in the parvocellular lamina. Only the function of the P system is abnormal in anisometropic amblyopia. Deficits in binocular processing are also more pronounced when tested with stimuli of high spatial frequency.

The critical period for anisometropic amblyopia begins when the unilateral optical blur exceeds the lessening bilateral neural blur, which improves as the visual system develops sensitivity to high spatial frequency. This critical period may have a later onset than strabismic amblyopia and may require a prolonged period of unilateral blur. Meridional (astigmatic) amblyopia does not develop during the first year of life and may not develop until age 3.

Strabismus can be artificially created in monkeys by the sectioning of an extraocular muscle. Some monkeys develop alternating fixation after this procedure; they maintain normal acuity in each eye. Examination of the striate cortex reveals cells with normal receptive fields and an equal number of cells responsive to stimulation of either eye. However, the cortex is bereft of binocular cells (see Fig 4-4). After one extraocular muscle is cut, some monkeys do not alternately fixate but constantly fixate with the same eye and the deviating eye develops amblyopia. An important factor in the development of strabismic amblyopia is interocular suppression due to image uncorrelation. Strabismus causes abnormal input to the striate cortex by preventing the synchronous firing provided by simultaneous correlated images from the two foveas. Another factor is the optical defocus of the deviated eye. The dominant eye is focused on the object of regard while the deviated eye is pointed in a different direction; for the deviated eye, an object may be too near or too far to be in focus. Either mechanism can cause asynchrony or inhibition of one set of signals in the striate cortex layer IV C. Few cells in the striate cortex can be driven by stimulation of the amblyopic eye.

The critical period for developing strabismic amblyopia appears to begin at approximately 4 months of age, during the time of ocular dominance segregation and sensitivity to binocular correlation.

It is remarkable that abnormal sensory input alone is sufficient to alter the normal anatomy of the visual cortex. Other areas of the cerebral cortex may also depend on sensory stimulation to form the proper anatomical circuits necessary for normal adult visual function. This notion underscores the importance of providing children with an adequate and healthy sensory environment.

Booth R, Fulton A. Amblyopia. In: Albert D, Jakobiec F, eds. *Principles and Practice of Ophthalmology*. 2nd ed. Philadelphia: Saunders; 2000:4340–4354.

Bron A, Tripathi RC, Tripathi BJ, et al. *Wolff's Anatomy of the Eye and Orbit*. 8th ed. London: Chapman and Hall; 1997:551–594.

Horton J. The central visual pathways. In: Hart WM, ed. *Adler's Physiology of the Eye: Clinical Applications*. 9th ed. St Louis: Mosby; 1992:728–767.

Shan Y, Moster ML, Roemer RA, et al. Abnormal function of the parvocellular visual system in anisometropic amblyopia. *J Pediatr Ophthalmol Strabismus.* 2000;37:73–78.

Tychsen L. Binocular vision. In: Hart WM, ed. *Adler's Physiology of the Eye: Clinical Applications.* 9th ed. St Louis: Mosby; 1992:773–853.

Abnormalities of Binocular Vision

When a manifest deviation of the eyes occurs, the corresponding retinal elements of the eyes are no longer directed at the same object. This places the patient at risk for two different visual phenomena: visual confusion and diplopia.

Confusion

Visual confusion is the simultaneous perception of two different objects projected onto corresponding retinal areas. The two foveal areas are physiologically incapable of simultaneous perception of dissimilar objects. The closest foveal equivalent is retinal rivalry, wherein the two perceived images rapidly alternate (Fig 4-5). Confusion may be a phenomenon of nonfoveal retinal areas only. Clinically significant visual confusion is rare.

Diplopia

Double vision, or *diplopia*, usually results from an acquired misalignment of the visual axes that causes an image to fall simultaneously on the fovea of one eye and on a nonfoveal point in the other eye. The object that falls on these noncorresponding points must be outside Panum's area to be seen double. The same object is seen as having two different locations in subjective space, and the foveal image is always clearer than the nonfoveal image of the nonfixating eye. The symptoms of diplopia depend on the age at onset, duration, and subjective awareness. The younger the child, the greater the ability to suppress, or inhibit, the nonfoveal image.

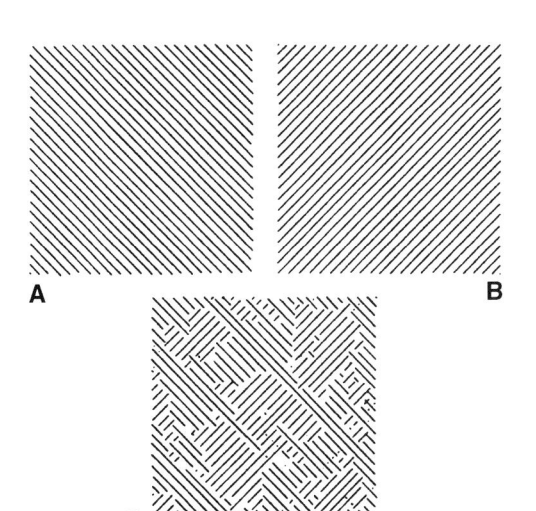

Figure 4-5 Rivalry pattern. **A,** Pattern seen by the left eye. **B,** Pattern seen by the right eye. **C,** Binocular vision. *(From von Noorden GK. Binocular Vision and Ocular Motility. 5th ed. St Louis: Mosby; 1996:13.)*

Central fusional disruption (horror fusionis) is an intractable diplopia that features both an absence of suppression and a loss of fusional amplitudes to maintain fusion. The angle of strabismus may be small or may vary. Horror fusionis can occur in a number of clinical settings: after disruption of fusion for a prolonged period; after head trauma; and, rarely, in long-standing strabismus. Management can be challenging.

> Lee MC. Acquired central fusional disruption with spontaneous recovery. *Strabismus.* 1998;6:175–179.

Sensory Adaptations in Strabismus

To avoid confusion and diplopia, the visual system can use the mechanisms of suppression and ARC (amblyopia is discussed in detail in Chapter 5). It is important to realize that pathological suppression, ARC, and amblyopia develop only in the immature visual system.

Suppression

Suppression is the alteration of visual sensation that occurs when the images from one eye are inhibited or prevented from reaching consciousness. *Pathological suppression* results from strabismic misalignment of the visual axes. Such suppression can be seen as an adaptation of a visually immature brain to avoid diplopia. *Physiologic suppression* is the mechanism that prevents physiologic diplopia from reaching consciousness.

The following is a useful classification of suppression for the clinician:

- *Central versus peripheral. Central suppression* is the term used to describe the mechanism that keeps the foveal image of the deviating eye from reaching consciousness, thereby preventing confusion. However, because the two foveas cannot simultaneously perceive dissimilar objects, this central scotoma of the nonfixating fovea is considered by many clinicians to be a *physiologic* form of suppression rather than a *pathological* one. In addition, this scotoma of the deviated eye can be documented immediately after the onset of ocular misalignment even in new-onset strabismus in a visually mature adult. Despite complaints of diplopia, adults with new-onset strabismus fixate with one eye at a time and demonstrate a small scotoma of the nonfixating fovea, preventing central visual confusion. This response to adult-onset strabismus supports the opinion that central suppression should be classified as physiologic rather than pathological because pathological suppression can develop only in an immature visual system. *Peripheral suppression* is the mechanism that eliminates diplopia by preventing awareness of the image that falls on the peripheral retina in the deviating eye, the image that resembles the image falling on the fovea of the fixating eye. This form of suppression is clearly pathological, developing as a cortical adaptation only within an immature visual system. Adults may be unable to develop peripheral suppression and therefore may be unable to eliminate the peripheral second image of the object viewed by the fixating eye (the *object of regard*) without closing or occluding the deviating eye.

- *Monocular versus alternating.* If suppression is unidirectional or always causes the image from the dominant eye to predominate over the image from the deviating eye, the suppression is *monocular*. This type of mechanism may lead to the establishment of strabismic amblyopia. If the process is bidirectional or switches over time between the images of the two eyes, the suppression is described as *alternating*.
- *Facultative versus obligatory.* Suppression may be considered *facultative* if present only when the eyes are in the deviated state and absent in all other states. Patients with intermittent exotropia, for instance, often experience suppression when the eyes are divergent but enjoy high-grade stereopsis when the eyes are straight. In contrast, *obligatory* suppression is present at all times, whether the eyes are deviated or aligned. The suppression scotomata in the deviating eye may be either *relative* (in the sense of permitting some visual sensation) or *absolute* (permitting no perception of light).

Tests of suppression

If a patient with strabismus and NRC does not have diplopia, suppression is present provided the sensory pathways are intact. In less clear-cut situations, several simple tests are available for clinical diagnosis of suppression. (See Subjective Testing for Suppression and Anomalous Retinal Correspondence, later in this chapter.)

Management of suppression

Therapy for suppression often involves the treatment of the strabismus itself:

- Proper refractive correction
- Occlusion to permit equal and alternate use of each eye and to overcome any amblyopia that may be present
- Alignment of the visual axes to permit simultaneous stimulation of corresponding retinal elements by the same object

Orthoptic exercises may be attempted to overcome the tendency of the image from one eye to suppress the image from the other eye when both eyes are open. These exercises are designed to make the patient aware of diplopia first, then of simultaneous perception, and then of fusion, both on an instrument and in free space. The role of orthoptics in the therapy of suppression is controversial. In treatment of patients with esotropia, antisuppression therapy can cause intractable diplopia as suppression disappears. Antisuppression therapy is safer in patients with intermittent exotropia, but the results have received mixed reviews. Patients with no fusion potential should never undergo antisuppression therapy.

Anomalous Retinal Correspondence

ARC can be described as a condition wherein the fovea of the fixating eye has acquired an anomalous common visual direction with a peripheral retinal element in the deviated eye. The two foveas have different visual directions. ARC is an adaptation that restores some sense of binocular cooperation. The period during which ARC may develop probably extends through the first decade of life.

52 • Pediatric Ophthalmology and Strabismus

Paradoxical diplopia can occur when ARC persists after surgery. When esotropic patients whose eyes have been set straight or nearly straight postoperatively report a crossed diplopic localization of foveal or parafoveal stimuli, they are experiencing paradoxical diplopia (Fig 4-6). Clinically, paradoxical diplopia is a fleeting postoperative phenomenon and rarely lasts longer than a few days to weeks. However, in rare cases this condition has persisted for much longer.

Testing for anomalous retinal correspondence

Testing is performed to determine how patients use their eyes in normal life and to seek out any vestiges of normal correspondence. As discussed earlier, ARC is a sensory adaptation to abnormal binocular vision. Because the depth of the sensory rearrangement can vary widely, an individual can test positively for both NRC and ARC. Tests that closely simulate everyday use of the eyes are more likely to give evidence of ARC. The more dissociative the test, the more likely the test will produce an NRC response unless the ARC is deeply rooted. Some of the more common tests, in order of least dissociating to most dissociating, are the Bagolini striated glasses, amblyoscope, red-glass test (dissociation increases with the density of the red filter), Worth four-dot test, and afterimage test. The farther down this test list the patient gives an anomalous localization response, the greater the depth of ARC. (See Subjective Testing for Suppression and Anomalous Retinal Correspondence, later in this chapter.)

Figure 4-6 Paradoxical diplopia. Diagram of esotropia and ARC wherein the deviation is being neutralized with a base-out prism. A red glass and base-out prism are placed over the right eye. The prism neutralizes the deviation by moving the retinal image of the penlight temporally, off the pseudofovea (P) to the true fovea (F). Because the pseudofovea is the center of orientation, the image is perceived to fall on temporal retina and is projected to the opposite field, thus resulting in crossed diplopia. *(From Wright KW, Spiegel PH. Pediatric Ophthalmology and Strabismus: The Requisites in Ophthalmology. St Louis: Mosby; 1999:219.)*

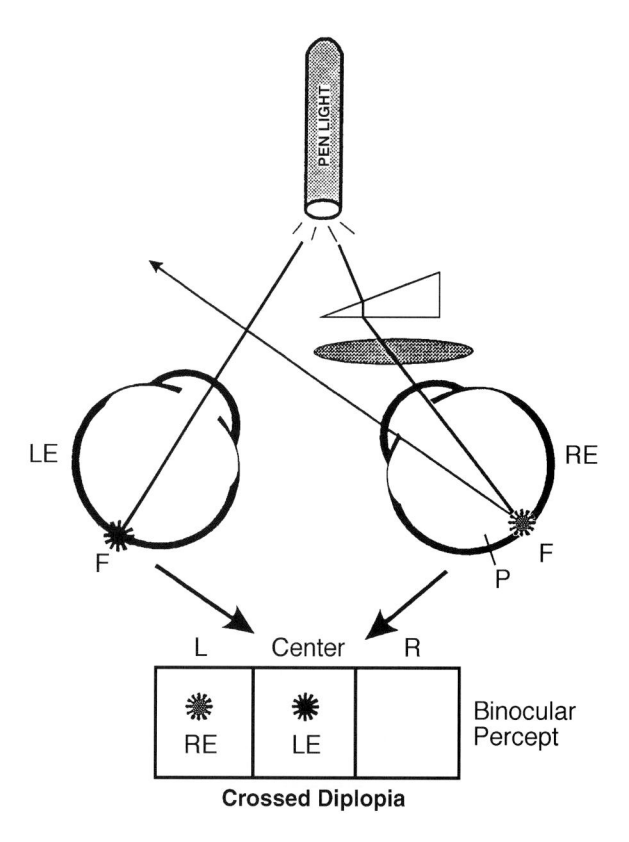

The tests for ARC can basically be divided into two groups: those that stimulate the fovea of one eye and an extrafoveal area of the other eye, and those that stimulate the foveal area in each eye. Note that ARC is a binocular phenomenon, tested for and documented in both eyes simultaneously. Eccentric fixation is a monocular phenomenon found on testing one eye alone, and it is not in any way related to ARC. In eccentric fixation, patients do not fixate with the fovea when the fellow eye is covered. On cover testing, the eye remains more or less deviated depending on how far the nonfoveolar area of fixation is from the fovea. Because some tests for ARC depend on separate stimulation of each fovea, the presence of eccentric fixation can significantly affect the test results.

Monofixation Syndrome

The term *monofixation syndrome* is used to describe a particular clinical presentation of the two preceding sensory adaptations. In this syndrome, both a small foveal suppression scotoma and a minute angle of ARC are present. The essential feature of this syndrome is the presence of peripheral fusion without central fusion.

A patient with monofixation syndrome usually has a small-angle esotropia, but there may be exotropia or even no manifest deviation. A small-angle strabismus (usually <8Δ) usually can be detected under binocular conditions. These patients are sometimes said to have *microtropias*. A central scotoma and peripheral fusion are present with binocular viewing. Amblyopia is a common finding; usually it is slight, but it may be profound. Fixation can be central or eccentric, stereo acuity is reduced, and horizontal fusional amplitudes are present. ARC is found on some sensory tests.

Patients with monofixation syndrome may have latent phoria in excess of a manifest microtropia. When this occurs, the alternate prism cover test measurement will exceed the simultaneous prism cover test measurement.

Monofixation syndrome may be a primary condition, although it is a favorable consequence of esotropia treatment with glasses, surgery, or both. This syndrome can also result from anisometropia or macular lesions. It can be the cause of unilaterally reduced vision when no obvious strabismus is present. If amblyopia is clinically significant, occlusion therapy is indicated.

Diagnosis

To accurately diagnose monofixation syndrome, the clinician must demonstrate both the absence of central binocular vision *(bifixation)* and the presence of peripheral binocular vision *(peripheral fusion)*. Documentation of a macular scotoma in the nonfixating eye during binocular viewing is needed to verify the absence of bifixation. Several binocular perimetric techniques have been described to plot the monofixation scotoma. However, they are rarely used clinically.

Vectographic projections of Snellen letters can be used clinically to document the facultative scotoma of the monofixation syndrome. Snellen letters are viewed through polarized analyzers (AO Vectograph Project-O-Chart slide) or goggles equipped with liquid crystal shutters (BVAT II BVS, Mentor O&O) in such a way that some letters are seen with only the right eye, some with only the left eye, and some with both eyes. Patients with monofixation syndrome delete letters that are imaged only in the nonfixating eye.

Testing stereo acuity is an important part of the monofixation syndrome evaluation. Any amount of gross stereopsis confirms the presence of peripheral fusion. Most patients with monofixation syndrome demonstrate 200–3000 seconds of arc stereopsis. However, because some patients with monofixation syndrome have no demonstrable stereopsis, other tests for peripheral fusion must be used in conjunction with stereo acuity measurement. Fine stereopsis (40 seconds of arc or better) is present only in patients with bifixation.

> Parks MM. The monofixation syndrome. *Trans Am Ophthalmol Soc.* 1969;67:609–657. *(This classic thesis outlines early studies of small-angle deviations and central versus peripheral binocular vision. The development of the various terms used to describe these conditions is also covered in detail.)*
>
> von Noorden GK. *Binocular Vision and Ocular Motility: Theory and Management of Strabismus.* 5th ed. St Louis: Mosby; 1996:182–330.

Subjective Testing for Suppression and Anomalous Retinal Correspondence

All tests are tainted by the inability of the testing conditions to reproduce the patient's condition of casual seeing. The more dissociative the test, the less the test simulates everyday use of the eyes. These tests should always be performed in conjunction with a cover test to decide whether a fusion response is due to orthophoria or ARC.

Red-glass (diplopia) test

The red-glass test involves stimulation of both the fovea of the fixating eye and an extrafoveal area of the other eye. First, the patient's deviation is measured objectively. Then a red glass is placed before the nondeviating eye while the patient fixates on a white light. This test can be performed both at distance and at near. Diplopia is present if the patient notes both a red light (through the glass) and a white light (Fig 4-7A and B). If only one light is seen (either red or white), suppression is present (Fig 4-7C). A 5Δ or 10Δ prism in front of the deviated eye can be used to move the image out of the suppression scotoma, causing the patient to experience diplopia. With NRC, the white image will be localized correctly: the white image is seen below and to the right of the left image (Fig 4-7D). With ARC, the white image will be localized incorrectly: it is seen directly below the image (Fig 4-7E).

The following responses are possible with the red-glass test:

- The patient may see a red light and a white light. If the patient has esotropia, the images appear uncrossed (eg, the red light is to the left of the white light with the red glass over the left eye). This response is known as *homonymous,* or *uncrossed, diplopia.* This can easily be remembered because the esotropic patient sees the red light on the same side as the red glass (Fig 4-7A). If the patient has exotropia, the images appear crossed (eg, the red light is to the right of the white light with the red glass over the left eye). This response is known as *heteronymous,* or *crossed, diplopia* (Fig 4-7B). If the measured separation between the two images equals the previously determined deviation, the patient has NRC.

CHAPTER 4: Sensory Physiology and Pathology • 55

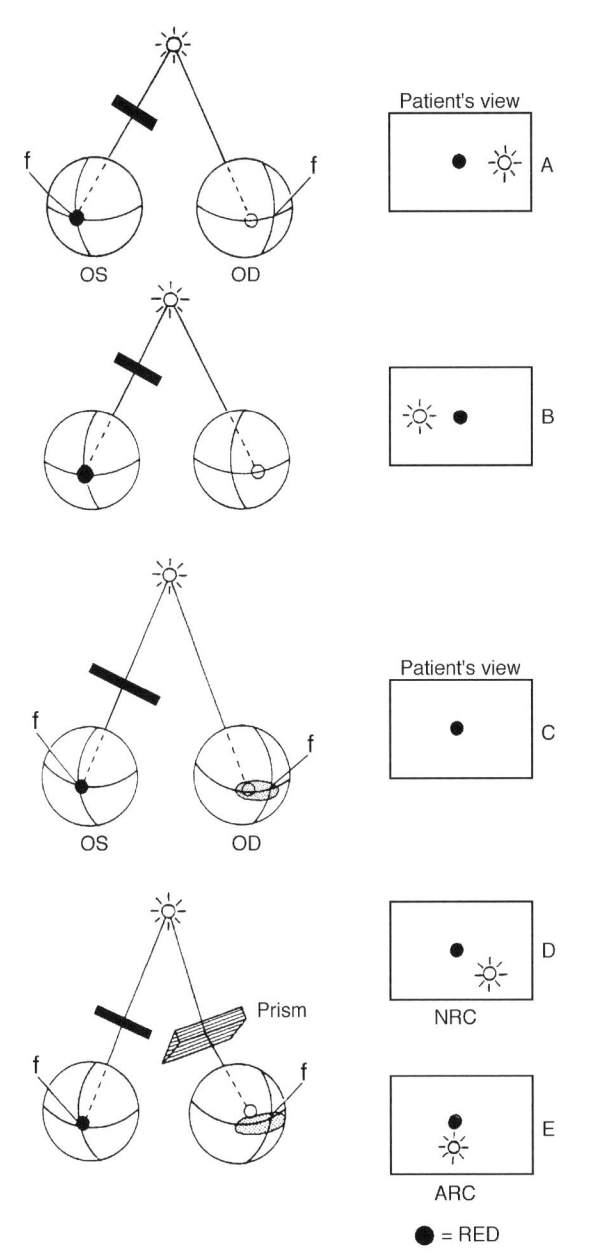

Figure 4-7 Red-glass test for suppression and ARC (see text for explanation). *(From von Noorden GK.* Binocular Vision and Ocular Motility: Theory and Management of Strabismus. *5th ed. St Louis: Mosby; 1996:256.)*

● = RED

- If the patient sees the two lights superimposed so that they appear pinkish despite a measurable esotropia or exotropia, an abnormal localization of retinal points is present. This condition is known as *harmonious anomalous retinal correspondence.*
- If the patient sees two lights (with uncrossed diplopia in esotropia and with crossed diplopia in exotropia), but the separation between the two images is found to be less than the previously determined deviation, the patient has *unharmonious anom-*

Worth four-dot test

In the *Worth four-dot test,* a red glass is worn in front of one eye and a green glass in front of the other (Fig 4-8). The eye behind the red glass can see red light but not green light because the red glass blocks this wavelength. Similarly, the eye behind the green glass can see green light but not red light. If a target consisting of two green lights, one red light, and one white light is viewed, the patient with normal ocular alignment will report a total of four lights. The white light is usually reported to undergo color rivalry; however, only one light is seen in the position of the white light. If the eye behind the green glass is suppressed, a total of two lights is reported. If the eye behind the red glass is suppressed, a total of three lights is reported. If the patient reports five lights, diplopia is present. A report of more than five lights is factitious. A polarized Worth four-dot test is now available, which is administered and interpreted much like the traditional test except that polarized glasses are worn rather than red and green ones. As with the red-glass test, the Worth four-dot test can produce a diplopic response in nonsuppression heterotropic NRC and either a diplopic or a fusion response in ARC, depending on the

Figure 4-8 The Worth four-dot test. **A,** Looking through a pair of red and green goggles, the patient views a box with four lights (one red, two green, one white) at 6 m and at 33 cm (with the four lights mounted on a flashlight). The possible responses are given in **B** to **E**. **B,** Patient sees all four lights: peripheral fusion with orthophoria or strabismus with anomalous retinal correspondence. Depending on ocular dominance, the light in the 6 o'clock position is seen as white or pink. **C,** Patient sees two red lights: suppression OS. **D,** Patient sees three green lights: suppression OD. **E,** Patient sees five lights. The red lights may appear to the right, as in this figure (uncrossed diplopia with esotropia) or to the left of the green lights (crossed diplopia with exotropia). (From von Noorden GK. Atlas of Strabismus. 4th ed. St Louis: Mosby-Year Book; 1983:71.)

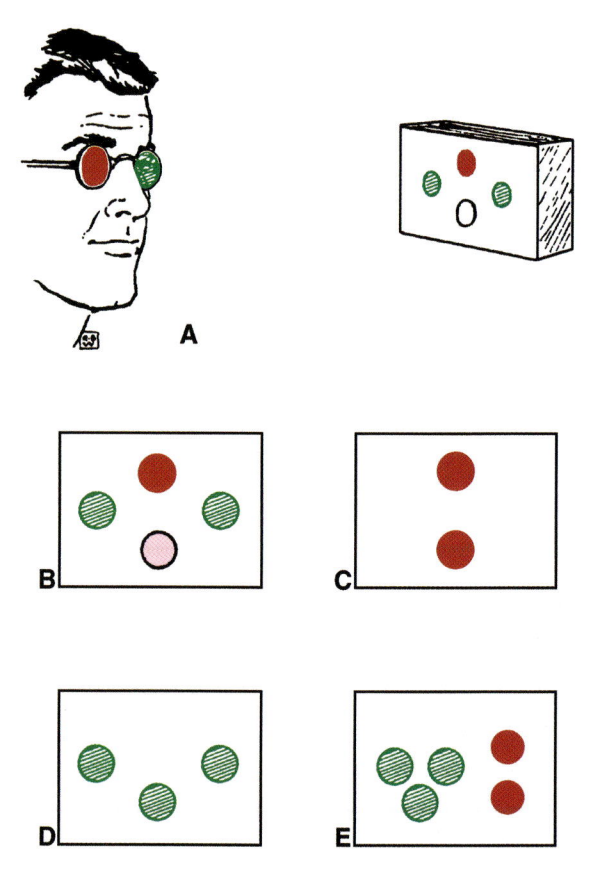

depth of the AKC adaptation. As mentioned earlier, this test must be performed in conjunction with cover testing.

When testing a patient for monofixation syndrome, the Worth four-dot test can be used to demonstrate both the presence of peripheral fusion and the absence of bifixation. The standard Worth four-dot flashlight projects onto a central retinal area of 1° or less when viewed at 10 feet, well within the 3°–5° scotoma characteristic of monofixation syndrome. Therefore, patients with monofixation syndrome will report two or three lights when viewing at 10 feet, depending on their ocular fixation preference. Bifixators will report four lights. As the Worth four-dot flashlight is brought closer to the patient, the dots begin to project onto peripheral retina outside of the central monofixation scotoma until a fusion response (four lights) is obtained. This usually occurs between 2 and 3 feet.

Bagolini glasses

Bagolini striated glasses are glasses of no dioptric power that have many narrow striations running parallel in one meridian. These glasses cause the fixation light to appear as an elongated streak, like micro-Maddox cylinders. The lenses are usually placed at 135° in front of the right eye and at 45° in front of the left eye. The advantages of the Bagolini glasses are that they afford the most lifelike testing conditions and permit the examiner to perform cover testing during the examination. Figure 4-9 summarizes some of the possible subjective results of this test. Note that in monofixation syndrome, the central scotoma is perceived as a gap in one of the lines surrounding the fixation light.

4Δ base-out prism test

The 4Δ base-out prism test is a diagnostic maneuver performed primarily to document the presence of a small facultative scotoma in a patient with monofixation syndrome. In this test, a 4Δ base-out prism is quickly placed before one eye and then the other during binocular viewing, and motor responses are observed (Fig 4-10). Patients with bifixation usually show a version (bilateral) movement away from the eye covered by the prism followed by a unilateral fusional convergence movement of the eye not behind the prism. A similar response occurs regardless of which eye the prism is placed over. Often, no movement is seen in patients with monofixation syndrome when the prism is placed before the nonfixating eye. A refixation version movement is seen when the prism is placed before the fixating eye, but the expected fusional convergence does not occur.

The 4Δ base-out prism test is the least reliable method used to document the presence of a macular scotoma. An occasional patient with bifixation recognizes diplopia when the prism is placed before an eye but makes no convergence movement to correct for it. Patients with monofixation syndrome may switch fixation each time the prism is inserted and show no movement, regardless of which eye is tested.

Afterimage test

The afterimage test is used to determine whether a patient has NRC or ARC. This test involves stimulation of the macula of each eye. Because the light flash stimulation is done for each eye separately, this test requires good foveal fixation with each eye. The presence of eccentric fixation in one eye significantly affects the results. This test involves the

58 • Pediatric Ophthalmology and Strabismus

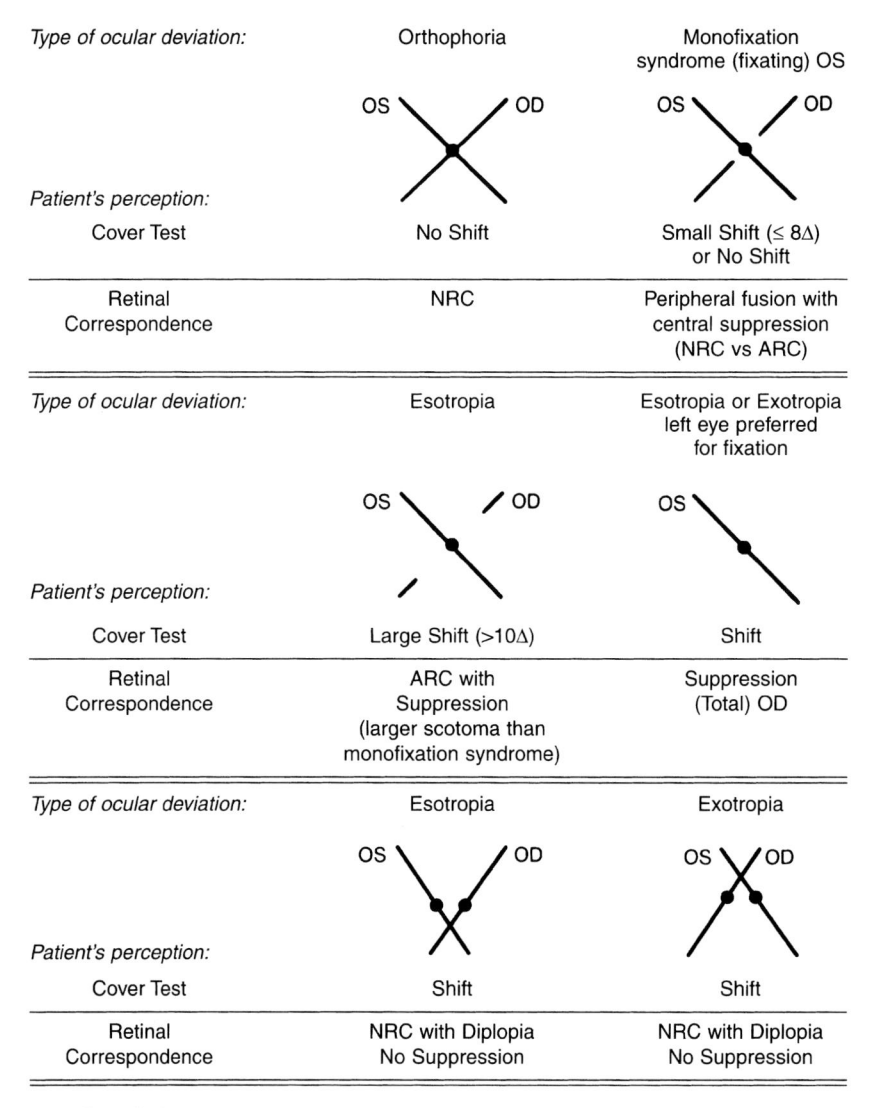

Type of ocular deviation:	Orthophoria	Monofixation syndrome (fixating) OS
Patient's perception: Cover Test	No Shift	Small Shift (≤ 8Δ) or No Shift
Retinal Correspondence	NRC	Peripheral fusion with central suppression (NRC vs ARC)
Type of ocular deviation:	Esotropia	Esotropia or Exotropia left eye preferred for fixation
Patient's perception: Cover Test	Large Shift (>10Δ)	Shift
Retinal Correspondence	ARC with Suppression (larger scotoma than monofixation syndrome)	Suppression (Total) OD
Type of ocular deviation:	Esotropia	Exotropia
Patient's perception: Cover Test	Shift	Shift
Retinal Correspondence	NRC with Diplopia No Suppression	NRC with Diplopia No Suppression

Figure 4-9 Bagolini striated glass test for retinal correspondence and suppression. For these figures, the Bagolini lens is oriented at 135° in front of the right eye and at 45° in front of the left eye. The perception of the oblique lines seen by each eye under binocular conditions is shown. Examples of the types of strabismus in which these responses are commonly found are given.

stimulation, or *labeling,* of each eye with a different linear afterimage, one horizontal and one vertical. Because suppression scotomata extend along the horizontal retinal meridian and may obscure most of a horizontal afterimage, the vertical afterimage is placed on the deviating eye and the horizontal afterimage on the fixating eye simply by having each eye fixate the linear light filament separately.

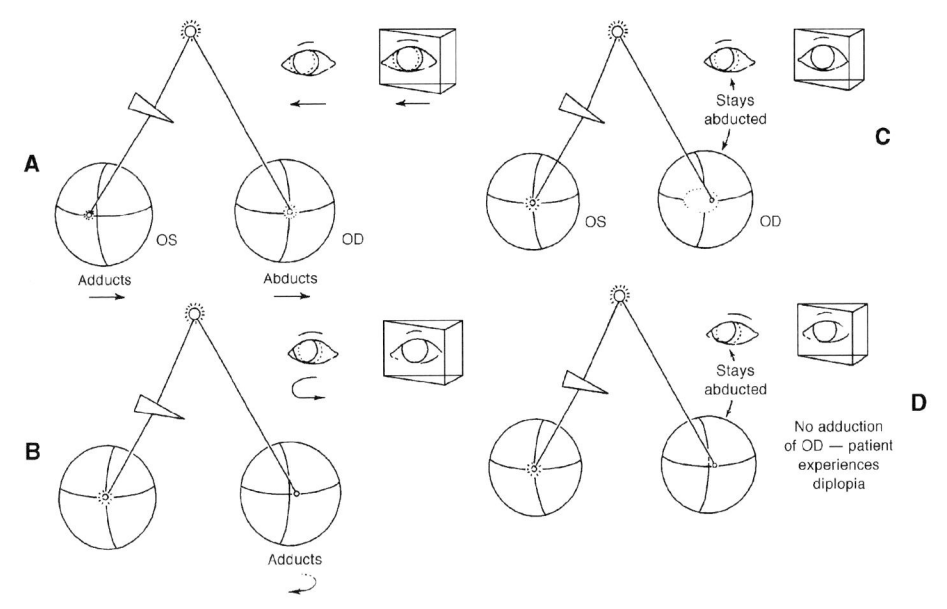

Figure 4-10 The 4Δ base-out prism test. **A,** When a prism is placed over the left eye, dextroversion occurs during refixation of that eye, indicating absence of foveal suppression in the left eye. If a suppression scotoma is present in the left eye, there will be no movement of either eye when placing the prism before the left eye. **B,** A subsequent slow fusional adduction movement of the right eye is observed, indicating absence of foveal suppression in the right eye. **C,** In a second patient, the right eye stays abducted, and the absence of an adduction movement **(B)** indicates foveal suppression in the right eye. **D,** Another cause for absence of the adduction movement is weak fusion, and such patients experience diplopia until refusion occurs spontaneously. *(From von Noorden GK. Present status of sensory testing in strabismus. In: Helveston EM, New Orleans Academy of Ophthalmology. Symposium on Strabismus: Transactions of the New Orleans Academy of Ophthalmology. St Louis: Mosby-Year Book; 1978:51.)*

The central zone of the linear light is occluded to allow the fovea to fixate and remain unlabeled. The patient is then asked to draw the relative positions of the perceived afterimages. Possible perceptions are the following (Fig 4-11):

- If the patient has NRC, the two afterimages will be seen as a cross with a single gap (which corresponds to the fovea of each eye) in the center.
- If the patient has an esotropia and ARC, the afterimages from both eyes will be seen as crossed.
- If the patient has a left exotropia and ARC, the afterimages from both eyes will be seen as uncrossed.

Amblyoscope testing

The amblyoscope provides another test that can determine whether a patient has NRC or ARC. With the amblyoscope, the examiner determines the *objective angle,* at which the targets imaged on the two foveas will produce no movement with alternate target presentation. If the images are seen superimposed, with the angle between the arms of the amblyoscope equal to the objective angle, correspondence is normal (Fig 4-12A); if

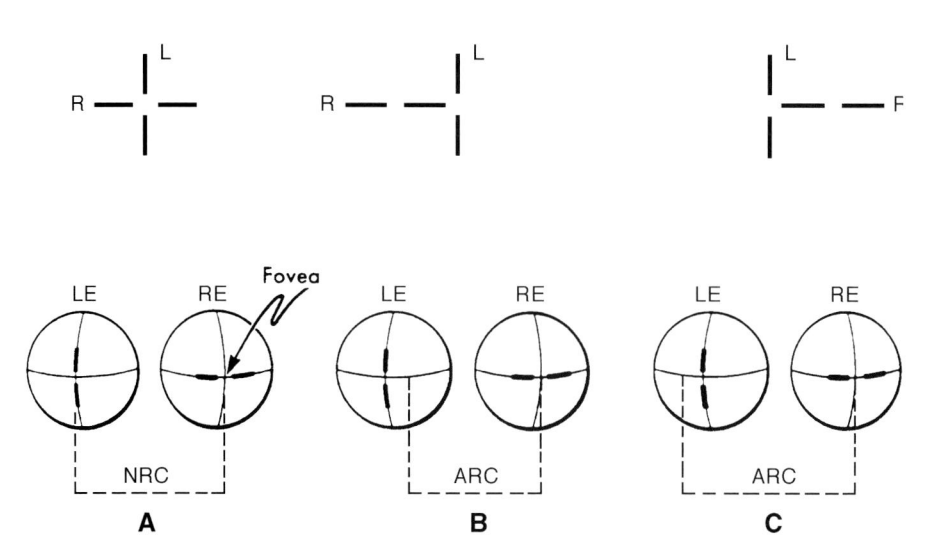

Figure 4-11 Afterimage test. **A,** Normal localization *(cross)* in normal correspondence *(NRC)*. **B,** Anomalous crossed localization *(ARC)* in a case of esotropia. **C,** Anomalous uncrossed localization in a case of exotropia.

not, correspondence is anomalous. The patient is then asked to superimpose the two targets. If superimposition occurs with the amblyoscope arms set at zero angle (arms parallel), the patient shows harmonious ARC (Fig 4-12B). If the arms are set somewhere between zero and the objective angle of squint, unharmonious ARC is theoretically present (Fig 4-12C). The reader is reminded that unharmonious ARC may be an artifact of the testing situation.

CHAPTER 4: Sensory Physiology and Pathology • 61

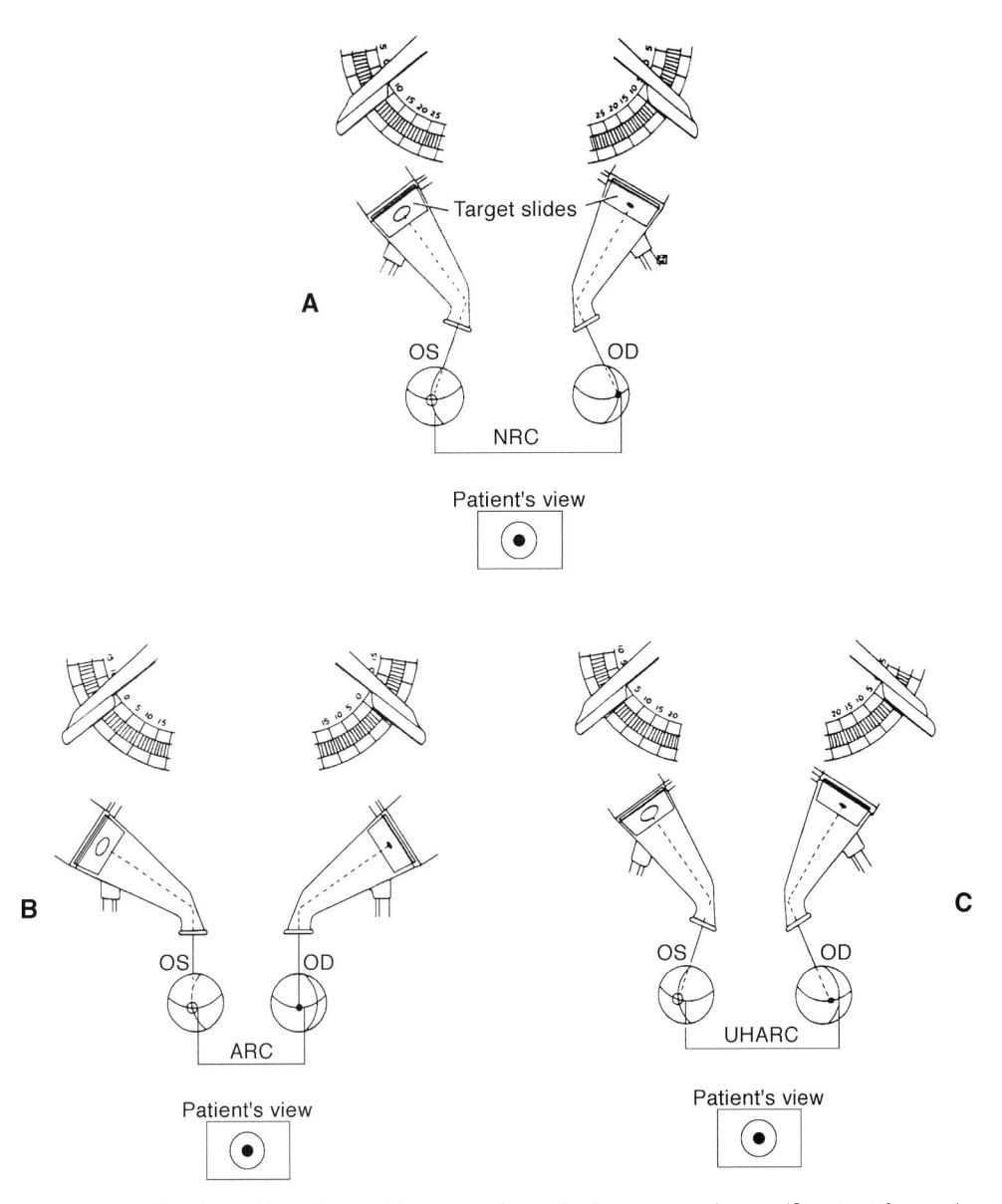

Figure 4-12 Testing with major amblyoscope for retinal correspondence. (See text for explanation of **A–C.**) NRC, normal retinal correspondence; ARC, anomalous retinal correspondence; UHARC, unharmonious anomalous retinal correspondence. *(From von Noorden GK.* Atlas of Strabismus. *4th ed. St Louis: Mosby-Year Book; 1983.)*

CHAPTER 5

Amblyopia

Amblyopia is a unilateral or, less commonly, bilateral reduction of best-corrected visual acuity that cannot be attributed directly to the effect of any structural abnormality of the eye or the posterior visual pathway. Amblyopia is caused by abnormal visual experience early in life resulting from one of the following:

- Strabismus
- Anisometropia or high bilateral refractive errors (isometropia)
- Visual deprivation

Amblyopia is responsible for more unilaterally reduced vision of childhood onset than all other causes combined, with a prevalence of 2%–4% in the North American population. This fact is particularly distressing because, in principle, nearly all amblyopic visual loss is preventable or reversible with timely detection and appropriate intervention. Children with amblyopia or at risk for amblyopia should be identified at a young age, when the prognosis for successful treatment is best. Screening for amblyopia can be performed in the primary care practitioner's office or in community-based vision screening programs. The role of photoscreening to identify amblyogenic risk factors in children who cannot be screened with visual acuity tests is being intensively investigated. A consensus about the best technology and the appropriate age to screen has not yet emerged, however.

Simons K. Photoscreening [editorial]. *Ophthalmology*. 2000;107:1619–1620.
Simons K. Preschool vision screening: rationale, methodology and outcome. *Surv Ophthalmol*. 1996;41:3–30.

Amblyopia is primarily a defect of central vision; the peripheral visual field nearly always remains normal. Experimental studies on animals and clinical studies of infants and young children support the concept of critical periods for sensitivity in developing amblyopia. These critical periods correspond to when the child's developing visual system is sensitive to abnormal input caused by stimulus deprivation, strabismus, or significant refractive errors. In general, the critical period for stimulus deprivation amblyopia occurs earlier than that for ocular misalignment or anisometropia. Furthermore, the time necessary for amblyopia to occur during the critical period is shorter for stimulus deprivation than for strabismus or anisometropia.

Although the neurophysiologic mechanisms that underlie amblyopia are far from clear, the study of experimental modification of visual experience in animals and laboratory testing of amblyopic humans has provided some insights. Animal models have revealed that a variety of profound disturbances of visual system neuron function may result from abnormal early visual experience. Cells of the primary visual cortex can completely lose their innate ability to respond to stimulation of one or both eyes, and cells that remain responsive may show significant functional deficiencies. Abnormalities also occur in neurons in the lateral geniculate body. Evidence concerning involvement at the retinal level remains inconclusive; if present, changes in the retina make at most a minor contribution to the overall visual defect.

Several findings from both animals and humans, such as increased spatial summation and lateral inhibition when light detection thresholds are measured using different-sized spots, suggest that the receptive fields of neurons in the amblyopic visual system are abnormally large. This disturbance may account for the *crowding phenomenon* (also known as *contour interaction*), whereby Snellen letters or equivalent symbols of a given size become more difficult to recognize if they are closely surrounded by similar forms, such as a full line or chart of letters. The crowding phenomenon sometimes causes the measured "linear" acuity of an amblyopic eye to drop several lines below that measured with isolated letters.

Daw NW. Critical periods and amblyopia. *Arch Ophthalmol.* 1998;116:502–505.
von Noorden GK. Amblyopia: a multidisciplinary approach. Proctor lecture. *Invest Ophthalmol Vis Sci.* 1985;26:1704–1716.

Classification

Amblyopia has traditionally been subdivided in terms of the major disorders that may be responsible for its occurrence.

Strabismic Amblyopia

The most common form of amblyopia develops in the consistently deviating eye of a child with ocular misalignment. Constant, nonalternating tropias (typically esodeviations) are most likely to cause significant amblyopia. Strabismic amblyopia is thought to result from competitive or inhibitory interaction between neurons carrying the nonfusible inputs from the two eyes, which leads to domination of cortical vision centers by the fixating eye and chronically reduced responsiveness to the nonfixating eye's input. It has been suggested, but not proved, that this same mechanism is responsible for eliminating diplopia in strabismic children through suppression. Amblyopia itself does not as a rule prevent diplopia, however. Older patients with long-standing deviations frequently develop double vision after strabismus surgery, despite the presence of substantially reduced amblyopic acuity.

Several features of typical strabismic amblyopia are uncommon in other forms of amblyopia. *Grating acuity*, the ability to detect patterns composed of uniformly spaced stripes, which normally corresponds closely to Snellen acuity, is often reduced considerably less than Snellen acuity in strabismic amblyopia. Apparently, the affected eye sees forms in a twisted or distorted manner that interferes more with letter recognition than with the simpler task of determining whether a grating pattern is present. This discrepancy must be considered when the results of tests based on grating detection, such as Teller card preferential looking (a method of estimating acuity in infants and toddlers), are interpreted.

When illumination is reduced, the acuity of an eye with strabismic amblyopia tends to decline less sharply than that of an organically diseased eye. This phenomenon is sometimes called the *neutral-density filter effect* after the device classically used to demonstrate it.

Eccentric fixation

Eccentric fixation refers to the consistent use of a nonfoveal region of the retina for monocular viewing by an amblyopic eye. Minor degrees of eccentric fixation, detectable only with special tests such as visuscopy, Haidinger's brushes, or Maxwell's spot, are seen in many patients with strabismic amblyopia and relatively mild acuity loss. Clinically evident eccentric fixation, detectable by observing the noncentral position of the corneal reflection from the amblyopic eye while it fixates a light with the dominant eye covered, generally implies visual acuity of 20/200 or worse. See Chapter 6 for discussions of clinical testing. Use of nonfoveal retina for fixation cannot in general be regarded as the primary cause of reduced acuity in affected eyes. The mechanism of this interesting phenomenon, long a source of speculation, remains unknown.

Anisometropic Amblyopia

Second in frequency to strabismic amblyopia, anisometropic amblyopia develops when unequal refractive error in the two eyes causes the image on one retina to be chronically defocused. This condition is thought to result partly from the direct effect of image blur on the development of visual acuity in the involved eye and partly from interocular competition or inhibition similar (but not necessarily identical) to that responsible for strabismic amblyopia. Relatively mild degrees of hyperopic or astigmatic anisometropia (1–2 D) can induce mild amblyopia. Mild myopic anisometropia (less than -3 D) usually does not cause amblyopia, but unilateral high myopia (-6 D) often results in severe amblyopic visual loss. Unless strabismus is associated, which is not uncommon, the eyes of a child with anisometropic amblyopia look normal to the family and primary care physician; detection and treatment are often delayed until school age, when the prognosis for recovery of vision is guarded.

Amblyopia Due to Bilateral High Refractive Errors (Isometropia)

A bilateral reduction in acuity that is usually relatively mild, isometropic amblyopia results from large, approximately equal, uncorrected refractive errors in both eyes of a young child. Its mechanism involves the effect of blurred retinal images alone. Hyperopia exceeding about 5 D and myopia in excess of 10 D carry a risk of inducing bilateral amblyopia. Uncorrected bilateral astigmatism in early childhood may result in loss of resolving ability limited to the chronically blurred meridians *(meridional amblyopia)*. The degree of cylindrical ametropia necessary to produce meridional amblyopia is not known, but most ophthalmologists recommend correction of greater than 2.00 D of cylinder.

Deprivation Amblyopia

The old terms *amblyopia ex anopsia* or *disuse amblyopia* are sometimes still used for deprivation amblyopia, which is usually caused by congenital or early acquired media opacities. This form of amblyopia is the least common but most damaging and difficult to treat. Amblyopic visual loss resulting from a unilateral lack of form vision tends to be worse than that produced by bilateral deprivation of similar degree because interocular effects add to the direct developmental impact of severe image degradation. Even in bilateral cases, however, acuity can be 20/200 or worse.

In children younger than 6 years, dense congenital cataracts that occupy the central 3 mm or more of the lens must be considered capable of causing severe amblyopia. Similar lens opacities acquired after age 6 are generally less harmful. Small polar cataracts, around which retinoscopy can be readily performed, and lamellar cataracts, through which a reasonably good view of the fundus can be obtained, may cause mild to moderate amblyopia or may have no effect on visual development. *Occlusion amblyopia* is a form of deprivation amblyopia caused by excessive therapeutic patching.

Diagnosis

Amblyopia is diagnosed when evidence of reduced visual acuity that cannot be explained entirely on the basis of physical abnormalities is found in association with a history or finding of a condition known to be capable of causing amblyopia. Characteristics of vision alone cannot be used to reliably differentiate amblyopia from other forms of visual loss. The crowding phenomenon, for example, is typical of amblyopia but not uniformly demonstrable. Afferent pupillary defects are characteristic of optic nerve disease but occasionally appear to be present with amblyopia. Amblyopia sometimes coexists with visual loss directly caused by an uncorrectable structural abnormality of the eye such as optic nerve hypoplasia or coloboma. When such a situation is encountered in a young child, it is appropriate to undertake a trial of occlusion therapy; improvement in vision confirms that amblyopia was indeed present.

Multiple assessments using a variety of tests or performed on different occasions are sometimes required to make a final judgment concerning the presence and severity of amblyopia. General techniques for visual acuity assessment in children are discussed in Chapter 6, but the clinician trying to determine the degree of amblyopic visual loss in a young patient should keep certain special considerations in mind. The *binocular fixation pattern*, which indicates strength of preference for one eye or the other under binocular viewing conditions, is a test for estimating the relative level of vision in the two eyes for children with strabismus who are under the age of about 3. This test is quite sensitive for detecting amblyopia, but results can be falsely positive, showing a strong preference when vision is equal or nearly equal in the two eyes, particularly with small-angle strabismic deviations.

The modified Snellen technique directly measures acuity in children 3–6 years old. Often, however, only isolated letters can be used, which may lead to underestimated amblyopic visual loss. Crowding bars may help alleviate this problem (Fig 5-1). In addition, the young child's brief attention span frequently results in measurements that fall short of the true limits of acuity; these results can mimic bilateral amblyopia or obscure or falsely suggest a significant interocular difference.

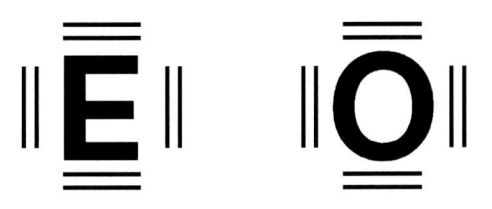

Figure 5-1 Crowding bars, or contour interaction bars, allow the examiner to test the crowding phenomenon with isolated optotypes. Bars surrounding the optotype mimic the full row of optotypes to the amblyopic child. *(Reproduced with permission from Coats DK, Jenkins RH. Vision assessment of the pediatric patient. Refinements. San Francisco: American Academy of Ophthalmology; 1997;1:1.)*

Treatment

Treatment of amblyopia involves the following steps:
- Eliminating (if possible) any obstacle to vision such as a cataract
- Correcting refractive error
- Forcing use of the poorer eye by limiting use of the better eye

Cataract Removal

Cataracts capable of producing amblyopia require surgery without unnecessary delay. Removal of significant congenital lens opacities during the first 2–3 months of life is necessary for optimal recovery of vision. In symmetrical bilateral cases, the interval between operations on the first and second eyes should be no more than 1–2 weeks. Acutely developing severe traumatic cataracts in children younger than 6 years should be removed within a few weeks of injury, if possible. Significant cataracts with uncertain time of onset also deserve prompt and aggressive treatment during childhood if recent development is at least a possibility (eg, in the case of an opacity that appears to have originated from a posterior lenticonus deformity). BCSC Section 11, *Lens and Cataract*, discusses the special considerations of cataract surgery in children; see also Chapter 22 of this volume.

Refractive Correction

In general, optical prescription for amblyopic eyes should correct the full refractive error as determined with cycloplegia. Because the amblyopic eye's ability to control accommodation tends to be impaired, it cannot be relied on to compensate for uncorrected hyperopia as would the normal child's eye. Sometimes, however, symmetrical decreases in plus lens power may be required to foster acceptance of spectacle wear by the child. Refractive correction for aphakia following cataract surgery in childhood must be provided promptly to avoid compounding the visual deprivation effect of the lens opacity with that of a severe optical deficit. Both anisometropic and isometropic amblyopia may improve considerably with refractive correction alone over several months.

Occlusion and Optical Degradation

Full-time occlusion of the sound eye, defined as occlusion for all or all but one waking hour, is the most powerful means of treating amblyopia by enforced use of the defective eye. This treatment is usually done with commercially available adhesive patches; the patch can either be left in place at night or removed at bedtime. Spectacle-mounted occluders or special opaque contact lenses can be used as an alternative to full-time patching if skin irritation or poor adhesion proves to be a significant problem, provided that close supervision ensures that the spectacles remain in place consistently. (Most skin-related problems can be eliminated by switching to a different brand of patch or by preparing the skin with tincture of benzoin or ostomy adhesive before application.) Full-time patching should generally be used only when constant strabismus eliminates any possibility of useful binocular vision because full-time patching runs a small risk of perturbing binocularity. Rarely, strabismus is thought to be due to full-time patching; it is not known whether strabismus would have occurred with other forms of amblyopia treatment. The child whose eyes are consistently or intermittently straight should be given some opportunity to see binocularly.

Part-time occlusion, defined as occlusion for 1–6 hours per day, may achieve the same results as full-time occlusion. The relative duration of patch-on and patch-off intervals should reflect the degree of amblyopia; for moderate to severe deficits, at least 6 hours per day is preferred. The child undergoing part-time occlusion should be kept as visually active as possible when the patch is in place, but no specific visual exercises have been proved to be of particular benefit.

Compliance with occlusion therapy for amblyopia declines with increasing age. The effectiveness of more acceptable part-time patching regimens in older children is being actively investigated. Furthermore, recent experimental work in older amblyopic children has shown that the addition of the neurotransmitter precursor levodopa/carbidopa to part-time occlusion regimens may extend the effective age range for amblyopia therapy.

Other methods of amblyopia treatment involve *optical degradation* of the better eye's image to the point that it becomes inferior to the amblyopic eye's, an approach often called *penalization*. Use of the amblyopic eye is thus promoted within the context of binocular seeing. A cycloplegic agent (usually atropine 1% drops or homatropine 5% drops) is administered once daily to the better eye so that it is unable to accommodate and experiences blur with near viewing and, if uncorrected hyperopia is present, with distance viewing. This form of treatment has recently been demonstrated to be as effective as patching for mild to moderate amblyopia (visual acuity of 20/100 or better in the amblyopic eye). Depending on the depth of amblyopia and the prior response to treatment, the hyperopic correction of the dominant eye can be reduced to *plano* to enhance the effect. Regular follow-up of patients whose amblyopia is being treated with cycloplegia is important to avoid reverse amblyopia in the previously preferred eye.

Atropinization offers the particular advantage of being difficult to thwart even if the child objects. Alternative methods of treatment based on the same principle involve prescribing excessive plus-power lenses (fogging) or diffusing filters. These methods avoid potential pharmacologic side effects and may be capable of inducing greater blur. If the child is wearing glasses, application of translucent tape or a Bangerter foil (a neutral-density filter) to the spectacle lens can be tried. Proper utilization (no peeking!) of spectacle-borne devices must be closely monitored.

Another benefit of atropinization and other nonoccluding methods in patients with straight eyes is that the eyes can work together, a great practical advantage in children with latent nystagmus and, theoretically, an advantage in all patients.

When a therapeutic approach other than occlusion is initiated, it must be established that the better eye's vision has in fact been sufficiently degraded. In the strabismic patient, this is easily done by noting an immediate switch of fixation preference. When the eyes are straight, preference for use of the amblyopic eye over its blurred fellow eye should be demonstrated with the aid of a vertical prism that optically induces ocular misalignment. Reduction of the preferred eye's measured acuity below the amblyopic eye's level does not by itself ensure that treatment will be effective.

> The Pediatric Eye Disease Investigator Group . A randomized trial of atropine vs. patching for treatment of moderate amblyopia in children. *Arch Ophthalmol.* 2002;120:268–278.

Complications of Therapy

Any form of amblyopia therapy introduces the possibility of overtreatment leading to amblyopia in the originally better eye. Full-time occlusion carries the greatest risk of this complication and requires close monitoring, especially in the younger child. The first follow-up visit after initiation of treatment should occur within 1 week for an infant and after an interval corresponding to 1 week per year of age for the older child (eg, 4 weeks for a 4-year-old). Subsequent visits can be scheduled at longer intervals based on early response. Part-time occlusion and optical degradation methods allow for less frequent observation, but regular follow-up is still critical. The parents of a strabismic child should be instructed to watch for a switch in fixation preference and to report its occurrence promptly. Iatrogenic amblyopia can nearly always be treated successfully with judicious patching of the better-seeing eye or by alternating occlusion. Sometimes, simply stopping treatment altogether for a few weeks leads to equalization of vision.

The desired endpoint of therapy for unilateral amblyopia is free alternation of fixation (although one eye may still be used somewhat more frequently than the other), linear Snellen acuity that differs by no more than one line between the two eyes, or both. The time required for completion of treatment depends on the following:

- Degree of amblyopia
- Choice of therapeutic approach
- Compliance with the prescribed regimen
- Age of the patient

More severe amblyopia, less complete obstruction of the dominant eye's vision, and older age are all associated with a need for more prolonged treatment. Full-time occlusion during infancy may reverse substantial strabismic amblyopia in 1 week or less. In contrast, an older child who wears a patch only after school and on weekends may require a year or more of treatment to overcome a moderate deficit.

Compliance issues

Lack of compliance with the inevitably unpleasant therapeutic regimen is a common problem that can prolong the period of treatment or lead to outright failure. If difficulties derive from a particular treatment method, a suitable alternative should be sought. Families who appear to lack sufficient motivation need to be counseled concerning the importance of the project and the need for firmness in carrying it out. They can be reassured that once an appropriate routine is established and maintained for a short time, the daily effort required is likely to diminish.

The problems associated with an unusually resistant child vary according to age. In infancy, restraining the child through physical methods such as arm splints or mittens or merely making the patch stick tighter with tincture of benzoin may be useful. For children older than 3 years, creating goals and offering rewards tends to work well, as does linking patching to play activities (eg, decorating the patch each day). Authoritative words directed specifically toward the child by the doctor may also help. The toddler period (1–3 years) is particularly challenging; sometimes, the best solution is to back off and renew efforts when the child turns 3. Prevent Blindness America has developed a program, *The Eye Patch Club*, that offers support and motivational materials for children with amblyopia and their families *(www.PreventBlindness.org)*.

Unresponsiveness

In some cases, even conscientious application of an appropriate therapeutic program fails to improve vision at all or beyond a certain level. Complete or partial unresponsiveness to treatment occasionally affects younger children but most often occurs in patients older than 5 years. Conversely, significant improvement in vision may be achievable with protracted effort even in adolescents. The decision whether to initiate or continue treatment in a prognostically unfavorable situation should consider the wishes of the patient and family. Primary therapy should generally be terminated if there is a lack of demonstrable progress over 3–6 months with good compliance.

Before it is concluded that intractable amblyopia is present, refraction should be carefully rechecked and the macula and optic nerve critically inspected for subtle evidence of hypoplasia or other malformation that might have been previously overlooked. Amblyopia associated with unilateral high myopia and extensive myelination of retinal nerve fibers is a specific syndrome in which treatment failure is particularly common.

Recurrence

When amblyopia treatment is discontinued after fully or partially successful completion, approximately half of patients show some degree of recurrence, which can nearly always be reversed with renewed therapeutic effort. Backsliding can be prevented by instituting an acuity maintenance regimen such as patching for 1–3 hours per day, optical penalization with spectacles, or pharmacologic penalization with atropine 1 or 2 days per week. If the need for maintenance is established, it must be continued until stability of visual acuity is demonstrated with no treatment other than regular spectacles. This may require periodic monitoring until age 8–10. As long as vision remains stable, intervals of up to 6 months between follow-up visits are acceptable.

> Keech RV. Practical management of amblyopia. In: *Focal Points: Clinical Modules for Ophthalmologists.* San Francisco: American Academy of Ophthalmology; 2000: vol 18, no 2.
> Lambert SR, Boothe RG. Amblyopia: basic and clinical science perspectives. In: *Focal Points: Clinical Modules for Ophthalmologists.* San Francisco: American Academy of Ophthalmology; 1994: vol 12, no 8.
> Preferred Practice Patterns Committee, Pediatric Ophthalmology Panel. *Amblyopia.* San Francisco: American Academy of Ophthalmology; 1997.

CHAPTER 6

Diagnostic Techniques for Strabismus and Amblyopia

History and Characteristics of the Presenting Complaint

The motility examination begins with the patient's history. Because children become increasingly impatient during an examination, an experienced ophthalmologist will take advantage of the opportunity to observe the child while taking the history. The ophthalmologist should attempt to establish rapport with the patient and, if examining a child, with the parent(s) as well. See Introduction: Rapport With Children: Tips for a Productive Examination for a detailed discussion on examining the child.

Especially when the patient is a child, it is important to obtain information regarding the mother's pregnancy, paying close attention to maternal health, gestational age at the time of birth, birth weight, and neonatal history. The physician should also ask about the child's developmental milestones.

It is desirable to document the age of onset of a deviation or symptom. Old photographs are invaluable for this purpose. Baby pictures, grade-school snapshots, graduation photographs, and driver's license pictures can provide critical information. In addition, the physician should seek to answer the following questions about the deviation or symptom:

- Did its onset coincide with trauma or illness?
- Is the deviation constant or intermittent?
- Is it present for distance, near, or both?
- Is it unilateral or alternating?
- Is it present only when the patient is inattentive or fatigued?
- Does one eye have a tendency to close when the patient is outside in bright sunlight?
- Is the deviation associated with double vision?

Earlier treatment should be reviewed, including any previous management such as amblyopia therapy, spectacle correction, use of miotics, orthoptic therapy, or prior eye muscle surgery. While obtaining the history, the physician should observe the patient continually, noting such behaviors as head posturing, head movement, attentiveness, and motor control.

Past and present medications should be recorded, along with drug sensitivities and allergic responses. Any history of thyroid or neurologic problems should be particularly emphasized. It is also important to document previous surgeries, anesthetic methods used and any problems, and a detailed family history of strabismus or other eye disorders.

Assessment of Visual Acuity

Distance Visual Acuity

Several tests are available for distance visual acuity determination. Snellen letters or numbers, the HOTV test, Lea symbols, the illiterate E test, and Allen pictures are the most commonly used tests for visual acuity. Table 6-1 lists the standards of acuity for various tests at different ages.

Visual acuity is determined, by convention, first for the right eye and then for the left. A patch or occluder is used in front of the left eye as the acuity of the right eye is checked, then vice versa. An adhesive patch is the most effective occluder but the most objectionable from the child's point of view. The line with the smallest figures in which the majority of letters can be read accurately is recorded; if the patient misses a few of the figures on a line, a notation is made. If the patient does not have corrective lenses, a pinhole may be used to estimate the best visual acuity potential. However, the use of pinholes in children is cumbersome and often inconclusive.

Patients with poor vision may need to walk to the chart until they can see the big E or equivalent (20/400 line). In such cases, visual acuity is recorded as the distance in feet (numerator) over the size of the letter (denominator)—for example, if the patient is able to read the big E at 5 feet, the acuity would be recorded as 5/400. Because the selection of large figures is limited, it is advisable to confirm measurements slightly closer to the chart using figures that can be changed.

The visual acuity assessment in children is often difficult, and the clinician must resort to various means of evaluation. In preverbal or nonverbal children, acuity can be evaluated by the *CSM method.* C refers to the location of the corneal light reflex as the patient fixates the examiner's light under monocular conditions (opposite eye covered). Normally, the reflected light from the cornea is near the *center* of the cornea, and it should be positioned symmetrically in both eyes. If the fixation target is viewed eccentrically, fixation is termed *uncentral* (UC). S refers to the *steadiness* of fixation on the

Table 6-1 Normal Visual Acuity Using Various Tests in Children

Age (Years)	Vision Test	Normal
0–2	Visual evoked potential (VEP)	20/30 (age 1)
0–2	Preferential looking	20/30 (age 2)
0–2	Fixation behavior	CSM (see text)
2–5	Allen pictures	20/40–20/20
2–5	HOTV	20/40–20/20
2–5	E-game	20/40–20/20
5+	Snellen	20/30–20/20

examiner's light as it is held motionless and as it is slowly moved about. The S evaluation is also done under monocular conditions. *M* refers to the ability of the strabismic patient to *maintain* alignment first with one eye, then with the other, as the opposite eye is uncovered. Maintenance of fixation is evaluated under binocular conditions. Inability to maintain fixation with either eye with the opposite eye uncovered is presumptive evidence of a difference in acuity between the two eyes. Thus, preverbal or nonverbal patients with strong fixation preference in one eye should be suspected of having amblyopia in the other eye. An eye that has eccentric fixation and nystagmoid movements when attempting fixation would have its visual acuity designated uncentral, unsteady, and unmaintained (UC, US, UM).

In a child with straight eyes, it is impossible to tell if he or she will maintain fixation with either eye unless the *induced tropia test* is used. This test is performed by placing a 10Δ–15Δ base-down prism over one eye to induce a vertical deviation. An alternative method includes the use of a prism of greater strength held base-out. The patient is then tested for the ability to maintain fixation with either eye under binocular, albeit dissociated, viewing conditions. It is important to determine whether each eye can maintain fixation through smooth pursuit or a blink; strong fixation preference for one eye indicates amblyopia in the nonpreferred eye.

Occasionally, avoidance movements can be demonstrated when the good eye is occluded. The patient may attempt to maneuver around the occluder when the good eye is covered but not when the poorly seeing eye is covered. A child with poor vision in the right eye, for example, might be noted to "fix and follow" (F and F) more poorly using that eye and to object to occlusion of the left eye.

The visual acuity of preschool age and older children can be tested using the illiterate E test (the *E-game*), letters, numbers, or symbols, all generically referred to as *optotypes*. Children being tested with the E-game are asked to point their hand or fingers in the direction of the E. This test can be difficult to use because of developmental status and confusion of right versus left even among normal children. Visual acuity testing with Snellen letters or numbers requires the child to name each letter or number, whereas visual acuity testing with the HOTV test or with Lea symbols can be done by matching, a cognitively easier task. Whenever possible, a line of optotypes or single optotypes surrounded by *contour interaction bars* ("crowding bars") should be used to prevent the overestimation of visual acuity of an amblyopic eye that often occurs with isolated optotypes (see Chapter 5, Fig 5-1). Allen pictures should be used only if the child cannot be tested with any other class of optotypes; Allen pictures do not provide any contour interaction, and their overall size and the width of their underlying components fail to conform to accepted parameters of optotype design.

The type of test used should be identified along with the results to facilitate comparisons with measurements taken at other times. Most pediatric ophthalmologists consider Snellen acuity most reliable, followed by HOTV, Lea symbols, the illiterate E test, Allen pictures, and fixation behavior. The most reliable test that the child can perform should be used. Preferential looking techniques using Teller acuity cards can be a useful adjunctive test for comparing visual acuity between fellow eyes in infants and preverbal children.

Patients with latent nystagmus may show better visual acuity with both eyes together than with one eye occluded. To assess distance monocular visual acuity in this situation, it may be helpful to fog the eye not being tested with a lens that is +5.00 D greater than the refractive error in that eye.

Near Visual Acuity

Tests of near visual acuity include reading cards with graduated, small standardized print. With a near card, visual acuity at 14 inches (35 cm) is recorded. Again, both uncorrected and corrected visual acuity are determined. Because of inaccuracy related to viewing distance, near visual acuities should never be compared with distance acuities in children.

Assessment of Eye Movements

Generally, versions are tested first. The examiner should pay particular attention to the movements of both eyes into the nine diagnostic positions of gaze. Limitations of movement into these positions and asymmetry of excursion of the two eyes should be noted. Spinning the child, or provoking the doll's head phenomenon, may be helpful in eliciting the vestibular-stimulated eye movements. If versions are not full, duction movements should be tested for each eye separately. BCSC Section 5, *Neuro-Ophthalmology,* also discusses testing of the ocular motility system.

The examiner must use ingenuity to keep the patient's attention, and such tricks as brightly colored toys, pictures, and storytelling about the objects are essential. A well-prepared examiner always has several toys or pictures at hand (see Introduction: Rapport With Children: Tips for a Productive Examination).

Tests of Ocular Alignment

Ocular alignment tests can be grouped into four basic types: cover tests, corneal light reflex tests, dissimilar image tests, and dissimilar target tests.

Cover tests

Eye movement capability, image formation and perception, foveal fixation in each eye, attention, and cooperation are all necessities for cover testing. If the patient is unable to maintain constant fixation on an accommodative target, the results of cover testing may not be valid, and this battery of tests therefore should not be used.

There are three types of cover tests: the cover-uncover test, the alternate cover test, and the simultaneous prism and cover test. All can be performed with fixation at distance or near. Some deviations (eg, intermittent exotropia) may be more evident at distance; others (eg, accommodative esotropia) may be more evident at near.

The monocular *cover-uncover test* is the most important test to detect the presence of manifest strabismus and to differentiate a phoria from a tropia (Fig 6-1). As one eye is covered, the examiner watches carefully for any movement in the opposite, *noncovered* eye; such movement indicates the presence of a tropia. Movement of the *covered* eye in one direction just after the cover is applied and a movement in the opposite direction (a fusional movement) as the cover is removed indicates a phoria that becomes manifest

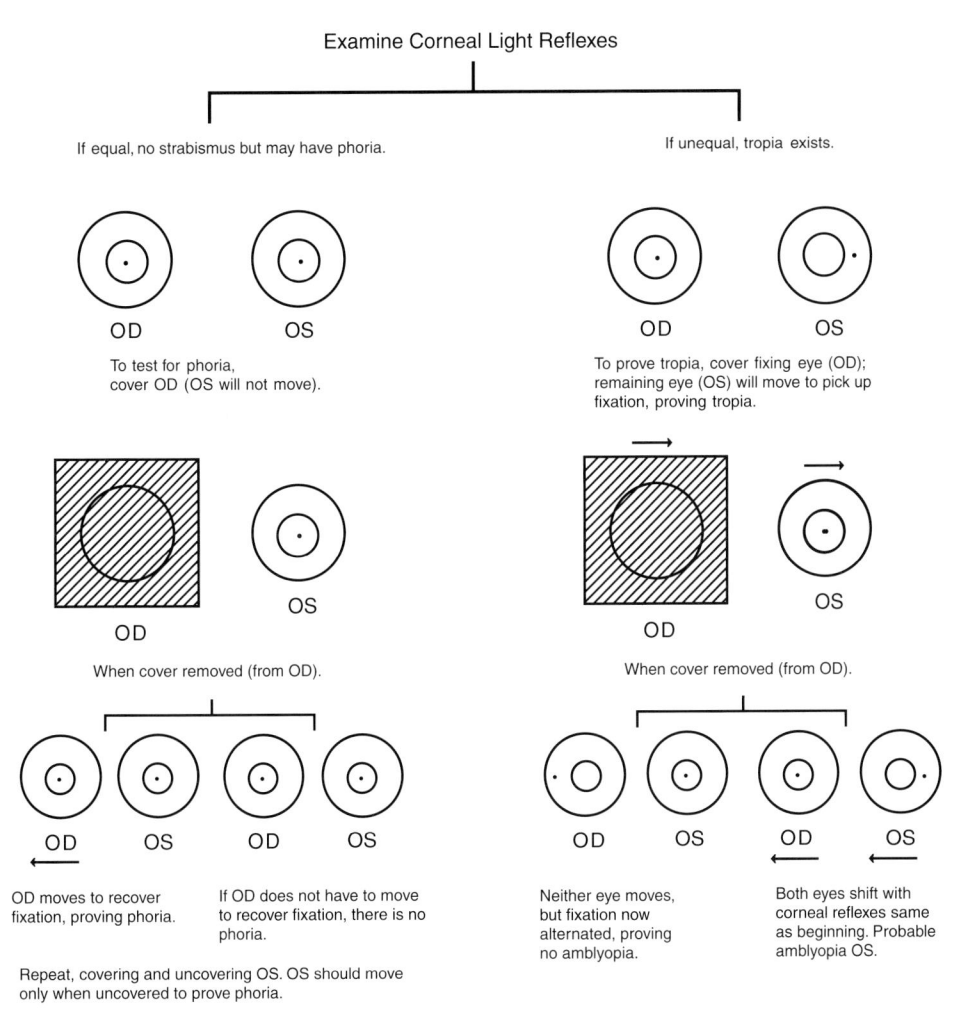

CHAPTER 6: Diagnostic Techniques for Strabismus and Amblyopia • 75

Figure 6-1 The monocular cover-uncover test.

only when binocularity is interrupted. If the patient has a phoria, the eyes will be straight before and after the cover-uncover test; the deviation that appears during the test is a result of interruption of binocular vision and the inability of the fusional mechanism to operate. A patient with a tropia, however, starts out with a deviated eye and ends up (after the test) with either the same or the opposite eye deviated (if the opposite eye is the deviated one, the condition is termed *alternating heterotropia*). Some patients may have straight eyes and start out with a phoria prior to the cover-uncover test; however, after prolonged testing—and therefore prolonged interruption of binocular vision—dissociation into a manifest tropia can occur.

The *alternate cover test (prism and cover test)* measures the total deviation, both latent and manifest (Fig 6-2). This test does not specify how much of each type of deviation is present (ie, it does not separate the phoria from the tropia). The cover is placed alternately

76 • Pediatric Ophthalmology and Strabismus

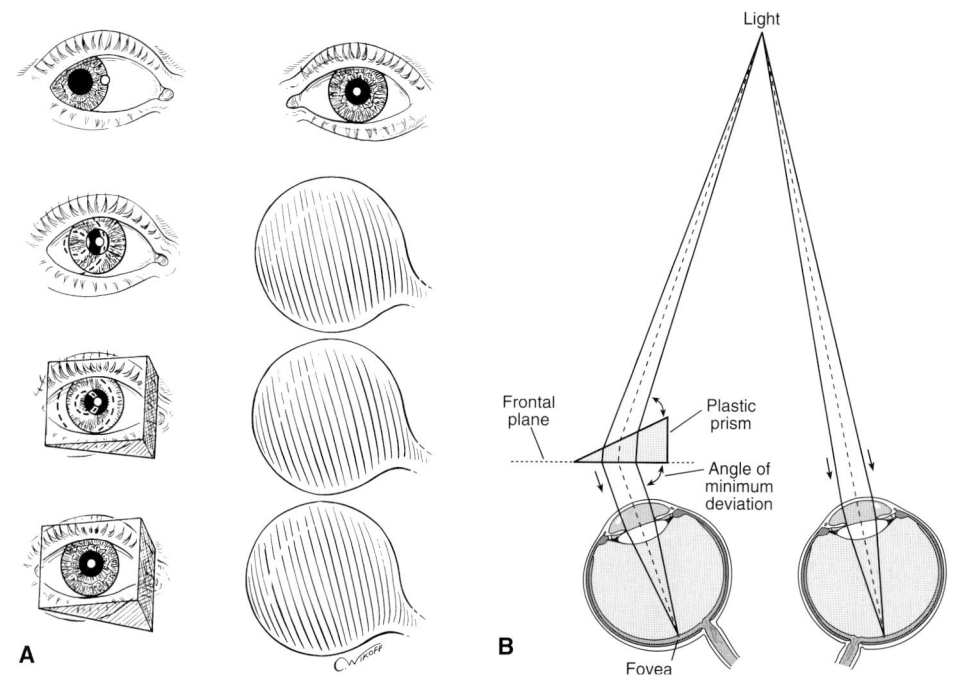

Figure 6-2 A, In the top row, the child is seen to have a right exotropia. In the second row the cover test shows movement of the right eye to fixate when the left eye is covered. In the third row, a small prism introduced before the right eye begins to neutralize the deviation. In the bottom row, the correct prism has been introduced and no more movement is seen when the cover is alternated between eyes. **B,** The diagram shows how the prism eliminates movement on cover testing by aligning rays of light from the fixation target with the fovea in the exotropic right eye. The size of the prism gives a measurement of the exotropia. *(Reproduced with permission from Simon JW, Calhoun JH. A Child's Eyes: A Guide to Pediatric Primary Care. Gainesville, FL: Triad Publishing Co; 1997:72.)*

in front of each eye several times to dissociate the eyes and maximize the deviation; it is important to quickly transfer the occluder from one eye to the other to prevent fusion. This test should be done at both distance and near fixation, with and without glasses. Once dissociation is achieved, the amount of deviation is measured using prisms to eliminate the eye movement as the cover is alternately switched from eye to eye. It may be necessary to use both horizontally and vertically placed prisms. The amount of prism power required is the measure of deviation. Two horizontal or two vertical prisms should not be stacked on each other because this can induce significant measurement errors. A more accurate method to measure large deviations is to place prisms in front of each eye. However, it is acceptable to stack a horizontal and a vertical prism before the same eye if necessary.

Whereas the alternate cover test measures the total deviation (phoria and tropia), the *simultaneous prism and cover test* is helpful in determining the actual heterotropia when both eyes are uncovered (tropia alone). The test is performed by covering the fixating eye at the same time the prism is placed in front of the deviating eye. The test is repeated using increasing prism powers until the deviated eye no longer shifts. Again, the power of the prism is the measure of the deviation. This test has special application in monofixation syndrome, which may include a small-angle heterotropia. Patients with this condition may reduce the amount of deviation measured in the alternate cover test by exerting at least partial control over a coexisting phoria through peripheral fusion when both eyes are open. In this instance, the simultaneous prism and cover test measures the amount of tropia in a deviation that has a superimposed phoria. This test may be useful to assess the deviation under real-life conditions with both eyes viewing.

   Wilson ME. *Ocular Motility Evaluation of Strabismus and Myasthenia Gravis.* [videotape]. San Francisco: American Academy of Ophthalmology; 1993.

Corneal light reflex tests

Corneal light reflex tests are useful in assessing ocular alignment in patients who cannot cooperate sufficiently to allow cover testing or who have poor fixation. The main tests of this type are the Hirschberg, modified Krimsky, Brückner, and major amblyoscope methods.

Hirschberg's method is based on the premise that 1 mm of decentration of the corneal light reflection corresponds to about 7°, or 15Δ, of ocular deviation of the visual axis. Therefore, a light reflex at the pupillary margin is about 2 mm from the pupillary center (with a 4 mm pupil), which corresponds to 15°, or 30Δ, of deviation. A reflex in the mid-iris region is about 4 mm from the pupillary center, which is roughly 30°, or 60Δ, of deviation; similarly, a reflex at the limbus is about 45°, or 90Δ, of deviation (Fig 6-3).

Krimsky's method uses reflections produced on both corneas by a penlight. The original method involved placing prisms in front of the deviating eye. More common modifications involve prisms held before the fixing eye or split between the two eyes. By adjusting the prisms so as to center the corneal reflection in the deviated eye, it is possible to approximate and quantitate the near deviation (Fig 6-4). A simple method to estimate the distance deviation by either the Hirschberg or Krimsky method has been described

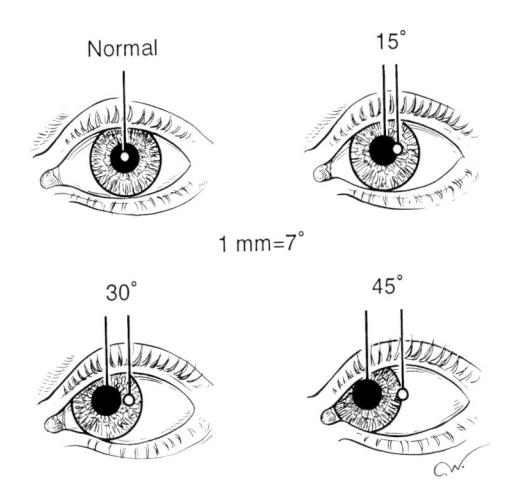

Figure 6-3 Hirschberg test. The extent to which the corneal light reflex is displaced from the center of the pupil provides an approximation of the angular size of the deviation (in this example, a left esotropia). *(Reproduced with permission from Simon JW, Calhoun JH. A Child's Eyes: A Guide to Pediatric Primary Care. Gainesville, FL: Triad Publishing Co; 1997:72.)*

Figure 6-4 Krimsky test. The right exotropia in the top picture is measured by the size of the prism required to center the pupillary reflexes, as shown at bottom. *(Reproduced with permission from Simon JW, Calhoun JH. A Child's Eyes: A Guide to Pediatric Primary Care. Gainesville, FL: Triad Publishing Co; 1997:72.)*

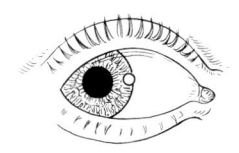

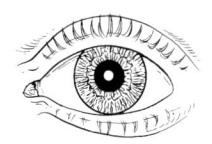

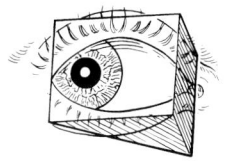

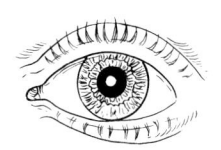

by Wisnicki and Guyton. Their method may be helpful for comparing the deviations at near and distance fixation in patients with poor fixation in one eye.

> Wisnicki HJ, Guyton DL. A modified corneal light reflex test with distance fixation. *Am J Ophthalmol.* 1986;102:661–662.

The *Brückner* test is performed by using the direct ophthalmoscope to obtain a red reflex simultaneously in both eyes. If strabismus is present, the deviated eye will have a lighter and brighter reflex than the fixating eye. Note that this test detects, but does not measure, the deviation. This test also identifies opacities in the visual axis and moderate to severe anisometropia. The Brückner test is primarily used by primary care practitioners to screen for strabismus and anisometropia.

The *major amblyoscope method* uses separate target illumination, which can be moved to center the corneal light reflection. The amount of deviation is then read directly from the scale of the amblyoscope.

Dissimilar image tests

These tests are based on the patient's response to diplopia created by two dissimilar images. The three major types are the Maddox rod test, the double Maddox rod test, and the red glass test.

The *Maddox rod test* uses a specially constructed device consisting of a series of parallel cylinders. It converts a point source of light into a line image. The optical properties of the cylinders cause the streak of light to be situated 90° to the orientation of the parallel cylinders. Because fusion is precluded by the Maddox rod, heterophorias and heterotropias cannot be differentiated. The Maddox rod can be used to test for horizontal, vertical, and (when used in conjunction with another Maddox rod) cyclodeviations.

To test for horizontal deviations, the Maddox rod is placed in front of the right eye with the cylinders in the horizontal direction. The patient fixates a point source of light and then sees a vertical line with the right eye and a white light with the left eye. If the light superimposes the line, orthophoria is present; if the light is on the left side of the line, an esodeviation is present; and if the light is on the right side of the line, an exodeviation is present. A similar procedure with the cylinders aligned vertically is used to test for vertical deviations. To measure the amount of deviation, the examiner holds prisms of different powers until the line superimposes the point source. The Maddox rod test is not a satisfactory test for horizontal deviations, however, because accommodative convergence cannot be controlled.

The *double Maddox rod test* is used for determination of cyclodeviations. A Maddox rod is placed in front of each eye in a trial frame or phoropter with the rods aligned vertically so that the patient sees horizontal line images. The patient or examiner rotates the axes of the rods until the lines are perceived to be parallel. To facilitate the patient's recognition of the two lines, it is often helpful to dissociate the lines by placing a small prism base-up or base-down in front of one eye. The degrees of deviation and the direction (incyclo or excyclo) can be determined by the angle of rotation that causes the line images to appear horizontal and parallel. Traditionally, a red Maddox rod was placed before the right eye and a white Maddox rod before the left, but recent evidence suggests the different colors can cause fixation artifacts that do not occur if the same color is used bilaterally.

> Simons K, Arnoldi K, Brown MH. Color dissociation artifacts in double Maddox rod cyclo-deviation testing. *Ophthalmology*. 1994;101:1897–1901.

In the *red glass test,* a red glass is placed in front of the right eye. This test is used for the same purpose as the Maddox rod test but is not applicable to cyclodeviations. As in the Maddox rod test, prisms are used to eliminate the horizontal or vertical diplopia, and the amount of deviation is recorded.

Dissimilar target tests

Dissimilar target tests are based on the patient's response to the dissimilar images created by each eye viewing a different target; the deviation is measured first with one eye fixating and then with the other. Several tests of this type have been devised, but the three most frequently encountered are the Lancaster red-green projection test, the Hess screen test, and the major amblyoscope test.

The *Lancaster red-green test* uses red-green goggles that can be reversed, a red slit projector, a green slit projector, and a screen ruled into squares of 7 cm. At the test distance of 2 m, each square subtends 2°. The patient's head is held steady; by convention, the test is begun with the red filter in front of the right eye. The examiner projects a red slit onto the screen, and the patient is asked to place the green slit so that it appears to coincide with the red slit. The relative positions of the two streaks are then recorded. The test is repeated for the diagnostic positions of gaze (these positions are discussed later in the chapter), and the goggles are then reversed so that the deviation with the fellow eye fixating can be recorded. The Lancaster red-green test is used primarily in patients with diplopia caused by incomitant strabismus and requires that the patient have normal retinal correspondence.

The *Hess screen test* is also useful in evaluating patients with paretic or paralytic strabismus who have normal retinal correspondence. The test uses red-green goggles, a special screen that has a red dot (or light) in 8 inner positions and 16 outer positions, and a green slit projector. At a test distance of 50 cm, the patient is asked to place the green slit light so that it appears to coincide with the individual red dots (or lights). The relative positions are connected by a straight line; usually, just the eight inner dots (or lights) and the central point of fixation are plotted. The goggles are then reversed so the deviation with the other eye fixating can be recorded.

Major amblyoscope testing uses dissimilar targets that the patient is asked to superimpose. If the patient has normal retinal correspondence, the horizontal, vertical, and torsional deviations can be read directly from the calibrated scale of the amblyoscope.

Confounding Factors in Ocular Alignment Assessment

Two potential pitfalls in the evaluation of ocular alignment are the conditions of pseudostrabismus and angle kappa. *Pseudostrabismus* is the appearance of strabismus despite normal alignment. The most common form is pseudoesotropia, which results from coverage of the nasal sclera by the wide, flat nasal bridge and epicanthal folds so common in infancy. Because no real deviation exists, both corneal light reflex testing and cover testing results are normal. The appearance of crossing should gradually improve during infancy and early childhood. If it does not, repeat examination is warranted.

Angle kappa is the angle between the visual axis and the anatomical pupillary axis of the eye. If the fovea is temporal to the pupillary axis (as is usually the case), the corneal light reflection will be slightly nasal to the center of the cornea. This is termed *positive angle kappa*, which simulates exodeviation. If the position of the fovea is nasal to the pupillary axis, the corneal light reflection will be slightly temporal to the center of the cornea. This is termed *negative angle kappa*, which simulates esodeviation (Fig 6-5). One cause for a positive angle kappa is retinopathy of prematurity with temporal dragging of the macula. Although affected patients appear to be exotropic, the eye continues to appear abducted even when fixating under monocular conditions.

Positions of Gaze

The *primary position of gaze* is the position of the eyes when fixating straight ahead on an object at infinity. For practical purposes, infinity is considered to be 20 ft (6 m), and for this position the head should be straight. If the patient has vertical strabismus, the definition of primary position is expanded to include the eyes fixating straight ahead on a distant object with the head tilted to the right and to the left (see Three-Step Test, later in the chapter).

Cardinal positions are those six positions of gaze in which the prime mover is one muscle of each eye, together called *yoke muscles* (see Chapter 3, Fig 3-3). *Midline positions* are straight up and straight down from primary position. These latter two gaze positions help determine the elevating and depressing capabilities of the eye, but they do not isolate any one muscle because two elevator and two depressor muscles affect midline gaze positions.

The phrase *diagnostic positions of gaze* has been applied to the composite of these nine gaze positions: the six cardinal positions, straight up and down, and primary position. Several schemes have been devised to record the results of ocular alignment and motility in the various diagnostic positions of gaze, as well as those obtained with the head tilted to the right and to the left (Fig 6-6).

A and V patterns should be noted at this point. An *A pattern* refers to an esotropia greatest in upgaze or an exotropia greatest in downgaze; a *V pattern* denotes an esotropia

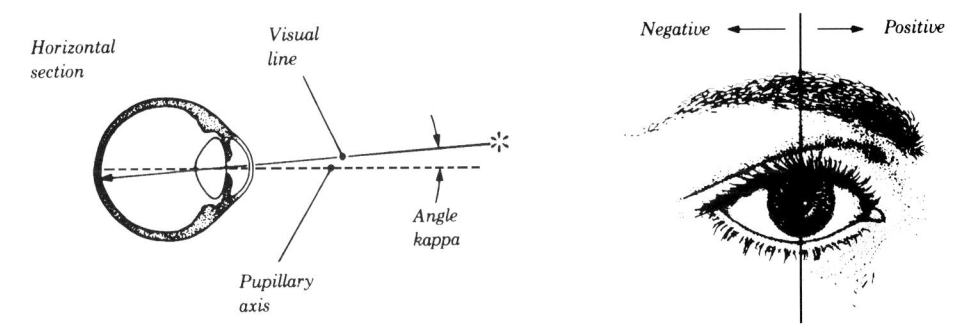

Figure 6-5 Angle kappa. A positive angle kappa simulates exotropia whereas a negative angle kappa simulates esotropia. *(Reprinted from Parks MM. Ocular Motility and Strabismus.* Hagerstown, MD: Harper & Row; 1975.)

greatest in downgaze or an exotropia greatest in upgaze. The patient should be observed carefully for any chin elevation or depression. See Chapter 10 for a full discussion of A and V patterns.

Convergence

Alignment at near is usually measured at 13 inches (33 cm) directly in front of the patient in the horizontal plane. Comparison of the alignment in the primary position at both distance and near fixation helps assess the accommodative convergence (synkinetic near) reflex. The *near point of convergence* is determined by placing a fixation object at 40 cm in the midsagittal plane of the patient's head. As the subject fixates on the object, it is moved toward the subject until one eye loses fixation and turns out. The point at which this action occurs is the near point of convergence. The eye that is able to maintain fixation is considered to be the dominant eye. The normal near point of convergence is 8–10 cm or less.

AC/A ratio

The *accommodative convergence/accommodation (AC/A) ratio* is defined as the amount of convergence measured in prism diopters per unit (diopter) change in accommodation. There are two methods of clinical measurement.

- The *gradient method* arrives at the AC/A ratio by the change in deviation in prism diopters divided by the change in lens power. An accommodative target must be used, and the working distance (typically at 1/3 m or 6 m) is held constant. Plus or minus lenses (eg, +1, +2, +3, −1, −2, −3) are used to vary the accommodative requirement. This method measures the *stimulus AC/A ratio*, which is not necessarily identical to the *response AC/A ratio*. The latter can be determined only with the use of an optometer that records the change in accommodation actually produced.
- The *heterophoria method* employs the distance–near relationship, measuring the distance and near deviations. A similar alignment is normally present for distance and near fixation. If the patient is more exotropic or less esotropic at near, too

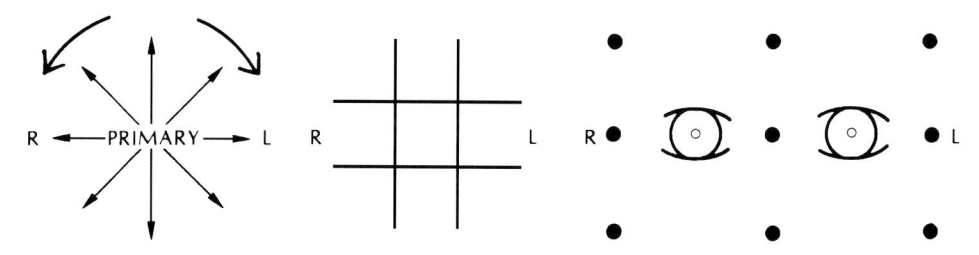

Figure 6-6 Three examples of methods for recording the results of ocular alignment testing.

little convergence, or a low AC/A ratio, is present; if the patient is more esotropic or less exotropic at near, a high AC/A ratio is present. In accommodative esotropia, an increase of esotropia of 10Δ or more from distance to near fixation is considered to represent a high AC/A ratio.

An abnormally high AC/A ratio can be managed either optically or pharmacologically. For example, plus lens spectacles for hyperopia reduce accommodation and therefore reduce accommodative convergence. This principle is the mainstay of the medical management of esotropia. Bifocals reduce or eliminate the need to accommodate for near fixation. This optical management is used for excess convergence at near—that is, an esodeviation greater at near. Underplussed or overminused spectacles create the need for greater-than-normal accommodation. This excess accommodation creates more accommodative convergence and is occasionally used to reduce an exodeviation.

Long-acting cholinesterase inhibitors (eg, echothiophate iodide) can be used to decrease accommodative convergence. These drugs act directly on the ciliary body, facilitating transmission at the myoneural junction. They reduce the central demand for accommodative innervation and thus reduce the amount of convergence induced by accommodation.

Fusional Vergence

Vergences move the two eyes in opposite directions. Fusional vergences are motor responses used to eliminate horizontal, vertical, or torsional image disparity. They can be grouped by the following functions:

- *Fusional convergence* eliminates bitemporal retinal disparity and controls an exophoria
- *Fusional divergence* eliminates binasal retinal disparity and controls an esophoria.
- *Vertical fusional vergence* controls a hyperphoria or hypophoria.
- *Torsional fusional vergence* controls incyclophoria or excyclophoria.

Fusional vergences can be measured by using a haploscopic device, a rotary prism, or a bar prism, gradually increasing the prism power until diplopia occurs. Accommodation must be controlled during fusional vergence testing. Fusional vergences can be changed by a number of mechanisms:

- *Involuntary by patient:* As a tendency to deviate evolves, the patient gradually develops a larger-than-normal fusional vergence for that deviation. Very large fusional vergences are common in compensated long-standing vertical deviations and in exodeviations.
- *Visual acuity:* Improved acuity improves the fusional vergence mechanism. The treatment of reduced vision may change a symptomatic intermittent deviation to an asymptomatic phoria.
- *State of awareness:* Fatigue, illness, or drug and alcohol ingestion may decrease the fusional vergence mechanism, converting a phoria to a tropia.
- *Orthoptics:* The magnitude of the fusional vergence mechanism may be increased by exercises. This treatment works best for near fusional convergence, particularly for the relief of the syndrome of convergence insufficiency.
- *Optical stimulation of fusional vergence:* (1) In controlled accommodative esotropia, reducing the strength of the hyperopia or bifocal correction induces an esophoria that stimulates fusional divergence. (2) Prisms to control diplopia may be gradually reduced to stimulate a compensatory fusional vergence.

Tests of Binocular Sensory Cooperation

Assessment of the vergence system indicates the extent to which the two eyes can be directed at the same object. Sensory binocularity involves the use of both eyes together to form one perception. In general, normal sensory binocularity depends on normal fusional vergence. Ideally, testing should therefore be performed before binocularity is disrupted by occlusion of either eye. Two classes of tests are commonly used to assess sensory binocularity: Worth four-dot testing (and its equivalents) and stereo acuity testing.

Worth four-dot testing

The mechanics of Worth four-dot testing are described in Chapter 4. Only patients who are using the two eyes together can appreciate all four lights being projected (see Fig 4-8). If the right eye is suppressed, as often occurs if that eye is deviated, the patient will report seeing three green lights because the white light appears green. If the left eye is suppressed, the patient will report seeing two red lights because the white light appears red. If alternate eyes are suppressed, the patient may see two red and three green lights alternating. Patients with diplopia may report seeing five lights simultaneously.

Use of the Worth four-dot test at distance illuminates a smaller, more central portion of the retina; testing at closer distances illuminates a progressively larger, more peripheral portion. Distance testing can reveal small suppression scotomata that may be inapparent on testing at near. Results of testing should be reported as fusion or suppression of one eye at distance and at near. Many cases of small-angle strabismus (eg, that associated with monofixation syndrome) may combine fusion at near with suppression of one eye at distance. A polarized version of the Worth four-dot test is also available.

Stereo acuity testing

Worth four-dot testing is best at detecting suppression, but stereo acuity testing assesses the use of the two eyes for binocular depth perception. Stereopsis occurs when the two retinal images, slightly disparate because of the normally different views provided by the horizontal separation of the two eyes, are cortically integrated. There are two types of stereopsis tests: *contour* and *random dot*. Contour stereopsis tests involve actual horizontal separation of the targets presented to each eye (with polarized or red-green glasses) such that monocular clues to depth are present at lower stereo acuity levels; random dot stereopsis tests circumvent the problem of monocular clues by embedding the stereo figures in a background of random dots.

In the *Stereo Fly* test (a contour stereopsis test), a card with superimposed images of a fly is shown to the patient. Ability to detect the elevation of the fly's wings above the plane of the card indicates stereopsis. Because the separation of the superimposed images is 3500 seconds of arc, this test is one of gross stereopsis. Other figures included on the same card contain less separated images. Thus, quantitation of finer stereo acuity may be possible in cooperative patients.

Several different types of random dot stereopsis tests are clinically useful. The *Randot test*, in which polarized glasses are worn, can measure stereo acuity to 20 seconds of arc. The *Random Dot "E" test* employs a preferential looking strategy to test stereopsis and is used extensively in pediatric vision screening programs. Red-green glasses are used in the *TNO test* to provide separation of the images seen by each eye. The *Lang stereopsis tests* do not require glasses to produce a random dot stereoscopic effect and therefore may be useful in young children who object to wearing glasses.

Stereopsis can also be measured at distance using the AO Vectograph Project-O-Chart slide or the BVAT (Binocular Visual Activity Acuity Test). Distance stereo acuity measurements may be helpful in monitoring control of intermittent exotropia.

Special Motor Tests

Special motor tests include forced ductions, active force generation, and saccadic velocity. These are also discussed with illustrations in BCSC Section 5, *Neuro-Ophthalmology*.

- *Forced ductions* are performed by using forceps to move the eye into various positions, thus determining resistance to passive movement. This test is usually performed at the time of surgery but can sometimes be performed preoperatively with topical anesthesia in cooperative patients.
- *Active force generation* assesses the relative strength of a muscle. The patient is asked to move the eye in a given direction while the observer grasps the eye with an instrument. If the muscle tested is paretic, the examiner feels less than normal tension.
- *Saccadic velocity* can be recorded using a special instrument that graphically records the speed and direction of eye movement. This test is useful to differentiate paralysis from restriction. A paralyzed muscle generates a reduced saccadic velocity throughout the movement of the involved eye, whereas a restricted muscle produces an initially normal velocity that rapidly decelerates when the eye reaches the limit of its movement.

The field of single binocular vision may be tested on either a Goldmann perimeter or a tangent screen. These tests are useful for following the recovery of a paretic muscle or to measure the outcome of surgery to alleviate diplopia. A small white test object is followed by both eyes in the various cardinal positions throughout the visual field. When the patient indicates that the test object is seen double, this point is plotted. The examiner then repeats the same procedure until the entire visual field has been plotted, noting the area in which the patient reported single vision and the area of double vision. The field of binocular fixation normally measures about 45°–50° from the fixation point except where it is blocked by the nose (Fig 6-7).

Three-Step Test

Cyclovertical muscle palsies, especially those involving the superior oblique muscles, are often responsible for hyperdeviations. The three-step test is an algorithm that can be used to help identify the paretic cyclovertically acting muscle. As helpful as this test is, it is not always diagnostic and can be misleading, especially in patients in whom more than one muscle is paretic, in patients who have undergone strabismus surgery, and in the presence of restrictions.

The examiner must be familiar with the anatomy and motor physiology of the extraocular muscles in order to understand the test. Briefly, there are eight cyclovertically acting muscles: four work as depressors (two in each eye), and four work as elevators (again, two in each eye). The two *depressors* of each eye are the *inferior rectus* and *superior oblique muscles*; the two *elevators* of each eye are the *superior rectus* and the *inferior oblique muscles*. The three-step test is performed as follows (Fig 6-8):

Step 1

Determine which eye is hypertropic by using the cover-uncover test (see Fig 6-1 and the discussion earlier in this chapter). Step 1 narrows the number of possibly underacting muscles from eight to four. In the example shown in Figure 6-8, the right eye has been found to be hypertropic. This means that the paresis will be found in either the depressors of the right eye (RIR, RSO) or the elevators of the left eye (LIO, LSR).

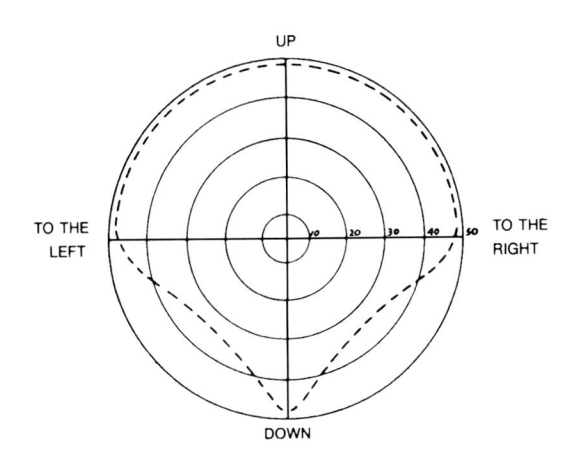

Figure 6-7 The normal field of single binocular vision.

86 • Pediatric Ophthalmology and Strabismus

STEP 1

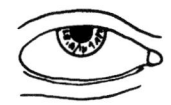

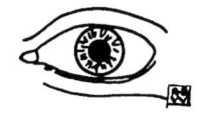

Possible paretic muscles: RSO, RIR, LSR, LIO

STEP 2

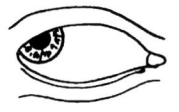

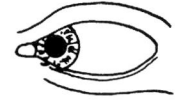

RIGHT GAZE
RIR and LIO
eliminated

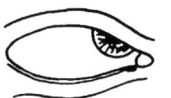

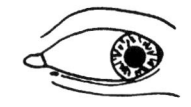

LEFT GAZE
RSO or LSR
are possible paretic muscles

STEP 3

(for left-gaze
deviation only)

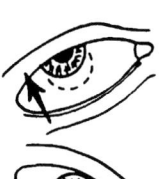

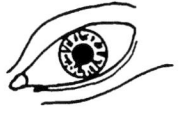

RSO is paretic

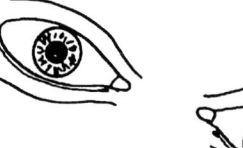

LSR not paretic

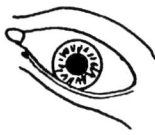

Figure 6-8 When an isolated cyclovertical muscle palsy is present, the three-step test can be used to identify the paretic muscle. *Step 1,* The cover test has been used to determine that patient has a *right hypertropia.* This step eliminates four of the cyclovertically acting muscles, in this case leaving the right superior oblique (RSO), right inferior rectus (RIR), left superior rectus (LSR), and left inferior oblique (LIO) to be tested further. *Step 2,* The prism and cover test shows that the right hypertropia is greater with left gaze than with right gaze. This finding eliminates the RIR and LIO and implicates the RSO and LSR as possible paretic muscles. *Step 3,* Head tilt to the right followed by head tilt to the left. *Top,* If the RSO is paretic, the deviation is larger on right head tilt (*dotted line* indicates normal position, and *arrow* shows abnormal movement). *Bottom,* If the LSR were paretic, the deviation would have been larger on left head tilt. In this example, the three-step test result is consistent with a right superior oblique muscle palsy. *(Illustration modified from von Noorden GK.* Atlas of Strabismus. *4th ed. St Louis: Mosby; 1983:149.)*

Step 2

Determine whether the vertical deviation is greater in right gaze or in left gaze. At the end of step 2, the two remaining possible muscles (one in each eye) are both intortors or extortors and both superior or inferior muscles (one rectus and one oblique). Note that in Figure 6-8, the increased left-gaze deviation eliminates two inferior muscles and implicates two superior muscles.

Step 3

Known as the *Bielschowsky head-tilt test*, the final step involves tilting the head to the right and then to the left. Head tilt to the right stimulates intorsion of the right eye (RSR, RSO) and extorsion of the left eye (LIR, LIO). Head tilt to the left stimulates extorsion of the right eye (RIR, RIO) and intorsion of the left eye (LSR, LSO). Normally, the two intortors and the two extortors of each eye have *opposite* vertical actions that cancel each other. If one intortor or one extortor is paretic, it cannot act vertically and the vertical action of the other ipsilateral torting muscle becomes manifest.

Figure 6-8 illustrates the results if step 2 above had demonstrated that the deviation was greater in left gaze and the RSO was the paretic muscle.

> Parks MM. Isolated cyclovertical muscle palsy. *Arch Ophthalmol.* 1958;60:1027–1035.
> von Noorden GK. *Atlas of Strabismus.* 4th ed. St Louis: Mosby; 1983:149.

Cycloplegic Refraction

One of the most important tests in the evaluation of any patient with complaints pertinent to binocular vision and ocular motility is refraction with cycloplegic agents. *Cyclopentolate* (1.0%) is the preferred drug for routine use in children, especially when combined with phenylephrine, which has no cycloplegic effect itself. Use of 0.5% strength is suggested in infants, and the clinician should be aware that some adverse psychological effects have been observed in children receiving cyclopentolate. *Homatropine* (5.0%) and *scopolamine* (0.25%) are occasionally used instead of cyclopentolate, but neither is as rapid-acting or effective. *Tropicamide* (0.5% or 1.0%), which is used in conjunction with phenylephrine (2.5%) for routine dilation, is usually not strong enough for effective cycloplegia in children. Some ophthalmologists use a combination of cyclopentolate and tropicamide to achieve maximum dilation. Although many ophthalmologists advocate *atropine* 1.0% drops or ointment, it causes prolonged blurring and is more often associated with toxic or allergic side effects (see below). Nonetheless, 1% atropine drops (once per day to one eye only) are being used safely and with increasing frequency for the treatment of amblyopia (see Chapter 5).

Table 6-2 shows the schedule of administration and duration of action for commonly used cycloplegics. The duration of action varies highly, and the pupillary effect occurs earlier and lasts longer than does the cycloplegic effect, so a dilated pupil does not necessarily indicate complete cycloplegia. For patients with accommodative esodeviations, frequent repeated cycloplegic examinations are essential. Retinoscopic measurements should be made along the patient's visual axis.

88 • Pediatric Ophthalmology and Strabismus

Table 6-2 Administration and Duration of Cycloplegics

Medication	Administration Schedule	Duration of Mydriatic Action
Tropicamide	1 drop q 5 min × 2; wait 30 min	4–8 hr
Cyclopentolate	1 drop q 5 min × 2; wait 30 min	8–24 hr
Scopolamine	1 drop q 5 min × 2; wait 1 hr	1–3 d
Homatropine	1 drop q 5 min × 2; wait 1 hr	1–3 d
Atropine*	1 drop tid × 3 days; then 1 drop morning of appointment	1–2 wk

* Some physicians think that atropine ointment is a safer vehicle for delivery of the drug, given once a day × 3 days.

Side effects

Adverse reactions to cycloplegic agents include allergic (or hypersensitivity) reaction with conjunctivitis, edematous eyelids, and dermatitis. These reactions are more frequent with atropine than with any of the other agents. Hypnotic effect can be seen with scopolamine and occasionally with cyclopentolate or homatropine.

Systemic intoxication from atropine manifests in fever, dry mouth, flushing of the face, rapid pulse, nausea, dizziness, delirium, and erythema. Treatment is discontinuation of the medicine with supportive measures as necessary. If the reaction is severe, physostigmine may be given. Remember, one drop of 1.0% atropine = 0.5 mg of atropine.

Zimmerman TJ, Kooner KS, Sharir M, et al. *Textbook of Ocular Pharmacology*. Philadelphia: Lippincott Williams & Wilkins; 1997.

Prism Adaptation Test

The prism adaptation test represents the formalization of a simple clinical practice that has been used for many years, especially in Europe. For a variety of reasons, strabismus surgery in Europe is often delayed until the second half of the first decade of life. In the interim, to help the child obtain binocular fusion while awaiting surgical alignment of the eye, the patient is often fitted with prisms of sufficient magnitude to permit alignment of the visual axes. In many cases, this step provokes a restoration of sensory binocular cooperation in a form of fusion and even stereopsis. This technique then actually simulates orthotropia, offering some predictive value of whether fusion may be restored when the patient undergoes surgical alignment.

In some patients, however (especially those with acquired esotropia), placement of such prisms increases the deviation. In such cases, anomalous retinal correspondence based on the objective angle may drive the eyes to maintain this adaptive alignment even with prismatic correction. After wearing such prisms, the patient returns with a greater angle of deviation corresponding to the addition of the prisms. The Prism Adaptation Study has concluded that these patients may require significantly more surgery than other patients in order to correct deviation. In some cases, patients who obtain fusion with this prism therapy may simply be weaned off the prisms if the angle of their deviation is not too large, and surgery may thereby be avoided. For patients in whom prism therapy results in an increase in the deviation rather than in fusion, some practitioners recommend successively increasing the prism until orthophoria with correction is obtained and then performing surgery for this maximal deviation rather than for the smaller deviation. This last concept of prism adaptation can be used to determine the target angle in cases of acquired esotropia.

> Repka MX, Connett JE, Scott WE. The one-year surgical outcome after prism adaptation for the management of acquired esotropia. *Ophthalmology.* 1996;103:922–928.

CHAPTER 7

Esodeviations

Esodeviations, the most common type of strabismus, account for more than 50% of ocular deviations in the pediatric population. An esodeviation is a latent or manifest convergent misalignment of the visual axes. Three commonly recognized forms of esodeviation are grouped according to variations in fusional capabilities:

- *Esophoria* is a latent esodeviation that is controlled by fusional mechanisms so that the eyes remain properly aligned under normal binocular viewing conditions.
- *Intermittent esotropia* is an esodeviation that is intermittently controlled by fusional mechanisms but spontaneously becomes minifest, particularly with fatigue or illness
- *Esotropia* is an esodeviation that is not controlled by fusional mechanisms, so the deviation is constantly manifest.

Esodeviations can result from innervational, anatomical, mechanical, refractive, genetic, and accommoative causes. Table 7-1 lists the major types of esodeviation.

Pseudoesotropia

Infants often have a wide, flat nasal bridge with prominent medial epicanthal folds and a small interpupillary distance. Thus, they may appear esotropic when in fact their eyes are straight. Because no real deviation exists, both corneal light reflex testing and cover testing results are normal. The appearance of crossing should gradually improve during infancy and early childhood. If it does not, repeat examination is warranted. It is important to remember that even though a child may indeed have a pseudoesodeviation as an infant, an intermittent esodeviation can be present. A report from a parent that one eye does not seem to "track" with the other eye should therefore not be taken lightly. In such a case, the child's alignment should be reexamined without delay.

Infantile (Congenital) Esotropia

Classic Congenital (Essential Infantile) Esotropia

Onset at birth is often the history of the esotropia given by the parents; however, the exact date is not precisely established in most cases. Documented presence of esotropia

Table 7-1 Types of Esodeviation

Pseudoesotropia

Infantile (congenital) esotropia
  Classic congenital (essential infantile) esotropia
  Nystagmus and esotropia
    Ciancia syndrome
    Manifest latent nystagmus
    Nystagmus blockage syndrome

Accommodative esotropia
  Refractive (normal AC/A)
  Nonrefractive (high AC/A)
  Partially accommodative

Nonaccommodative acquired esotropia
  Basic
  Acute
  Cyclic
  Sensory deprivation
  Divergence insufficiency and divergence paralysis
  Spasm of the near synkinetic reflex
  Surgical (consecutive)

Incomitant esotropia
  Sixth nerve (abducens) paresis
  Medial rectus restriction
    Thyroid ophthalmopathy
    Medial orbital wall fracture
  Duane syndrome and Möbius syndrome

by age 6 months has arbitrarily been accepted as the definition of congenital esotropia by most ophthalmologists. This criterion has been used in clinical studies.

A family history of esotropia or strabismus is often present, but well-defined genetic patterns are unusual. Other than their ocular misalignment, children with early-onset esotropia are usually normal. This type of esotropia, however, occurs in up to 30% of children with neurologic and developmental problems, including cerebral palsy and hydrocephalus.

Equal visual acuity associated with alternation of fixation from one eye to the other is common in children with esotropia. Also frequent is cross-fixation, in which a large-angle esotropia is associated with the use of the adducted eye for fixation of objects in the contralateral temporal field (Fig 7-1). Amblyopia may be present when a constant in-turning of only one eye occurs with or without cross-fixation.

The misalignment is often apparent, characteristically larger than 30D. The child's ability to abduct each eye may be difficult to confirm but can frequently be elicited with the doll's head maneuver, by rotating the child, or by observation with one eye patched. Associated vertical deviations, such as overaction of the inferior oblique muscles and dissociated vertical deviation, become common over time. Inferior oblique muscle overaction and dissociated vertical deviation may occur in more than 50% of patients with congenital esotropia but are not commonly recognized until age 1 year or older.

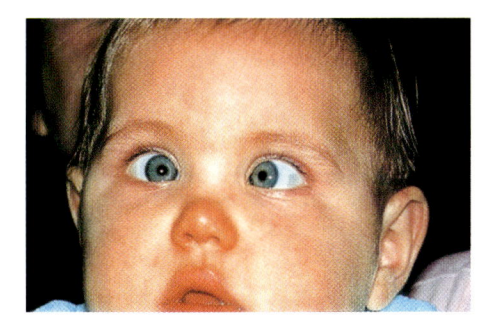

Figure 7-1 Classic congenital esotropia. *(Reproduced from Archer SM. Esotropia. In:* Focal Points: Clinical Modules for Ophthalmologists. *San Francisco: American Academy of Ophthalmology; 1994: vol 12, no 12.)*

Asymmetry of monocular horizontal smooth pursuit is normal in infants up to age 6 months, with nasal-to-temporal smooth pursuit less well developed than temporal-to-nasal smooth pursuit. Patients with congenital esotropia have persistent monocular smooth pursuit asymmetry that does not resolve.

> Birch EE, Fawcett S, Stager D. Co-development of VEP motion response and binocular vision in normal infants and infantile esotropes. *Invest Ophthalmol Vis Sci.* 2000;41:1719–1723.

Management

Cycloplegic refraction characteristically reveals 1–2 D of hyperopia, which is the normal refractive error in young children. Significant astigmatism or myopia may be present and require correction. Repeat refractions are important because an accommodative component is sometimes discovered with follow-up of these children. Because accommodative esotropia can occur as early as age 4 months and often responds to hyperopic correction, significant refractive errors (>+2.50 D of sphere) are corrected by prescribing the full cycloplegic retinoscopy findings. A small-angle esotropia that is also varying or intermittent may be more likely to respond to hyperopic correction than a large-angle, constant esotropia. An atropine refraction may be useful in some hyperopic patients with esotropia to ensure that all the hyperopia has been identified; this practice also ensures that esotropes who are surgical candidates receive a confirmation refraction prior to surgery.

Ocular alignment is rarely achieved without surgery in the child with early-onset esotropia. However, surgery should be undertaken only after correction of significant refractive errors and treatment of amblyopia because failure to correct these problems may compromise a stable surgical alignment of the eyes. It is wise to repeat the measurement of the amount of esotropia shortly before surgery because many infants show a significant increase compared with their first evaluation.

Most ophthalmologists agree that surgery should be undertaken early. The eyes should be aligned by age 24 months to stimulate some form of sensory binocular co-operation or fusion. However, operation for congenital esotropia is frequently performed in healthy children at age 6 months to try to maximize binocular visual function such as stereopsis, and some ophthalmologists advocate surgery as early as age 13 weeks to achieve a superior sensory outcome.

The child's psychological and motor development may improve and accelerate after the eyes are straightened. Bonding difficulties that may accompany abnormal ocular alignment and psychological damage from lack of eye contact and from the surgical procedure itself are probably minimized by early correction. Improved techniques have minimized the risk of general anesthesia such that anesthetic concerns need not dictate the age at which surgery is performed.

Two main surgical approaches have been suggested for this type of esotropia. The most common procedure for infantile esotropia is recession of both medial rectus muscles. Recession of a medial rectus muscle combined with resection of the ipsilateral lateral rectus muscle is an acceptable alternative. Some surgeons operate on three or even four horizontal rectus muscles at the time of the initial surgery if the deviation is larger than 50Δ. Associated overaction of the inferior oblique muscles is often treated at the time of the initial surgery via inferior oblique muscle-weakening procedures. No single approach for correction of esotropia has been uniformly successful, and later operations for undercorrections, or less frequently for overcorrections, may be needed. Chapter 13 discusses surgical procedures in greater detail.

Botulinum toxin injections into the medial rectus muscles have been investigated by several ophthalmologists as an alternative to traditional incisional surgery. Although results have been promising, many children require multiple injections and long-term sensory and motor outcomes have not been superior to those from incisional surgery. A prospective randomized clinical trial comparing the two techniques is lacking.

Alignment within 8Δ of orthophoria has been suggested as an acceptable goal because it frequently results in stable microstrabismus or monofixation with peripheral fusion, central suppression, and excellent appearance. Recent information, however, suggests that orthotropia and small-angle esotropia (≤8Δ) are superior outcomes to small-angle exotropia. Small-angle strabismus generally represents a stable functional surgical outcome even though bifoveal fusion is not achieved. Untreated patients do not improve spontaneously and may develop secondary contractures of the extraocular tissues.

> Birch EE, Stager DR, Everett ME. Random dot stereo acuity following surgical correction of infantile esotropia. *J Pediatr Ophthalmol Strabismus.* 1995;32:231–235.
> Kushner BJ. Botulinum toxin management of essential infantile esotropia [editorial]. *Arch Ophthalmol.* 1997;115:1458–1459.
> Kushner BJ, Fisher M. Is alignment within 8 prism diopters of orthotropia a successful outcome for infantile esotropia surgery? *Arch Ophthalmol.* 1996;114:176–180.
> McNeer KW, Tucker MG, Spencer RF. Botulinum toxin management of essential esotropia in children. *Arch Ophthalmol.* 1997;115:1411–1418.
> Pediatric Eye Disease Investigator Group. The clinical spectrum of early-onset esotropia: experience of the Congenital Esotropia Observational Study. *Am J Ophthalmol.* 2002;133: 102–108.
> von Noorden GK. A reassessment of infantile esotropia. XLIV Edward Jackson memorial lecture. *Am J Ophthalmol.* 1988;105:1–10.

Nystagmus and Esotropia

Some patients with early-onset esotropia also have nystagmus. Three patterns of nystagmus and esotropia have been described. Patients with the *Ciancia syndrome* have a very-large-angle constant esotropia and often show a pattern of cross-fixation. Nystagmus is minimal with the fixing eye in adduction; however, nystagmus increases with attempted abduction of the fixing eye. Abduction is usually limited, and the nystagmus is similar to exaggerated end-position nystagmus on attempted abduction. Patients with Ciancia syndrome are often undercorrected after surgery and may require large bilateral medial rectus recessions.

> Ciancia AO. On infantile esotropia with nystagmus in abduction. *J Pediatr Ophthalmol Strabismus.* 1995;32:280–288.

Patients with *latent nystagmus* show no nystagmus under binocular viewing conditions; with occlusion of one eye, a jerk nystagmus develops in both eyes with the fast phase toward the viewing eye. If nystagmus is present when both eyes are open but only one eye is being used for vision (the other is suppressed), the patient is said to have *manifest latent nystagmus.* This nystagmus is also jerk in type and may increase with monocular occlusion. Quantitative eye movement recording shows characteristic waveforms that distinguish latent nystagmus and manifest latent nystagmus from congenital nystagmus. Patients with latent nystagmus and manifest latent nystagmus frequently have an underlying esotropia but may also have other types of strabismus. To improve visual acuity, the patient with manifest latent nystagmus may adopt a face turn to place the fixing eye in adduction, where the amplitude of nystagmus is reduced.

Nystagmus blockage syndrome is a type of congenital nystagmus in which the angle of esotropia and the amplitude of nystagmus are inversely related. The nystagmus intensity is greatest when the eyes are straight, and it is damped or blocked by convergence of the eyes that leads to an esodeviation. The diagnosis is based on the appearance of nystagmus with attempted abduction of either eye, a head turn in the direction of the uncovered eye with occlusion of the fellow eye, and damping of nystagmus with convergence of the eyes that results in an esodeviation.

> Dell'Osso LF, Ellenberger C Jr, Abel LA, et al. The nystagmus blockage syndrome. Congenital nystagmus, manifest latent nystagmus, or both? *Invest Ophthalmol Vis Sci.* 1983;24: 1580–1587.

Accommodative Esotropia

All accommodative esodeviations are acquired, with the following characteristics:

- Onset generally between 6 months and 7 years, averaging 2½ years of age (can be as early as age 4 months)
- Usually intermittent at onset, becoming constant
- Often hereditary
- Sometimes precipitated by trauma or illness
- Frequently associated with amblyopia
- Diplopia may occur but usually disappears as patient develops facultative suppression scotoma in the deviating eye

Types of accommodative esotropia are listed in Table 7-1 and discussed below.

Refractive Accommodative Esotropia

Two main mechanisms contribute to refractive accommodative esotropia: uncorrected hyperopia and insufficient fusional divergence. The uncorrected hyperopia forces the patient to accommodate to sharpen the retinal image, thus leading to increased convergence. If the patient's fusional divergence mechanism is insufficient to deal with the increased convergence tonus, esotropia results. The angle of esotropia is generally between 20Δ and 30Δ and approximately equal at distance and near fixation. The amount of hyperopia averages +4.00 D, with a range of +3.00 to +10.00 D.

Treatment of refractive accommodative esotropia consists of amblyopia therapy if necessary and correction of the full amount of hyperopia as determined under cycloplegia with cyclopentolate or atropine. Bifocals may be required if the patient has a residual esotropia at near. Significant delay in the initiation of treatment following the onset of esotropia increases the likelihood that a portion of the esodeviation will fail to respond to antiaccommodative therapy. A gradual reduction of hyperopic correction may be possible over time if the patient can maintain control of the ensuing esophoria. This reduction stimulates the development of increased fusional divergence amplitudes, which in some patients may allow discontinuation of spectacle therapy in the future.

Parents must understand the importance of *full-time wear* of spectacle correction. A common cause of treatment failure or partial response to antiaccommodative management is inconsistent spectacle wear. Atropine 1.0% ointment or drops applied to both eyes at bedtime may facilitate initial compliance.

Therapy with miotic agents (echothiophate iodide or isoflurophate) has been advocated as a substitute for glasses. However, because of potential ocular and systemic side effects from these medications, their use is usually confined to children who are uncooperative in wearing glasses at all or who spend long hours playing near the water in the summer.

Surgical correction may be required when a patient with refractive accommodative esotropia fails to regain fusion with glasses or subsequently develops a nonaccommodative component to the deviation. However, the ophthalmologist must rule out latent uncorrected hyperopia before proceeding with surgery.

Nonrefractive Accommodative Esotropia

Patients with nonrefractive accommodative esotropia have an abnormal relationship between accommodation and accommodative convergence (ie, a high AC/A ratio). Excess convergence tonus results from accommodation, and esotropia develops in the setting of insufficient fusional divergence. Because more accommodation is required at near fixation than at distance, the angle of esotropia is greater at near. It can be reduced by +3.00 D bifocal lenses. Measurement of the angle of esotropia with fixation targets that require appropriate accommodation is critical to making the diagnosis of this type of esotropia. The refractive error in these patients averages +2.25 D sphere but can range from myopic to highly hyperopic. Thus, patients with refractive and nonrefractive accommodative esotropia may show overlap in their amount of hyperopia.

No consensus exists on the best management of nonrefractive accommodative esotropia. Several options are available:

- *Bifocals.* The most commonly used treatment option for nonrefractive accommodative esotropia is bifocal spectacles. If bifocals are employed, they should initially be prescribed in the executive or 35 mm flattop style with a power of +2.50 or +3.00 D. The top of the segment should cross the pupil, and the vertical height of the bifocal should not exceed that of the distance portion of the lens. Detailed instructions concerning the bifocal should be given to the optician. Progressive bifocal lenses have been used successfully, but conventional bifocals are preferred. If progressive bifocals are used, they should be fitted higher than adult lenses (about 4 mm) and with maximum bifocal power (+3.50 D). An ideal response to bifocal glasses is restoration of normal binocular function (fusion and stereopsis) at both distance and near fixation. An acceptable response is fusion at distance with less than 10Δ of residual esotropia through the bifocal at near fixation.
- *Long-acting cholinesterase inhibitors.* Ophthalmologists who use long-acting cholinesterase inhibitors suggest starting with maximum strength (0.125% echothiophate iodide drops) in both eyes once daily for 6 weeks. If such treatment is effective, strength or frequency should be decreased to the minimum effective dose. Parents must be warned about the potentially serious side effects of these drugs, including deletion of pseudocholinesterase from the blood, which makes the patient highly susceptible to depolarizing muscle relaxants such as succinylcholine. Echothiophate iodide can also cause iris cysts to form; some ophthalmologists prescribe phenylephrine drops concurrently to reduce the risk of cyst formation.
- *Surgery.* If a nonaccommodative esodeviation develops in the setting of full control of accommodation at distance and near, surgery may be indicated based on the size of the residual deviation and the patient's potential for binocular function. Some ophthalmologists also advocate medial rectus muscle recessions for the near deviation so that the child, usually an adolescent, can discontinue bifocal wear and maintain control of the esodeviation with single-vision glasses or contact lenses. Progressive power bifocals or bifocal contact lenses may be an alternative to surgery in such children. Despite recent controversy regarding surgery as an alternative to glasses for patients with fully accommodative esotropia, most ophthalmologists do not recommend surgery in this setting.

For the long-term management of both refractive and nonrefractive accommodative esotropia, it is important to remember that measured hyperopia usually increases until age 5–7 years. Therefore, if esotropia with glasses increases, the cycloplegic refraction should be repeated and the full correction prescribed. After age 5–7 years, hyperopia may decrease, and the full cycloplegic refraction in place will thus blur vision. The ophthalmologist should seek the minimum hyperopic correction to provide optimal alignment and best visual acuity.

If glasses or drugs correct all or nearly all of the esotropia and some degree of sensory binocular cooperation or fusion is present, the clinician may begin to reduce the strength of glasses or drugs to create a small esophoria when the patient reaches age 5 or 6. This reduction may stimulate the fusional divergence mechanism to redevelop normal magnitude. An increase in the fusional divergence combined with the natural decrease of both the hyperopia and the high AC/A ratio may enable the patient to maintain straight eyes without glasses, bifocals, or drugs. For example, in the case of a 5-year-old who has worn glasses since age 2 for esotropia and has a visual acuity of 20/25 in both eyes:

>Hyperopia 4.00 D OU
>>with +4.00 D OU: orthophoria at distance and near
>>>after 6–12 months of spectacle wear: with +3.00 D OU: E = E′ = 6Δ
>
>Prescribe +3.00 OU

Further reductions may be possible if the child maintains good visual acuity, has control of the esophoria, and does not have astehnopic symptoms.

Another example is an 8-year-old child who presents with new onset of esotropia at age 3 years:

>Hyperopia 2.00 D OU
>>with +2.00 D OU: E = 4Δ; E′ = 24Δ
>>+2.50 D bifocals prescribed: E = E′ = 4Δ
>
>At age 6 hyperopia remains 2.00 D
>>with +2.00 D add: E = 4Δ; E′ = 8Δ
>>with +1.50 D add: E = 4Δ; E(T)′ = 12Δ
>
>Prescribe +2.00 D sphere OU with +2.00 D add

Further bifocal reductions may be possible as long as the child maintains an asymptomatic esophoria. If the amount of hyperopia increases and is prescribed in new glasses, the bifocal add can sometimes be reduced by the same amount that the hyperopia increased without affecting the resultant lens power through the bifocal. This change increases the chance that the child will eventually be able to discontinue bifocal use.

Partially Accommodative Esotropia

Patients with partially accommodative esodeviations show a reduction in the angle of esotropia with glasses but maintain a residual esotropia despite treatment of amblyopia and provision of full hyperopic therapy. Sometimes, partially accommodative esotropia results from decompensation of a fully accommodative esotropia, but in other instances the child may have had esotropia that subsequently developed an accommodative element. An interval of weeks to months between the onset of accommodative esotropia and the application of full cycloplegic refraction often results in some residual esotropia even after the proper glasses are worn. Hence, prompt treatment of accommodative esotropia may offer substantial benefits. Patients with pure refractive accommodative esotropia who have been made orthotropic with glasses are less likely to develop a nonaccommodative component to their esodeviation than patients with the type of accommodative esotropia with a high AC/A ratio.

Treatment of partially accommodative esotropia consists of amblyopia management and prescription of the full hyperopic correction. Strabismus surgery may be warranted for the nonaccommodative portion. The amount of surgery should be conservative for those with a history of amblyopia because of an increased risk of consecutive exotropia. It is important that the patient and parents understand before surgery that its purpose is to produce straight eyes *with* glasses—not to allow the child to discontinue wearing glasses altogether.

Mulvihill A, MacCann A, Flitcroft I, et al. Outcome in refractive accommodative esotropia. *Br J Ophthalmol.* 2000;84:746–749.

Watanabe-Numata K, Hayasaka S, Watanabe K, et al. Changes in deviation following correction in children with fully refractive accommodative esotropia. *Ophthalmologica.* 2000; 214:309–311.

Nonaccommodative Acquired Esotropia

Basic (Acquired) Esotropia

Esotropia that develops after age 6 months and that is not associated with an accommodative component is called *basic*, or *acquired*, *esotropia*. As with infantile esotropia, an accommodative factor is usually absent, the amount of hyperopia is not significant, and the near deviation is the same as the distance deviation. Although most children with this form of esotropia are otherwise healthy, central nervous system lesions must be considered. Therapy consists of amblyopia treatment and surgical correction as soon as possible after the onset of the deviation.

When planning surgery for patients with acquired esotropia, some ophthalmologists advocate prism adaptation. Prism adaptation is a process of prescribing the full hyperopic correction if indicated and adding Press-On prisms to neutralize any residual esodeviation. The patient wears the glasses with the Press-On prisms for 1 or 2 weeks and is then reexamined. If the esodeviation increases with the prisms, new prisms are prescribed to neutralize the deviation. In some patients, the esodeviation increases as the patient "eats up" the prism. Surgery is then planned for the full prism-adapted deviation. This process of prism adaptation may reduce the undercorrection rate associated with acquired or decompensated accommodative esotropia, and it has been shown to produce a better motor outcome after surgery than that of the control group in a randomized clinical trial (see Prism Adaptation Test in Chapter 6).

Acute Esotropia

Occasionally, an acquired esotropia is acute in onset. In such cases, the patient immediately becomes aware of the deviation and frequently has diplopia. A careful motility evaluation is important to rule out an accommodative or paretic component. Artificial disruption of binocular vision, such as may follow treatment of an ocular injury or patching for amblyopia, is one of the known causes of acute esotropia. Physical and emotional stress, illness, and aging are other postulated causes. Because the onset of comitant esotropia in an older child may indicate an underlying neurologic disorder, neurologic evaluation may be indicated. Most patients with acute onset of esotropia have a history of normal binocular vision, and therefore the prognosis for restoration of single binocular vision with prisms and surgery is good. Prisms may be used during a period of observation before surgery is performed.

Cyclic Esotropia

Cyclic esotropia is rare, with an estimated incidence of 1:3000–1:5000 strabismus cases. Onset typically occurs during the preschool years, although a congenital case and several adult cases have been reported. The esotropia is present intermittently, usually every other day (48-hour cycle). Variable cycles and 24-hour cycles have also been documented. Most patients with cyclic esotropia become constantly esotropic with time. In some ways, cyclic esotropia resembles accommodative esotropia with a similar time of onset, moderate hyperopia, and a moderate angle of esotropia.

Amblyopia is occasionally present in cases of cyclic esotropia, and V patterns are common (see Chapter 10). On the days when the cyclic esodeviation is not present, the patient has normal binocular vision and good stereo acuity.

Treatment of cyclic esotropia addresses the amblyopia and hyperopia. Some cases resolve with full hyperopic correction; others continue the cyclic deviation and require surgery. Hyperopic correction and standard surgery for residual esotropia have resulted in functional cure. Phenobarbital and amphetamines have reportedly altered the frequency of the esotropic cycles in some patients.

Helveston EM. Cyclic strabismus. *Am Orthopt J.* 1973;23:48–51.

Sensory Deprivation Esodeviation

Monocular organic lesions such as cataract, corneal scarring, optic atrophy, or prolonged blurred or distorted retinal images may cause an esodeviation. Anisometropia with amblyopia is common in this type of esodeviation.

Obstacles preventing clear and focused retinal images and symmetrical visual stimulation must be identified and remedied as soon as possible. Animal and clinical data indicate that restoration of normal, symmetrical inputs must be accomplished at an early age if irreversible amblyopia is to be avoided. After all obstacles to balanced sensory inputs have been removed, any secondary amblyopia is treated. Surgery for residual esotropia may be indicated. The surgical management of these cases is similar to that of early-onset esotropia, except when good visual acuity cannot be restored as a result of irreversible amblyopia or organic defects. In such situations, esotropia surgery should generally be performed only on the abnormal eye.

Divergence Insufficiency

The characteristic finding of divergence insufficiency is an esodeviation, generally in adult patients, that is greater at distance than at near. The deviation does not change with vertical or horizontal gaze, and fusional divergence is reduced. *Divergence paralysis* may represent a more severe form of divergence insufficiency. Because true paralysis of divergence cannot generally be documented, the term *divergence insufficiency* is preferred. Divergence insufficiency can be divided into a primary isolated form and a secondary form associated with other neurologic abnormalities stemming from pontine tumors or severe head trauma. A thorough clinical evaluation can frequently distinguish between the two forms of divergence insufficiency. Primary isolated divergence insufficiency is frequently a benign condition: symptoms resolve in 40% of patients within several months. Patients with secondary divergence insufficiency may obtain relief from symptoms with treatment of the underlying neurologic disorder (eg, corticosteroids for temporal arteritis, treatment of intracranial hypertension). Management of diplopia consists of base-out prisms and, rarely, surgery (lateral rectus resections).

> Jacobson DM. Divergence insufficiency revisited: natural history of idiopathic cases and neurologic associations. *Arch Ophthalmol.* 2000;118:1237–1241.

Spasm of the Near Synkinetic Reflex

Spasm of the near reflex is a spectrum of abnormalities of the near response. Thus, patients can present with varying combinations of excessive convergence, excessive accommodation, and miosis. The etiology is generally thought to be functional, related to psychological factors, but rarely it can be associated with organic disease. Patients may present with acute, persistent esotropia alternating at other times with orthotropia. The characteristic movement is the substitution of a convergence movement for a gaze movement on horizontal versions. Monocular abduction is normal in spite of marked abduction limitation on versions. Pseudomyopia may occur. Treatment, which may be problematic, has consisted of cycloplegic agents such as atropine or homatropine, plus lenses for patients with significant hyperopia, and bifocals.

> Goldstein JH, Schneekloth BB. Spasm of the near reflex: a spectrum of anomalies. *Surv Ophthalmol.* 1996;40:269–278.

Surgical (Consecutive) Esodeviation

Esodeviation following surgery for exodeviation frequently improves spontaneously. Treatment includes base-out prisms, plus lenses or miotics (especially if the patient is hyperopic), alternate occlusion, and, finally, surgery. Unless the deviation is very large or symptomatic, surgery should be postponed for several months because of the possibility of spontaneous improvement.

A slipped or lost lateral rectus muscle produces varying amounts of esotropia, depending on the amount of slippage. Surgical exploration and reattachment of the muscle to the globe is required. Transposition procedures may be necessary when lost muscles cannot be found. For slipped muscles, advancement of the muscle on the globe is required. (See Chapter 13, Figs 13-11 and 13-12, and the discussion in the text accompanying those illustrations.)

Incomitant Esodeviation

The term *incomitant esodeviation* is used when esodeviation varies in different fields of gaze.

Sixth Nerve (Abducens) Paralysis

Paralysis of the lateral rectus muscle causes an incomitant esodeviation. Sixth nerve paralysis occurring at birth has been reported but is uncommon. Congenital sixth nerve paralysis is thought to be caused by the increased intracranial pressure associated with the birth process and usually resolves spontaneously. Sixth nerve palsy occurs much more frequently in childhood than in infancy. Older patients may complain of double vision and often have a head turn toward the side of the paretic sixth nerve to maintain fusion. Approximately one third of these cases are associated with intracranial lesions and may have associated neurologic findings. Other cases may be related to infectious or immunologic processes that involve cranial nerve VI. Spontaneous benign lesions usually resolve over several months.

The vision in both eyes is usually equal unless strabismic amblyopia or associated structural defects are found. The esotropia increases in gaze toward the paretic lateral rectus muscle. Saccadic velocities show slowing of the affected lateral rectus muscle, and active force generation tests document the weakness of that muscle. Versions show limited or no abduction of the affected eye.

A careful history should be taken to define antecedent infections, head trauma, or other possible inciting factors for sixth nerve palsy. Neurologic evaluation and computed tomography or magnetic resonance imaging are indicated when neurologic signs or symptoms are present.

Patching may be required to maintain vision in the esotropic eye in children in the amblyopia age range, especially if the child has no head turn to maintain binocular fusion. Fresnel Press-On prisms are useful to correct the diplopia in primary position. Spontaneous resolution may occur in more than half of patients with traumatic palsies, particularly if the paresis is unilateral. Injection of botulinum toxin into the antagonist medial rectus muscle has successfully aligned the eye by temporarily paralyzing the medial rectus muscle. The botulinum treatment may be helpful in preventing contracture of the medial rectus muscle while the patient is observed for several months prior to surgical intervention. In patients with unilateral or bilateral traumatic sixth nerve palsies, botulinum toxin injection does not appear to improve the rate of recovery.

Surgery is indicated when spontaneous resolution does not take place after 6 months or more of follow-up and after exclusion of intracranial lesions. A large recession of the antagonist medial rectus muscle with resection of the lateral rectus muscle is often a successful first operation. In a patient in whom previous surgery has resulted in orthotropia or esophoria in primary position but a limited field of single binocular vision in the direction of the paretic lateral rectus muscle, the surgeon may consider a posterior fixation with or without recession of the contralateral medial rectus muscle. Adjustable sutures are helpful in paralytic strabismus if the patient can cooperate with this technique. In cases of total paralysis, muscle transposition procedures, perhaps in conjunction with botulinum toxin injection into the ipsilateral medial rectus muscle, may be required.

See additional discussions in Chapter 11, Special Forms of Strabismus, and Chapter 14, Chemodenervation Treatment of Strabismus and Blepharospasm Using Botulinum Toxin. See also BCSC Section 5, *Neuro-Ophthalmology*.

Foster RS. Vertical muscle transposition augmented with lateral fixation. *J AAPOS.* 1997; 1:20–30.

Holmes JM, Beck RW, Kip KE, et al. Botulinum toxin treatment versus conservative management in acute traumatic sixth nerve palsy or paresis. *J AAPOS.* 2000;4:145–149.

Rosenbaum AL, Kushner BJ, Kirschen D. Vertical rectus transposition and botulinum toxin (Oculinum) to medial rectus for abducens palsy. *Arch Ophthalmol.* 1989;107:820–823.

Other Forms of Incomitant Esodeviation

Medial rectus muscle restriction

Medial rectus muscle restriction may result from thyroid myopathy, medial orbital wall fracture, or excessively resected medial rectus muscle (see Chapter 13).

Duane syndrome and Möbius syndrome

See discussions in Chapter 11, Special Forms of Strabismus, and BCSC Section 5, *Neuro-Ophthalmology.*

Preferred Practice Patterns Committee, Pediatric Panel. *Esotropia.* San Francisco: American Academy of Ophthalmology; 1997.

CHAPTER 8

Exodeviations

An *exodeviation* is divergent strabismus that can be latent (controlled by fusion) or manifest. Although the exact etiology of most exodeviations is unknown, proposed causes include anatomical and mechanical factors within the orbit as well as abnormalities of innervation such as excessive tonic divergence. Some families show a hereditary basis for exodeviation.

> Wilson ME. Exotropia. In: *Focal Points: Clinical Modules for Ophthalmologists.* San Francisco: American Academy of Ophthalmology; 1995: vol 13, no 11.

Pseudoexotropia

The term *pseudoexotropia* refers to an appearance of exodeviation when in fact the eyes are properly aligned. Pseudoexotropia may result from the following:
- Positive angle kappa without other ocular abnormalities (see discussion of angle kappa in Chapter 6)
- Wide interpupillary distance
- Positive angle kappa together with ocular abnormalities such as temporal dragging of the macula in retinopathy of prematurity

Exophoria

Exophoria is an exodeviation controlled by fusion under conditions of normal binocular vision. Exophorias are detected when binocular vision is interrupted, as during an alternate cover test. Exophoria may be asymptomatic if the angle of strabismus is small and fusional convergence amplitudes are adequate. Prolonged, detailed visual work or reading may bring about asthenopia. Treatment is usually not necessary unless an exophoria progresses to an intermittent exotropia.

Intermittent Exotropia

With the possible exception of exophoria at near, the most common type of exodeviation is intermittent exotropia, which is latent at some times and manifest at others (Fig 8-1).

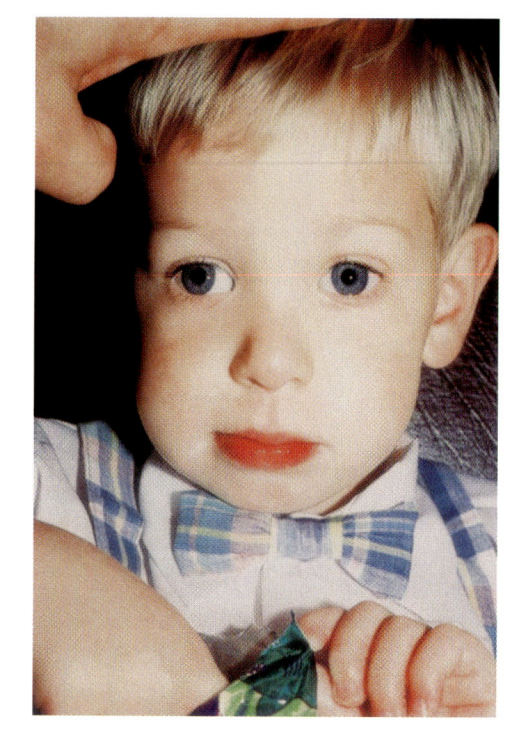

Figure 8-1 A 3-year-old boy with intermittent exotropia. *(Reproduced with permission from Wilson ME. Exotropia. In: Focal Points: Clinical Modules for Ophthalmologists. San Francisco: American Academy of Ophthalmology; 1995: vol 13, no 11.)*

Clinical Characteristics

The onset of intermittent exotropia usually occurs early, before age 5, but it may be detected for the first time much later in childhood. Because proper eye alignment with intermittent exotropia requires that compensatory fusional factors be active, the deviation often becomes manifest during times of visual inattention, fatigue, or stress. Parents of affected children often report that exotropia occurs late in the day with fatigue or during illness, daydreaming, drowsiness upon awakening, or when the child is being scolded. Exposure to bright lights often causes a reflex closure of one eye.

In childhood, deviation of the eyes is usually larger for distance viewing than for near, and exotropia manifests more frequently when the visual target is remote. In adults, the near and distance exodeviation tend to be more equal in magnitude even if fusional control remains good. Intermittent exotropias can be associated with small hypertropias, A and V patterns, and oblique muscle dysfunction, all of which are discussed in Chapters 9 and 10. Inferior oblique muscle overaction can be detected in about one third of patients.

In some patients, untreated intermittent exotropia progresses toward constant exotropia. As exotropia progresses, tropic episodes occur at lower levels of fatigue and last longer than previously. Children younger than 10 years may develop sensory adaptations. Initial awareness of diplopia during manifest exotropia is often replaced by the cortical adaptations of suppression and abnormal retinal correspondence. However, normal retinal correspondence with high-grade or reduced stereo acuity remains when the eyes are straight. Amblyopia is uncommon unless the exotropia progresses to constant or nearly constant exotropia at an early age or unless another amblyogenic factor such as anisometropia is present.

Clinical Evaluation

The clinical evaluation begins with a detailed history to try to pinpoint the age of onset of the strabismus and to determine whether the exotropia is progressing toward constancy. The clinician records how often and under what specific circumstances the manifest exotropia occurs. Control of the exodeviation exhibited throughout the examination can be categorized as:

- *Good control:* Exotropia manifests only after cover testing, and the patient resumes fusion rapidly without blinking or refixating.
- *Fair control:* Exotropia manifests after fusion is disrupted by cover testing, and the patient resumes fusion only after blinking or refixating.
- *Poor control:* Exotropia manifests spontaneously and may remain manifest for an extended time.

Prism and alternate cover testing should be used to evaluate the exodeviation at fixation distances of 20 feet and 14 inches. A far distance measurement at 100–200 feet (at the end of a long hallway or out a window) may bring out an even larger deviation. For patients with significantly more exodeviation in the distance than at near, a near prism and cover test after 1 hour of monocular occlusion to eliminate the effects of *tenacious proximal fusion* may help to distinguish between patients with a truly high accommodative convergence/accommodation (AC/A) ratio and a pseudo-high AC/A ratio. Tenacious proximal fusion is a proximal vergence aftereffect that occurs in some patients with intermittent exotropia; this aftereffect is due to a slow-to-dissipate fusion mechanism that prevents intermittent exotropia from manifesting at near fixation with a brief cover test. A patient with a pseudo-high AC/A ratio would have roughly equal distance and near measurements after occlusion; a patient with a truly high AC/A ratio would continue to have significantly less exodeviation at near. The abnormality of the AC/A ratio can be confirmed by testing with +3.00 D lenses at near or −2.00 D lenses at distance.

> Kushner BJ, Morton GV. Distance/near differences in intermittent exotropia. *Arch Ophthalmol.* 1998;116:478–486.

Classification

Intermittent exotropia has traditionally been classified into four groups, based on the difference between alternating prism and cover test measurements at distance and at near and the change in near measurement produced by unilateral occlusion or +3.00 D lenses:

- *Basic* type exotropia is present when the exodeviation is approximately the same at distance and near fixation.
- *Divergence excess* type consists of an exodeviation that is greater at distance fixation than at near and can be subdivided into two subtypes.

- *True divergence excess* type refers to those deviations that remain greater at distance than at near even after a period of monocular occlusion. Some of these patients prove to have a high gradient AC/A ratio when tested at near with +3.00 D lenses.
- *Simulated divergence excess* type refers to a deviation that is initially greater at distance fixation than at near but that becomes about the same after one eye is occluded for 1 hour (to remove the effect of tenacious proximal fusion).
- The *convergence insufficiency* type is present when the exodeviation is greater at near than at distance. This type excludes isolated convergence insufficiency, which is discussed later in this Chapter.

As indicated above, sensory testing usually reveals excellent stereopsis with normal retinal correspondence when the exodeviation is latent and suppression with abnormal retinal correspondence when the exodeviation is manifest. However, if the deviation manifests rarely, diplopia may persist during those manifestations. It is useful to measure stereopsis at 20 feet as well as at 14 inches because reduced distance stereopsis may indicate poor control of a distance exodeviation.

Nonsurgical Management

Corrective lenses are prescribed for significant myopic, astigmatic, and hyperopic refractive errors. Correction of even mild myopia may improve control of the exodeviation. Mild to moderate degrees of hyperopia are not routinely corrected in children with intermittent exotropia for fear of worsening the deviation. However, some patients with more than 4.0 D of hyperopia (or more than 1.5 D of hyperopic anisometropia) may actually gain better control of the exodeviation after optical correction. Children with severe hyperopia may be unable to sustain the necessary accommodation for a clear image, and the lack of accommodative effort produces a blurred retinal image and manifest exotropia. Optical correction may improve retinal image clarity and help control the exodeviation.

>Haldi B, Mets MB. Nonsurgical treatment of strabismus. In: *Focal Points: Clinical Modules for Ophthalmologists.* San Francisco: American Academy of Ophthalmology; 1997: vol 15, no 4.

Some ophthalmologists use additional minus lens power, usually 2–4 D beyond refractive error correction, to temporarily stimulate accommodative convergence to help control the exodeviation. This therapy may cause asthenopia in school-age children, but it can be effective as a temporizing measure to promote fusion and avoid surgery during the most visually immature years, when surgical overcorrection can lead to amblyopia and loss of stereopsis.

>Caltrider N, Jampolsky A. Overcorrecting minus lens therapy for treatment of intermittent exotropia. *Ophthalmology.* 1983;90:1160–1165.

A rare but distinct group of patients with intermittent exotropia have a true high AC/A ratio measured by the gradient method after fusional aftereffects have been eliminated with 60 minutes of unilateral patching. Conventional surgery may cause overcorrection to an esotropia at near. Minus lenses and bifocals may eliminate the need for surgery by effectively controlling the deviation in this small group of patients.

> Kushner BJ. Diagnosis and treatment of exotropia with a high accommodation convergence-accommodation ratio. *Arch Ophthalmol.* 1999;117:221–224.

Part-time patching of the dominant (nondeviating) eye 4–6 hours per day, or alternate daily patching when no strong ocular preference is present, can be an effective treatment for small to moderate-sized deviations, although the benefit produced is often temporary. The exact mechanism by which patching improves control of intermittent exotropia is not known; presumably, patching disrupts suppression and is characterized as a *passive orthoptic treatment*.

> Freeman RS, Isenberg SJ. The use of part-time occlusion for early onset unilateral exotropia. *J Pediatr Ophthalmol Strabismus.* 1989;26:94–96.

Active orthoptic treatments that consist of antisuppression therapy/diplopia awareness and fusional convergence training can be used alone or in combination with patching, minus lenses, and surgery. For deviations of 20Δ or less, orthoptic treatment has been reported to have a long-term success rate comparable to that of surgery. Other authors have found no benefit and recommend surgery for any poorly controlled deviation.

Fusional convergence training works best for patients old enough to cooperate and who have a remote near point of convergence or poor fusional amplitudes. Diplopia awareness and antisuppression therapy provide the patient with a sensory biofeedback mechanism (diplopia) that stimulates the fusional vergence system. These methods are more controversial but may still be appropriate when suppression is dense, especially when the deviation is 20Δ or less and the patient is old enough to cooperate. Because the data on fusional convergence training are conflicting, further study is needed to determine which patients might benefit. In addition, the pre- and postoperative role of orthoptic treatment remains unclear.

Base-in prisms can be used to promote fusion in intermittent exotropia, but this treatment option is seldom chosen for long-term management because it can cause a reduction in fusional vergence amplitudes.

Surgical Treatment

Many patients with intermittent exotropia ultimately require surgery, which is customarily performed when progression toward constant exotropia is documented despite the use of appropriate nonsurgical treatments. No consensus exists regarding specific indications, however. Some surgeons advocate very early surgery for any intermittently manifested deviation of 15Δ or more in the belief that realignment before suppression is firmly established will lead to long-term stability of proper alignment. Other surgeons prefer a more conservative approach, reserving surgery for patients whose condition has progressed to nearly constant exotropia. The conservative group often advises withholding surgery whenever possible in very young patients to avoid the amblyopia and loss of fine stereopsis that could result from overcorrection and subsequent development of monofixation syndrome. These risks are minimized with close postoperative follow-up, however. The best sensory outcomes are probably achieved with motor alignment before age 7, before 5 years of strabismus duration, and while the deviation is still intermittent.

> Abroms AD, Mohney BG, Rush DP, et al. Timely surgery in intermittent and constant exotropia for superior sensory outcome. *Am J Ophthalmol.* 2001;131:111–116.

Symmetrical recession of both lateral rectus muscles is the most common surgical procedure for intermittent exotropia. Recession of one lateral rectus muscle combined with resection of the ipsilateral medial rectus muscle is an acceptable alternative and may be preferred for patients with basic type intermittent exotropia. Some strabismus surgeons use unilateral lateral rectus muscle recession, particularly in patients with smaller exodeviations.

> Kushner BJ. Selective surgery for intermittent exotropia based on distance/near differences. *Arch Ophthalmol.* 1998;116:324–328.
>
> Olitsky SE. Early and late postoperative alignment following unilateral lateral rectus recession for intermittent exotropia. *J Pediatr Ophthalmol Strabismus.* 1998;35:146–148.

Management of surgical overcorrection

A temporary overcorrection of up to 10Δ–15Δ is desirable after bilateral lateral rectus muscle recessions. Persistent overcorrection (beyond 3–4 weeks) may require treatment with base-out prisms (usually Fresnel Press-On prisms) or alternate patching to prevent amblyopia or relieve diplopia. Corrective lenses or miotics should be considered if hyperopia is moderate. Bifocals can be used for a high AC/A ratio. Unless deficient ductions suggest a slipped or lost muscle, a delay of 4–6 months is recommended before reoperation because spontaneous improvement is common. Following a bilateral lateral rectus muscle recession, medial rectus muscle recessions can be performed, provided the lateral rectus muscle ductions are normal. Unilateral lateral rectus muscle recession/medial rectus muscle resection surgery can be followed by medial rectus muscle recession/lateral rectus muscle resection surgery on the other eye. Botulinum toxin injection into one medial rectus muscle may be effective in the management of consecutive esotropia, particularly when fusion is present.

Management of surgical undercorrection

Mild to moderate residual exodeviation is often treated by observation alone if fusional control is good. However, manifest exotropia commonly returns in time. Therefore, some surgeons recommend aggressive base-in prism management for undercorrections with a gradual weaning of the prism dosage. Postoperative patching and orthoptic treatment using the same techniques listed under nonsurgical treatment can be applied to surgical undercorrections. In small doses, botulinum toxin injection has also been used to treat surgical undercorrections, but supportive data are limited. Indications for reoperation in undercorrected patients are the same as for initial surgery. If lateral rectus muscle recessions have been performed bilaterally, medial rectus muscle resections are often chosen when reoperation is needed. Unilateral lateral rectus muscle recession/medial rectus muscle resection is often followed by a similar recess/resect procedure of the other eye. The surgical dose-response curve appears to be similar to that for the initial surgery. Therefore, the surgical dosage can often be selected as though the surgery were a primary operation.

Constant Exotropia

Constant exotropia is encountered more often in older patients manifesting sensory exotropia or decompensated intermittent exotropia. This usually large-angle exotropia may be associated with an *X pattern*, possibly as a result of overaction of all four oblique muscles. The deviation in an X pattern exotropia increases in both upgaze and downgaze.

Surgical treatment for constant exotropia consists of appropriate recessions of lateral rectus muscles with or without tightening of the medial rectus muscles. Oblique muscle surgery may be required. In some cases, the patient has been aware of an enlarged field of peripheral vision because of rapid alternation of fixation and notices the change when the eyes are straight.

Congenital Exotropia

Congenital exotropia presents before age 6 months with a large-angle constant exotropia, often associated with neurologic impairment or craniofacial disorders (Fig 8-2). The prevalence of systemic and other ocular disease is at least as high in patients with congenital exotropia as with congenital esotropia. The potential for high-grade stereopsis and bifoveal fixation is poor. Early surgery may help to establish peripheral fusion, but the literature provides few supportive data for this possibility. Late consecutive esotropia,

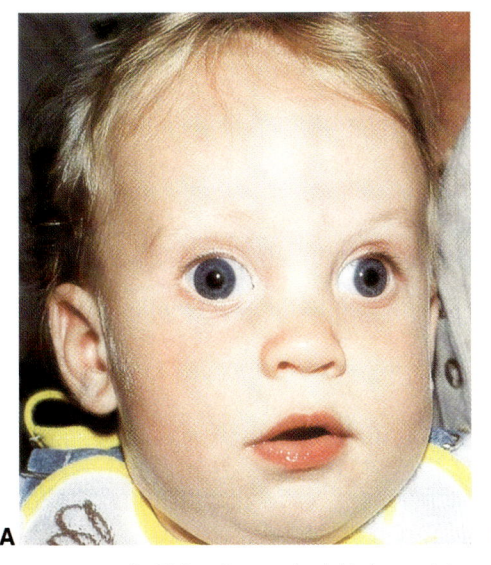

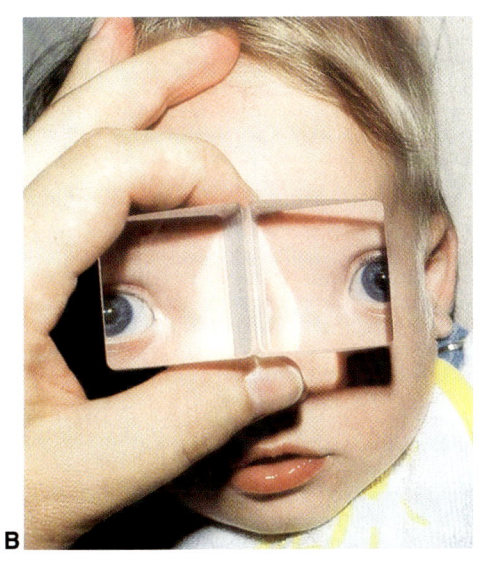

Figure 8-2 A, This 10-month-old infant with congenital exotropia also shows moderate motor developmental delay. **B,** Krimsky testing uses two 45Δ prisms placed base-to-base in the frontal plane to measure 90Δ of exotropia. *(Reprinted with permission from Wilson ME. Exotropia. In: Focal Points: Clinical Modules for Ophthalmologists. San Francisco: American Academy of Ophthalmology; 1995: vol 13, no 11.)*

recurrent exotropia, and dissociated vertical deviation are all common, even with early successful surgical alignment.

>   Biglan AW, Davis JS, Cheng KP, et al. Infantile exotropia. *J Pediatr Ophthalmol Strabismus.* 1996;33:79–84.
>   Hunter DG, Ellis FJ. Prevalence of systemic and ocular disease in infantile exotropia: comparison with infantile esotropia. *Ophthalmology.* 1999;106:1951–1956.

Sensory Exotropia

Any condition that reduces visual acuity in one eye can cause sensory exotropia. The causes include anisometropia, corneal or lens opacities, optic atrophy or hypoplasia, and macular lesions. It is not known why some persons become esotropic after unilateral visual loss and others become exotropic. Both sensory esotropia and sensory exotropia are common in children, but exotropia predominates in older children and adults.

If the eye with sensory exotropia can be visually rehabilitated, peripheral fusion may sometimes be reestablished after surgical realignment, provided the sensory exotropia has not been present for an extended period. Loss of fusional amplitudes, known as *central fusional disruption,* or *horror fusionis,* can lead to constant and permanent diplopia when adult-onset sensory exotropia has been present for several years prior to visual rehabilitation and realignment. In these patients, intractable diplopia may persist, even with well-aligned eyes.

Consecutive Exotropia

Consecutive exotropia is defined as exotropia that follows previous strabismus surgery for esotropia. Treatment of consecutive exotropia depends on many factors, including the size of the deviation, the type and amount of surgery that preceded its development, the presence of duction limitations, lateral incomitance, and the level of visual acuity in each eye. The planning of strabismus surgery is discussed in Chapter 13.

Exotropic Duane (Retraction) Syndrome

Duane syndrome can present with exotropia, usually accompanied by a face turn away from the affected eye. Adduction is most often markedly deficient; other signs include eyelid narrowing, globe retraction, and characteristic upshoots and downshoots. See Chapter 11 for further discussion of Duane syndrome.

Neuromuscular Abnormalities

A constant exotropia may result from third nerve palsy, internuclear ophthalmoplegia, or myasthenia gravis. These conditions are discussed in detail in BCSC Section 5, *Neuro-Ophthalmology.*

Dissociated Horizontal Deviation

Dissociated strabismus may contain vertical, horizontal, and torsional components. When the dissociated abduction movement is prominent, it is called *dissociated horizontal deviation.* Although not a true exotropia, dissociated horizontal deviation can be confused with a constant or intermittent exotropia. Dissociated vertical deviation and latent nystagmus often coexist with dissociated horizontal deviation (Fig 8-3). Treatment usually consists of unilateral or occasionally bilateral lateral rectus recession in addition to any necessary oblique muscle or dissociated vertical deviation surgery.

> Wilson ME, Hutchinson AK, Saunders RA. Outcomes from surgical treatment for dissociated horizontal deviation. *J AAPOS.* 2000;4:94–101.

Convergence Insufficiency

Characteristics of convergence insufficiency include asthenopia, blurred near vision, and reading problems in the presence of poor near fusional convergence amplitudes and a remote near point of convergence. The patient, typically an older child or adult, may have an exophoria at near but, by definition, should not have an exotropia. Rarely, accommodative spasms may occur if voluntary accommodation and convergence are stimulated in an effort to overcome the convergence insufficiency. Convergence insufficiency, as discussed here, should not be confused with the convergence insufficiency type of intermittent exotropia discussed above.

Treatment of convergence insufficiency usually involves orthoptic exercises. Base-out prism reading can be used to stimulate fusional convergence. Stereograms, "pencil push-ups," and other near point exercises are often used. If these exercises fail, base-in prism reading glasses may be needed. Medial rectus muscle resection, unilateral or bilateral, has been used in rare cases when nonsurgical treatments have been unsatisfactory, but surgery carries a substantial risk of diplopia in distance viewing. Patients with combined convergence and accommodative insufficiency may benefit from plus lenses and base-in prisms for reading.

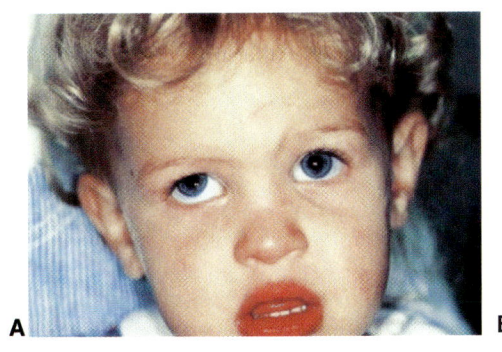

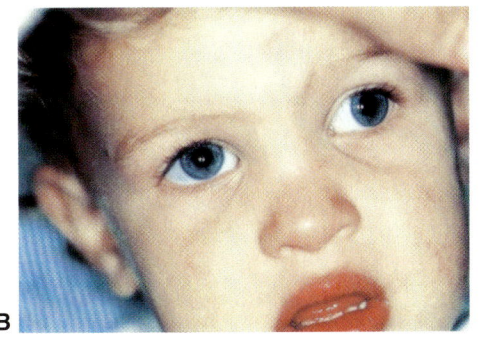

Figure 8-3 Dissociated strabismus complex. **A,** When the patient fixates with the left eye, a prominent dissociated vertical deviation is shown in the right eye. **B,** However, when the patient fixates with the right eye, a prominent dissociated horizontal deviation (DHD) is shown in the left eye. *(Reproduced with permission from Wilson ME. Exotropia. In: Focal Points: Clinical Modules for Ophthalmologists. San Francisco: American Academy of Ophthalmology; 1995: vol 13, no 11.)*

Convergence Paralysis

Convergence paralysis, a condition distinct from convergence insufficiency and usually secondary to an intracranial lesion, is characterized by normal adduction and accommodation with exotropia and diplopia on attempted near fixation only. Convergence paralysis differs from convergence insufficiency in its relatively acute onset and the patient's inability to overcome any base-out prism introduced with a rotary prism. Convergence paralysis usually results from a lesion in the corpora quadrigemina or the nucleus of cranial nerve III and may be associated with Parinaud syndrome.

Treatment is limited to providing base-in prisms at near to alleviate the diplopia. Occasionally, accommodation also is weakened, particularly in a chronically ill patient, and plus lenses may also be required at near. These patients have little if any fusional vergence amplitudes at near, and it may not be possible to restore comfortable single binocular vision. Occlusion of one eye at near is indicated in such cases, and eye muscle surgery is contraindicated.

> Cooper J, Medow N. Major review: intermittent exotropia; basic and divergence excess type. *Binocul Vis Eye Muscle Surg Q.* 1993;8:185–216.
>
> Ing MR, Nishimura J, Okino L. Outcome study of bilateral lateral rectus recession for intermittent exotropia in children. *Trans Am Ophthalmol Soc.* 1997;95:433–443; discussion 443–452.
>
> Kushner BJ. Exotropic deviations: a functional classification and approach to treatment. 18th Richard G. Scobee Memorial Lecture. *Am Orthoptic J.* 1988;38:81–93.

CHAPTER 9

Vertical Deviations

A vertical deviation (vertical misalignment of the visual axes) may be comitant or, more usually, incomitant (noncomitant). Either form of vertical deviation can occur alone or be associated with a horizontal deviation. Such an association is the more typical setting for comitant vertical deviations, which usually are small.

The majority of vertical deviations are incomitant. They are produced by so-called *dysfunctional overactions* or *underactions* of the superior and inferior oblique muscles, paresis or contracture of one or more of these cyclovertical muscles, or mechanical restriction of vertical movement. Although nearly every vertical paretic deviation is incomitant at onset, it may become comitant with time in the absence of any associated mechanical restrictions, as might occur with a blowout fracture or thyroid ophthalmopathy. However, in most (some say all) vertical deviations, some differences in the magnitude of deviation in various gaze positions are found.

A vertical deviation is described according to the direction of the vertically deviating nonfixating eye. If the right eye is higher than the left and the left eye is fixating, this is called a *right hypertropia*. If the nonfixating right eye is lower than the fixating left eye, this is called a *right hypotropia*. If alternating fixation is present, the deviation is usually named for the hyperdeviating eye.

The following references are excellent sources of in-depth current information on the entities discussed in this chapter, as well as other topics in strabismus:

> Rosenbaum AL, Santiago AP. *Clinical Strabismus Management: Principles and Surgical Techniques.* Philadelphia: Saunders; 1999.
> Spector RH. Vertical diplopia. *Surv Ophthalmol.* 1993;38:31–62.
> von Noorden GK. *Binocular Vision and Ocular Motility: Theory and Management of Strabismus.* St Louis: Mosby; 1996.

Inferior Oblique Muscle Overaction

Primary overaction of the inferior oblique muscle is so named because it is not associated with superior oblique muscle paralysis.

Clinical Features

This type of overaction may be mechanical, innervational, or both; the cause is not well understood. Primary inferior oblique muscle overaction has been reported to develop between ages 1 and 6 years in approximately two thirds of patients with congenital eso-

116 • Pediatric Ophthalmology and Strabismus

tropia. This entity also is associated with acquired esotropia or exotropia and occasionally occurs in patients with no other form of strabismus. *Secondary overaction* of the inferior oblique muscle accompanies a palsy or paresis of its antagonist superior oblique muscle.

The eye in adduction is overelevated (Fig 9-1); this is apparent with the eyes in lateral gaze and the abducting eye fixating. Alternate cover testing under these conditions shows that the higher eye refixates with a downward movement and that the lower eye does so with an upward movement. When inferior oblique overaction is bilateral, which eye is higher and which is lower reverses in the opposite lateral gaze. These features differentiate inferior oblique overaction from dissociated vertical deviation (DVD, see below), in which neither eye refixates with an upward movement whether adducted, abducted, or in primary position. Additionally, a V-pattern horizontal deviation is common with overacting inferior oblique muscles but not with DVD.

Management

With clinically significant hyperdeviation of the adducted eye, a weakening procedure on the inferior oblique muscle (recession, disinsertion, or myectomy) is indicated (see Chapter 13). Structural variations in this muscle may affect the surgical result. Anteriorization (anterior displacement) of the inferior oblique muscle has been used to correct both marked overaction of the inferior oblique muscles and DVD when both are present simultaneously. Caution is advisable because excessively anterior reattachment can restrict elevation.

De Angelis D, Makar I, Kraft SP. Anatomic variations of the inferior oblique muscle: a potential cause of failed inferior oblique weakening surgery. *Am J Ophthalmol.* 1999;128: 485–488.

Stager DR. Costenbader Lecture. Anatomy and surgery of the inferior oblique muscle: recent findings. *J AAPOS.* 2001;5:203–208.

Superior Oblique Muscle Overaction

Unlike inferior oblique muscle overaction, superior oblique muscle overaction is usually not divided into primary and secondary forms because pareses of the inferior rectus and inferior oblique muscles are uncommon. Therefore, for clinical purposes, almost all cases of bilateral superior oblique muscle overaction can be considered primary.

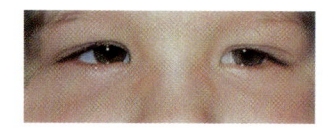

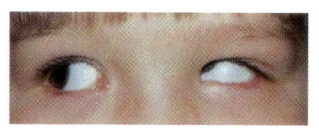

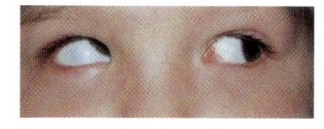

Figure 9-1 Small esotropia with marked overaction of both inferior oblique muscles. Note the elevation of each eye in adduction.

Clinical Features

A hypotropia often occurs in primary position with unilateral or asymmetrical bilateral overaction of the superior oblique muscles. The lower eye is the one with the unilaterally or more prominent bilaterally overacting superior oblique muscle. An associated horizontal deviation, most often exotropia, may be present, and the overacting superior oblique muscle also causes depression with resulting hypotropia in adduction (Fig 9-2).

Management

In a patient with a clinically significant ocular deviation or A pattern secondary to bilateral superior oblique overaction, a bilateral superior oblique weakening procedure (tenotomy or tendon lengthening by insertion of a silicone expander or nonabsorbable suture) is indicated. Both procedures are effective in patients who have reduced binocularity. However, many surgeons are reluctant to perform superior oblique weakening in patients with bifixation and normal stereopsis, in whom the resulting uncontrolled torsional and sometimes asymmetrical vertical effect can cause torsional diplopia or symptoms of secondary superior oblique palsy with head tilt.

Wright KW, Ryan SJ. *Color Atlas of Ophthalmic Surgery: Strabismus*. Philadelphia: Lippincott; 1991:210–216.

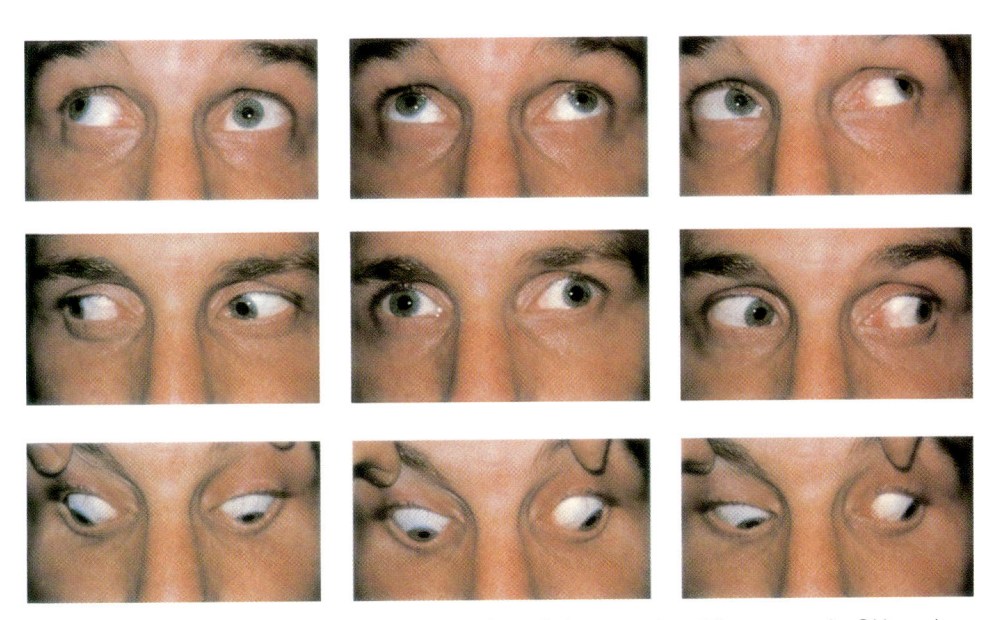

Figure 9-2 Exotropia with A pattern, overaction of the superior oblique muscle OU, and underaction of the inferior oblique muscle OU. Note depression of adducting eye in lateral gaze and in side gaze down, with slight limitation of elevation of the adducting eye in gaze to the side and up.

Dissociated Vertical Deviation

DVD is a common innervational disorder found in two thirds or more of patients with congenital esotropia. The cause is unknown, but DVD appears to be associated with early disruption of binocular development. Recent work has suggested that DVD may be the result of compensating mechanisms for latent nystagmus and of the dorsal light reflex.

Clinical Features

Either eye may spontaneously and slowly drift upward and outward, with simultaneous extorsion, when an eye is occluded or during periods of visual inattention without occlusion (Fig 9-3). The vertical movement usually predominates and is called *DVD*. Sometimes the principal dissociated movement is one of abduction, in which case the term *dissociated horizontal deviation* is used. Dissociated horizontal deviation is only occasionally seen without simultaneous DVD.

As the vertically deviated eye moves down to refixate when the previously fixating fellow eye is occluded, the latter makes no downward movement. Note that in true hypertropia, when the hypertropic eye refixates, the occluded fellow eye moves downward into a hypotropic position of equal magnitude. In contrast, eyes with DVD have no corresponding hypotropia of the fellow eye when the hypertropic eye refixates. In this respect, Hering's law of equal innervation appears not to apply to DVD, but this has been questioned.

The condition usually is bilateral although frequently asymmetrical. DVD may occur spontaneously *(manifest DVD)* or only when one eye is occluded *(latent DVD)*. In addition to dissociated horizontal deviation, latent nystagmus and horizontal strabismus are often associated with DVD. A prior history of congenital esotropia is particularly common. A coexisting vertical deviation, in which Hering's law does apply, can also occur. Some patients attempt to compensate by tilting the head in an effort to lessen the magnitude of the deviation and to improve motor control.

Measurement of DVD is difficult and imprecise. Each eye is tested separately in cases of bilateral DVD. One method uses base-down prism in front of the deviating eye under an occluder. The occluder is then switched to the fixating eye. Base-down prism is added until the deviating eye shows no downward movement. Results are similar when a red Maddox rod is used to generate a horizontal stripe viewed by the dissociated higher eye while the other eye fixates on a small light and vertical prism power is used to eliminate the separation of the light and the line. Another method, using a modified form of the

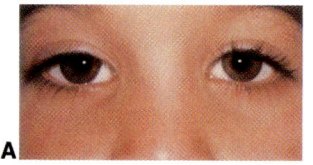

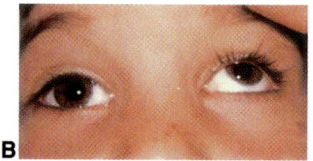

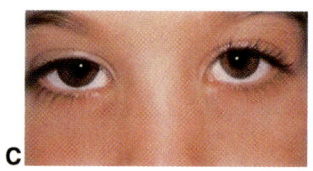

Figure 9-3 Dissociated vertical deviation, left eye. **A,** Binocular gaze. **B,** A large left hyperdeviation immediately after the eye is uncovered. **C,** Left eye drifts back down toward horizontal.

Krimsky test, is particularly useful in evaluating patients who cannot fixate with the deviating eye. The deviation can also simply be graded on a 1+ (least) to 4+ (most) scale. The earlier discussion of inferior oblique muscle overaction describes the features that distinguish this condition from DVD.

Management

Treatment for DVD is indicated if the vertical deviation occurs spontaneously, is frequent, and is cosmetically significant. Nonsurgical treatment, which changes the fixation pattern by patching or by optical means, is most effective in unilateral or highly asymmetrical bilateral DVD. Surgical treatment often improves the condition but rarely eliminates it (see Chapter 13). It is important to differentiate DVD from overaction of the inferior oblique muscles because the surgical approaches to these two conditions are different.

> Brodsky MC. Dissociated vertical divergence: a righting reflex gone wrong. *Arch Ophthalmol.* 1999;117:1216–1222.
> Burke JP, Scott WE, Kutschke PJ. Anterior transposition of the inferior oblique muscle for dissociated vertical deviation. *Ophthalmology.* 1993;100:245–250.
> Guyton DL. Dissociated vertical deviation: etiology, mechanism, and associated phenomena. Costenbader Lecture. *J AAPOS.* 2000;4:131–134.
> Santiago AP, Rosenbaum AL. Dissociated vertical deviation and head tilts. *J AAPOS.* 1998;2: 5–11.

Superior Oblique Muscle Palsy (or Paresis)

The most common isolated cyclovertical muscle palsy encountered by the ophthalmologist is the fourth, or trochlear, nerve palsy. The palsy may be congenital, resulting from a defect in the nucleus or the motor portion of cranial nerve IV, or acquired, most commonly as a result of closed head trauma or, rarely, central nervous system vascular problems, diabetes, or brain tumors. The palsy may be unilateral or bilateral. Markedly asymmetrical bilateral palsies that initially appear to be unilateral have prompted the term *masked bilateral*. The examiner should maintain a high index of suspicion for possible bilaterality when evaluating patients with superior oblique muscle palsy. Direct trauma to the tendon or the trochlear area is an unusual cause of unilateral superior oblique palsy.

To differentiate congenital from acquired palsies, it is helpful to examine old family photographs to detect a compensatory head tilt extending back to childhood. Facial asymmetry from long-standing childhood head tilting and large vertical fusional amplitudes also indicate chronicity. In addition, patients with a congenital palsy more frequently demonstrate a long, redundant, or "floppy" superior oblique tendon at the time of surgery. Congenital cases are usually unilateral, and acquired cases are more often bilateral. The distinction is important because acquired palsies that cannot be reasonably attributed to known instances of trauma suggest the possibility of serious intracranial lesions and the need for often extensive neurologic investigation.

Clinical Features

In unilateral cases, the patient may present with hypertropia. Either the normal or the affected eye can be preferred for fixation. Abnormal head positions are common, usually a head tilt toward the shoulder opposite the side of the paresis. Amblyopia is uncommon in acquired pareses but may be present in congenital ones. Extorsion and a complaint of apparent tilting of objects are common in acquired cases.

The possibility of bilaterality should always be considered. To differentiate bilateral from unilateral superior oblique paresis, the following criteria are used:

- *Bilateral cases* usually show a V-pattern esotropia in downgaze (see Chapter 10). Extorsion, when measured by the double Maddox rod test, is usually at least 5° and is highly diagnostic when 10° or more. The Bielschowsky head-tilt test (see Chapter 6) yields positive results on tilt to each side—that is, right head tilt shows a right hypertropia and left head tilt a left hypertropia. The ductions attributable to the superior oblique muscles are usually diminished in bilateral cases. Signs of bilaterality in cases initially thought to be unilateral include bilateral objective fundus extorsion, esotropia in downgaze, and even the mildest degree of inferior oblique overaction on the presumed uninvolved side.
- *Unilateral cases* usually show little esotropia in downgaze; torsion, measured by the double Maddox rod test, shows less than 10° excycloduction; the head tilt test yields positive results for the involved side only; and the actions of the superior oblique muscle may be normal or diminished.

The diagnosis of superior oblique muscle palsy is supported by results of the three-step test, double Maddox rod testing to measure torsion, and careful analysis of the ductions and versions. However, it should be remembered that three-step test results can be abnormal in some cases of DVD or entities involving restriction and therefore can be misleading.

Measurement of the ocular deviation in all nine diagnostic gaze positions, as well as with right and left head tilt, is important in diagnosing and planning treatment for superior oblique muscle palsy (Fig 9-4). Versions should be examined, with attention paid to the principal actions of the involved superior oblique muscle, the antagonist inferior oblique muscle, and depression of the involved eye (because of possible limitation due to contracture of the ipsilateral superior rectus muscle). Some ophthalmologists document any changes in the deviation by means of the Hess screen or Lancaster red-green test, or plot the field of binocular single vision, to follow patients with superior oblique muscle palsy.

Management

Indications for treatment are abnormal head position, significant vertical deviation, or diplopia. Prisms may be used to overcome diplopia in small, symptomatic, comitant or nearly comitant deviations that lack a symptomatic torsional component.

When surgery is indicated, the clinician must analyze both the versions and the diagnostic gaze position measurements. Common surgical strategies are discussed below and in Chapter 13.

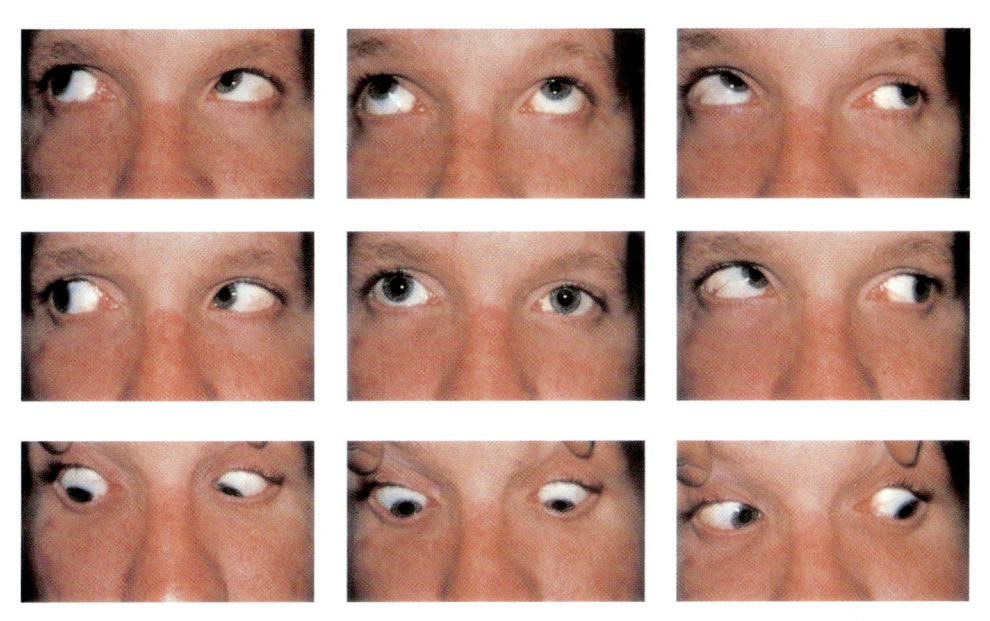

Figure 9-4 Right superior oblique palsy shown in nine positions of gaze. There is a right hypertropia that increases on left gaze. Note accompanying overaction of the right inferior oblique. Observations and measurements should be made in these positions and in right and left head tilt.

Unilateral superior oblique paralysis

When the antagonist inferior oblique muscle is overacting and the deviation in primary position is no greater than 15Δ, weakening of the inferior oblique muscle usually is the preferred first approach. The amount of deviation in primary position that is corrected by any weakening technique is proportional to the degree of overaction of the inferior oblique muscle. Correcting mild overaction may yield only 5Δ–8Δ of primary gaze correction. Operating on a moderate to severely overacting muscle often can achieve 10Δ–15Δ of correction.

If the deviation is greater than 15Δ with an overacting antagonist inferior oblique muscle, one should consider adding a second muscle to the procedure. Possibilities include recessing the contralateral inferior rectus muscle or tucking the tendon of the weak superior oblique muscle if it is significantly lax. In suitable patients, inferior rectus muscle recession has the additional advantage of facilitating use of an adjustable suture. A basic guideline: each millimeter of recession of a vertical rectus muscle results in approximately 3Δ of vertical correction.

If the antagonist inferior oblique muscle is not overacting, either the yoke contralateral inferior rectus muscle should be recessed or the ipsilateral superior oblique tendon should be tucked. The ability to determine the quantity of a superior oblique tendon tuck comes with experience. An attempt should be made to tuck the tendon until a positive forced duction test result is created for elevation in adduction just as the inferior limbus crosses an imaginary line drawn between the medial and lateral canthi.

The surgical plan should include recession of the ipsilateral superior rectus muscle if a forced duction test shows limited depression on the side of the deviation. This finding is more common in long-standing superior oblique palsy. Much of the previously mentioned "spread of comitance" that occurs over time in superior oblique muscle paresis results from ipsilateral superior rectus muscle contracture. For example, with right superior oblique muscle weakness, the hypertropia is usually greatest in left gaze. In cases with contracture of the ipsilateral superior rectus muscle, the deviation in right gaze is more like the deviation in primary position and left gaze.

The deficient depression caused by ipsilateral superior rectus muscle contracture can also produce a depression deficiency in abduction. On version testing, this deficiency may appear to represent superior oblique muscle *overaction* in the normal eye. If the surgeon is misled by this appearance and performs superior oblique tenotomy on the normal eye, thus iatrogenically converting a unilateral superior oblique paresis to a bilateral one, disabling torsional diplopia can result.

If the deviation is greater than 35Δ in primary position, three-muscle surgery may be required. This treatment might include recession of the overacting antagonist inferior oblique muscle, superior oblique tendon tuck, and ipsilateral superior rectus recession or contralateral inferior rectus recession, as dictated by forced duction test results.

Whatever the approach, it is important to avoid overcorrection of a long-standing unilateral superior oblique muscle in an adult patient: overcorrection will be aggravated with time and often causes disabling symptoms resembling the original problem.

Bilateral superior oblique paralysis

Surgery is performed on both eyes, graded for unequal severity if necessary. Bilateral inferior oblique muscle weakening is appropriate but may not be completely effective. Other options are inferior rectus muscle recession, the Harada-Ito procedure, and tucking of the superior oblique tendon.

As noted above, inferior rectus muscle recession can be adjusted and is easily graded; care is required to avoid postoperative recession of the lower eyelid margin. The Harada-Ito procedure is preferred in bilateral cases with predominantly torsional complaints. This operation involves anterior and temporal displacement of the anterior portions of the superior oblique tendons to a location adjacent to the lower edge of the lateral rectus muscle several millimeters posterior to that muscle's insertion. The procedure corrects the extorsion and abducting weakness of the superior oblique muscle in downgaze but not the vertical deviation in primary position. Some surgeons prefer superior oblique tendon tucking, but this risks the possibility of Brown syndrome on one or both sides in order to obtain a sufficient effect.

Harada M, Ito Y. Surgical correction of cyclotropia. *Jpn J Ophthalmol.* 1964;8:88–96.

Helveston EM, Mora JS, Lipsky SN, et al. Surgical treatment of superior oblique palsy. *Trans Am Ophthalmol Soc.* 1996;94:315–334.

Siatkowski RM. Third, fourth, and sixth nerve palsies. In: *Focal Points: Clinical Modules for Ophthalmologists.* San Francisco: American Academy of Ophthalmology; 1996: vol 14, no 8.

Brown Syndrome

The motility disorder described by Brown in 1950 as the *superior oblique tendon sheath syndrome* is now known simply as *Brown syndrome*. The characteristic restriction of elevation in adduction was originally thought to be caused by shortening of the anterior sheath of the superior oblique. Brown and others later abandoned this theory.

Brown syndrome occurs in congenital or acquired form and may be constant or intermittent. Prominent causes of acquired Brown syndrome include local trauma in the region of the trochlea and systemic inflammatory conditions. Acquired Brown syndrome is more likely to be intermittent and to resolve spontaneously than congenital Brown syndrome, although the latter may do so over many years, sometimes becoming intermittent before resolving completely. Restriction of the superior oblique tendon at the trochlear pulley is central to all forms of Brown syndrome. This condition is bilateral in approximately 10% of cases.

Clinical Features

Well-recognized clinical features of Brown syndrome include deficient elevation in adduction (Fig 9-5) that improves with abduction (ie, rotation of the eye out of the field of vertical action of the superior oblique muscle). Attempts at midline elevation usually cause divergence. This finding is an important point of difference from inferior oblique palsy. In adduction, the palpebral fissure widens and a downshoot of the involved eye is often seen, and can be distinguished from superior oblique muscle overaction because downshoot in the latter condition occurs less abruptly as adduction is increased. This finding, along with positive forced duction testing results, differentiates Brown syndrome from inferior oblique muscle palsy (discussed below).

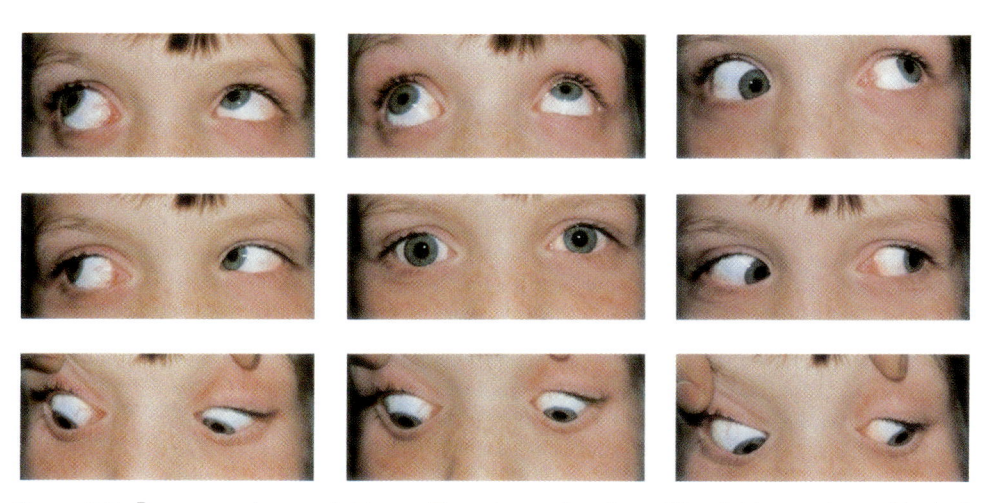

Figure 9-5 Brown syndrome, right eye. There is no elevation of the right eye when adducted; in this patient, the right eye is depressed when adducted. Elevation also is limited in straight-up gaze, and even slightly in up and right gaze. The characteristic divergence in straight-up gaze should be noted.

Brown syndrome can be graded as mild, moderate, or severe. In the mild form, no hypotropia is present in primary position and no downshoot of the eye occurs in adduction. Moderate cases have a downshoot in adduction but still no primary gaze hypotropia. Severe Brown syndrome cases have both a downshoot in adduction and a primary gaze hypotropia, often accompanied by a chin-up head posture and sometimes by a face turn away from the affected eye.

Occasionally, patients present with a manifest hypotropia and no compensatory head posturing. These patients often have associated horizontal strabismus and are at greater risk for amblyopia. Mild and moderate forms make up about two thirds of all Brown syndrome cases. Such cases are usually left untreated because strabismus is absent in primary position.

An unequivocally positive forced duction test demonstrating restricted passive elevation in adduction is essential for the diagnosis of Brown syndrome. Retropulsion of the globe during this determination stretches the superior oblique tendon and accentuates the restriction in Brown syndrome. When inferior rectus muscle fibrosis or inferior orbital blowout fracture (the principal entities to be differentiated) produces a restrictive elevation deficiency, the limitation to passive elevation is accentuated by forceps-induced proptosis of the eye rather than by retropulsion. In addition, the elevation deficiency produced by inferior rectus fibrosis or blowout fracture is usually more marked in abduction than in adduction.

Management

Observation alone remains the most common form of management for all but the most severe cases. Range-of-motion eye exercises, oral corticosteroids, and corticosteroids injected near the trochlea have produced improvement in selected patients. When Brown syndrome is associated with rheumatoid arthritis or other systemic inflammatory diseases, resolution may occur as systemic treatment brings the underlying disease into remission. Sinusitis has also led to Brown syndrome, and it has been suggested that patients presenting with acute-onset Brown syndrome of undetermined cause undergo CT of the orbits and paranasal sinuses to investigate this possibility.

Surgical treatment is indicated in cases of primary position hypotropia, anomalous head posture, or both wherein spontaneous resolution seems unlikely. Brown's originally advocated sheathectomy has been abandoned in favor of ipsilateral superior oblique tenotomy. However, iatrogenic superior oblique muscle palsy may occur postoperatively. Although the occurrence rate of this sequel has been reported to be 44%–82%, careful preservation of the intermuscular septum during tenotomy can reduce the rate to approximately 20%. This modified tenotomy often produces an early undercorrection that gradually improves with time.

To further reduce the incidence of superior oblique muscle palsy after tenotomy, some surgeons perform simultaneous ipsilateral inferior oblique muscle weakening. More recently, surgeons have performed a guarded tenotomy using an inert spacer formed from a solid silicone retinal band sewn to the cut ends of the superior oblique tendon. This procedure eliminates the need for simultaneous inferior oblique muscle weakening but sometimes results in a downgaze deficiency from adhesions to the nasal border of the superior rectus muscle. Care must be taken to place the silicone spacer nasal to the superior rectus muscle and to avoid direct contact of the spacer with sclera by preserving the intermuscular septum.

> Crawford JS. Surgical treatment of true Brown's syndrome. *Am J Ophthalmol.* 1976;81: 289–295.
> Helveston EM. The influence of superior oblique anatomy on function and treatment. The 1998 Bielschowsky Lecture. *Binocul Vis Strabismus Q.* 1999;14:16–26.
> Wright K. Brown's syndrome: diagnosis and management. *Trans Am Ophthalmol Soc.* 1999;97:1023–1109.

Inferior Oblique Muscle Palsy

Damage to the inferior division of cranial nerve III and especially to the branch that supplies the inferior oblique muscle has been proposed as a possible cause of inferior oblique muscle paralysis. However, the exact cause is unknown. The condition is rare, and whether it exists is controversial. It has not been associated with any other neurologic abnormalities.

Clinical Features

As with Brown syndrome, elevation is deficient in an adducted position. An A pattern is usually present, and the superior oblique muscle usually overacts. The diagnosis of inferior oblique muscle palsy is supported by findings of the three-step test. When the three-step results are not clear, such cases may in fact represent asymmetrical or unilateral primary superior oblique muscle overaction with secondary underaction of the inferior oblique muscle. Forced ductions are free when the adducted eye is elevated (Table 9-1).

Management

Indications for treatment of inferior oblique muscle palsy are abnormal head position, vertical deviation in primary gaze, and diplopia. Management consists of either ipsilateral superior oblique weakening or contralateral superior rectus muscle recession.

Monocular Elevation Deficiency (Double Elevator Palsy)

The term *double elevator palsy* implies a paralysis of the inferior oblique and superior rectus muscles of the same eye. However, double elevator palsy has become an umbrella

Table 9-1 Comparison of Inferior Oblique Muscle Palsy With Brown Syndrome

	Inferior Oblique Muscle Palsy	Brown Syndrome
Forced ductions	Negative	Positive
Strabismus pattern	A pattern	V pattern
Superior oblique muscle overaction	Usually present	None or minimal

term for any strabismus manifesting deficient elevation in all horizontal orientations of the eye. Because this motility pattern is well known to be caused by inferior rectus muscle restriction as well as paresis of one or both elevator muscles, double elevator muscle palsy is a misleading name and has been replaced by *monocular elevation deficiency.*

Clinical Features

Monocular elevation deficiency is characterized by limitation of elevation in adduction as well as in abduction on both versions and ductions (elevation is often more reduced in abduction than in primary gaze and improves somewhat in adduction, in contrast with Brown syndrome); hypotropia of the involved eye that increases in upgaze; chin-up position with fusion in downgaze or straight head with amblyopia in the hypotropic eye; and ptosis or pseudoptosis in primary position (Fig 9-6). An element of true ptosis is present in 50% of patients. Up to one third of such patients also show the Marcus Gunn jaw-winking phenomenon.

Three types of monocular elevation deficiency are found:

With inferior rectus restriction

These deficiencies are diagnosed by:

- Positive forced ductions in elevation
- Normal force generations (no muscle paralysis)
- Normal elevation saccades

With elevator weakness

These deficiencies are diagnosed by:

- Free forced ductions
- Reduced elevation force generation
- Reduced saccadic velocities for elevation of the affected eye (often with Bell's phenomenon preserved, indicating a supranuclear cause)

Combination

Combination deficiencies have inferior rectus restriction and also weak elevators. They are diagnosed by:

- Positive forced ductions for elevation
- Reduced force generation of the elevators of the involved eye (evidence of paralysis)
- Reduced vertical (upward) saccadic velocities in the involved eye

Patients with inferior rectus muscle restriction often have an extra or deeper lower eyelid fold on the affected side and a very poor or absent Bell's phenomenon.

Management

Indications for treatment include a large vertical deviation in primary position with or without ptosis and an abnormal head position, usually chin up. If inferior rectus muscle

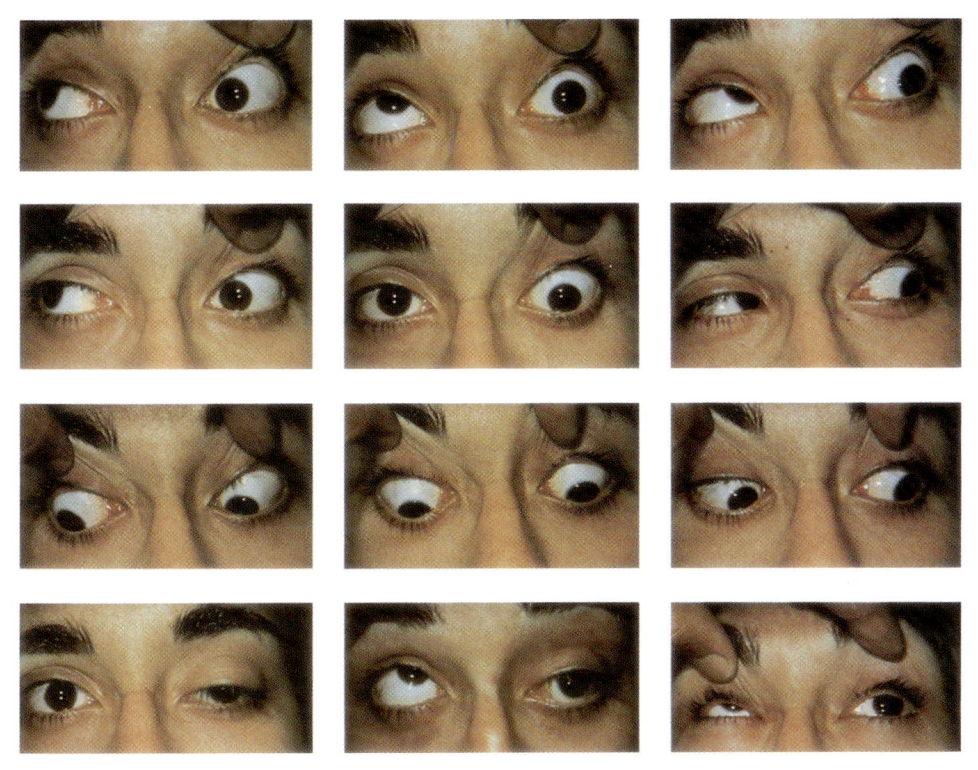

Figure 9-6 Monocular elevation deficiency of the left eye. *Top three rows*, no voluntary elevation of the left eye above horizontal. *Bottom left,* ptosis of the left upper eyelid when fixating with the right eye, persisting when fixating with the left eye *(bottom center).* The bottom center photograph also shows the marked secondary overelevation of the right eye when fixating with the left eye. *Bottom right,* a partially intact Bell's phenomenon with the left eye elevating above the horizontal on forced eyelid closure.

restriction is present, this muscle should be recessed. If there is no restriction, the medial rectus and the lateral rectus muscles should be transposed toward the superior rectus muscle *(Knapp procedure).*

> Raab EL. Double elevator palsy. In: Roy FH, ed. *Master Techniques in Ophthalmic Surgery.* Baltimore: Williams & Wilkins; 1995:267–274.

Orbital Floor Fractures

Blunt facial trauma is the usual cause of orbital floor fractures; auto accidents account for the majority. Fracture of the orbital floor can be part of more extensive fractures of the midface or can occur without similar consequences to the orbital rim or the zygomatic complex. The latter type of injury is considered due to a sudden hydraulic effect as intraorbital pressure increases acutely from a direct impact, which closes the orbital entrance without injury to its rim (blowout fracture).

Clinical Features

The clinical features of orbital floor fractures are as follows:

- Ecchymosis of the involved eye
- Diplopia in some or all positions of gaze immediately following injury (may persist in upgaze or downgaze)
- Paresthesia or hypoesthesia of the infraorbital area, secondary to damage of the infraorbital nerve, a sign more meaningful if present after the initial swelling subsides
- Enophthalmos, either early or late
- Entrapment of the inferior rectus muscle, inferior oblique muscle, or surrounding tissues
- Hypotropia in the primary position that increases with upgaze and may decrease or become a hypertropia in downgaze, suggesting combined mechanical restriction to elevation and inferior rectus paresis or pseudoparesis (Fig 9-7)
- Limited horizontal rotations, especially abduction, from an associated medial orbital wall fracture, resulting in entrapment of the medial rectus muscle

In the presence of limited elevation or depression, forced duction testing indicates the presence of restriction. Saccadic eye movement testing sometimes helps to determine whether the eye is additionally or entirely limited in movement because of a paretic process. Orbital CT and MRI of the involved soft tissues are useful to indicate the extent of the fracture and the degree of damage. Ocular injury frequently is associated, requiring a complete eye examination.

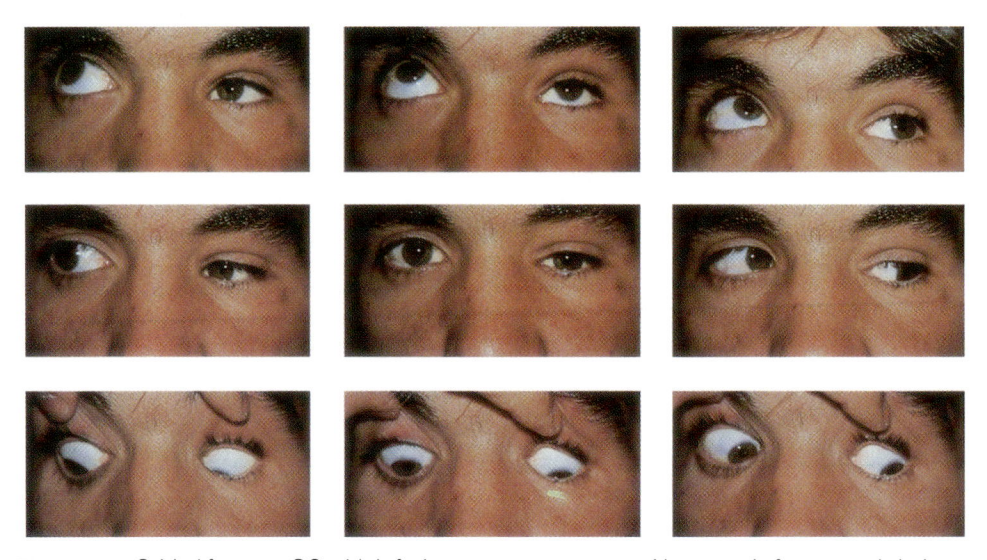

Figure 9-7 Orbital fracture OS with inferior rectus entrapment. Note ptosis from enophthalmos and limitation of elevation OS.

Management

Surgical management of orbital floor fractures is controversial. Some clinicians advocate immediate exploration once the diagnosis is made; others recommend waiting for orbital edema and hematoma to subside (usually within 5–10 days) before considering surgery. Some ophthalmologists wait up to 3–6 months before exploration if the hypotropia persists.

Damage to the inferior rectus muscle with resulting weakness may be caused by direct trauma to the muscle or its nerve and can occur either at the time of injury or at the time of the repair of an orbital floor fracture.

Inferior rectus muscle paralysis without prior trauma is a rare but recognized occurrence. If inferior rectus muscle paresis is present without entrapment, a hypertropia is usually seen in primary position. If paresis is present with entrapment, the patient may have very little deviation or even a slight hypotropia in primary position, which decreases in downgaze.

If entrapment is present, exploration of the fracture and release of the inferior rectus muscle and surrounding tissues may limit the subsequent damage. The initial management of inferior rectus muscle paresis without entrapment is observation because the paresis may reverse with time. If recovery does not take place within 6 months of the injury, muscle surgery may be indicated.

Residual strabismus generally can be corrected using standard eye muscle surgical techniques. For partial inferior rectus muscle paresis, a resection of the affected muscle combined with a recession of the ipsilateral superior rectus muscle can be performed. Alternatively, a recession of the contralateral inferior rectus muscle with or without the addition of a posterior fixation suture can be used to limit downgaze and match the duction deficiency of the injured eye. This approach is particularly useful when diplopia occurs in the reading position but no deviation is present in primary position (see also BCSC Section 7, *Orbit, Eyelids, and Lacrimal System*). Transposition of the ipsilateral medial and lateral rectus muscles to the inferior rectus muscle (inverse Knapp procedure) can be performed for complete inferior rectus muscle paralysis.

> Bonsagi ZC, Meyer DR. Internal orbital fractures in the pediatric age group—characterization and management. *Ophthalmology*. 2000;107:829–836.
> Manson PN, Iliff N. Early repair for selected injuries. In: Dutton JJ, Slamovits T, eds. Viewpoints. Management of blowout fractures of the orbital floor. *Surv Ophthalmol*. 1991; 35:280–292.
> Putterman AM. The conservative approach. In: Dutton JJ, Slamovits T, eds. Viewpoints. Management of blowout fractures of the orbital floor. *Surv Ophthalmol*. 1991;35:292–298.

CHAPTER 10

A and V Patterns

Horizontal deviations that change in magnitude with upgaze and downgaze—A patterns and V patterns—are incomitant subtypes of horizontal strabismus. An *A pattern* is present when a horizontal deviation shows a more convergent (less divergent) alignment in upgaze compared with downgaze. *V pattern* describes a horizontal deviation that is more convergent (less divergent) in downgaze compared with upgaze. Other less common variations of vertically incomitant horizontal strabismus include Y, λ, ◇, and X patterns.

Clinical Features

According to the traditional (and somewhat arbitrary) definition, an A pattern is considered clinically significant only when it measures 10Δ or more of difference between upgaze and downgaze, each approximately 25° from the primary position. A clinically significant V pattern is one that measures 15Δ or more of difference. Accordingly, we encounter V-pattern esotropia, V-pattern exotropia, A-pattern esotropia, and A-pattern exotropia.

An A or V pattern is associated with 15%–25% of all strabismus cases. Each of the conditions noted below has been considered a cause of A and V patterns. The ophthalmologist should pay careful attention to these anatomical or innervational anomalies in planning surgical correction.

- *Oblique muscle dysfunction.* Inferior oblique muscle overaction is associated with V patterns (Figs 10-1, 10-2), and superior oblique muscle overaction is associated with A patterns (Fig 10-3).
- *Horizontal rectus muscle dysfunction.* For example, increased lateral rectus muscle action in upgaze, or increased medial rectus muscle action in downgaze, produces a V pattern. Decreased horizontal rectus muscle action in these respective gazes produces an A pattern.
- *Vertical rectus muscle dysfunction.* For example, if the superior rectus muscles are primarily underacting, their tertiary adducting effect in upgaze will decrease, resulting in a V pattern. Similar underaction of the inferior rectus muscle results in an A pattern.

Patients with upward- or downward-slanting palpebral fissures may also show A and V patterns. Most likely, the pattern is due to altered force vectors of the extraocular muscles; the alteration is caused by an underlying variation in orbital configuration, reflected in the orientation of the fissures.

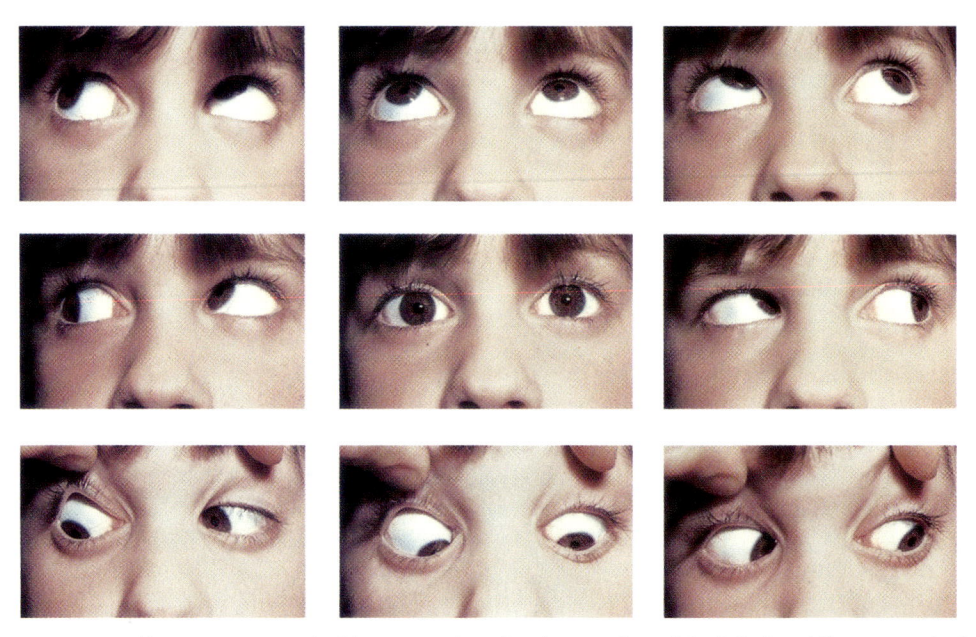

Figure 10-1 V-pattern esotropia. Note overelevation (overaction of the inferior oblique muscles) and limitation of depression (underaction of the superior oblique muscles) of each eye when in adduction.

Similarly, patients with Apert or Crouzon syndrome (see discussion of craniosynostosis in Chapter 25) frequently show a V-pattern exotropia or esotropia with marked elevation of the adducting eye, resembling the pattern caused by overacting inferior oblique muscles. The cause of this unusual motility disorder may be a combination of mechanical factors (eg, extorsion of the entire bony orbit) and structural abnormalities (abnormal size, number, or insertion of muscles). Surgical correction can be difficult. In addition, facial surgery for these conditions may produce a large eye alignment shift, usually in an esotropic direction.

A and V patterns are diagnosed via measurement of the patient's alignment while he or she is fixating on an accommodative target at distance. Proper refractive correction is necessary during measurement. Underactions and overactions of the oblique muscles are detected by study of the versions. Any compensatory head position (chin up or chin down) is noted.

Management

Clinically significant patterns (defined above) typically are treated surgically, most often in combination with correction of the underlying horizontal deviation. The following are guidelines to help the clinician plan surgical correction of A- and V-pattern deviations:
- Primary and reading positions are functionally the most important positions of gaze.
- Surgery to eliminate the horizontal deviation in primary position should be independently selected.

CHAPTER 10: A and V Patterns • 133

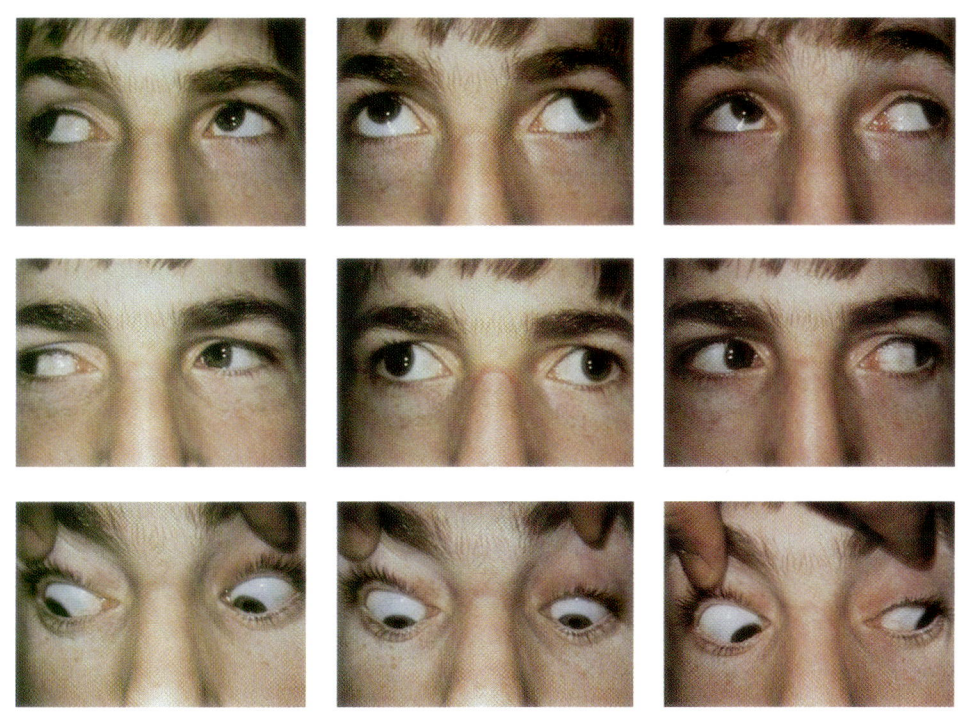

Figure 10-2 V-pattern exotropia with moderate overaction of inferior oblique muscles OU. There is no apparent underaction of either superior oblique muscle.

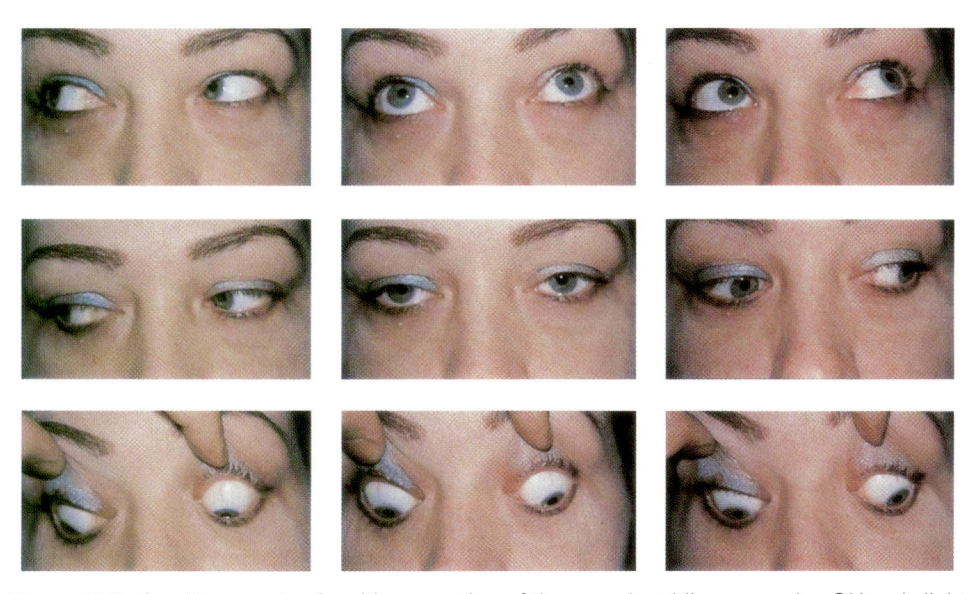

Figure 10-3 A-pattern exotropia with overaction of the superior oblique muscles OU and slight underaction of only the left inferior oblique muscle, with depression of the adducted right eye. Asymmetry of oblique muscle over- and underactions is not uncommon and usually is ignored in correcting A or V patterns when the discrepancy is minimal.

- Patients with large A or V patterns usually also have significant corresponding oblique muscle dysfunction.
- Most surgeons use the presence or absence of significant oblique dysfunction to determine their surgical approach. If the pattern is consistent with which oblique muscles are overacting (see above), oblique muscle weakening is included in the surgical plan.
- Most surgeons think that horizontal rectus muscle displacement (see below) is indicated when there is no oblique dysfunction (Fig 10-4), but this approach is not a substitute for oblique muscle surgery when overaction is present.
- Weakening the inferior oblique muscles or tucking the superior oblique tendons corrects up to 15Δ–25Δ of V pattern, but the tuck procedure is somewhat unpredictable.
- Inferior oblique muscle weakening tends to be self-adjusting, improving the V pattern without overcorrection.
- Bilateral superior oblique tenotomies correct up to 35Δ–45Δ of A pattern (ie, they produce 35Δ–45Δ of eso shift in downgaze).

Horizontal rectus muscles can be vertically displaced to correct A- or V-pattern strabismus that is not associated with oblique muscle dysfunction, as shown in Figure 10-5. The amount of displacement usually is one half to a full tendon width. Some surgeons vertically displace the tendon without keeping its reattachment parallel to the limbal tangent; this increases the effect on the pattern.

The *medial rectus muscles* are always moved toward the direction of vertical gaze where the *convergence* is greater or *divergence* is less (ie, upward in A patterns and downward in V patterns). The *lateral rectus muscles* are moved toward the direction of vertical

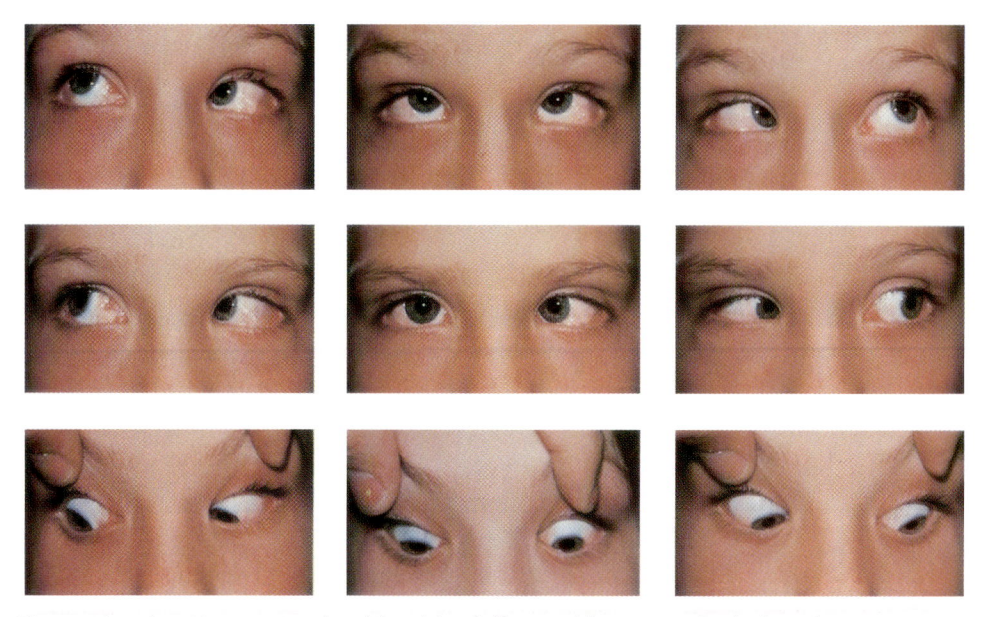

Figure 10-4 A-pattern esotropia with minimal, if any, oblique muscle dysfunction.

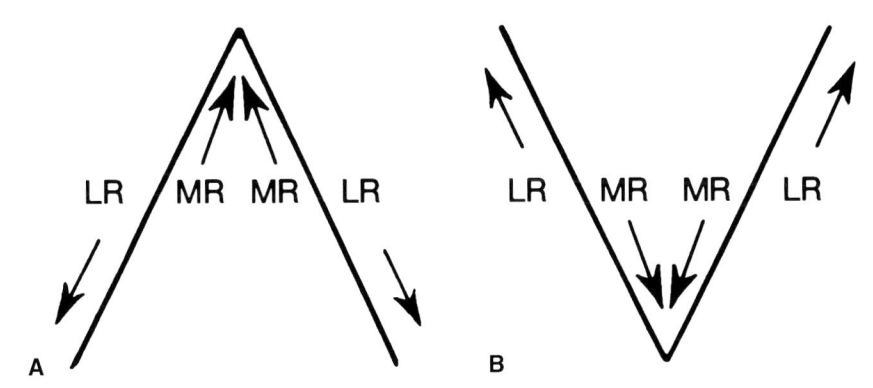

Figure 10-5 Direction of displacement of medial rectus (MR) and lateral rectus (LR) muscles in operations to treat V-pattern deviations **(A)** and A-pattern deviations **(B)**. *(Reprinted from von Noorden GK.* Binocular Vision and Ocular Motility. *5th ed. St Louis; Mosby; 1996:388.)*

gaze in which the *divergence* is greater or *convergence* is less (ie, upward in V patterns and downward in A patterns). These rules apply whether the horizontal recti are weakened or tightened.

When recession-resection surgery is indicated in an A pattern, displacement of the medial rectus muscle upward and the lateral rectus muscle downward has no net vertical or torsional effect in the primary position, but in upgaze the medial rectus muscle will be relaxed and the lateral rectus muscle tightened, thereby decreasing the A pattern. Similarly, for V patterns, the medial rectus muscle is displaced downward and the lateral rectus muscle upward. In downgaze, the medial rectus muscle will be relaxed and the lateral rectus muscle will be tightened, thereby decreasing the V pattern without a vertical or torsional effect.

A useful mnemonic for these procedures is MALE: *m*edial rectus muscles to the *a*pex, *l*ateral rectus muscles to the *e*mpty space. For more precise consideration of the muscle mechanics, remember that the surgeon moves the muscle in the direction in which the muscle's horizontal effect is to be lessened (eg, medial rectus muscles downward for V pattern).

Horizontal displacement of the vertical rectus tendons has been proposed as an alternative treatment. The superior rectus muscles are moved temporally and the inferior rectus muscles nasally for an A pattern, and the opposite approach is used for a V pattern. Although such procedures are theoretically appealing, they are rarely used because horizontal deviations, calling for horizontal rectus muscle procedures, usually are present. One indication for the vertical rectus muscle approach is one of the patterns associated with a negligible deviation in the primary position, an unusual but possible occurrence.

Sample Treatment Plans for the Various Patterns

V-Pattern Esotropia

If inferior oblique muscle overaction is present, the inferior oblique muscles should be weakened and the deviation in primary position should be corrected with the appropriate horizontal rectus muscle procedure.

If significant inferior oblique muscle overaction is not present, the procedure of choice is bilateral medial rectus muscle recession with downward displacement, bilateral resection of the lateral rectus muscles with upward displacement, or a recession-resection operation moving the medial rectus muscle downward and the lateral rectus muscle upward, depending on the pertinent factors in the case (eg, prior surgery, unimprovable vision in one eye).

V-Pattern Exotropia

The same scheme as is used for V-pattern esotropia should be followed, except that the opposite horizontal deviation is present and horizontal surgery is chosen accordingly.

A-Pattern Esotropia

If superior oblique muscle overaction is present, these muscles should be weakened with bilateral tenotomies or tendon-lengthening procedures. Weakening of the superior oblique muscle corrects up to 40Δ–45Δ of excess divergence in downgaze, if present. There is a risk of induced torsional imbalance, especially in patients with fusion capacity.

The effect of bilateral superior oblique weakening on primary position horizontal alignment remains somewhat controversial. Some surgeons think that the loss of abducting forces resulting from bilateral superior oblique weakening increases convergence in primary position by 10Δ–15Δ. These surgeons suggest adjusting horizontal surgery to compensate for this expected change. Other surgeons think that superior oblique tenotomy or other weakening procedures have no significant effect on primary position alignment and thus that no adjustment of horizontal surgery is warranted. With this issue in mind, the ophthalmologist must plan appropriate surgery for the associated horizontal deviation. Because the amount of horizontal surgery required is difficult to predict when superior oblique tenotomies are completed, adjustable sutures on the horizontal muscles may be helpful.

> Biglan AW. Pattern strabismus. In: Rosenbaum AL, Santiago AP, eds. *Clinical Strabismus Management: Principles and Surgical Techniques.* Philadelphia: Saunders; 1999:202–215.
> Diamond GR, Parks MM. The effect of superior oblique weakening procedures on primary position horizontal alignment. *J Pediatr Ophthalmol Strabismus.* 1981;18:35–38.
> von Noorden GK. *Binocular Vision and Ocular Motility: Theory and Management of Strabismus.* 5th ed. St Louis: Mosby; 1996:376–391.

Without superior oblique overaction, the treatment of choice is horizontal rectus muscle surgery with the appropriate displacement.

A-Pattern Exotropia

The appropriate plan, depending on whether or not the superior oblique muscles are overacting, can be inferred by extension of the schemes outlined above.

CHAPTER 11

Special Forms of Strabismus

The following general reference is a valuable summary of current knowledge concerning many eye movement disorders in children.

> Cassidy L, Taylor D, Harris C. Abnormal supranuclear eye movements in the child: a practical guide to examination and interpretation. *Surv Ophthalmol.* 2000;44:479–506.

Duane Syndrome

Duane syndrome is a spectrum of motility disturbances, all of which feature retraction of the globe in actual or attempted adduction. Horizontal movement is usually somewhat limited in either direction. Upshoot or downshoot *(leash phenomenon)* of the affected eye in attempted adduction is common in more severe cases.

A defect in development occurring in the fourth week of gestation appears to be the cause of Duane syndrome, according to studies of patients prenatally exposed to thalidomide. Although most affected patients have Duane syndrome alone, many associated systemic defects have been observed, including Goldenhar syndrome (hemifacial microsomia, ocular dermoids, ear anomalies, preauricular skin tags, and upper eyelid colobomas) and Wildervanck syndrome (sensorineural hearing loss, Klippel-Fiel anomaly with fused cervical vertebrae). Most cases of Duane syndrome are sporadic, but about 5%–10% show autosomal dominant inheritance.

A higher prevalence in females is reported in most series of patients with Duane syndrome. Discordance in monozygotic twins raises the possibility that intrauterine environment may be important. The many nonfamilial cases and the predilection for the left eye also suggest nongenetic factors.

In the few anatomical studies performed, the nucleus of the sixth cranial nerve has been absent and an aberrant branch of the third cranial nerve has innervated the lateral rectus muscle. Electromyographic studies have shown paradoxical innervation of the lateral rectus muscle (innervation on attempted adduction and reduced innervation on attempted abduction). Anomalous synergistic innervation of the medial, inferior, and superior rectus muscles and the oblique muscles has been demonstrated as well. Although considered an innervational anomaly, tight and broadly inserted medial rectus muscles and fibrotic lateral rectus muscles, with corresponding forced duction abnormalities, are often encountered at surgery.

> Hotchkiss MG, Miller NR, Clark AW, et al. Bilateral Duane's retraction syndrome. A clinical-pathologic case report. *Arch Ophthalmol.* 1980;98:870–874.

Clinical Features

The most widely employed classification of Duane syndrome specifies three groups, which for clinical purposes may only represent differences in severity of the limited horizontal rotations: type I consists of poor abduction, frequently with primary position esotropia (Fig 11-1); type II consists of poor adduction and exotropia (Fig 11-2); and type III consists of both poor abduction and poor adduction, with esotropia, exotropia, or no primary position deviation (Fig 11-3). About 15% of cases are bilateral; the type and severity need not be the same in each eye. Consideration of the direction of the strabismus in primary gaze is more useful than identifying the type for designing management strategies.

Many patients with Duane syndrome have some position of gaze in which the eyes are properly aligned, allowing the development of binocular vision. Amblyopia and significant refractive errors occur but less often than was originally reported.

Duane syndrome with esotropia and deficient abduction is the most common form (50%–80% in several series). Parents often misconstrue what actually is the normal eye as turning in excessively, not realizing that the involved eye is not abducting. Careful observation for globe retraction on adduction, particularly viewing from the side of the patient, obviates a neurologic investigation for a sixth nerve palsy, although retraction

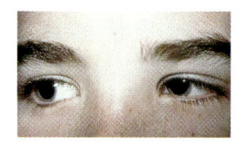

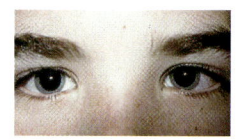

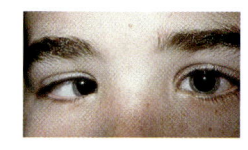

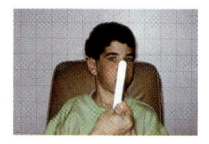

Figure 11-1 Type I Duane syndrome with esotropia, left eye, showing limitation of abduction and almost full adduction. Retraction of the globe on adduction. *Extreme right*, compensatory left face turn. *(Photographs courtesy of Edward L. Raab, MD.)*

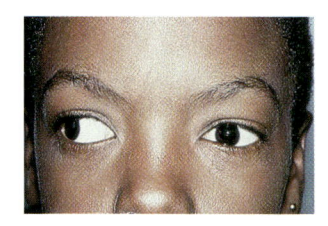

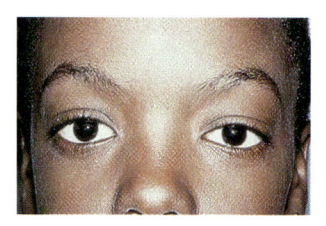

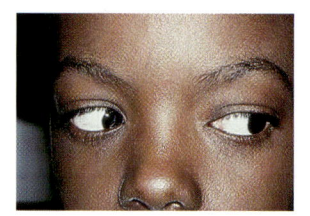

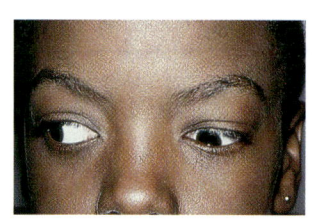

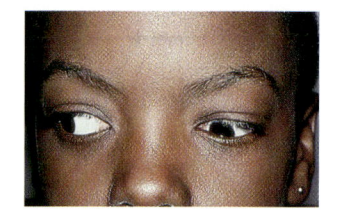

Figure 11-2 Type II Duane syndrome with exotropia, left eye. *Top row*, full abduction and marked limitation of adduction. *Bottom row*, variable up- or downshoot of the left eye with extreme right gaze effort. The typical primary position exotropia is not present in this patient. *(Photographs courtesy of Edward L. Raab, MD.)*

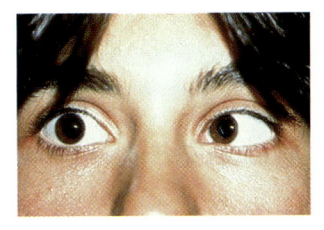

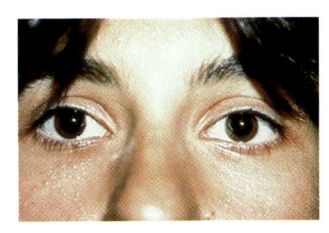

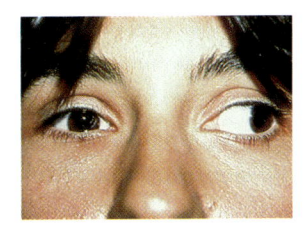

Figure 11-3 Type III Duane syndrome, right eye. Severe limitation of abduction and adduction, with palpebral fissure narrowing even though adduction cannot be accomplished. No deviation in the primary position. *(Photographs courtesy of Edward L. Raab, MD.)*

can be hard to appreciate in an infant. Another indicator pointing away from sixth cranial nerve palsy is the lack of correspondence between the absent or typically modest primary position esotropia and the usually profound abduction deficit (a comparison useful in ruling out paralysis in other entities as well). A further point of differentiation is that, even in esotropic Duane syndrome, a small-angle exotropia frequently is present in gaze away from the affected eye, a finding not present in lateral rectus muscle paralysis.

Management

Because any surgical approach results in partial improvement at best, surgery is reserved primarily for cases with primary position deviations, an abnormal head position, marked globe retraction, or large upshoots or downshoots.

For Duane syndrome with esotropia, recession of the medial rectus muscle on the involved side has been the most often used procedure to correct primary position deviation and eliminate the head turn. Abduction is not improved by this operation, but overcorrection is rare. Adding recession of the opposite medial rectus is recommended for deviations over 20 D in primary position. Although primary position overcorrection by medial rectus recession is not a significant risk, postoperative exotropia when the involved eye is adducted, either newly created or as an increase in existent exotropia, is possible. Recession of the lateral rectus muscle of the uninvolved eye can offset this effect.

Resection of the lateral rectus muscle for Duane syndrome with esotropia is not favored because of the likelihood that globe retraction will worsen. Transposition of the vertical rectus muscles (with or without additional scleral fixation) has been advocated to improve abduction. The value of botulinum injection into the medial rectus muscle to improve abduction is controversial.

The recommended surgery for Duane syndrome with exotropia and deficient adduction is comparable to that for esotropic Duane syndrome: recession of the lateral rectus on the involved side for small deviations and of both lateral recti for large deviations, with avoidance of resection of the medial rectus. The latter aspect is especially important when an up- or downshoot is present on attempted adduction because this finding indicates severe cocontraction.

Patients with Duane syndrome who have poor abduction and adduction often have straight eyes in or near the primary position and little, if any, head turn. No surgery improves the globe excursion. Severe globe retraction may be helped by recession of both the medial and the lateral rectus muscles, which also may benefit the induced anomalous vertical excursion. Other suggested procedures for the vertical excursion are splitting the lateral rectus muscle in a Y configuration and a posterior fixation procedure on this muscle. Improvement from either of these procedures has not been dramatic.

> DeRespinis PA, Caputo AR, Wagner RS, et al. Duane's retraction syndrome. *Surv Ophthalmol.* 1993;38:257–288.
>
> Foster RS. Vertical muscle transposition augmented with lateral fixation. *J AAPOS.* 1997;1: 20–30.
>
> Jampolsky A. Duane syndrome. In: Rosenbaum AL, Santiago AP, eds. *Clinical Strabismus Management: Principles and Surgical Techniques.* Philadelphia: Saunders; 1999:325–346.

Third Cranial Nerve (Oculomotor) Palsy

The causes of third cranial nerve palsy in children include congenital (40%–50%), traumatic, inflammatory, and (infrequently) neoplastic lesions. Third cranial nerve palsy can also occur after viral infection and with migraine.

In adults, third cranial nerve palsy may be caused by intracranial aneurysm, diabetes, neuritis, trauma, infection, or, rarely, tumor. Many patients with aneurysm are poor surgical candidates and are not referred for ocular muscle surgery. Diabetic third cranial nerve palsy generally resolves spontaneously within 3–4 months. Thus, the majority of adults referred for surgical treatment have palsy due to trauma.

Clinical Features

Exodeviation occurs in third cranial nerve palsy, whether congenital or acquired. Third cranial nerve palsy is generally associated with a hypotropia of the paretic eye. These findings would be expected because the remaining unopposed muscles are the lateral rectus (abductor) and the superior oblique (depressor).

Because the visual system is still developing in pediatric patients, amblyopia is a common finding and must be treated aggressively. In congenital and traumatic cases, the clinical findings and treatment may be complicated by aberrant regeneration (misdirection) of the damaged nerve, presenting as anomalous eyelid elevation, pupil constriction, or depression of the globe on attempted adduction (see BCSC Section 5, *Neuro-Ophthalmology*, for further discussion and extensive illustration).

Management

Before surgical correction is planned, it is advisable to wait 6–12 months for spontaneous recovery. Third cranial nerve palsies present difficult surgical challenges because multiple extraocular muscles as well as the levator may be involved. Replacing all of the lost vector forces on the globe is impossible; therefore, the goals of surgery must be thoroughly discussed with patients so that their expectations are realistic. Adequate alignment for binocular function in primary position and in slight downgaze for reading may be all that can be expected.

Although good primary position alignment can be achieved in most patients, surgery should be undertaken cautiously in patients with complete palsy and previously good binocular visual function because elevation of the eyelid and incomplete realignment without useful single binocular fields may produce incapacitating diplopia. Patients with at least partial recovery are much better candidates for good functional as well as cosmetic results. Prism adaptation testing has shown that adult patients who can achieve single binocular vision with prisms of any power before surgery are most likely to do well with surgical therapy. The occurrence rate of diplopia in patients under age 8 years is small because of the ability of the young binocular visual system to suppress conflicting visual information.

Planning for the appropriate surgical procedure is dictated by the number and condition of the involved muscles and the presence of noticeable paradoxical rotations. Frequently, a large recession-resection procedure on the horizontal rectus muscles to correct the exodeviation, with supraplacement to correct the hypotropia, is effective, especially with incomplete paralysis.

Some surgeons use superior oblique tenotomy instead of supraplacement of the horizontal rectus muscles for hypotropia correction when the palsy is complete. Transfer of the tendon to the upper nasal quadrant of the globe has been employed; however, anomalous and disfiguring eye movements can result from this procedure.

> Mudgil AV, Repka MX. Ophthalmologic outcome after third cranial nerve palsy in childhood. *J AAPOS*. 1999;3:2–8.
> Schumacher-Feero LA, Uyoo KW, Solari FM, et al. Third cranial nerve palsy in children. *Am J Ophthalmol*. 1999;128:216–221.
> Siatkowski RM. Third, fourth, and sixth nerve palsies. In: *Focal Points: Clinical Modules for Ophthalmologists*. San Francisco: American Academy of Ophthalmology; 1996: vol 14, no 8.

Graves Eye Disease (Thyroid Ophthalmopathy)

Graves eye disease is also discussed in several other volumes of the BCSC as thyroid ophthalmopathy (consult the *Master Index*). Additional terms used elsewhere in the literature include *thyroid orbitopathy* and *thyroid-related immune orbitopathy*. European literature uses the eponym *von Basedow* rather than *Graves*. The eye and the orbit can be affected in a variety of ways that are discussed in BCSC Section 7, *Orbit, Eyelids, and Lacrimal System*. Only motility disturbances are covered in this volume.

The myopathy is not caused by thyroid dysfunction. Rather, both conditions probably result from a common autoimmune disease. Therefore, patients may be euthyroid, hyperthyroid, or hypothyroid at the time of diagnosis, or they may have a history of past thyroid dysfunction. Smoking can aggravate thyroid orbital inflammation. Some patients with Graves disease also have myasthenia gravis (see below), complicating the clinical findings. (See also Chapter 4 of BCSC Section 7, *Orbit, Eyelids, and Lacrimal System*.)

Clinical Features

Severe restrictive myopathy may occur with Graves disease. The muscles affected, in decreasing order of severity and frequency, are the inferior rectus, medial rectus, superior rectus, and lateral rectus. Forced duction test results are almost always positive in one or more directions.

The patient presents most often with some degree of proptosis, hypotropia, or esotropia (Fig 11-4). Thyroid ophthalmopathy is a common cause of acquired vertical deviation in adults, especially females, but is rare in children.

Edema, inflammation, and fibrosis are present because of lymphocytic infiltration of the extraocular muscles. These conditions result in massive enlargement of affected extraocular muscles and may not only restrict motility but also cause compressive optic neuropathy. Detection of this muscle enlargement by orbital ultrasound imaging, CT, or MRI helps confirm the diagnosis of Graves eye disease.

Management

Indications for strabismus surgery include diplopia, abnormal head position, or a stable deviation. Extraocular muscle surgery may eliminate diplopia in primary gaze but rarely restores normal motility because of the restrictive myopathy, the need for very large recessions to allow the eye to be in primary position, and the replacement of muscle tissue by fibrous scar.

It is important to establish stability of the strabismus measurements before surgery is performed; waiting for at least 3 months is recommended. In the meantime, prisms may alleviate diplopia in primary position or for reading, but they are not necessarily effective in other positions of gaze. One recent study investigated performance of surgery prior to the achievement of stability but beyond the period of acute inflammation. The results were favorable, although half of the patients required repeat operation.

Recession of the affected muscles is the primary surgical treatment. Strengthening procedures are performed rarely because they usually worsen restriction. Adjustable strabismus sutures can be helpful in these difficult cases. Because late overcorrection is com-

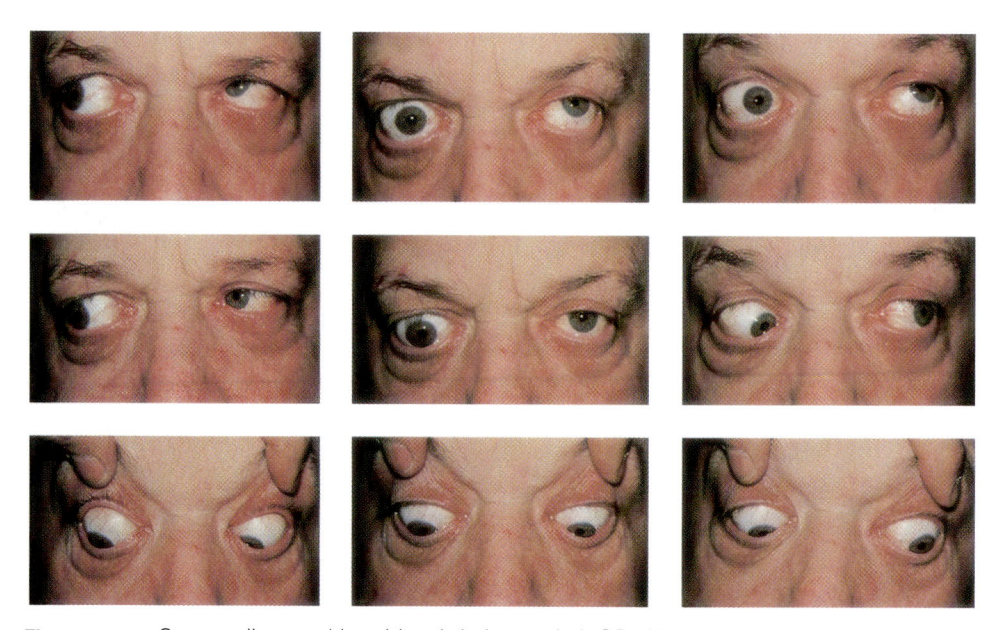

Figure 11-4 Graves disease (thyroid ophthalmopathy) OD. Note right eyelid retraction and restrictive right hypotropia with very limited elevation of the right eye.

mon, especially with large inferior rectus recessions, slight initial undercorrection is desirable. Limited depression of the eyes after large inferior rectus recessions can prevent bifocal use by patients after surgery.

Proptosis can become worse after muscle recessions. If the need for orbital decompression is foreseeable, it is usually preferable to postpone strabismus surgery until the former has been accomplished. Likewise, eyelid surgery usually is performed at a later time because upper eyelid retraction may be improved when the patient no longer strains to elevate the eye.

Large recessions of very tight inferior rectus muscles can cause lower eyelid retraction severe enough to require eyelid surgery later despite extensive dissection around the muscle. Separate treatment of the lower eyelid retractors at the time of the strabismus surgery has led to some success at preventing lower eyelid retraction.

> Coats DK, Paysse EA, Plager DA, et al. Early strabismus surgery for thyroid ophthalmopathy. *Ophthalmology*. 1999;106:324–329.
>
> Cockerham KP, Kennerdel JS. Thyroid-associated orbitopathy. In: *Focal Points: Clinical Modules for Ophthalmologists*. San Francisco: American Academy of Ophthalmology; 1997: vol 15, no 1.
>
> Meyer DR, Simon JW, Kansora J. Primary infratarsal lower eyelid retractor lysis to prevent eyelid retraction following inferior rectus recession. *Am J Ophthalmol*. 1996;122:331–339.

Chronic Progressive External Ophthalmoplegia

Clinical Features

Chronic progressive external ophthalmoplegia (CPEO) usually begins in childhood with ptosis and slowly progresses to total paralysis of the eyelids and extraocular muscles. CPEO may be sporadic or familial. Although a true pigmentary retinal dystrophy usually is absent, constricted fields and electrodiagnostic abnormalities can occur. Defects in mitochondrial DNA have been found in some patients. The triad of retinal pigmentary changes, CPEO, and cardiomyopathy (especially heart block) is called *Kearns-Sayre syndrome*. BCSC Section 2, *Fundamentals and Principles of Ophthalmology*, discusses this condition in greater detail.

Management

Treatment options are limited. Cautious surgical elevation (suspension) of the upper eyelids is sometimes indicated to lessen a severe chin-up head position.

Myasthenia Gravis

Onset of myasthenia gravis may occur at any age, although it is uncommon in children. The disease may be purely ocular, or it may occur as part of a major systemic disorder, with other skeletal muscles involved as well. BCSC Section 5, *Neuro-Ophthalmology*, discusses both the ocular and the systemic aspects of myasthenia gravis in depth.

Clinical Features

The principal ocular manifestation is extraocular muscle weakness, including the levator muscle. Marked variability of motility measurements and ptosis should suggest the presence of the disease. Affected muscles fatigue rapidly, so that ptosis typically increases when the patient is required to look upward for 30 seconds. In the sleep test, the ptosis often resolves after 20–30 minutes with the eyelids closed in a dark room. The presence of *Cogan twitch*, an overshoot of the eyelid when the patient looks straight ahead after looking down for several minutes, is also diagnostic.

In the Tensilon test, a preliminary dose of 0.2 mL edrophonium chloride is injected intravenously. The patient's eyelids and eye movements are observed. If function improves obviously (Fig 11-5), no additional drug is needed. If no adverse reaction or improvement occurs, 0.2 mL increments are injected intravenously to a total of 1.0 mL. Atropine for IV administration is kept available as an antidote should a severe adverse cholinergic reaction occur. A similar test using neostigmine (Prostigmin), administered intramuscularly following pretreatment with atropine, has been described for use in children because the neostigmine effect is prolonged, allowing more time for measurement of changes in alignment, which is difficult with edrophonium because of the latter's brief action.

Orbital cooling by the external application of ice for 2–5 minutes improves function of the levator and other affected extraocular muscles, giving a rapid and apparently reliable method of establishing this diagnosis without the need for drug administration.

Electromyography shows decreased electrical activity of involved muscles after prolonged voluntary innervation and increased activity (including saccadic velocity) after the administration of edrophonium or neostigmine. Documentation of abnormalities in single-fiber electromyography or the presence of circulating antiacetylcholine receptor antibodies is necessary in difficult cases.

Management

Ocular myasthenia gravis is frequently resistant to the usual systemic myasthenia treatment. If and when the ocular deviation has stabilized, standard eye muscle surgery can be helpful in restoring binocular function in at least some gaze positions.

Table 11-1 compares Graves disease with CPEO and myasthenia gravis.

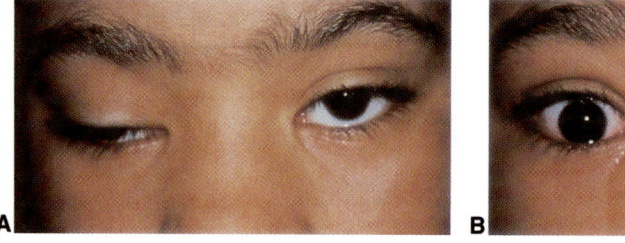

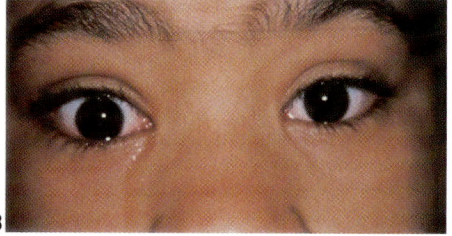

Figure 11-5 Myasthenia gravis. **A,** Bilateral ptosis with right hypotropia and right exotropia. **B,** Following Tensilon injection, the eye shows orthophoria, normal eyelid elevation, and the lacrimation that frequently accompanies Tensilon injection.

Table 11-1 Differentiation of Conditions Producing Ptosis and Extraocular Muscular Involvement

	Graves Disease (Thyroid Ophthalmopathy)	Chronic Progressive External Ophthalmoplegia (CPEO)	Myasthenia Gravis
Age	Any age	Any age	Any age
Muscle preferentially involved	Inferior rectus Medial rectus muscles	Levator Extraocular muscles	Levator Extraocular muscles
Fatiguability	No, unless coexistent myasthenia gravis	No	Yes
Response to Tensilon	No, unless coexistent myasthenia gravis	No	Yes
Other eye signs	External eye signs	Pigmentary retinopathy Optic neuropathy	No
Forced ductions	Restriction	Restriction if long-standing	Normal
Clinical course	May resolve or progress	Slowly progressive	Fluctuation May have generalized weakness
Eyelids	Retraction	Ptosis	Ptosis
Diplopia	Yes	No	Yes
Other signs and symptoms	Tachycardia, arrhythmia, tremor, weight loss, diarrhea, heat intolerance	Heart block Manifestation of Kearns-Sayre syndrome	Dysphagia, jaw weakness, limb weakness, dyspnea

Ellis FD, Hoyt CS, Ellis FJ, et al. Extraocular muscle responses to orbital cooling (ice test) for ocular myasthenia gravis diagnosis. *J AAPOS*. 2000;4:271–281.

Golnik KC, Pena R, Lee AG, et al. An ice test for the diagnosis of myasthenia gravis. *Ophthalmology*. 1999;106:1282–1286.

Mullaney P, Vajsar J, Smith R, et al. The natural history and ophthalmic involvement in childhood myasthenia gravis at the Hospital for Sick Children. *Ophthalmology*. 2000; 107:504–510.

Congenital Fibrosis Syndrome

Congenital fibrosis syndrome is a rare group of congenital disorders characterized by varying amounts of restriction of the extraocular muscles and replacement of the muscles by fibrous tissue. The spectrum ranges from isolated fibrosis of a single muscle to bilateral involvement of all extraocular muscles (Fig 11-6).

The cause of congenital fibrosis syndrome is unknown, although orbital inflammation has been implicated in some types. Diagnosis depends on finding limited voluntary motion, with restriction confirmed by forced duction testing. The congenital origin is an important distinction from thyroid ophthalmopathy.

146 • Pediatric Ophthalmology and Strabismus

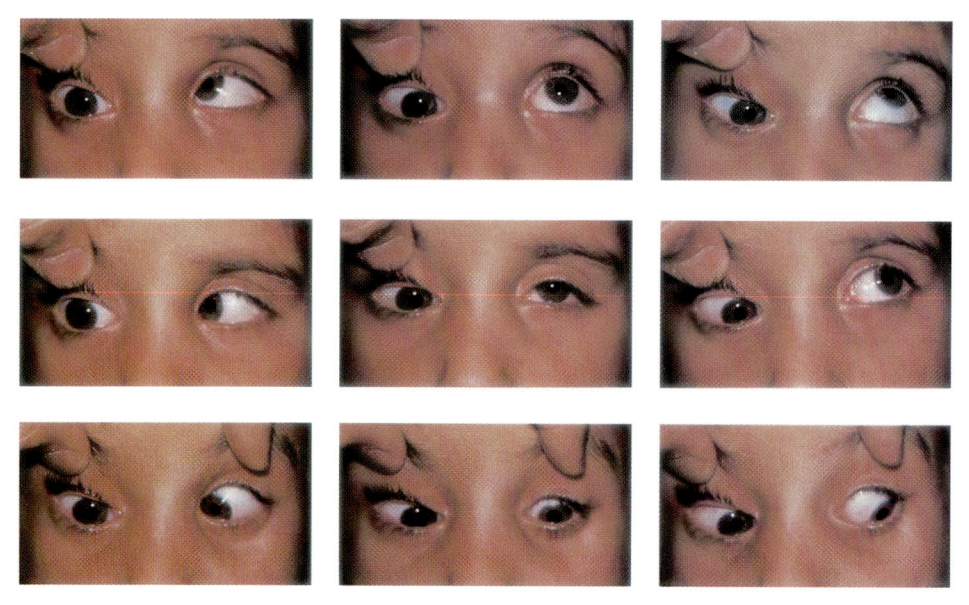

Figure 11-6 Congenital fibrosis syndrome, right eye, involving all extraocular muscles.

Clinical Features

General fibrosis is the most severe form, involving all the extraocular muscles of both eyes, including the levator palpebrae superioris, with ptosis. General fibrosis is usually autosomal dominant but may be autosomal recessive.

Congenital unilateral fibrosis with enophthalmos and ptosis is nonfamilial, with fibrosis of all the extraocular muscles and the levator on one side.

Congenital fibrosis of the inferior rectus muscle alone may be unilateral or bilateral and sporadic or familial. This condition is commonly inherited as an autosomal dominant trait, and its genetic locus is known.

Strabismus fixus involves the horizontal recti, usually the medial rectus muscles, with severe esotropia. Occasionally, the lateral recti are affected. The condition usually is sporadic and can be acquired, often in highly myopic patients.

Vertical retraction syndrome involves the superior rectus muscle, with inability to depress the eye.

Management

Surgery is difficult and requires release of the restricted muscles (ie, weakening procedures). Fibrosis of the adjacent tissues may be present as well. A good surgical result aligns the eyes in primary position, but full ocular rotations cannot be restored and the outcome is unpredictable.

> Traboulsi EI, Jaafar MS, Kattan HM, et al. Congenital fibrosis of the extraocular muscles: report of 24 cases illustrating the clinical spectrum and surgical management. *Am Orthoptic J.* 1993;43:45–53.

Möbius Syndrome (Sequence)

Clinical Features

Möbius syndrome is a rare condition characterized by the association of both sixth and seventh nerve palsies, the latter causing masklike facies. Patients may also manifest gaze palsies that can be attributed to abnormalities in the pontine paramedian reticular formation, indicating that the lesion is not only nuclear. (See BCSC Section 5, *Neuro-Ophthalmology*, for discussion of the pontine paramedian reticular formation.) Many patients also show limb, chest, and tongue defects, and some geneticists think that Möbius syndrome is one of a family of syndromes in which hypoplastic limb anomalies are associated with orofacial and cranial nerve defects. Poland syndrome (absent pectoralis muscle) occurs in some patients with Möbius syndrome.

Both abduction and adduction may be limited; in some patients, adduction is better with convergence than with versions, similar to a gaze paresis. Some patients appear to have palpebral fissure changes on adduction, and a few have vertical muscle involvement. The patient may have an esotropia or straight eyes in primary position.

Management

Medial rectus recession has been advocated, but in the presence of a significant limitation of adduction, a conservative approach is indicated.

Miller M, Stromland K. The Möbius sequence: a relook. *J AAPOS*. 1999;3:199–201.

Internuclear Ophthalmoplegia

Interconnecting the ocular motor nuclei in the pons and midbrain is a prominent group of fibers called the *medial longitudinal fasciculus*, located dorsally on either side of the brain stem midline. The medial longitudinal fasciculus passes between the sixth nerve nuclei, below and lateral to the fourth and third nerve nuclei. This group of fibers integrates the nuclei of the cranial nerves governing ocular motility and has major connections with the vestibular nuclei. An intact medial longitudinal fasciculus is essential for the production of conjugate eye movements.

Clinical Features

Injury to the medial longitudinal fasciculus results in a typical pattern of disconjugate movement called *internuclear ophthalmoplegia*. In this condition, the ipsilateral eye adducts slowly and incompletely or not at all while the abducting eye exhibits a characteristic horizontal nystagmus. Both eyes adduct normally on convergence. Some degree of skew deviation may be present.

Bilateral internuclear ophthalmoplegia is an abnormality of the ocular motor system in patients with demyelinating disease, but it may also occur in patients who have had a cerebrovascular accident or brain tumor.

Management

If a large deviation persists after 6 months, medial rectus muscle resection and contralateral lateral rectus muscle recession (to limit exotropia in lateral gaze) can be helpful in eliminating diplopia, particularly in bilateral cases.

Congenital Ocular Motor Apraxia

Congenital ocular motor apraxia is a rare disorder of ocular motility, sometimes associated with strabismus. It is more common in males than in females and may be familial.

The pathogenesis of this condition is not known. It has been associated with premature birth. Developmental delay, especially of motor milestones, may be present. Central nervous system abnormalities, including bilateral lesions of the frontoparietal cortex, agenesis of the corpus callosum, hydrocephalus, and Joubert syndrome, also have been associated. Several case reports have identified mass lesions of the cerebellum that compress the rostral part of the brain stem. Assessment of children with ocular motor apraxia by neuroimaging of the skull as well as a complete systemic and developmental evaluation is prudent.

Clinical Features

Findings include an inability to generate normal voluntary horizontal saccades. Instead, changes in horizontal fixation are made by a head thrust that overshoots the target, followed by a rotation of the head back in the opposite direction once fixation is established. The initial thrust serves to break fixation and may be associated with a blink that serves the same purpose. Vertical saccades and random eye movements are intact, but vestibular and optokinetic nystagmus are impaired. Reading can be difficult. The head thrust may improve in later childhood.

The differential diagnosis of acquired ocular motor apraxia subsumes conditions that affect the generation of voluntary saccades, including metabolic and degenerative diseases such as Huntington chorea.

Cogan DG. Congenital ocular motor apraxia. *Can J Ophthalmol.* 1966;1:253–260.

Harris CM, Shawkat F, Russell-Eggitt I, et al. Intermittent horizontal saccade failure ("ocular motor apraxia") in children. *Br J Ophthalmol.* 1996;80:151–158.

Special Settings for Strabismus

In addition to the unique varieties of ocular motility disturbances discussed above, there are several more or less familiar clinical settings in which strabismus is one of the consequences. These are mentioned briefly here.

Refractive surgery creating monovision, to facilitate visual clarity at distance and near without spectacles or contact lenses in adults in the presbyopic age range, can result in dissimilar sensory input to the two eyes sufficient to cause loss of motor control of the extraocular muscles and disruption of fusion in predisposed patients.

Surgery for retinal detachment can lead to scarring of the fascial tissues covering the globe, with restricted rotations. Corrective surgery can be extremely difficult, especially if it is deemed necessary to remove the elements attached to the globe as part of the repair of the detachment. The presence of the operating retinal surgeon for guidance during the strabismus correction can be valuable.

The recently introduced modality of macular translocation surgery can cause torsional diplopia and other binocular sensory disturbances.

Aqueous drainage devices for otherwise unresponsive glaucoma can cause scarring and interference with ocular rotations, as has been noted for retinal detachment surgery. Treatment may require removal of the device and relocation or substitution of another size or type, a dilemma if it has been functioning well.

The extraocular muscles can be damaged after retrobulbar injection of anesthetic agents. Such damage may result from direct mechanical injury of the muscle or from a toxic effect of the anesthetic agent. Rotation deficiency should be managed according to the principles outlined for extraocular muscle paralysis, including the allowance of several months to permit spontaneous recovery. Because of the usual placement of these injections, the vertical rectus and inferior oblique muscles are the most vulnerable.

Laceration of the medial rectus muscle has been described as a complication of endoscopic sinus surgery. In the most severe form, an entire section of the muscle can be excised inadvertently. Restoration of function can be an extremely difficult surgical challenge.

> Penne RB, Flanagan JC, Stefanyszyn MA, et al. Ocular motility disorders secondary to sinus surgery. *Ophthal Plast Reconstr Surg.* 1993;9:52–61.
> Trotter WL, Kaw P, Meyer DR, et al. Treatment of subtotal medial rectus myectomy complicating functional endoscopic sinus surgery. *J AAPOS.* 2000;4:250–253.

CHAPTER 12

Childhood Nystagmus

The child with nystagmus presents a difficult diagnostic challenge. The primary goal of the ophthalmic evaluation is to determine whether the nystagmus is a sign of a significant neurologic abnormality necessitating immediate intervention, an ocular abnormality that may affect visual development, or a simple motor defect compatible with good visual function.

In most children with nystagmus, the condition has an ophthalmic cause that can be determined by simple office examination techniques. Further diagnostic evaluation is usually unnecessary (Table 12-1).

BCSC Section 5, *Neuro-Ophthalmology*, discusses the neurologic implications of nystagmus, and Section 4, *Ophthalmic Pathology and Intraocular Tumors*, covers some of the tumors mentioned in Table 12-1.

> Lavery MA, O'Neill JF, Chu FC, et al. Acquired nystagmus in early childhood: a presenting sign of intracranial tumor. *Ophthalmology*. 1984;91:425–435.
> Newman NM. Discussion of acquired nystagmus in early childhood: a presenting sign of intracranial tumor. *Ophthalmology*. 1984;91:435.

Nomenclature

Nystagmus is an involuntary, rhythmic to-and-fro oscillation of the eyes. Parents often describe their child's eyes as dancing, jiggling, or jumping. The two most common types of childhood nystagmus are pendular and jerk. *Pendular nystagmus* is a to-and-fro movement of the eyes with equal velocity in each direction. *Jerk nystagmus* denotes a movement of unequal speed and, by convention, the fast component defines the direction of the nystagmus. Therefore, a right jerk nystagmus has a slow movement to the left and a fast movement (jerk) to the right.

The nystagmus movement can be further classified according to the frequency (number of oscillations per unit of time) and the amplitude (the angular distance traveled during the movement). Finally, the movements may be horizontal, vertical, rotary, oblique, or circular.

Characteristics of the nystagmus movement may change with different gaze direction. It is not uncommon for a pendular nystagmus to become jerk on extreme gaze, and certain gaze positions can affect the amplitude and frequency. This is especially true of jerk nystagmus, which typically has a *null point* (the gaze location where the nystagmus is minimal) located in the gaze opposite the fast phase component *(Alexander's law)*.

152 • Pediatric Ophthalmology and Strabismus

Table 12-1 **Common Intracranial Tumors in Childhood**

Type	Location
Glial tumors	
Astrocytoma	Cerebellum
	Brain stem
	Hypothalamus
	Optic nerve/chiasm
Ependymoma	Fourth ventricle
Neural tumors	
Medulloblastoma	Cerebellum
Neuroblastoma	
Congenital tumors	
Germinomas	
Craniopharyngioma	Suprasellar, chiasmal
Arachnoid cysts	

Thus, a right jerk nystagmus becomes much worse on right gaze and improves significantly on left gaze. A patient with a right jerk nystagmus would therefore develop a right head turn, left gaze preference (Fig 12-1).

Evaluation

History

Many forms of nystagmus are inherited, either as a direct genetic abnormality or because of an association with other ocular diseases (Table 12-2). A thorough family history is therefore important in the initial evaluation. Questions should be asked about other types of inherited ocular diseases, systemic diseases, or syndromes known to affect visual development. Examination of family members with nystagmus can provide valuable prognostic information about the anticipated visual function in affected children. Although nystagmus can be inherited as an autosomal dominant or recessive trait, the most common form is an X-linked disorder.

Events at the time of delivery can significantly affect the developing visual system and, if severe enough, can result in nystagmus. Inquiries as to whether there were problems with labor and delivery, maternal infections, and prematurity can illuminate the cause of nystagmus. In children older than 3 months, parental observations about head tilts, head movements, gaze preference, and viewing distances can aid in diagnosis and possible future management.

Ocular Examination

The ophthalmic evaluation should concentrate on visual acuity testing, pupillary responses, ocular motility, and funduscopic examination.

CHAPTER 12: Childhood Nystagmus • 153

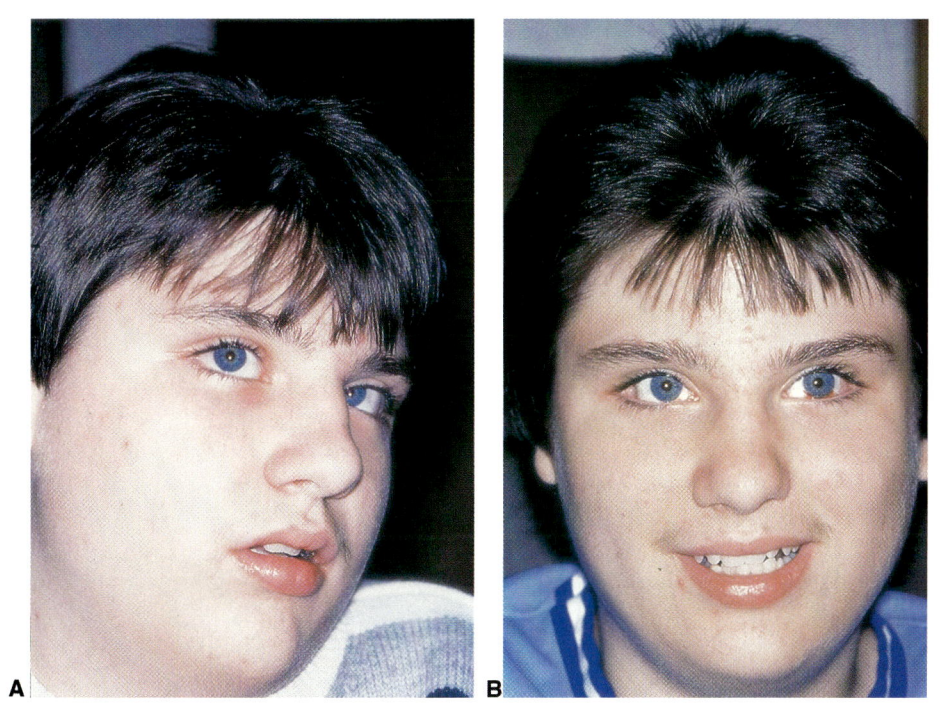

Figure 12-1 A, Patient with left face turn, right gaze preference due to a left beating jerk nystagmus. Visual acuity was 20/30 in right gaze and 20/60 facing straight. **B,** After nystagmus surgery consisting of recession of the left medial and right lateral rectus, and resection of the right medial and left lateral rectus, the face turn was eliminated. *(Photographs courtesy of Edward G. Buckley, MD.)*

Table 12-2 Ocular Conditions Associated With Nystagmus

Ocular coloboma
  Optic nerve
  Retinal
Congenital cataract
Congenital glaucoma
Retinoblastoma
Cicatricial retinopathy of prematurity
Iridocorneal dysgenesis
Aniridia
Retinal dysplasia
Congenital toxoplasmosis
Congenital "macular coloboma"
Leber congenital amaurosis
Bilateral optic nerve hypoplasia/atrophy
Albinism
  Ocular albinism
  Oculocutaneous albinism
Achromatopsia
Congenital stationary night blindness
Congenital retinoschisis

Visual acuity testing

The level of visual function can be helpful in determining the cause of nystagmus. Patients with nystagmus and nearly normal visual acuity usually have congenital motor nystagmus, which is a benign entity. Markedly decreased visual acuity usually implies either retinal or optic nerve abnormalities.

Visual acuity should be measured at distance and near as well as under binocular conditions, allowing children to use whatever head position or movement they choose. This last measurement is crucial in establishing the true functional visual performance. Near visual acuity is usually better than distance and can give a measure of the difficulty the child is likely to experience in a school setting. Many children with 20/400 or worse distance acuity can read at the 20/40 to 20/60 level by viewing the material at close range. Glasses or other devices can enable these children to attend regular schools.

In preverbal children, the optokinetic response to vertically moving targets can be useful in predicting further visual function. If a vertical optokinetic nystagmus (OKN) response can be superimposed on the child's underlying nystagmus, the visual function is usually 20/400 or better. Preferential looking can also be a useful test but often must be performed vertically in patients with a horizontal nystagmus.

Pupils

Pupils should be assessed for asymmetry, direct reaction to light, afferent defect, reaction to darkness, and anatomical structure. Sluggish or absent response to light indicates severe anterior visual pathway abnormalities such as optic nerve or retinal dysfunction. Responses can be normal in mild abnormalities such as macular hypoplasia, rod monochromatism, and primary motor nystagmus. An afferent pupillary defect also suggests an optic nerve or retinal cause, though with asymmetrical involvement.

A particularly useful pupillary response, when present, is the paradoxical pupillary constriction to darkness. The normal response to darkness is the immediate dilation of the pupil. If instead of dilating the pupils paradoxically constrict, optic nerve or retinal disease is present (Table 12-3). In addition to pupillary responses, iris structure should be assessed. Defects such as colobomas may indicate similar optic nerve or retinal defects. Iris transillumination defects are the hallmark of ocular albinism, which is associated with macular hypoplasia, poor vision, and nystagmus. Absence of the iris, or *aniridia*, is also associated with macular hypoplasia and nystagmus.

Table 12-3 Differential Diagnosis of Paradoxical Pupillary Phenomena

Congenital stationary night blindness
Congenital achromatopsia
Optic nerve hypoplasia
Leber congenital amaurosis
Best disease
Albinism
Retinitis pigmentosa

Ocular motility

Patients with nystagmus often have strabismus, either as a result of poor vision or as an attempt to dampen the nystagmus by converging. Some children with nystagmus fixate with the eye in adduction and turn their heads to look across their noses. This maneuver can be used at distance or near to improve visual acuity. The combination of a nystagmus and esotropia has been termed *nystagmus blockage syndrome.* This presents characteristically as an esotropia that "eats up prism" on attempted measurement. This syndrome also exhibits an increased jerk nystagmus on attempted lateral gaze. Any child with an esotropia should be examined carefully for this type of underlying nystagmus.

Fundus

Funduscopic evaluation should concentrate on abnormalities of the optic nerve and macula. Optic nerve or macular hypoplasia is common in children with nystagmus. Although many of the retinal disorders are associated with visible abnormalities, in some of the disorders the fundus appears normal or retinal pigmentary changes are subtle (Table 12-4). In patients with nystagmus and normal-appearing posterior poles, electrophysiologic testing may be necessary to identify the cause.

> Barricks ME, Flynn JT, Kushner BJ. Paradoxical pupillary response in congenital stationary night blindness. *Arch Ophthalmol.* 1977;95:1800–1804.
>
> Buckley EG. The clinical approach to the pediatric patient with nystagmus. *Int Pediatr.* 1990;5:225–231.

Childhood Nystagmus Types

Congenital Nystagmus

Congenital motor nystagmus

Congenital motor nystagmus (Table 12-5) is a binocular conjugate nystagmus that is usually uniplanar and horizontal, and it commonly remains horizontal on up- and downgaze. Congenital motor nystagmus can be pendular, jerk, circular, or elliptical, and more than one type may exist in the same individual. The characteristic waveform of congenital motor jerk nystagmus is a slow phase with an exponential increase in velocity. Congenital motor nystagmus is dampened by convergence and therefore is often associated with an

Table 12-4 Conditions Associated With Decreased Vision and Minimal Fundus Changes

> Leber congenital amaurosis
> Rod monochromacy
> Blue-cone monochromacy
> Hereditary optic atrophy
> Optic nerve hypoplasia
> Ocular albinism
> Congenital stationary night blindness

esotropia (nystagmus blockage syndrome). A *null point,* or *neutral zone,* may be present where the intensity of oscillations is diminished and the visual acuity improves. If the null point is not in primary position, anomalous head postures may be assumed to dampen the nystagmus and provide the best visual acuity. Head bobbing or movement may also be present at first, though this usually decreases with age. Oscillopsia is rare (Fig 12-2).

Approximately two thirds of patients with congenital motor nystagmus with a jerk waveform exhibit a paradoxical inversion of the OKN response. Normally, if a patient with right jerk nystagmus views an OKN drum rotating to the patient's left (eliciting a pursuit left, jerk right response), the right jerk nystagmus will increase. However, patients with congenital motor nystagmus exhibit either a damped right jerk nystagmus or possibly even a left jerk nystagmus. This paradoxical response of left jerk instead of right jerk nystagmus occurs only in congenital motor nystagmus.

Table 12-5 Characteristics of Congenital Nystagmus

Bilateral
Conjugate
Horizontal
Worsens with attempted fixation
Improves with convergence
Null point often present with head position
Two thirds of patients have "inverted" OKN response
Oscillopsia usually not present

Figure 12-2 Left jerk nystagmus. **A,** Electronystagmographic evaluation of congenital motor nystagmus shows exponential increase in velocity of the slow phase. **B,** Manifest latent nystagmus shows a waveform with an exponential decrease in velocity of the slow phase.

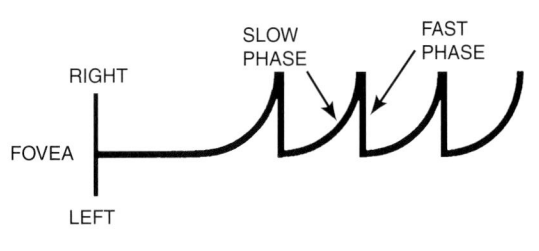

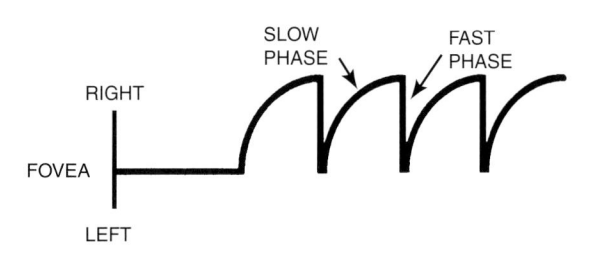

Some cases of congenital motor nystagmus may be inherited as an autosomal dominant, recessive, or X-linked trait. Purely congenital motor nystagmus is not associated with other central nervous system abnormalities. Visual function is quite good and can be near normal. Patients develop a preferred gaze position to utilize a null location. This head position becomes more obvious as the child reaches school age.

Sensory defect nystagmus

Sensory defect nystagmus, another congenital form, is secondary to an abnormality in the afferent visual pathway. Inadequate image formation results in failure of development of the normal fixation reflex. If visual loss is present at birth, the resulting nystagmus begins in the first 3 months of life. The severity of the nystagmus usually depends on the severity of the visual loss. All waveforms may be present, but pendular nystagmus is most common. On lateral gaze, the nystagmus may become jerk. Searching, slow, wandering, or conjugate eye movements may also be observed. Sensory defect is the most common cause of nystagmus in the pediatric population.

Optic nerve disorders such as hypoplasia and coloboma, and retinal diseases such as albinism, achromatopsia, stationary night blindness, X-linked juvenile retinoschisis, and Leber congenital amaurosis, can all give rise to nystagmus. In general, the character of the nystagmus typically reflects the severity of the visual loss in the perinatal period. Searching nystagmus defined as roving or drifting, typically horizontal movement of the eyes without fixation is usually observed in children whose vision is worse than 20/200. Pendular nystagmus occurs when the visual acuity is better than 20/200 in at least one eye. Jerk nystagmus is often associated with visual acuity between 20/60 and 20/100.

Periodic alternating nystagmus

Periodic alternating nystagmus is an unusual form of congenital motor jerk nystagmus that periodically changes direction. Typically, the motion starts with a jerk nystagmus in one direction that lasts for 60–90 seconds and then slowly begins to dampen. A period of no nystagmus lasts anywhere from 10 to 20 seconds, and then the nystagmus begins to jerk in the opposite direction. The nystagmus continues to jerk in the opposite direction for 60–90 seconds, and then the process repeats itself. Some children adopt an alternate head position to take advantage of the changing null position. The cause of congenital periodic alternating nystagmus is unknown, but it has been associated with oculocutaneous albinism.

Latent nystagmus

Latent nystagmus is a congenital conjugate horizontal jerk nystagmus that occurs under conditions of monocular fixation. When one eye is occluded, a jerk nystagmus develops in both eyes with the fast phase directed toward the uncovered eye. Thus, a left jerk nystagmus of both eyes occurs when the right eye is covered. When the left eye is covered, both eyes show right jerk nystagmus. This nystagmus is the only form that reverses direction with a change in fixation. Asymmetries in amplitude, frequency, and velocity of the nystagmus can also be present, depending on which eye is covered.

Latent nystagmus is often noted in early childhood, especially in patients with congenital esotropia and dissociated vertical deviation. The cause is unknown. Because a nystagmus is induced when an eye is covered, binocular visual acuity is better than monocular, and occlusion must be avoided during monocular tests of vision. Use of polarizing lenses and a polarized chart, blurring of the nontested eye with a +5.00 D sphere, or repositioning of the occluder several inches in front of the eye not being tested can be effective.

A latent nystagmus may become manifest *(manifest latent nystagmus)* when both eyes are open but only one eye is being used for vision (ie, the other eye is suppressed or amblyopic). Just as with latent nystagmus, occlusion of the preferred eye results in a change in the direction of the jerk nystagmus. Electronystagmographic evaluation of latent and manifest latent nystagmus reveals a similar waveform with an exponential decrease in velocity of the slow phase. This pattern is the opposite of congenital motor nystagmus, which shows an exponential increase in velocity of the slow phase (see Fig 12-2). Latent nystagmus may be superimposed on congenital motor nystagmus.

> Dell'Osso LF, Schmidt D, Daroff RB. Latent, manifest latent, and congenital nystagmus. *Arch Ophthalmol.* 1979;97:1877–1885.

Acquired Nystagmus

Spasmus nutans

Spasmus nutans is an acquired nystagmus that occurs in children 3–24 months old. Spasmus nutans is usually associated with a triad of findings including nystagmus, head nodding, and torticollis. The nystagmus is generally bilateral; however, it can be monocular, asymmetrical, and variable in different gaze positions. It is a small-amplitude, high-frequency nystagmus *(shimmering)* and often difficult to see. It can be horizontal, vertical, or rotary and is occasionally intermittent. In most cases, spasmus nutans is a benign disorder, but a nystagmus form characteristic of spasmus nutans has been associated with chiasmal or suprachiasmal tumors in children with other central nervous system abnormalities. When doubt persists about the cause of presumed spasmus nutans, neuroradiologic investigation is warranted. Spasmus nutans occasionally can be familial and has been present in monozygotic twins. It usually disappears by age 3–4 years.

> Arnoldi KA, Tychsen L. Prevalence of intracranial lesions in children initially diagnosed with disconjugate nystagmus (spasmus nutans). *J Pediatr Ophthalmol Strabismus.* 1995;32:296–301.
>
> Garty BZ, Weitz R, Mimouni M, et al. Spasmus nutans as a presenting sign of diencephalic syndrome [letter]. *J Pediatr.* 1985;107:484.
>
> Koenig SB, Naidich TP, Zaparackas Z. Optic glioma masquerading as spasmus nutans. *J Pediatr Ophthalmol Strabismus.* 1982;19:20–24.
>
> Norton EWD, Cogan DG. Spasmus nutans: a clinical study of twenty cases followed two years or more since onset. *Arch Ophthalmol.* 1954;52:442–446.

See-saw nystagmus

An unusual but dramatic type of nystagmus, see-saw nystagmus has both vertical and torsional components. The name derives from the action of the playground device. If the eyes were placed on a see-saw, one at either end, they would "roll down the plank" as the see-saw rose, with the high eye intorting and the low eye extorting. As the direction of the see-saw changed, so would that of the eye movement. Thus, the eyes make alternating movements of elevation and intorsion followed by depression and extorsion.

This type of nystagmus is often associated with a lesion in the rostral midbrain or the suprasellar area. In children, the most likely intracranial tumor is a craniopharyngioma. Confrontation visual fields may elicit a bitemporal visual field defect. Neuroradiologic evaluation is necessary. The treatment for see-saw nystagmus is to remove the inciting cause.

> Daroff RB. See saw nystagmus. *Neurology.* 1963;3:306–311.

Nystagmus retractorius (dorsal midbrain syndrome)

Convergence-retraction nystagmus is a part of the dorsal midbrain syndrome associated with paralysis of upward gaze, defective convergence, and light–near dissociation. Unlike other types of childhood nystagmus, this form may be noticed only under particular circumstances. It is best elicited on attempted fast upgaze, when cocontraction of all the horizontal extraocular muscles occurs and the eyes are pulled into the orbit (hence the term *retractorius*). The eyes often converge on attempted upgaze as well. Voluntary convergence, however, is minimal. There is an associated pupillary abnormality with marked light–near dissociation. In the pediatric age group, convergence-retraction nystagmus is most commonly secondary to congenital aqueductal stenosis or a pinealoma.

Opsoclonus

Opsoclonus is an extremely rare eye movement disorder that is not a true nystagmus but a bizarre ocular oscillation. Opsoclonus is rapid, involuntary, and multivectorial. It can be present intermittently and often has a very-high-frequency, low-amplitude movement. The movements are so fast and chaotic that they are not easily confused with other forms of infantile nystagmus. The most common cause of opsoclonus is probably an acute cerebellar ataxia of childhood. The child presents with "dancing eyes and dancing feet." Opsoclonus can be a sign of occult neuroblastoma, a consequence of epidemic encephalitis of viral origin, or an effect of hydrocephalus.

Downbeat nystagmus

Downbeat nystagmus is a jerk nystagmus with the fast component downward. It obeys Alexander's law and is maximum in downgaze and down to the left and right. Downbeat nystagmus often has a null position in upgaze. When congenital, this condition is associated with good vision and normal neurologic findings. An acquired hereditary form of downbeat nystagmus may precede spinal cerebellar degeneration. More commonly, downbeat nystagmus is acquired. Structural abnormalities at the craniocervical junction produce compression of the caudal brain stem. The most common of these abnormalities is the Arnold-Chiari malformation. In this condition, the cerebellar tonsils herniate through the foramen magnum. At this point, they compress the brain stem, resulting in downbeat nystagmus. Decompression of this area often results in complete resolution. Pharmacologic agents such as lithium, tranquilizers, and anticonvulsants may also cause this condition.

> Schulman JA, Shults WT, Jones JM Jr. Monocular vertical nystagmus as an initial sign of chiasmal glioma. *Am J Ophthalmol.* 1979;87:87–90.

Monocular nystagmus

Monocular nystagmus has been reported to occur in severely amblyopic and blind eyes. The oscillations are pendular, chiefly vertical, slow, small in amplitude, and irregular in frequency. Monocular nystagmus is often difficult to detect, and it may be rare in infants and small children.

> Farmer J, Hoyt CS. Monocular nystagmus in infancy and early childhood. *Am J Ophthalmol*. 1984;98:504–509.
>
> Yee RD, Jelks GW, Baloh RW, et al. Uniocular nystagmus in monocular visual loss. *Ophthalmology*. 1979;86:511–522.

Dissociated nystagmus

Dissociated nystagmus (nystagmus in the abducting eye) occurs in several instances. The nystagmus seen with internuclear ophthalmoplegia is most common. Surgical weakening of the medial rectus muscle has also been reported to cause a nystagmus of the contralateral abducting eye similar to that seen with internuclear ophthalmoplegia. With internuclear ophthalmoplegia, however, a slowing of saccades in the adducting eye also occurs (which is not the case with pseudointernuclear ophthalmoplegia after surgical paresis of the medial rectus muscle). Myasthenia gravis may also simulate an internuclear ophthalmoplegia with nystagmus of the abducting eye.

> Cogan DG. Dissociated nystagmus with lesions in the posterior fossa. *Arch Ophthalmol*. 1963;70:361–368.
>
> von Noorden GK, Tredici TD, Ruttum M. Pseudo-internuclear ophthalmoplegia after surgical paresis of the medial rectus muscle. *Am J Ophthalmol*. 1984;98:602–608.

Differential Diagnosis

Figure 12-3 lists the signs and symptoms of various forms of horizontal nystagmus in children along with guidelines for testing and systemic associations.

Treatment

Prisms

Prisms, extraocular muscle surgery, or both can be used to reduce compensatory head positions and to improve visual acuity. Prisms can optically improve head positions by shifting the image into the null zone area or improve visual acuity by stimulating convergence. Prisms can be used as the sole treatment or as a trial to predict surgical success. To correct head positions, prisms are placed to shift the image into the null point area. Fresnel Press-On prisms are ideal for this because powers of 10Δ–20Δ are often necessary. Each prism is mounted with the apex pointing to the direction of the null zone. For example, with a left head turn and a null zone in right gaze, prisms before the right eye should be oriented base-in and prisms before the left eye should be oriented base-out. This shifts the image to the right by decreasing the amount of turn the patient requires to gain the same visual benefit. If this technique improves the head position, strabismus surgery is also likely to be effective.

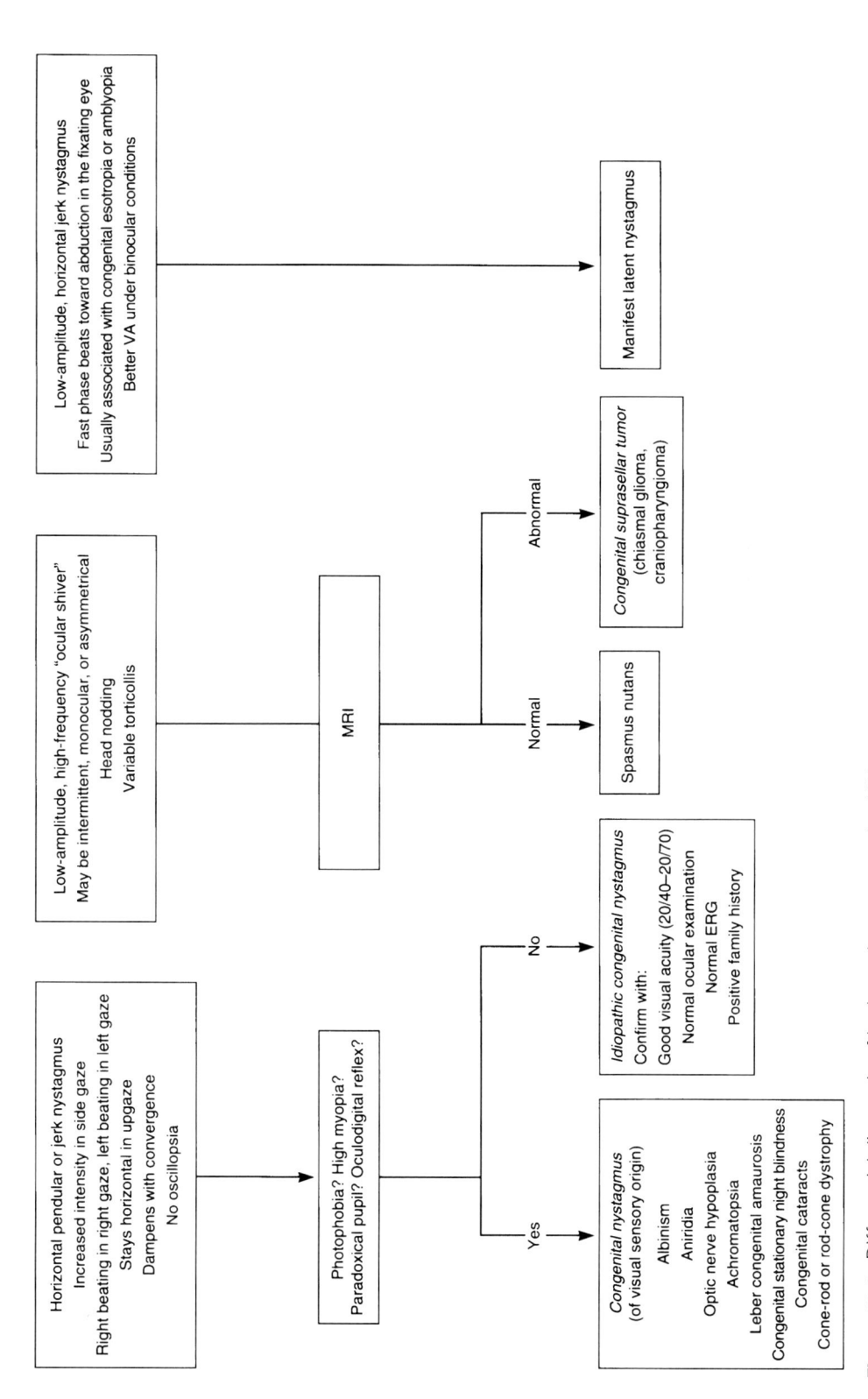

Figure 12-3 Differential diagnosis of horizontal nystagmus in children. *(Modified from Brodsky MC, Baker RS, Hameed LM. Pediatric Neuro-Ophthalmology. New York: Springer-Verlag; 1995:339.)*

Base-out prism spectacles can be used to improve visual acuity by stimulating fusional convergence, which dampens the nystagmus. In this situation, base-out prisms are placed in front of both eyes in amounts ranging from 5Δ to 10Δ. A trial of Fresnel prisms can be used before incorporating these into spectacles. The ideal amount is determined by trial and error.

Nystagmus Surgery

Surgery for nystagmus is indicated to correct a head turn by shifting the null point to the primary position and to improve visual acuity by decreasing nystagmus intensity and broadening the null zone. The types of surgery typically recommended are a recess-resect procedure performed on both eyes *(Kestenbaum-Anderson)* or a four-horizontal-muscle recession. In the Kestenbaum-Anderson procedure, the eyes are surgically rotated toward the direction of the head turn and away from the null zone or preferred position of gaze. For example, if a patient with congenital nystagmus has a left face turn and null zone in right gaze, the eyes are surgically rotated to the left by recession of the right lateral and left medial rectus muscles, and resection of the right medial and left lateral rectus muscles. This, in effect, makes it harder for the patient to look into right gaze, thereby dampening the nystagmus more toward the primary position.

The amount of resection-recession performed using the Kestenbaum-Anderson procedure has been modified to improve long-term results. Table 12-6 describes the original Kestenbaum-Anderson procedure for horizontal rectus muscle surgery to both eyes plus two different modifications. Each eye undergoes a recess-resect procedure to move the eyes in the same direction. *The total amount of surgery for each eye (as measured in millimeters) is equal in order to rotate each globe an equal amount.* Each of the modifications recommends greater amounts of surgery by increasing Parks' original figures by 40% or 60%. Measurements are rounded off to the nearest 0.5 mm at surgery. For head turns of 30°, the 40% augmented procedure is recommended; for face turns of 45°, the 60% augmentation procedure is used. The augmented procedures may cause restriction of motility, which is usually necessary to achieve a satisfactory result.

If vertical torticollis is present with congenital nystagmus, chin-up or -down posturing may be ameliorated by surgery on the vertical rectus muscles. As with horizontal nystagmus, the eyes are rotated away from the null point. Thus, if a chin-up, gaze-down posture is present, the inferior rectus muscles are recessed and the superior rectus muscles

Table 12-6 **Kestenbaum-Anderson Procedure and Modifications**

Procedure	Kestenbaum	40% Augmented	60% Augmented
Recess medial rectus	5.0 mm	7.0 mm	8.0 mm
Resect medial rectus	6.0 mm	8.4 mm	9.6 mm
Recess lateral rectus	7.0 mm	9.8 mm	11.2 mm
Resect lateral rectus	8.0 mm	11.2 mm	12.8 mm
Total surgery	13.0 mm	18.2 mm	20.8 mm
R + R	(5+8) = (6+7)	(7+11.2) = (8.4+9.8)	(8+12.8) = (9.6+11.2)

are resected. The amount of surgery varies but usually is 5–7 mm of recession and resection on each eye.

An alternative to the standard Kestenbaum-Anderson procedure is a recession of all the horizontal rectus muscles to a position posterior to the equator. This usually requires 8–10 mm of recession of both medial rectus muscles and 10–12 mm of recession of both lateral rectus muscles. This approach may be especially beneficial in improving visual function when head position is not a problem.

Surgery for nystagmus blockage syndrome involves recession of the medial rectus muscles, usually with amounts that are slightly larger than normal. This can be combined with a posterior fixation suture to enhance the effect.

For patients with nystagmus, head turn, and strabismus, the above procedures can be modified. The described nystagmus surgery often is performed on the dominant fixating eye; surgery on the nondominant eye is adjusted to account for the strabismus. For example, a patient who is right eye dominant and has a right head turn and left gaze preference would undergo a right medial rectus recession and right lateral rectus resection in the amounts indicated in Table 12-6. The left eye would then either receive no surgery or much less correction so as not to recreate the esotropia.

Flynn JT, Dell'Osso LF. The effects of congenital nystagmus surgery. *Ophthalmology*. 1979; 86:1414–1425.

Kestenbaum A. Nouvelle opération du nystagmus. *Bull Soc Ophtalmol Fr*. 1953;6:599–602.

Nelson LB, Ervin-Mulvey LD, Calhoun JH, et al. Surgical management for abnormal head position in nystagmus: the augmented modified Kestenbaum procedure. *Br J Ophthalmol*. 1984;68:796–800.

Roberts EL, Saunders RA, Wilson ME. Surgery for vertical head position in null point nystagmus. *J Pediatr Ophthalmol Strabismus*. 1996;33:219–224.

Zubcov AA, Stark N, Weber A, et al. Improvement of visual acuity after surgery for nystagmus. *Ophthalmology*. 1993;100:1488–1497.

CHAPTER 13

Surgery of the Extraocular Muscles

Both the experienced and the beginning strabismus surgeon should become familiar with the basic references and surgical atlases listed below. The following discussion does not specifically refer to these works, but the reader should turn to them when additional information is needed. See also Chapters 1 and 2 of this volume.

> Calhoun JH, Nelson LB, Harley RD. *Atlas of Pediatric Ophthalmic Surgery*. Philadelphia: Saunders; 1987.
>
> Del Monte MA, Archer SM. *Atlas of Pediatric Ophthalmology and Strabismus Surgery*. New York: Churchill Livingstone; 1993.
>
> Helveston EM. *Surgical Management of Strabismus*. 4th ed. St Louis: Mosby; 1993.
>
> Price RL, Beauchamp GR. *Strabismus Surgery: Rectus Recession and Resection* [videotape]. San Francisco: American Academy of Ophthalmology; 1989.
>
> Rosenbaum AL, Santiago AP. *Clinical Strabismus Management*. Philadelphia: Saunders; 1999.
>
> von Noorden GK. *Burian-von Noorden's Binocular Vision and Ocular Motility: Theory and Management of Strabismus*. 5th ed. St Louis: Mosby; 1996.
>
> Wright KW. *Color Atlas of Strabismus Surgery: Strabismus*. Irvine, CA: Wright; 2000.

A thorough knowledge of the anatomy of the extraocular muscles and surrounding fascia, along with an understanding of their motor physiology, is essential to planning and executing strabismus surgery. Lifelong problems for the patient can be avoided by the use of appropriate surgical technique guided by knowledge of the anatomy of the extraocular muscles and surrounding fascia. Similarly, the surgeon should become familiar with the appropriate types of surgical instruments, sutures, and needles used in strabismus surgery. The references mentioned above are excellent resources for this understanding.

The history and a detailed motility evaluation (often repeated at a subsequent visit to corroborate the initial findings), in conjunction with a complete ocular examination, provide the information necessary to plan the correct surgery. Evaluation may include sensory testing, forced duction testing, active force generation testing, saccadic velocities, and diplopia visual fields. Preoperative planning must address the patient's and family's expectations as well as those of the surgeon, and risks and complications must be discussed. Such communication is the basis of informed patient consent.

Indications for Surgery

Surgery is performed to improve function, appearance, and well-being. The indications for surgery may be subtle or obvious. Asthenopia, a vague but real sense of ocular fatigue, is common in patients with phorias or intermittent tropias. Occasionally, subconjunctival scar tissue from prior muscle surgery may warrant additional surgical revision to improve appearance or to relieve mechanical restriction.

Double vision in one or all fields of gaze is often the complaint of patients with adult-onset strabismus, and eliminating diplopia is one of the goals of strabismus surgery. If some degree of fusion can be achieved, postsurgical ocular alignment will be improved. Alignment of the visual axes can restore stereopsis in some patients or allow the development of a certain amount of stereopsis in others, especially if the preoperative deviation is intermittent or of recent onset.

Some patients assume an abnormal head position to relieve diplopia (eg, with superior oblique or lateral rectus muscle weakness) or to improve vision (eg, with nystagmus and an eccentric null point). Surgical treatment may not only increase the field of useful vision but reduce habitual head posturing. Correcting an abnormal head position or eliminating an ocular deviation can, in turn, improve the patient's self-image and sense of well-being. Strabismus is not a variation of normal; therefore, correcting it is reconstructive rather than cosmetic surgery, even if enhanced fusion is not feasible.

> Coats DK, Paysse EA, Towler MA, et al. Impact of large angle horizontal strabismus on ability to obtain employment. *Ophthalmology*. 2000;107:402–405.
>
> Hertle RW. Clinical characteristics of surgically treated adult strabismus. *J Pediatr Ophthalmol Strabismus*. 1998;35:138.
>
> Satterfield D, Keltner JL, Morrison TL. Psychosocial aspects of strabismus. *Arch Ophthalmol*. 1993;111:1100.

Surgical Techniques for the Muscles and Tendons

Weakening Procedures

Table 13-1 defines the various weakening procedures and describes when each would be used.

Strengthening Procedures

To strengthen or enhance the effect of a muscle or tendon, surgeons usually use the resection technique:

- Absorbable sutures are placed at a predetermined distance posterior to the muscle insertion
- The muscle anterior to the position of the sutures is excised (resected)
- The shortened muscle is reattached to the globe at or near the original insertion

This technique is commonly used on any of the rectus muscles and rarely used to strengthen either of the oblique muscles. For detailed descriptions of the techniques, see the basic references listed at the beginning of the chapter.

A rectus muscle can also be strengthened by *advancing* the insertion nearer the limbus, a technique especially useful if the muscle has been previously recessed. Advancement of a muscle to a position anterior to its original anatomical insertion is rarely

Table 13-1 Weakening Procedures Used in Strabismus Surgery

Procedure	Used for
Myotomy: cutting across a muscle *Myectomy:* removing a portion of muscle	Used by some surgeons to weaken the inferior oblique muscles
Marginal myotomy: cutting partway across a muscle, usually following a maximal recession	To weaken a rectus muscle further
Tenotomy: cutting across a tendon *Tenectomy:* removing a portion of tendon	Both used routinely to weaken the superior oblique muscle; recently, silicone spacers have been interposed by some surgeons to control the weakening effect
Recession: removal and reattachment of a muscle (rectus or oblique) so that its insertion is closer to its origin	The standard weakening procedure for rectus muscles
Denervation and extirpation: the ablation of the entire portion of the muscle, along with its nerve supply, within Tenon's capsule	Used only on severely or recurrently overacting inferior oblique muscles
Recession and anteriorization: movement of the muscle's insertion anterior to its original position	Also used only on the inferior oblique muscle, to change its action from elevation to depression; particularly useful when an inferior oblique muscle overaction and dissociated vertical deviation (DVD) both exist
Posterior fixation suture (fadenoperation): attachment of a rectus muscle to the sclera 11–18 mm posterior to the insertion using a nonabsorbable suture; this procedure is difficult to perform	Used to weaken a muscle in its field of action by decreasing its mechanical advantage; often used in conjunction with recession; sometimes used in DVD, nystagmus, high AC/A esotropia, and noncomitant strabismus

performed because the muscle may become visible under the conjunctiva. The anterior half of the superior oblique tendon may be advanced temporally and toward the limbus, in the Harada-Ito procedure, to reduce excyclotorsion in patients with superior oblique muscle paresis.

The *tucking procedure* can be performed on the superior oblique tendon to enhance its effect, especially for superior oblique muscle paresis. However, tucking the superior oblique tendon may produce an iatrogenic Brown syndrome. For step-by-step techniques, see the basic references listed at the beginning of the chapter.

Adjustable Suture Techniques

Adjustable strabismus sutures have been used for many years in one form or another to improve the outcome of strabismus surgery. The purpose of adjustable strabismus sutures is to increase the likelihood of reaching the desired surgical alignment with one operation, thereby decreasing the need for staged operations and reoperations. Adjustable suture techniques do not solve the problem of long-term alignment (or permanence of the surgical results), which depends on the potential for fusion, the establishment of focused and comparable retinal images in both eyes, and the effect of tonic and innervational forces acting on the extraocular muscles.

Improved synthetic suture materials, refined surgical techniques, and the continued unpredictability of strabismus surgery have stimulated increased use of adjustable suture techniques. Various types of adjustable suture techniques have been described; some are included below.

Postoperative (two-stage) adjustment

Strabismus surgery is completed in the operating room using externalized sutures and knots so that the position of the muscle can be altered during the postoperative period as needed to obtain alignment.

Operation/reoperation

The strabismus surgery is completed using only short-acting or reversible anesthetic agents and externalized sutures and knots. The patient is examined a short time after surgery and reanesthetized for the final tying or adjustment of the sutures as indicated by the postoperative evaluation. This method has been used successfully in children. However, because a second general anesthesia is required, this technique offers little advantage over standard nonadjustable surgery with possible reoperation.

Topical anesthesia

The surgery is completed with the patient awake. Drugs that might affect ocular motility are avoided, and the patient's dynamic ocular motility and ocular alignment are observed and adjusted at the time of surgery. This technique requires a cooperative patient and is not appropriate for most patients who have significant scarring and need a reoperation, persons with thyroid ophthalmopathy, and almost all children. (Anesthesia is discussed later under Anesthesia for Extraocular Muscle Surgery.)

Pull-over (stay) sutures

A temporary suture is attached to the limbus and secured to periocular skin to fix the eye in a selected position during postoperative healing. This technique is particularly useful in cases with severely restricted rotations.

Transposition Procedures

Transposition procedures involve moving the extraocular muscles out of their original planes of action. These procedures are generally reserved for treatment of paralytic strabismus, small vertical and horizontal deviations, and A and V patterns. The usual indications for transposition procedures include paralysis of cranial nerves III and VI as well as monocular elevation deficiency. See the basic references at the beginning of this chapter for detailed descriptions of these techniques.

Considerations in Planning Surgery for Strabismus

Incomitance
Deviations that vary in different gaze positions require special alterations in technique to make the postoperative alignment more nearly comitant.

Vertical incomitance
If a horizontal deviation in the primary position is significantly different in upgaze and downgaze, an A or a V pattern is present (see Chapter 10). Surgical treatment may include surgery on the oblique muscles or displacement (upward or downward) of the horizontal rectus muscles.

Horizontal incomitance
If the deviation in left and right gaze is significantly different from the deviation in primary gaze, a paresis or restriction may be present. If the restriction is stable, surgical correction as illustrated in the following example might be considered:

XT = 20Δ	XT = 30Δ	XT = 40Δ
right gaze	primary position	left gaze

The surgeon might do one of the following:

- Perform a recession of each lateral rectus muscle, the left more than the right, to achieve greater reduction of the exotropia in the field of action of the left lateral rectus (ie, left gaze).
- Perform a greater recession of the left lateral rectus muscle and lesser resection of the left medial rectus muscle than the standard amount to achieve greater effect in left gaze.

Lateral incomitance
Standard amounts of surgery for intermittent exotropia may result in overcorrection if measurements in side gaze are substantially less than in primary position. For example:

XT = 15Δ	XT = 30Δ	XT = 15Δ
right gaze	primary position	left gaze

Some surgeons recommend reducing the amount of recession of each lateral rectus slightly in these patients.

> Moore S. The prognostic value of lateral gaze measurements in intermittent exotropia. *Am Orthopt J.* 1969;19:69–71.

Prior Surgery
It is technically easier and therefore preferable to operate on muscles that have not undergone prior surgery. However, each case must be considered individually. In cases of

mechanical restriction from excessive resection/scarring or weakness from excessive recession, these problems must be relieved by reoperation on the involved muscle to obtain optimal surgical results. Previous operative reports may be helpful in surgical planning. If retinal detachment surgery has been performed in the past, consultation with the retinal surgeon is advisable. In some cases, it may be preferable to operate on the other eye.

Cyclovertical Strabismus

In many patients with vertical strabismus, the deviation is different in right and left gaze. In some patients, the vertical deviation is different between upgaze to one side and downgaze to that side. In general, surgery should be performed on those muscles whose field of action is in the same field as the greatest vertical deviation. For example, in a patient with a right hypertropia that is greatest down and to the patient's left, the surgeon should strongly consider either strengthening the right superior oblique muscle or weakening the left inferior rectus muscle. If the right hypertropia is the same in left upgaze, straight left, and left downgaze, then any of the four muscles whose greatest vertical action is in left gaze may be chosen for surgery. In this example, the left superior rectus muscle or right superior oblique muscle could be strengthened, or the left inferior rectus muscle or right inferior oblique muscle could be weakened. Larger deviations may require surgery on more than one muscle.

Visual Acuity

Surgery is normally delayed until the vision has been made equal or nearly so by whatever means are appropriate, including spectacles and amblyopia therapy.

Guidelines for Strabismus Surgery

Two surgeons are unlikely to perform a specific surgical procedure in exactly the same fashion. Thus, the amount of dissection, the measurement and placement of sutures in the muscle and sclera, and the conjunctival incision will vary slightly between surgeons, even when both are following the same surgical table. Nonetheless, the beginning surgeon will find these guidelines a useful starting point for routine strabismus surgery.

Each surgeon must standardize his or her approach by continually reviewing the results and adjusting the amount of surgery to achieve the best possible outcomes. Thus, the surgery should be planned according to the surgeon's own ocular motility measurements and judgment.

Esodeviation

Symmetrical surgery

The amounts of medial rectus recession often performed in each eye of patients with specified deviations are given in Table 13-2. Some surgeons would advocate medial rectus muscle recessions of 6.5–7.0 mm for 60Δ–80Δ of esotropia; others avoid these very large recessions and favor operating on three or four muscles for large angles.

Monocular recess-resect procedures

The same figures given in Table 13-2 may be used, selecting the appropriate number of millimeters for each muscle as shown in Table 13-3. For example, for an esotropia of 30Δ, the surgeon would recess the medial rectus muscle 4.5 mm and resect the lateral rectus muscle 7.0 mm.

Exodeviation

Symmetrical surgery

The surgical guidelines for exodeviation are listed in Table 13-4. Some surgeons advocate bilateral lateral rectus muscle recessions of 9.0 mm or greater for deviations larger than 45Δ. Others advocate surgery on a third muscle for large-angle exotropias.

Table 13-2 Symmetrical Surgery for Esodeviation

Angle of Esotropia	Recess MR OU	or	Resect LR OU
15Δ	3.0 mm		4.0 mm
20Δ	3.5 mm		5.0 mm
25Δ	4.0 mm		6.0 mm
30Δ	4.5 mm		7.0 mm
35Δ	5.0 mm		8.0 mm
40Δ	5.5 mm		9.0 mm
50Δ	6.0 mm		9.0 mm

Table 13-3 Monocular Recess-Resect Procedures for Esodeviation

Angle of Esotropia	Recess MR	and	Resect LR
15Δ	3.0 mm		4.0 mm
20Δ	3.5 mm		5.0 mm
25Δ	4.0 mm		6.0 mm
30Δ	4.5 mm		7.0 mm
35Δ	5.0 mm		8.0 mm
40Δ	5.5 mm		9.0 mm
50Δ	6.0 mm		9.0 mm

Table 13-4 Symmetrical Surgery for Exodeviation

Angle of Exotropia	Recess LR OU	or	Resect MR OU
15Δ	4.0 mm		3.0 mm
20Δ	5.0 mm		4.0 mm
25Δ	6.0 mm		5.0 mm
30Δ	7.0 mm		6.0 mm
40Δ	8.0 mm		6.0 mm

Monocular recess-resect procedures

As with esodeviations, the surgical table can be used for monocular procedures as well as for symmetrical surgery, reading across according to the angle of deviation (Table 13-5). For example, for an exodeviation of 15Δ, the surgeon would recess the lateral rectus muscle 4.0 mm and resect the antagonist medial rectus muscle 3.0 mm. Monocular surgery of large-angle exotropia is likely to result in a limitation of abduction.

> Price RL, Beauchamp GR. *Strabismus Surgery: Rectus Recession and Resection* [videotape]. San Francisco: American Academy of Ophthalmology; 1989.

Value of immediate overcorrection in exodeviation

The surgical dosages listed in Table 13-4 for bilateral lateral rectus recessions tend to produce a small overcorrection of exotropia in the early postoperative period. Available evidence suggests that a small temporary esotropia during the first few days or weeks after surgery may yield the most favorable long-term result. Many patients have diplopia during the time they are esotropic, and they should be advised of this possibility.

> Raab EL, Parks MM. Recession of the lateral recti. Early and late postoperative alignment. *Arch Ophthalmol.* 1969;82:203–208.

Oblique Muscle-Weakening Procedures

Weakening the inferior oblique muscle

In cases that show a marked asymmetry of the overactions of the inferior oblique muscles with no superior oblique muscle paresis, unilateral surgery on the muscle with the most marked overaction is often followed by a significant degree of overaction in the fellow eye. Therefore, some surgeons recommend bilateral inferior oblique-weakening procedures, which can be graded if recessions are performed for bilateral overaction, even if asymmetrical. A good symmetrical result is the rule, and overcorrections are rare. Inferior oblique muscles that are not overacting should not undergo a surgical weakening procedure.

Secondary overaction of the inferior oblique muscle occurs in some patients who have superior oblique muscle paresis. In this situation, the greatest vertical deviation appears in the field of action of the ipsilateral inferior oblique muscle. A weakening of

Table 13-5 Monocular Recess-Resect Procedures for Exodeviation

Angle of Exotropia	Recess LR	and	Resect MR
15Δ	4.0 mm		3.0 mm
20Δ	5.0 mm		4.0 mm
25Δ	6.0 mm		5.0 mm
30Δ	7.0 mm		6.0 mm
40Δ	8.0 mm		6.0 mm
50Δ	9.0 mm		7.0 mm
60Δ	10.0 mm		8.0 mm
70Δ	10.0 mm		9.0 mm
80Δ	10.0 mm		10.0 mm

that inferior oblique muscle could be expected to correct up to 15Δ of vertical deviation in primary position. The amount of vertical correction is roughly proportional to the degree of preoperative overaction (see Chapter 9).

Frequently, a weakening procedure is performed on each inferior oblique muscle for V-pattern strabismus. Such surgery can be expected to cause 15Δ or more of eso shift in upgaze (decrease of an exodeviation or increase of an esodeviation), but weakening procedures have almost no effect on primary position or downgaze.

> Price RL, Beauchamp GR. *Strabismus Surgery: Oblique Procedures* [videotape]. San Francisco: American Academy of Ophthalmology; 1989.
> Stager DR, Parks MM. Inferior oblique weakening procedures. Effect on primary position horizontal alignment. *Arch Ophthalmol.* 1973;90:15–16.

Weakening the superior oblique muscle

Unilateral weakening of a superior oblique muscle is not commonly performed except as part of the treatment for Brown syndrome (see also the discussion of Brown syndrome in Chapter 9). This procedure may also be performed for an isolated inferior oblique muscle weakness, which is rare.

Bilateral weakening of the superior oblique muscle is often performed, with or without horizontal muscle surgery, for A-pattern deviations. This surgery can be expected to cause an eso shift of up to 30Δ–40Δ in downgaze, little change in primary position, and almost no effect in upgaze. In surgery on patients with normal binocularity, the possibility of creating diplopia from vertical or torsional strabismus must be considered.

Vertical Rectus Muscle Surgery for Hypotropia and Hypertropia

Because vertical deviations have many causes (eg, cyclovertical muscle palsy, mechanical restriction), no single approach for surgical correction can be recommended for all situations. Surgical planning must be individualized according to suspected cause and size of deviation. However, for small, largely comitant vertical deviations, recession or resection of vertical rectus muscles is frequently advocated. The atlases cited at the beginning of the chapter offer more specific guidance concerning selection of muscles and determination of the size of the recession or resection.

Dissociated vertical deviation

When treatment of dissociated vertical deviation is indicated, one of several surgical methods can be used. A recession of the superior rectus muscle, possibly on a "hangback" suture, of 6–10 mm is considered effective. Bilateral superior rectus muscle recession may be indicated whenever either eye can fixate. If only one eye can fixate, unilateral surgery is possible. Resection of the inferior rectus muscle for dissociated vertical deviation ranges from 4 mm for small deviations to 8 mm for large angles. This technique may advance the lower eyelid, especially if careful dissection is not performed. Some surgeons favor the fadenoperation or posterior fixation suture on the superior rectus muscle(s), often combined with recession.

Recession of the inferior oblique muscle with anteriorization of its insertion to a point adjacent to the lateral border of the inferior rectus has been found effective in reducing or eliminating dissociated vertical deviation; the mechanical tethering/depressing effect is important. This procedure is especially useful when a patient has both dissociated vertical deviation and a component of inferior oblique overaction.

Other Rectus Muscle Surgery

Vertical displacement of the horizontal rectus muscles for A and V patterns

Vertical displacement of two horizontal rectus muscles (one-half tendon width) produces about 15∆ of additional weakening of those muscles in the direction of gaze they are displaced. The muscles should thus be displaced in the direction of the desired additional weakening effect, whether the muscles were weakened or strengthened. The medial rectus muscle should be moved toward the apex of the A or V pattern (up in A pattern, down in V pattern). The lateral rectus muscle should be moved toward the open end of the A (down) or V (up).

This guideline applies whether surgery is performed on one or both eyes. For example, a patient with a V-pattern exotropia might undergo recession of both lateral recti with upward transposition or a recession of one lateral rectus with upward transposition along with a resection of the ipsilateral medial rectus with downward transposition.

> Knapp P. A and V patterns. In: Burian HM, ed. *Symposium on Strabismus.* St Louis: Mosby; 1971:242–254.
>
> Metz HS, Schwartz L. The treatment of A and V patterns by monocular surgery. *Arch Ophthalmol.* 1977:95:251–253.

Lateral rectus muscle paralysis

The treatment of lateral rectus muscle paralysis varies according to the degree of weakness of the lateral rectus muscle and the degree of contracture of the antagonist ipsilateral medial rectus muscle. Apart from the use of botulinum toxin, there are basically two treatment options:

- Resection of the lateral rectus muscle with recession of the ipsilateral medial rectus muscle (recess-resect procedure)
- Transposition of the vertical recti, perhaps with recession of the ipsilateral medial rectus muscle

Transposition procedures are more effective than recess-resect surgery in cases with severe paralysis, but anterior segment ischemia may be a risk, especially if medial rectus recession is added (see below). Some surgeons prefer to isolate and preserve the ciliary vessels; others avoid simultaneous surgery on the medial rectus. Options to be considered include augmenting the effect of the transposition by resecting the transposed muscles or by attaching them to the sclera along the border of the lateral rectus muscle, 16 mm posterior to the limbus. Another option is botulinum injection of the medial rectus.

> Brooks SE. Transposition procedures. In: *Focal Points: Clinical Modules for Ophthalmologists.* San Francisco: American Academy of Ophthalmology; 2001: vol 19, no 10.
>
> Brooks SE, Olitsky SE, deB Ribeiro G. Augmented Hummelsheim procedure for paralytic strabismus. *J Pediatr Ophthalmol Strabismus.* 2000;37:189–195.
>
> Foster RS. Vertical muscle transposition augmented with lateral fixation. *J AAPOS.* 1997;1: 20–30.

McKeown CA, Lambert HM, Shore JW. Preservation of the anterior ciliary vessels during extraocular muscle surgery. *Ophthalmology.* 1989;96:498–506.

Anesthesia for Extraocular Muscle Surgery

Topical anesthetic drops alone (eg, tetracaine 0.5%, proparacaine 0.5%, cocaine 4%) can be used effectively in cooperative patients for certain procedures. Lid blocks are not necessary if the eyelid speculum is not spread to the point of causing pain. Topical anesthesia is effective for making incisions in the conjunctiva and Tenon's capsule, placing sutures into the muscle, and disinserting the muscle from the globe. Such anesthesia is not effective in controlling the pain produced by pulling on or against a muscle. Topical anesthesia is effective for simple recession procedures but is not as effective for resection procedures or for recession procedures involving restricted muscles or difficult exposure.

Both *local infiltration* and *retrobulbar anesthesia* produce freedom from pain for most extraocular muscle procedures. Such anesthesia should be considered in adults for whom general anesthesia may pose an undue hazard. The administration of a short-acting hypnotic by an anesthesiologist just before retrobulbar injection greatly improves patient comfort. Because injected anesthesia may influence alignment during the first few hours after surgery, suture adjustment is best delayed for at least half a day following surgery.

General anesthesia is necessary for children and is frequently used for adults as well, particularly those requiring bilateral surgery. Neuromuscular blocking agents such as succinylcholine, which are often administered to facilitate intubation for general anesthesia, can temporarily affect the results of a traction test.

France NK, France TD, Woodburn JD Jr, et al. Succinylcholine alteration of the forced duction test. *Ophthalmology.* 1980;87:1282–1287.

Conjunctival Incisions

Fornix Incision

The fornix incision is made in either the superior or (more frequently) the inferior oblique quadrants. The incision is located on bulbar conjunctiva, not actually in the fornix, 1–2 mm to the limbal side of the cul-de-sac. The incision is parallel to the fornix, approximately 8 mm in length. The incision begins from an imaginary line dropped into the cul-de-sac from the midcornea and extends either nasally or temporally. It is usually possible to avoid making two contiguous incisions, which tend to become connected. All six extraocular muscles can be approached, if necessary, through an inferotemporal and a superonasal conjunctival incision.

Bare sclera is exposed by incising Tenon's capsule perpendicular to the conjunctival incision in its midportion. The muscle is engaged from this bare scleral exposure. The conjunctival incision is pulled or stretched over the point of the hook that has passed under the muscle belly.

When properly placed, the two-plane incision can be self-closed by gently massaging the conjunctiva into the fornix. Some surgeons prefer to close the incision with conjunctival sutures.

> Parks MM. Fornix incision for horizontal rectus muscle surgery. *Am J Ophthalmol.* 1968;65:907–915.

Limbal or Peritomy Incision

The initial incision through conjunctiva and Tenon's capsule to the sclera is made in an oblique quadrant, close to and radial to the limbus, on the side of the eye nearest the muscle. The combined layer of conjunctiva and Tenon's capsule is then cleanly severed from the limbus. A second radial incision is made in the other quadrant so that the combined conjunctiva/Tenon's capsule flap can be retracted to expose the muscle for surgery. At the completion of surgery, the flap is reattached to its original position with a single suture in each corner. If the conjunctiva is tight, contributing to a restriction of motility, it can be recessed at the end of surgery.

> von Noorden GK. The limbal approach to surgery of the rectus muscles. *Arch Ophthalmol.* 1968;80:94–97.

Complications of Strabismus Surgery

Unsatisfactory Alignment

The most common complication of surgery for strabismus is unsatisfactory postoperative alignment. With the above guidelines, undercorrections are more common than overcorrections. In some cases, it is apparent to both the patient and the surgeon in the immediate postoperative period that the alignment is not satisfactory. Even satisfactory initial alignment may not be permanent, however. Among the reasons for this unpredictability are poor fusion, poor vision, altered accommodation, and contracture of scar tissue. In many patients, the cause of the unstable alignment is unknown. Reoperations are often necessary.

Refractive Changes

Changes in refractive error are most common when strabismus surgery is performed on two rectus muscles of one eye. An induced with-the-rule astigmatism of low magnitude usually resolves within several months.

> Thompson WE, Reinecke RD. The changes in refractive status following routine strabismus surgery. *J Pediatr Ophthalmol Strabismus.* 1980;17:372–374.

Diplopia

Diplopia is common following strabismus surgery in older children and especially in adults. The surgery can move the image of the object of regard in the deviating eye out of a suppression scotoma. In the hours to several months following surgery, various responses can occur:

- Fusion of the two images can occur, obviating the need for a suppression scotoma.
- A new suppression scotoma may form, which corresponds to the new angle of alignment.
- Diplopia may persist.

If the initial strabismus was acquired before age 10, the ability to suppress is generally well developed, and a new suppression scotoma can usually be established to match the postoperative alignment, especially on the same side of the midline. Prolonged postoperative diplopia is therefore uncommon unless the patient's strabismus is overcorrected. If strabismus was first acquired in adulthood, however, the diplopia that was symptomatic before surgery is likely to persist unless fusion is regained. Prisms may be helpful in preoperatively assessing the fusion potential and the risk of bothersome postoperative diplopia.

Further treatment is indicated for patients, mainly adults, whose symptomatic diplopia persists more than 3–4 weeks following surgery, especially if it is severe and in the primary position. Patients with unequal visual acuities can frequently be taught to ignore the dimmer, fuzzier, nondominant image by closing the nondominant eye intermittently. If vision is equal or nearly so, Press-On prisms should be tried, generally with the full correction in a single prism over the nonpreferred eye, tilted to correct both vertical and horizontal deviations. If diplopia is eliminated, gradually decreasing the prisms or replacing them with permanent ground-in prism split between both eyes may provide long-term relief. If this approach fails, additional surgery or botulinum toxin injection may be needed (see Chapter 14).

Perforation of the Sclera

A needle may perforate into the suprachoroidal space or through the choroid and retina. In most cases, this perforation creates no problem other than a chorioretinal scar. However, perforation can lead to vitreous hemorrhage, retinal detachment, or endophthalmitis (Fig 13-1). Presumably, inadvertent perforation of the sclera with a suture pass provides access for infection within the globe. Some surgeons advocate laser or cryotherapy over the site of the perforation. Periodic fundus examination is advised, with

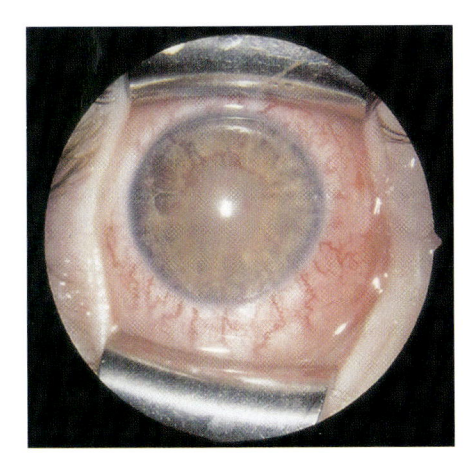

Figure 13-1 Endophthalmitis following muscle surgery of the right eye. Although rare, this complication can occur following scleral perforation.

further treatment as indicated. Topical antibiotics are generally used during the immediate postoperative period.

> Awad AH, Mullaney PB, Al-Hazmi AA, et al. Recognized globe perforation during strabismus surgery: incidence, risk factors, and sequelae. *J AAPOS.* 2000;4:150–153.
>
> Simon JW, Lininger LL, Scherage JL. Recognized scleral perforation during eye muscle surgery: incidence and sequelae. *J Pediatr Ophthalmol Strabismus.* 1992;29:273–275.

Postoperative Infections

Serious infection is uncommon following strabismus surgery. Some patients develop mild conjunctivitis, which may be caused by allergy to suture material or postoperative medications as well as by infectious agents. Preseptal or orbital cellulitis with proptosis, eyelid swelling, chemosis, and fever are also rare complications of strabismus surgery (Fig 13-2). These conditions usually develop 2–3 days after surgery and generally respond well to systemic (especially parenteral) antibiotics. Rarely, frank endophthalmitis has also been reported after strabismus surgery, which is identical to endophthalmitis following other types of ophthalmic surgery in its presentation, diagnosis, and treatment. Patients should be warned of the signs and symptoms of orbital cellulitis and endophthalmitis prior to discharge so that they will seek emergency consultation if those signs or symptoms develop.

> Kivlin JD, Wilson ME Jr. Periocular infection after strabismus surgery. Periocular Infection Study Group. *J Pediatr Ophthalmol Strabismus.* 1995;32:42–49.

Foreign Body Granuloma and Allergic Reaction

Occasionally, a foreign body granuloma develops several weeks after surgery, often at the suture site. The granuloma is characterized by a localized, elevated, slightly hyperemic, slightly tender mass, usually less than 1 cm in diameter. The granuloma may respond to topical corticosteroids. Surgical excision may be necessary if the granuloma persists (Fig 13-3).

Some suture materials may incite a vigorous allergic reaction, but such reactions are rare today because gut suture has largely been replaced in strabismus surgery (Fig 13-4).

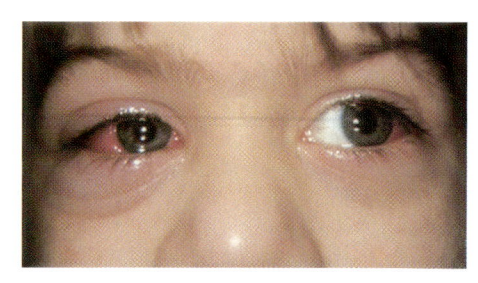

Figure 13-2 Orbital cellulitis, right eye, 2 days after bilateral recession of lateral rectus muscles. Typically noted 2 or 3 days postoperatively, the infection usually responds quickly to antibiotics, especially if given parenterally.

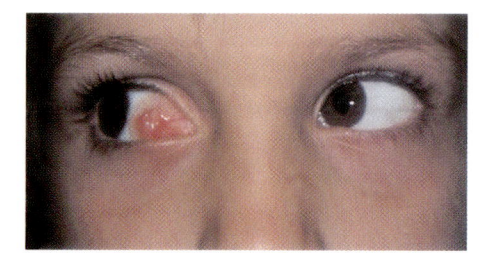

Figure 13-3 Severe postoperative granuloma over the right medial rectus persists 1 year after medial rectus recessions OU.

Conjunctival Inclusion Cyst

If any conjunctival epithelium is buried during muscle reattachment or closure of the incision, a conjunctival cyst may appear (Fig 13-5). This noninflamed translucent mass under the conjunctiva appears several days to several years after surgery. The cyst may disappear spontaneously. Persistent cases may require surgical excision when symptoms warrant.

Conjunctival Scarring

Improved alignment may occasionally be overshadowed by unsightly scarring of the conjunctiva and Tenon's capsule. The tissues may remain hyperemic or salmon pink instead of returning to their usual whiteness. This complication may result from the following factors:

- *Advancement of thickened Tenon's capsule too close to the limbus.* In resection procedures, pulling the muscle forward may advance into view the thicker Tenon's capsule that normally lies over and between the muscles. This situation is especially likely in reoperations, when the Tenon's capsule around and anterior to the insertion may be hyperplastic.

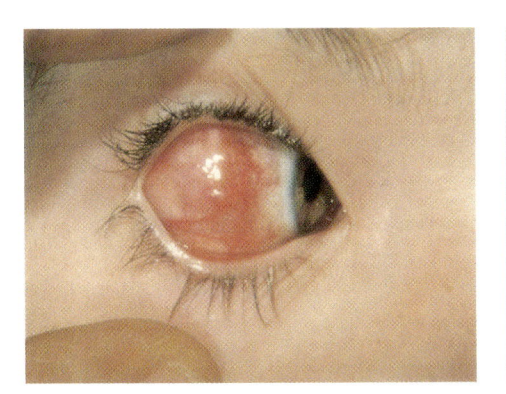

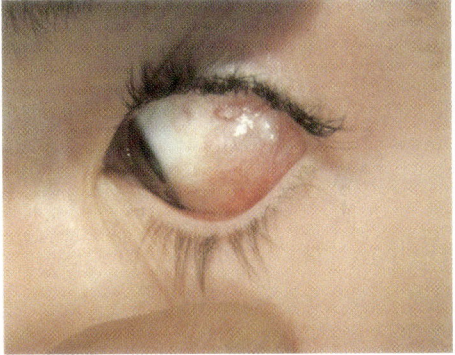

Figure 13-4 Chromic gut was used in the right eye and polyglycolic acid suture in the left eye. Right eye shows a severe allergic reaction 3 weeks postoperatively.

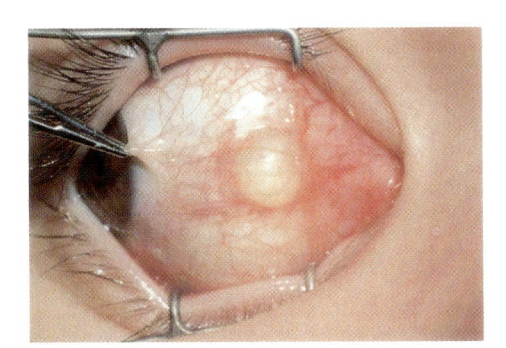

Figure 13-5 Postoperative conjunctival epithelial inclusion cyst following right medial rectus recession using fornix incision technique.

- *Advancement of the plica semilunaris onto bulbar conjunctiva.* In surgery on the medial rectus muscle using the limbal approach, the surgeon sometimes mistakes the plica semilunaris for a conjunctival edge and incorporates it or a portion of it into the closure. Although not strictly a conjunctival scar, the plica semilunaris, now pulled forward over bulbar conjunctiva, retains its normal fleshy color long after the remainder of the conjunctiva has returned to its normal color (Fig 13-6). A restrictive esotropia is also likely.

Adherence Syndrome

Violation of Tenon's capsule with prolapse of orbital fat into the sub–Tenon's space can cause formation of a pink fibrofatty scar of the muscle and globe, which may restrict motility. If an inadvertent rent in Tenon's capsule is recognized at the time of surgery, the prolapsed fat can be excised and the rent can be closed with absorbable sutures. Otherwise, the prognosis for normal motility is poor. Meticulous surgical technique usually prevents this serious complication.

Dellen

The term *dellen* (*delle*, singular), derived from the German word for "dents," refers to shallow depressions or corneal thinning just anterior to the limbus. Dellen occur when raised abnormal tissue on the bulbar conjunctiva prevents the eyelid from adequately resurfacing the cornea with tears during blinking (Fig 13-7). Fluorescein pools in these depressions but does not stain the stroma. Dellen occasionally occur when the limbal approach to muscle surgery is used. They should be followed carefully, and artificial tears or lubricants may be needed until the chemosis and conjunctival hemorrhage subside. Patching of the eye may be helpful.

Anterior Segment Ischemia

Most of the blood supply to the anterior segment of the eye comes through the anterior ciliary arteries that travel in the four rectus muscles. Simultaneous surgery on three of

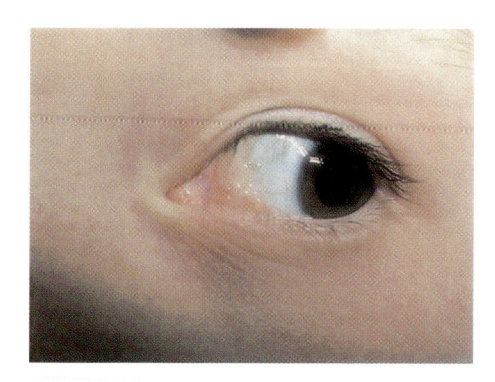

Figure 13-6 Involvement of plica semilunaris incision.

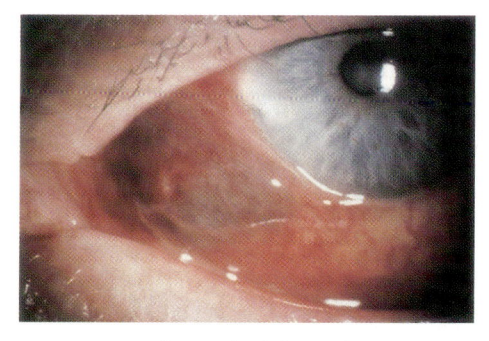

Figure 13-7 Corneal delle subsequent to postoperative subconjunctival hemorrhage.

these rectus muscles, or even two of them in patients with poor blood flow, may lead to anterior segment ischemia. This complication is characterized by corneal epithelial edema, folds in Descemet's membrane, and other signs of anterior uveitis (Fig 13-8). If severe, the complication may lead to phthisis bulbi. Treatment is directed at the anterior uveitis, which often responds to frequent administration of topical, subconjunctival, or systemic steroids.

It may be possible to recess or resect a rectus muscle while sparing its anterior ciliary vessels by using an operating microscope and vitrectomy microinstruments. Although difficult and time-consuming, this technique may be indicated in high-risk cases. Staging surgeries, with surgery of the third muscle performed several months after the first procedure, may also be helpful.

Saunders RA, Bluestein EC, Wilson ME, et al. Anterior segment ischemia after strabismus surgery. *Surv Ophthalmol.* 1994;38:456–466.

Change in Eyelid Position

Change in the position of the eyelids is most likely with surgery on the vertical rectus muscles. Pulling the inferior rectus muscle forward, as in a resection, pulls the lower eyelid up over the lower limbus; recessing the muscle pulls the lower eyelid down, exposing bare sclera below the lower limbus (Figs 13-9, 13-10). Surgery on the superior rectus muscle is less likely to affect the upper eyelid position when proper dissection is performed.

Eyelid position changes can be obviated somewhat by careful dissection. In general, all intermuscular septum and fascial connections between the eyelid and associated vertical rectus muscle must be severed at least 12–15 mm posterior to the muscle insertion (to the point at which the muscle disappears through Tenon's capsule). Some surgeons have advocated release of the lower eyelid retractors or advancement of the capsulopalpebral head to prevent lower eyelid retraction after inferior rectus muscle recession.

Kushner BJ. A surgical procedure to minimize lower-eyelid retraction with inferior rectus recession. *Arch Ophthalmol.* 1992;110:1011–1014.

Meyer DR, Simon JW, Kansora M. Primary infratarsal eyelid retractor lysis to prevent eyelid retraction after inferior rectus muscle recession. *Am J Ophthalmol.* 1996;122:331–339.

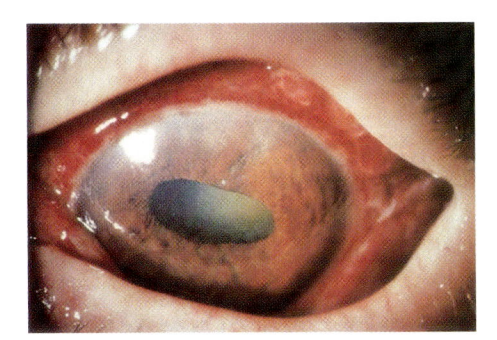

Figure 13-8 Superotemporal segmental anterior segment ischemia after simultaneous superior rectus muscle and lateral rectus muscle surgery following scleral buckling procedure.

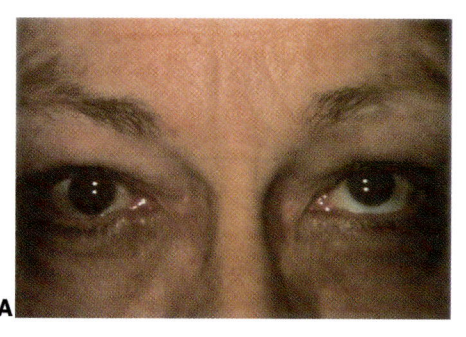

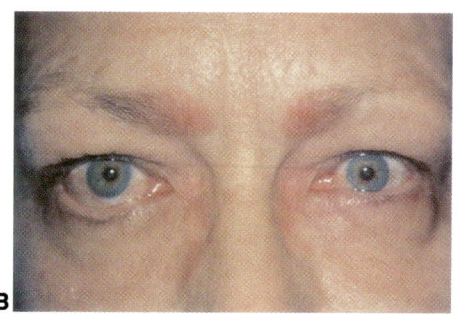

Figure 13-9 A, Preoperative photograph of patient who underwent recession of the right inferior rectus muscle, which pulled the right lower eyelid down, and a resection of the left inferior rectus muscle, which pulled the left lower eyelid up, causing postoperative asymmetry. **B,** Postoperative photograph.

Figure 13-10 One year after recession of the left inferior rectus muscle, with down-pulled left lower eyelid and conjunctival prolapse.

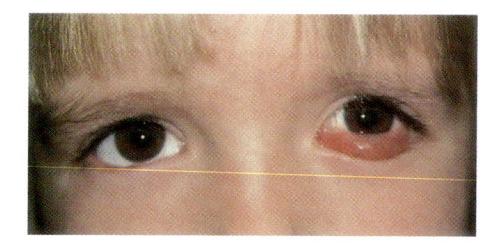

Lost Muscle

After a muscle is freed from its insertion, it sometimes slips out of the sutures or surgical instruments and is lost posteriorly in the orbit. The surgeon should immediately make every attempt to find the lost muscle, which retracts into its sleeve of Tenon's capsule. It is important to realize that a lost or retracted muscle usually does not remain next to the globe posterior to the equator but instead retracts into Tenon's capsule along the orbital wall. Generally, pulling Tenon's capsule forward in a "hand over hand" fashion brings the muscle into view. Malleable retractors and a headlight may be helpful. Care must be taken not to violate Tenon's capsule, in which case fibrofatty proliferation can occur (see earlier discussion, Adherence Syndrome).

When the diagnosis is made in the immediate postoperative period, the patient should be promptly returned to surgery for exploration and attempted retrieval of the lost muscle by a surgeon experienced with this potentially complex surgery. Muscle transposition surgery may be required if the lost muscle is not found, though anterior segment ischemia may be a risk.

Slipped Muscle

Occasionally an inadequately sutured muscle slips posteriorly within the muscle capsule during the postoperative period. Clinically, the patient manifests a weakness of that muscle with limited rotations and decreased saccades in its field of action. Surgery should be performed as soon as possible in order to replace the slipped muscle before further retraction and contracture take place. This problem can be prevented by adequately securing the muscle prior to tenotomy with full-thickness lock bites to include muscle tissue and not just capsule (Fig 13-11).

> Plager DA, Parks MM. Recognition and repair of the "lost" rectus muscle. *Ophthalmology.* 1990;97:131–137.
>
> Plager DA, Parks MM. Recognition and repair of the slipped rectus muscle. *J Pediatr Ophthalmol Strabismus.* 1988;25:270–274.

Postoperative Nausea and Vomiting

Nausea and vomiting are common following eye muscle surgery. The incidence and severity can be reduced using newer anesthetic agents and antiemetics.

Oculocardiac Reflex

The oculocardiac reflex is a slowing of the heart rate that is caused by traction on the extraocular muscles. In its most severe form, the reflex can produce asystole. The surgeon should be aware of the possibility of inducing the oculocardiac reflex when manipulating a muscle and should be prepared to release tension if the heart rate drops excessively. Intravenous atropine can protect against the oculocardiac reflex.

Malignant Hyperthermia

Malignant hyperthermia (MH) is an acute metabolic disorder that can be fatal if diagnosis and treatment are delayed. In its fully developed form, MH is characterized by extreme heat production. MH is often triggered by many inhalational anesthetics, by the muscle relaxant succinylcholine, and by local anesthetics of the amide type.

MH is a disorder of calcium binding by the sarcoplasmic reticulum of skeletal muscle. In the presence of an anesthetic triggering agent, unbound intracellular calcium increases, stimulating muscle contracture. As this increased metabolism outstrips oxygen delivery, anaerobic metabolism develops with lactate production and massive acidosis. Hyperthermia results from the hypermetabolic state. As cells are depleted of adenosine triphosphate, cell breakdown occurs with loss of potassium and myoglobin.

MH can occur as an isolated case or as a dominantly inherited disorder with incomplete penetrance. Other disorders associated with MH include strabismus, myopathies,

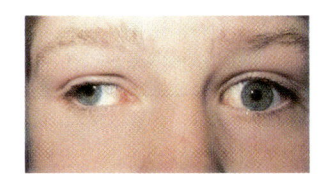

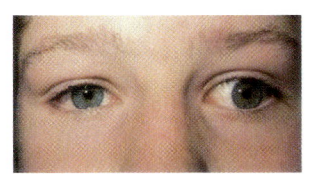

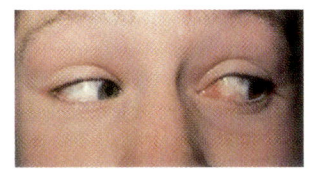

Figure 13-11 Slipped left medial rectus muscle. **Left,** Gaze right shows widening of palpebral fissure of left eye and inability to adduct. **Middle,** Exotropia in primary position with widened palpebral fissure. **Right,** Gaze left shows full abduction with normal width of fissure.

ptosis, and other musculoskeletal abnormalities. The incidence is variously reported as between 1:6000 and 1:60,000 and is thought to be higher in children. MH occurs in all age groups. Although the mortality rate used to be as high as 70%, it is probably lower than 10% with modern treatment.

Diagnosis

The diagnosis of MH is based on clinical signs and may be confirmed by laboratory studies. Muscle biopsy with in vitro halothane and caffeine contraction testing is the most specific test to confirm the clinical diagnosis. When the diagnosis is unconfirmed but the personal or family history is suspicious for MH, susceptibility testing may be warranted. If testing is not available, nontriggering anesthetic agents should be used and the patient treated as if MH is possible.

Clinical picture

Frequently, the earliest sign of MH is tachycardia that is greater than expected for the patient's anesthetic and surgical status. Other arrhythmias may also occur, as can unstable blood pressure. Other early signs include tachypnea, sweating, muscle rigidity, blotchy discoloration of skin, cyanosis, and dark urine. Onset may be manifested during the induction of anesthesia by trismus caused by masseter muscle spasm, although the significance of masseter spasm is controversial. Most of these patients do not develop MH, but they should be observed closely. If the patient is being monitored with capnography, elevated end-tidal carbon dioxide may be the presenting sign.

A later sign is a rise in temperature, which may reach extremely high levels. Other later signs include respiratory and metabolic acidosis, hyperkalemia, hypercalcemia, myoglobinuria and renal failure, skeletal muscle swelling, heart failure, disseminated intravascular coagulation, and cardiac arrest. Ideally, MH should be diagnosed and treated before the temperature rises significantly. Survival is greatly improved when treatment begins early.

Treatment

Early treatment of unexpected cases of MH cannot be overemphasized. Table 13-6 gives the protocol for treatment of MH. Once the condition is recognized, anesthetic agents should be discontinued, hyperventilation with oxygen started, and treatment with intravenous dantrolene begun. Dantrolene works to prevent release of calcium from the sarcoplasmic reticulum, preventing the excessive contractile response of muscle. Surgery should be terminated as soon as possible, even if incomplete. Temperature monitoring should be established along with an intra-arterial catheter for the monitoring of blood pressure and arterial blood gases. Electrolytes, electrocardiograms, urine output, prothrombin time, partial thromboplastin time, fibrinogen, and pulse oximetry should also be monitored. Central venous or pulmonary artery pressure may be monitored if indicated by the patient's condition.

Table 13-6 Malignant Hyperthermia Protocol

1. Stop the triggering agents immediately and conclude surgery as soon as possible.
2. Hyperventilate with 100% oxygen at high flow rates.
3. Administer
   a. Dantrolene: 2–3 mg/kg initial bolus with increments up to 10 mg/kg total. Continue to administer dantrolene until symptoms are controlled. Occasionally, a dose greater than 10 mg/kg may be needed.
   b. Sodium bicarbonate: 1–2, mEq/kg increments guided by arterial pH and pCO2. Bicarbonate will combat hyperkalemia by driving potassium into cells.
4. Actively cool patient:
   a. If needed, IV iced saline (not Ringer's lactate) 15 mL/kg q 10 minutes × 3. Monitor closely.
   b. Lavage stomach, bladder, rectum, and peritoneal and thoracic cavities with iced saline.
   c. Surface cool with ice and hypothermia blanket.
5. Maintain urine output. If needed, administer mannitol 0.25 gm/kg IV, furosemide 1 mg/kg IV (up to 4 doses each). Urine output greater than 2 mL/kg/hr may help prevent subsequent renal failure.
6. Calcium channel blockers *should not* be given when dantrolene is administered because hyperkalemia and myocardial depression may occur.
7. Insulin for hyperkalemia. Add 10 units of regular insulin to 50 mL of 50% glucose and titrate to control hyperkalemia. Monitor blood glucose and potassium levels.
8. Postoperatively: Continue dantrolene 1 mg/kg IV q6h × 72 hours to prevent recurrence. Lethal recurrences of MH may occur. Observe in an intensive care unit.
9. For expert medical advice and further medical evaluation, call the MHaus MH hotline consultant at (800) 644-9737. For nonemergency professional or patient information, call (800) 986-4287. E-mail address is mhaus@norwich.net.

CHAPTER 14

Chemodenervation Treatment of Strabismus and Blepharospasm Using Botulinum Toxin

Pharmacology and Mechanism of Action

Botox (purified botulinum toxin A) is a protein drug produced by the bacterium *Clostridium botulinum*. The toxin is injected directly into the orbicularis muscle or into selected extraocular muscles, often localized with a portable electromyographic device. Following injection, botulinum toxin is bound and internalized in 24–48 hours within local motor nerve terminals, where it remains for many weeks to interfere with the release of acetylcholine. Paralysis of the injected muscle begins within 2–4 days after injection and lasts clinically for at least 5–8 weeks in the extraocular muscle and for 3 or more months in the orbicularis muscle. An extraocular muscle lengthens while it is paralyzed by botulinum, and its antagonist contracts. These changes may produce long-term improvement in the alignment of the eyes.

Indications, Techniques, and Results

Strabismus Correction

Clinical trials have shown botulinum to be most effective when used in the following conditions:

- Small- to moderate-angle esotropia and exotropia (<40Δ)
- Postoperative residual strabismus (2–8 weeks following surgery or later)
- Acute paralytic strabismus (especially sixth nerve palsy) to block contracture of the antagonist while the palsy recovers
- Cyclic esotropia
- Active thyroid ophthalmopathy (Graves disease) or inflamed or prephthisical eyes, when surgery is inappropriate

Studies have shown this treatment to be disappointing in patients with large deviations, restrictive or mechanical strabismus (trauma or multiple reoperations), or secondary strabismus wherein a muscle has been overrecessed. Injection is ineffective in A and V patterns, dissociated vertical deviations, oblique muscle disorders, and chronic paralytic strabismus. Multiple injections are frequently required. As with surgical treatment, results are best when there is fusion to stabilize the alignment.

Results of treatment

The percentage of patients achieving a deviation of 10Δ or less at least 6 months after the last injection has ranged from 33% for large-angle exotropia to 72% for small-angle esotropia. Overcorrections are rare, and adults and children have responded similarly. The increased potency of surgical correction may be important, especially in larger-angle strabismus cases. The long-term recovery rate for patients with acute sixth nerve palsy who were treated with observation is similar to that of patients who received botulinum.

Complications

The most common side effects have been temporary ptosis, lasting from 3 weeks to 3 months (16% of adults and 25% of children), and induced vertical strabismus (17% of all patients). Rarely, these effects have persisted beyond 6 months (0.16% with slight residual ptosis and 2% with residual vertical strabismus of 2Δ or more). Other reported rare complications include scleral perforation (0.13%), retrobulbar hemorrhage (0.2%), pupillary dilation (0.6%), and permanent diplopia in one patient as a result of loss of suppression. Thus far in clinical use, no toxic systemic effects or loss of vision has been reported.

> Cohen DA, Savino PJ, Stern MB, et al. Botulinum injection therapy for blepharospasm: a review and report of 75 patients. *Clin Neuropharmacol.* 1986;9:415–429.
>
> Holmes JM, Beck RW, Kip KE, et al. Botulinum toxin versus conservative management in acute traumatic sixth nerve palsy or paresis. *J AAPOS.* 2000;4:145–149.
>
> McNeer KW, Tucker MG, Spencer RF. Management of essential infantile esotropia with botulinum toxin A: review and recommendations. *J Pediatr Ophthalmol Strabismus.* 2000; 37:63–67.
>
> Scott AB, Magoon EH, NcNeer KW, et al. Botulinum treatment of strabismus in children. *Trans Am Ophthalmol Soc.* 1989;87:174–184.

PART II

Pediatric Ophthalmology

INTRODUCTION TO PART II

Growth and Development of the Child's Eye

Children are different from adults in many significant ways. The infant eye, for example, is not simply a small adult eye. Because pathology in the infant eye may be indicated by variations in the size or proportions of its structures, the normal dimensions and proportions must be learned by ophthalmologists responsible for children's eye care.

The horizontal palpebral fissure at birth is almost as long as in childhood, yet a newborn's vertical fissure is only half the size of an adult's. The diameter of the eye at birth is about 66% of that in adulthood. The eye grows rapidly during the first 2 years of life; growth then slows until puberty. Infants often have astigmatism during their first months of life, and most young children are hyperopic. Absence of hyperopia during early childhood is usually a harbinger of myopia, which increases as growth progresses.

As the axial length of the eye increases (Fig I-1), the lens flattens (Fig I-2). At birth, the anteroposterior length of the eye is about 17 mm, increasing to approximately 24 mm in adulthood. The anterior chamber depth at birth is 2.3–2.7 mm, which is shallower than in adults because of the steep anterior lens surface in children.

The average corneal horizontal diameter is 9.5–10.5 mm in newborns and 12 mm in adults. The radius of corneal curvature is 6.6–7.4 mm in newborns and 7.4–8.4 mm in adults (Table I-1). Keratometry values change markedly in the first year of life, starting at approximately 52 D at birth and flattening to 42–44 D in adulthood. Thereafter, keratometry remains relatively stable (Fig I-3). The infant sclera is about half of its adult thickness and strength.

In newborns, additional pigment continues to be deposited in the anterior iris stroma for approximately a year after birth. In blue-eyed newborns, eye color may gradually darken to green or brown during the first months of life. Some normal children continue to show iris darkening to the age of 8 years. Pigment deposition may also increase after trauma or intraocular surgery. The dilator pupillae muscle is not well developed at birth, resulting in miotic pupils in infants. The fovea matures during the first months of life; myelinization of the optic nerve is usually completed shortly after birth. Only 3%–10% of infant eyes have asymmetrical cupping of their optic discs or optic discs whose cup/disc ratio is greater than 0.3.

Excellent visual acuities have been documented in infants. Visually evoked cortical potentials from the occipital cortex, recorded while the infant fixates on patterns of graded size, indicate that 6-month-old infants have already developed 20/20 visual acuity.

Figure I-1 Axial length plotted with respect to age. *Dots* represent mean values for age group indicated; *bars* represent standard deviations. *(Figures 1–3 reproduced by permission from Gordon RA, Donzis PB. Refractive development of of the human eye. Arch Ophthalmol. 1985;103:785–789. © 1985, American Medical Association.)*

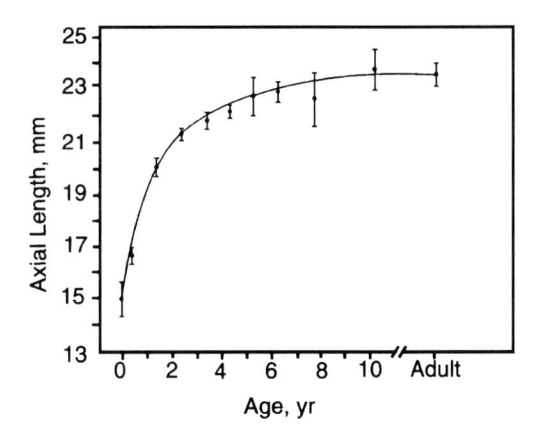

In the early months of life, behavioral tests such as the forced preferential looking test have documented somewhat lower visual acuities than indicated by electrophysiologic recordings. Normal children usually will not read the 20/20 line on an eye chart until the age of 3–6 years. Thus, tests that measure responses from the occipital cortex differ somewhat from tests that may also include responses from the visual association areas of the cortex.

The pediatric eye is a growing eye, which differentiates it in many ways from the adult eye. Furthermore, the developing immune system predisposes children to respond to inflammation and diseases differently than adults do. Similarly, because the central nervous system is in its formative period, it is particularly vulnerable to growth abnormalities and developmental interruptions. Thus, many interrelated influences are at work in pediatric ophthalmology. BCSC Section 2, *Fundamentals and Principles of Ophthalmology*, includes an extensive discussion of embryology and development.

Evaluation of the Child With Congenital or Juvenile Ocular Anomalies

Adult eye disorders usually result from senescence or trauma to previously normal ocular structures within a fully formed visual system. Not so with pediatric conditions. A serious congenital or developmental ocular abnormality should always alert the physician to search for other systemic problems. Cataracts or glaucoma are never routine in children; the presence of these common ocular disorders of advancing age in childhood is often a sign of a systemic syndrome such as Lowe syndrome, Down syndrome, Turner syndrome, galactosemia, diabetes, galactokinase deficiency, genetic abnormalities, or other disorders. Several principles should be kept in mind when evaluating any child with a serious ocular disorder.

First, take a detailed family history. It is not enough to ask whether anyone in the family has had retinoblastoma or Marfan syndrome; other family members may not know the syndrome names. The physician must be well acquainted with associated findings and ask questions about each—for example, a family history of other cancers in reti-

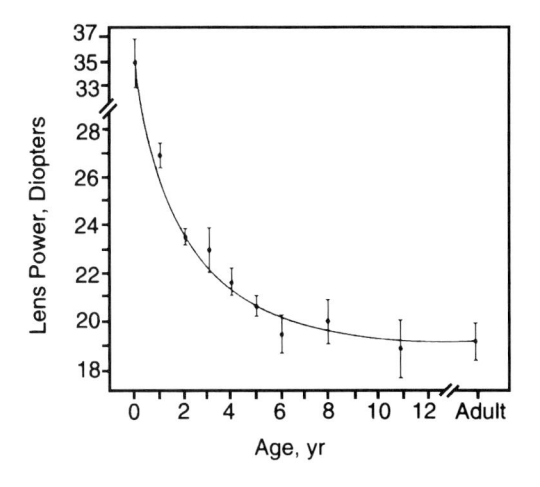

Figure I-2 Mean values *(dots)* and standard deviations *(bars)* for lens power as determined by modified SRK formula, plotted with respect to age.

Table I-1 Dimensions of Newborn and Adult Eyes

	Newborn	Adult
Anteroposterior length (mm)	17	24
Corneal horizontal diameter (mm)	9.5–10.5	12
Radius of corneal curvature (mm)	6.6–7.4	7.4–8.4

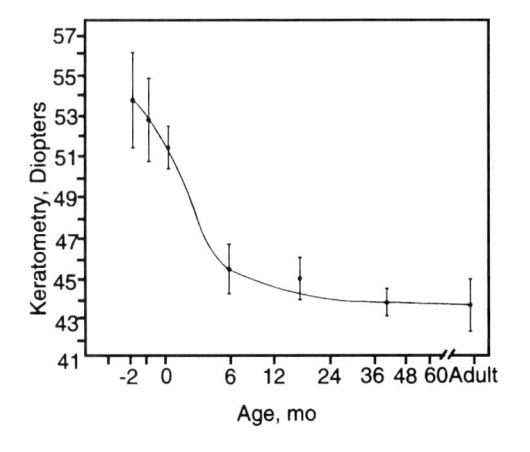

Figure I-3 Keratometry values plotted with respect to age on a logarithmic scale. Negative number represents months of prematuity; *dots,* mean value for age group indicated; and *bars,* standard deviations.

noblastoma or of sudden death in Marfan syndrome. Do not just ask about but also examine parents and family members. The mildest form of autosomal dominant coloboma is a small inferonasal chorioretinal scar that few people are aware they possess. Expression of autosomal dominant disorders varies extremely. A parent who carries the gene for autosomal dominant cataract may have good vision, but slit-lamp examination may reveal a lamellar cataract. For many parents who carry tuberous sclerosis and neurofibromatosis, to name just two conditions, diagnosis is possible only after the parents have a child who is severely affected. Furthermore, some dominant disorders demonstrate *anticipation.* This means each successive generation has a more severe form of the disease than the last. This is common in disorders caused by expanded repeats, such as fragile X syndrome and some neurodegenerative disorders with retinopathy and ataxia. Recurrence risk must be discussed with parents; this can only be done if the appropriate history and proper diagnosis are obtained. Often, the help of a geneticist is necessary.

Second, ask about and search for abnormalities of other organ systems. Any child with a coloboma and one other major organ system abnormality should undergo extended-band high-resolution karyotyping to look for deletions or rearrangements. Many congenital disorders result from disruption of embryogenesis at a certain fetal stage, and any organ developing at that time can be affected. Common abnormalities that occur with ocular anomalies include congenital heart defects, urogenital abnormalities, hearing loss, and developmental delays. In cases of severe bilateral ocular dysgenesis—such as microphthalmia, anophthalmia, persistent hyperplastic primary vitreous, optic nerve hypoplasia, and Peters anomaly—there is a very high association with coexisting brain abnormalities. After all, the eye is an extension of the brain. Many early-onset eye disorders are associated with very specific and life-threatening systemic anomalies. It often falls to the ophthalmologist to recognize these associations and recommend the appropriate workup. Some examples include evaluation for Joubert syndrome and Gaucher disease in children with oculomotor apraxia, monitoring for Wilms tumor in children with aniridia, and following renal function and glucose status in children with Bardet-Biedl or Alstrom syndromes, which must first be suspected and diagnosed in children who present with retinal degeneration and obesity.

Finally, all children with a serious ocular disorder must be referred to the appropriate community services. Children who do not see well walk later and more slowly reach other vision-dependent milestones. Directed therapy can help. In addition, parents who have received the difficult news that their child is visually impaired need the support system of such organizations. Such support is extremely important to the well-being of the child and family, and it falls to the ophthalmologist to be sure that such liaisons are in place.

CHAPTER 15

Congenital Anomalies

Many details and definitions pertaining to genetics, chromosomal anomalies, and developmental embryology are discussed and illustrated in BCSC Section 2, *Fundamentals and Principles of Ophthalmology*. See the glossary in this chapter for terms frequently associated with dysmorphology and congenital anomalies.

Major congenital anomalies occur in 2%–3% of live births. Causes include single genes, chromosomal anomalies, multifactorial disorders, environmental agents, and unidentified causes. The latter category, unknown causes, accounts for 50% or more of these malformations. Regardless of etiology, from a developmental point of view congenital anomalies may be organized into the following categories (examples are given in parentheses):

- *Agenesis:* developmental failure (anophthalmos)
- *Hypoplasia:* developmental arrest (optic nerve hypoplasia)
- *Hyperplasia:* developmental excess (distichiasis)
- Abnormal development (cryptophthalmos)
- Failure to divide or canalize (congenital nasolacrimal duct obstruction)
- *Dysraphia:* failure to fuse (choroidal coloboma)
- Persistence of vestigial structures (persistent fetal vasculature)

A *malformation* implies a morphologic defect present from the onset of development or a very early stage. A disturbance to a group of cells in a single developmental field may cause multiple malformations. Multiple causes may result in similar field defects and patterns of malformation. A single structural defect or factor can lead to a cascade, or domino effect, of secondary anomalies called a *sequence*. However, sequence does not always imply a single causative factor. The Pierre Robin group of anomalies (cleft palate, glossoptosis, micrognathia, respiratory problems) may represent a sequence caused by abnormal descent of the tongue and is noted in many syndromes (such as Stickler or fetal alcohol) and chromosomal anomalies. A *syndrome* is a recognizable and consistent pattern of multiple malformations known to have a specific cause, which is usually a mutation of a single gene, a chromosome alteration, or an environmental agent. An *association* represents defects noted to occur together in a statistically significant number of patients, such as the CHARGE association (ocular *c*oloboma, *h*eart defects, choanal *a*tresia, mental *r*etardation, and *g*enitourinary and *e*ar anomalies). An association may represent a variety of yet-unidentified causes. Two or more minor anomalies in combination significantly increase the chance of an associated major malformation.

Cohen MM Jr. *The Child with Multiple Birth Defects*. 2nd ed. New York: Oxford University Press; 1997.

Smith DW, Jones KL. *Smith's Recognizable Patterns of Human Malformation*. 5th ed. Philadelphia: Saunders; 1997.

Wyllie AH. The genetic regulation of apoptosis. *Curr Opin Genet Dev.* 1995;5:97–104.

Glossary

The following additional terms are frequently used in discussions of congenital anomalies and dysmorphology:

Apoptosis An orderly sequence of events in which cells shut down and self-destruct without causing injury to neighboring cells that are necessary for the development of the embryo. Persistent fetal vasculature is a likely example of a defect in apoptosis in the eye's development. Also called *programmed cell death*.

Congenital anomalies All forms of developmental defects present at birth, whether due to genetic, chromosomal, or environmental causes.

Deformation Abnormal form, shape, or position of a part of the body caused by a mechanical process such as intrauterine compression.

Developmental field A group of cells that respond as a coordinated unit to embryonic interaction defects in development, resulting in multiple malformations.

Disruption A morphologic defect resulting from the extrinsic breakdown of, or interference with, an originally normal developmental process.

Dysplasia Abnormal organization of cells into tissue(s) and its morphologic result; the process (and consequence) of abnormality of histogenesis (eg, collagen formation in the joints and zonular fibers of a patient with Marfan syndrome).

Neurocristopathy A constellation of malformations or a craniofacial syndrome involving structures that are primarily derived from neural crest cells (eg, Goldenhar syndrome).

Teratogen Any agent that can produce a permanent morphologic or functional abnormality. This category includes not only drugs and environmental agents such as ionizing radiation but also viruses and other pathogenic organisms (eg, rubella virus, *Toxoplasma gondii*) and metabolic abnormalities (eg, diabetes).

CHAPTER 16

Eyelid Disorders

Congenital eyelid disorders can result from abnormal differentiation of the eyelids and adnexa, developmental arrest, intrauterine environmental insults, and other unknown factors. Examples of these groups are discussed below. (BCSC Section 7, *Orbit, Eyelids, and Lacrimal System*, discusses the eyelids and their disorders and management in greater detail.)

Cryptophthalmos

Cryptophthalmos, a rare condition, results from failure of differentiation of eyelid structures. The skin passes uninterrupted from the forehead over the eye to the cheek and blends in with the cornea of the eye, which is usually malformed (Fig 16-1).

Congenital Coloboma of the Eyelid

The upper eyelid is usually involved in congenital coloboma of the eyelid. This condition varies from a small notch to the absence of the entire length of the eyelid, which may be fused to the globe (Fig 16-2). Eyelid colobomas are commonly associated with Goldenhar syndrome. The eye of an infant with a congenital coloboma should be observed for drying, but often the defect is well tolerated. Surgical closure of the eyelid defect is usually required eventually.

Ankyloblepharon

Fusion of part or all of the eyelid margins is known as *ankyloblepharon*. This condition may be dominantly inherited. A variant is *ankyloblepharon filiforme adnatum*, in which the eyelid margins are connected by fine strands (Fig 16-3). Treatment is surgical.

Congenital Ectropion

Eversion of the eyelid margin usually involves the lower eyelid secondary to a vertical deficiency of the skin. A lateral tarsorrhaphy may be needed for mild cases. More severe cases may require a skin flap or graft.

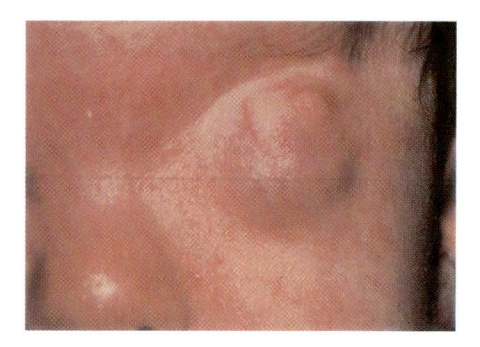

Figure 16-1 Cryptophthalmos, left eye.

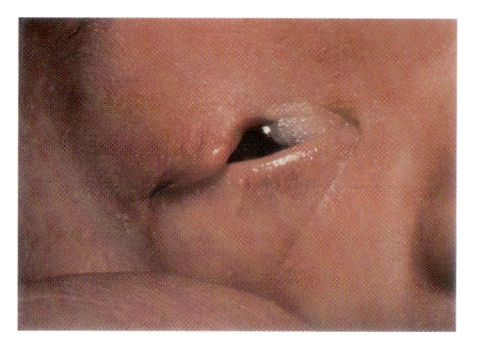

Figure 16-2 Congenital eyelid coloboma, right eye. The eyelid is fused to the globe.

Figure 16-3 Ankyloblepharon. The eyelid margins are fused by a fine strand. The eyelids were easily separated with blunt Wescott scissors in the office without anesthesia.

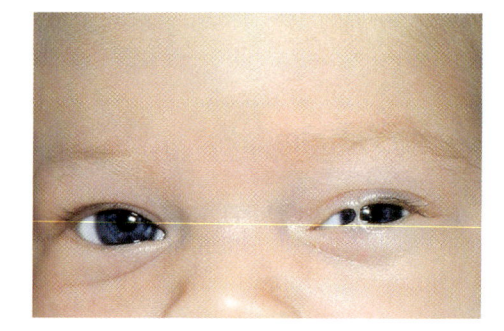

Congenital Entropion

Congenital entropion of the lower eyelid is uncommon, often asymptomatic, and usually associated with epiblepharon (see below). Surgery should be reserved for persistent cases that threaten the cornea. Congenital entropion of the upper eyelid usually results from congenital horizontal tarsal kink (see below) or microphthalmos.

Epiblepharon

A horizontal fold of skin adjacent to either the upper or the lower eyelid may turn the lashes against the cornea, most commonly by the lower eyelid. The cornea often tolerates this condition surprisingly well, and in the first several years of life epiblepharon resolves spontaneously. Severe cases require simple excision of the fold of skin/muscle.

Congenital Tarsal Kink

The origin of congenital tarsal kink is unknown. The child is born with the upper eyelid bent back and open. The upper tarsal plate often has an actual 180° fold. As with large congenital colobomas, the cornea may be exposed and traumatized by the bent edge, resulting in ulceration. Minor defects can be managed by manually unfolding the tarsus and taping the eyelid shut with a pressure dressing for 1–2 days. More severe cases require surgical incision of the tarsal plate or even excision of a V-shaped wedge from the inner surface to permit unfolding (Fig 16-4).

Distichiasis

A partial or complete accessory row of eyelashes growing out of or slightly posterior to the meibomian gland orifices is known as *distichiasis*. The abnormal lashes tend to be thinner, shorter, softer, and less pigmented than normal cilia and are therefore often well tolerated. Treatment is indicated if the patient is symptomatic or if corneal irritation is evident (Fig 16-5).

Euryblepharon

Enlargement of the lateral part of the palpebral aperture with downward displacement of the temporal half of the lower eyelid is known as *euryblepharon*. This condition gives the appearance of a very wide palpebral fissure or a droopy lower eyelid.

Epicanthus

Epicanthus, a crescent-shaped fold of skin running vertically between the eyelids and overlying the inner canthus, is shown in Figure 16-6. There are four types of epicanthus:
- *Epicanthus tarsalis:* the fold is most prominent in the upper eyelid
- *Epicanthus inversus:* the fold is most prominent in the lower eyelid
- *Epicanthus palpebralis*: the fold is equally distributed in the upper and lower eyelids
- *Epicanthus supraciliaris:* the fold arises from the brow and terminates over the lacrimal sac

Epicanthus may be associated with blepharophimosis or ptosis, or it may be an isolated finding. Surgical correction is required only occasionally.

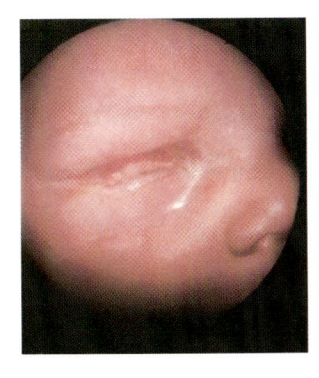

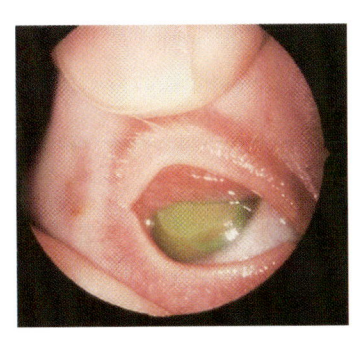

Figure 16-4 Congenital tarsal kink. Note large corneal epithelial defect.

Figure 16-5 Distichiasis. An accessory row of eyelashes exits from the meibomian gland orifices. *(Reproduced by permission from Byrnes GA, Wilson ME. Congenital distichiasis. Arch Ophthalmol. 1991;109:1752–1753. ©1991, American Medical Association.)*

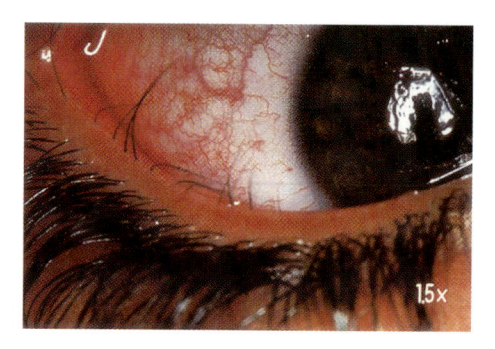

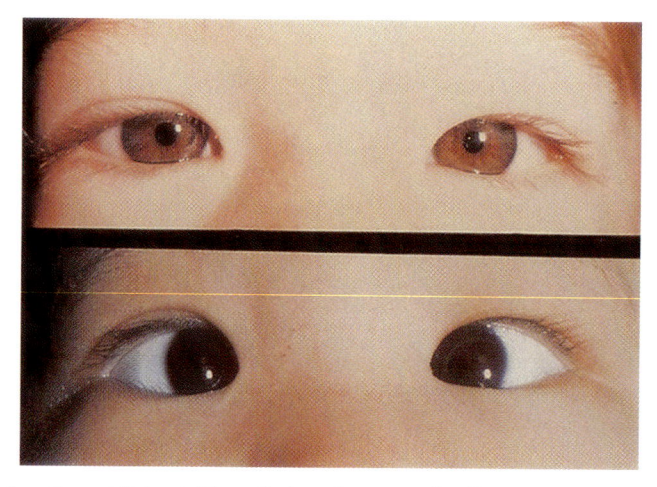

Figure 16-6 Epicanthus, bilateral. **Top,** Epicanthus tarsalis. **Bottom,** Epicanthus palpebralis. *(Reproduced by permission from Crouch E. The Child's Eye: Strabismus and Amblyopia. Slide script. San Francisco: American Academy of Ophthalmology; 1982.)*

Telecanthus

Wide intercanthal distance with a normal interpupillary distance is known as *telecanthus*. It is frequently associated with craniofacial syndromes such as Waardenburg syndrome. This condition tends to improve with time but can be corrected surgically if necessary. Telecanthus should not be confused with *hypertelorism* (increased separation between the bony orbits).

Palpebral Fissure Slants

In the normal eye, the lids are generally positioned so that the lateral canthus is about 1 mm higher than the medial canthus. Slight upward or downward slanting of palpebral fissures normally occurs on a familial basis or in groups such as persons of Asian descent. However, certain craniofacial syndromes frequently cause palpebral fissures to have a characteristic upward (eg, Down syndrome) or downward (eg, Treacher Collins syndrome) slant (see, Fig 28-3).

Blepharophimosis, Epicanthus Inversus, Telecanthus, and Ptosis (Kohn-Ramono Syndrome)

Kohn-Ramono syndrome frequently occurs as an isolated but often autosomal dominant disorder. The palpebral fissures are shortened horizontally and vertically *(blepharophimosis)* with poor levator function and no eyelid fold (Fig 16-7). The normal horizontal palpebral fissure length is 25–30 mm but is reduced to 18–22 mm in this syndrome. Repair of the ptosis, usually with frontalis slings, is often needed early in life. Because the epicanthus and telecanthus may improve with age, repair of these defects should be delayed.

Ptosis (Blepharoptosis)

Ptosis describes eyelid droop; the condition can be congenital or acquired. Acquired ptosis has been classified according to its various causes (Table 16-1). Evaluation of ptosis involves a thorough history that includes the date of onset and reviews any ocular disorders in the family. A complete examination, including slit-lamp examination and refraction, should be performed. Astigmatic errors may be associated with ptosis and may

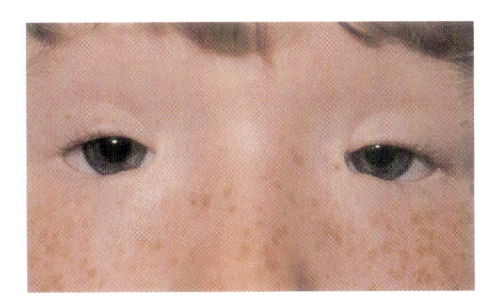

Figure 16-7 Blepharophimosis, epicanthus inversus, telecanthus, and ptosis.

Table 16-1 Classification of Ptosis

> **Pseudoptosis**
> **Congenital ptosis**
> **Acquired ptosis**
>   *Myogenic*
>   Myasthenia gravis
>   Progressive external ophthalmoplegia
>   *Neurogenic*
>   Horner syndrome
>   Third nerve palsy
>   *Mechanical*

cause amblyopia; the errors may persist after eyelid surgery. The eyelid is evaluated by description of the upper fold, and the amount of ptosis is documented by measurement of the height of the palpebral fissure. Levator function is measured while the effect of the frontalis muscle is blocked. Both tear function and corneal sensitivity should be evaluated because exposure and drying will be compounded by surgical repair. If Bell's phenomenon is poor, the cornea can decompensate quickly after ptosis repair. A documentary photograph of the patient is desirable.

Correction of ptosis in a child can often be delayed until the patient is several years old, although consistent chin-up head posturing justifies very early surgery. In rare cases, a completely closed eyelid must be elevated to avoid occlusion amblyopia. Surgical techniques include levator resection, tucking of the levator aponeurosis, and eyelid suspension anchored into the frontalis muscle. When levator function is less than 4 mm, frontalis suspension surgery is usually performed. Some surgeons prefer autogenous fascia lata for frontalis suspension surgery. However, others report good results with silicone rods or human donor fascia lata. Autogenous fascia cannot be obtained until the patient is 3 or 4 years old. One study reported a 50% recurrence rate by 8–10 postoperative years when human donor fascia lata was used. The long-term success using autogenous fascia lata has not been adequately studied.

Marcus Gunn Jaw Winking

In the typical Marcus Gunn jaw-winking syndrome, there is a congenital trigemino-oculomotor synkinesis. This results in ptosis, and the ptotic eyelid is elevated with jaw movement. Discussion with the family regarding their concerns about the ptosis versus the eyelid excursion is important. The eyelid excursion is the greater concern in some patients, and they may elect to sacrifice the levator and use a sling to elevate the eyelid.

> Kohn R. *Textbook of Ophthalmic Plastic and Reconstructive Surgery*. Philadelphia: Lea & Febiger; 1988:58–76.
> Meyer DR. Congenital ptosis. In: *Focal Points: Clinical Modules for Ophthalmologists*. San Francisco: American Academy of Ophthalmology; 2001: vol 19, no 2.
> Wilson ME, Johnson RW. Congenital ptosis. Long-term results of treatment using lyophilized fascia lata for frontalis suspensions. *Ophthalmology*. 1991;98:1234–1237.

CHAPTER 17

Infectious and Allergic Ocular Diseases

Intrauterine and Perinatal Infections of the Eye

Maternally transmitted congenital infections cause ocular damage in three ways:

- Through direct action of the infecting agent, which damages tissue
- Through a teratogenic effect resulting in malformation
- Through a delayed reactivation of the agent after birth, with inflammation that damages developed tissue

These infections can cause continuous tissue damage; therefore, long-term evaluation is required to determine their full impact. Most perinatal disorders have an exceedingly broad spectrum of clinical presentation, ranging from silent disease to life-threatening tissue and organ damage. Only the common types of congenital infections are included in this chapter. They can be remembered by the acronym *TORCHES*: *t*oxoplasmosis; *r*ubella; *c*ytomegalic inclusion disease; *h*erpesviruses, including *E*pstein-Barr; *s*yphilis.

> Stamos JK, Rowley AH. Timely diagnosis of congenital infections. *Pediatr Clin North Am.* 1994;41:1017–1033.

Toxoplasmosis

The etiologic agent of toxoplasmosis, *Toxoplasma gondii*, is an obligate intracellular protozoan. Cats are the definitive host, wherein the organism resides in the intestinal mucosa in the form of an oocyst. Once secreted into the environment, the oocyst can be ingested by many animals, including humans. Humans can also acquire the disease secondarily by ingesting undercooked infected meat such as pork, lamb, or even chicken.

The ingested cyst has a predilection for muscle, including the heart, and neural tissue, including the retinas. Encysted organisms can remain dormant indefinitely or the cyst can rupture, releasing hundreds of thousands of the proliferative phase of the protozoan called *tachyzoites*. The stimulus for local reactivation of an infected cyst is unknown.

Systemic infection in humans is common and usually goes undiagnosed. Symptoms may include fever, lymphadenopathy, and sore throat. The proportion of antibody titer–positive persons in North America increases with age from less than 10% in early childhood to greater than 80% in octogenarians.

Toxoplasmosis can be acquired congenitally via transplacental transmission from an infected mother to the fetus. This can result in varying degrees of retinitis, hepatosplenomegaly, intracranial calcifications, microcephaly, and developmental delay.

Ocular manifestations include retinitis, sometimes with associated choroiditis, iritis, and anterior uveitis (Fig 17-1). The active area of retinal inflammation is usually thickened and cream-colored with an overlying vitritis. The area may be at the edge of an old flat atrophic scar, frequently in the macular area, or adjacent to the scar (a so-called *satellite lesion*). Most cases of apparently acquired *Toxoplasma* retinitis probably represent reactivation of a congenital infection.

Diagnosis

Diagnosis is primarily a clinical one based on the characteristic retinal lesions. It can be supported by a positive enzyme-linked immunoassay for *Toxoplasma* antibody. Any positivity, even undiluted, is significant, but the rate of false-positive results is very high. In the infant, maternal IgM does not cross the placenta, so finding IgM in the infant serum is evidence of congenital infection in the infant. (See Chapter 4 of BCSC Section 4, *Ophthalmic Pathology and Intraocular Tumors*, and Chapter 9 of BCSC Section 9, *Intraocular Inflammation and Uveitis.*)

> Dodds EM. Ocular toxoplasmosis: clinical presentations, diagnosis, and therapy. In: *Focal Points: Clinical Modules for Ophthalmologists.* San Francisco: American Academy of Ophthalmology; 1999: vol 17, no 10.
>
> Montoya JG, Parmley S, Liesenfeld O, et al. Use of the polymerase chain reaction for diagnosis of ocular toxoplasmosis. *Ophthalmology.* 1999;106:1554–1563.

Treatment

Ocular inflammation from reactivated toxoplasmosis does not require treatment unless it threatens vision. Vision can be compromised by the location of the reactivation adjacent to the macula or optic nerve or because of significant vitritis. If the lesion is in the periphery of the eye and does not affect vision, it will likely quiet on its own in 1–2 months. If the macula or optic nerve is involved or if massive vitritis threatens vision, treatment may be indicated. Systemic treatment involves use of oral corticosteroids to quiet the inflammation in combination with one or more antimicrobial drugs aimed at the proliferating organisms. Steroids should never be used alone without antimicrobial coverage.

The commonly used antimicrobials are:

- Pyrimethamine—can cause bone marrow suppression, so its use is always accompanied by concomitant therapy with folinic acid. Patients should undergo weekly blood and platelet counts while on this drug. Pyrimethamine is usually used in combination with one of the following two agents:
  - Sulfadiazine—a sulfa drug with a long history for treatment of toxoplasmosis
  - Clindamycin—also effective against *Toxoplasma;* patients should be monitored for development of severe diarrhea from pseudomembranous colitis
- Trimethoprim-sulfamethoxazole—combination can be used if the other drugs are not available or not tolerated

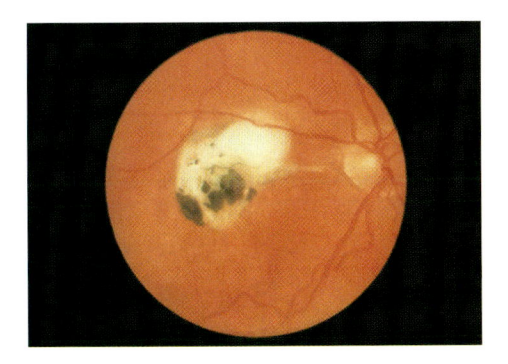

Figure 17-1 Toxoplasmosis, right eye.

- Atovaquone—newer antimicrobial that has been shown to be effective against *Toxoplasma* but is not a first-line therapy

Oral prednisone can be used judiciously to combat inflammation only while the patient is taking appropriate antimicrobial therapy.

> Dodds EM. Ocular toxoplasmosis: clinical presentations, diagnosis, and therapy. In: *Focal Points: Clinical Modules for Ophthalmologists.* San Francisco: American Academy of Ophthalmology; 1999: vol 17, no 12.
> Mets MB, Holfels E, Boyer KM, et al. Eye manifestations of congenital toxoplasmosis. *Am J Ophthalmol.* 1996;122:309–324.
> Remington JS, McLeod R, Thulliez P, et al. Toxoplasmosis. In: Remington JS, Klein JO, eds. *Infectious Diseases of the Fetus and Newborn Infant.* 5th ed. Philadelphia: Saunders; 2001.

Rubella (German Measles)

Congenital rubella syndrome is a well-defined combination of ocular, otologic, and cardiac abnormalities along with microcephaly and variable mental deficiency. The syndrome is caused by transplacental transmission of the rubella virus from an infected mother. The incidence of congenital rubella syndrome has decreased markedly in North America since widespread vaccination of children was instituted in the late 1960s, though rubella remains a cause of infant morbidity and mortality in less developed countries. The number of cases in the United States has decreased from 58,000 in 1969 to the 200–400 case/year range in 1998. Humans are the only known host.

Ocular abnormalities from rubella include a peculiar nuclear cataract (sometimes termed a *morgagnian cataract*), microphthalmos, and retinopathy varying from a subtle salt-and-pepper appearance to pseudo–retinitis pigmentosa (Fig 17-2).

Diagnosis is based on the characteristic clinical picture as described and is supported by serologic testing. The virus itself can be isolated from pharyngeal swabs and from the lens contents at the time of cataract surgery.

Lensectomy can be performed in the usual manner, though infected eyes are prone to excessive postoperative inflammation and subsequent secondary membrane formation. Topical steroids and mydriatics should be used aggressively.

> Cooper LZ, Alford CA. Rubella. In: Remington JS, Klein JO, eds. *Infectious Diseases of the Fetus and Newborn Infant.* 5th ed. Philadelphia: Saunders; 2001.

Wolff SM. The ocular manifestations of congenital rubella. *Trans Am Ophthalmol Soc.* 1972;70:577–614.

Zimmerman LE. Histopathologic basis for ocular manifestations of congenital rubella syndrome. *Am J Ophthalmol.* 1968;65:837–862.

Cytomegalovirus (Cytomegalic Inclusion Disease)

Cytomegalovirus (CMV) is a member of the herpesvirus family. CMV can cause a variety of human disease manifestations, both congenital and acquired, although symptomatic acquired infections occur almost exclusively in immunocompromised persons. Over 80% of adults in developed countries have antibodies to the virus.

Congenital infection with CMV is the most common congenital infection in humans, occurring in approximately 1% of cases, though over 90% of these remain asymptomatic. Transmission to the newborn can occur transplacentally, from contact with an infected birth canal during delivery, or perhaps from infected breast milk or maternal secretions. Congenital CMV disease is characterized by fever, jaundice, hematologic abnormalities, deafness, microcephaly, and periventricular calcifications.

Ophthalmic manifestations of congenital infection include retinochoroiditis, optic nerve anomalies, microphthalmos, cataract, and uveitis (Fig 17-3). The retinochoroiditis usually presents with bilateral focal involvement consisting of areas of retinal pigment epithelium atrophy and whitish opacities mixed with retinal hemorrhages. The retinitis can be progressive.

Figure 17-2 Fundus photograph of 6-year-old with rubella syndrome (ERG normal).

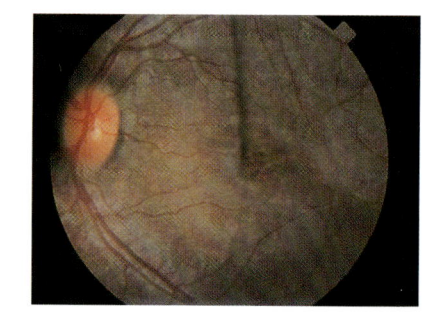

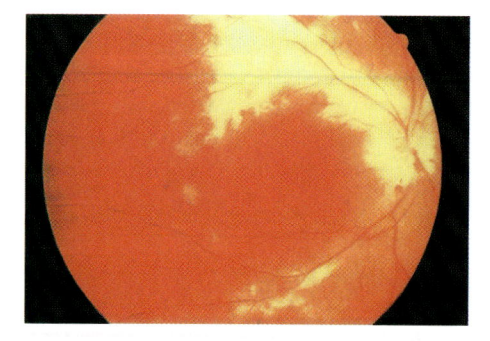

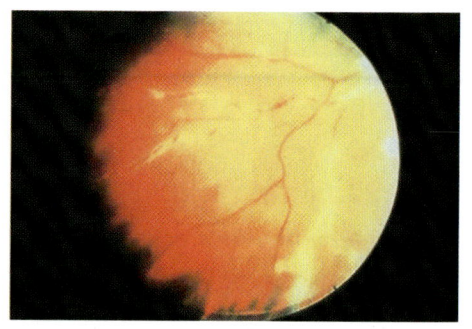

Figure 17-3 Active CMV retinochoroiditis in a premature infant, right eye.

CMV retinitis can be acquired in children who are immunocompromised (most frequently by AIDS) or iatrogenically following organ transplantation or chemotherapy. The retinitis is a diffuse retinal necrosis with areas of retinal thickening and whitening, hemorrhages, and venous sheathing. Vitritis may also be present.

Diagnosis is based on the clinical presentation in acquired disease and supplemented by serologic testing for antibody to CMV in congenital infection. The virus can be recovered from bodily secretions in infected infants.

Current treatment regimens include intravenous and intravitreal ganciclovir. Sustained-release intravitreal ganciclovir inserts are available. Oral valacyclovir can be used for acquired CMV retinitis that does not threaten vision.

Coats DK, Demmler GJ, Paysse EA, et al. Ophthalmologic findings in children with congenital cytomegalovirus infection. *J AAPOS*. 2000;4:110–116.

Stagno S. Cytomegalovirus. In: Remington JS, Klein JO, eds. *Infectious Diseases of the Fetus and Newborn Infant*. 5th ed. Philadelphia: Saunders; 2001.

Herpes Simplex

Herpes simplex virus (HSV) is a member of the herpesvirus family that includes two types of simplex virus (HSV-1 and HSV-2), herpes zoster, Epstein-Barr virus, and CMV. HSV-1 typically affects the eyes, skin, and mouth region and is transmitted by close personal contact. HSV-2 is typically associated with genital infection through venereal transmission and is responsible for most neonatal infections.

Congenital infection is usually acquired during passage through an infected maternal birth canal. The neonatal infection is confined to the central nervous system, skin, oral cavity, and eyes in one third of cases. It commonly manifests with vesicular skin lesions, ulcerative mouth sores, and keratoconjunctivitis. Disseminated disease occurs in two thirds of cases and can involve the liver, adrenal glands, and lungs. The mortality rate from disseminated disease is significant, and survivors usually have permanent impairment.

Eye involvement in congenital infection can include conjunctivitis, keratitis, retinochoroiditis, and cataracts. Keratitis can be epithelial or stromal. Retinal involvement can be severe, including massive exudates and retinal necrosis.

Diagnosis is based on the clinical presentation confirmed with viral cultures taken from vesicular fluid, conjunctival or corneal swabs, or from nasal secretions. Immunohistochemical and polymerase chain reaction testing are also available.

Treatment

Herpes conjunctivitis/keratitis is treated with topical antivirals such as trifluridine 1% drops nine times daily, vidarabine 3% ointment five times per day, and sometimes oral acyclovir. See Chapter 19 for further discussion of treatment of corneal disease. Disseminated disease requires intravenous antivirals such as acyclovir given under the direction of a specialist in pediatric infectious disease.

Diagnosis and treatment of acquired herpes simplex keratoconjunctivitis in children is similar to that in adults. See BCSC Section 8, *External Disease and Cornea*.

Arvin AM, Whitley RJ. Herpes simplex virus infections. In: Remington JS, Klein JO, eds. *Infectious Diseases of the Fetus and Newborn Infant.* 5th ed. Philadelphia: Saunders; 2001.

Overall JC. Herpes simplex virus infection of the fetus and newborn. *Pediatr Ann.* 1994;23:131–136.

Parrish CM. Herpes simplex virus eye disease. In: *Focal Points: Clinical Modules for Ophthalmologists.* San Francisco: American Academy of Ophthalmology; 1997: vol 15, no 2.

Schwartz GS, Holland EJ. Oral acyclovir for the management of herpes simplex virus keratitis in children. *Ophthalmology.* 2000;107:278–282.

Syphilis

Syphilis is caused by the spirochete *Treponema pallidum*, and sexual contact is the usual route of transmission. Fetal infection occurs following maternal spirochetemia. The longer the mother has had syphilis, the lower the risk of transmitting the disease to her child. If the mother has contracted primary or secondary disease, about one half of her offspring will be infected. In cases of untreated late maternal syphilis (the most common form), about 70% of infants are healthy.

Congenital syphilis should be considered in premature births of unexplained cause, large placenta, persistent rhinitis, intractable rash, unexplained jaundice, hepatosplenomegaly, pneumonia, anemia, generalized lymphadenopathy, and metaphyseal abnormalities or periostitis on radiograph. Congenitally acquired infection can lead to neonatal death or premature delivery. Early eye involvement in congenital syphilis is rare.

Chorioretinitis appears as a salt-and-pepper granularity of the fundus in some infants. An appearance of pseudoretinitis pigmentosa may ensue; rarely, anterior uveitis, glaucoma, or both may develop. In other cases, symptoms may not appear until late childhood or adolescence. Widely spaced, peg-shaped teeth; eighth nerve deafness; and interstitial keratitis constitute *Hutchinson triad*. Other manifestations include saddle nose, short maxilla, and linear scars around body orifices. Bilateral interstitial keratitis is the classic ophthalmic finding in older children and adults, occurring in approximately 10% of patients.

Diagnosis

The Centers for Disease Control and Prevention define confirmed congenital syphilis as when *T pallidum* is identified by dark-field microscopy. Congenital syphilis can be presumptively diagnosed by the combination of a positive result with the Venereal Disease Research Laboratory (VDRL) test and one or more of the following:

- Evidence of congenital syphilis on physical examination
- Long-bone radiographic evidence
- A positive result on VDRL testing of cerebrospinal fluid
- Otherwise unexplained elevation of cerebrospinal fluid protein or cell count
- Quantitative nontreponemal serologic titer four times greater than the mother's
- A positive FTA-ABS-19s-IgM test result

Treatment

Treatment for congenital syphilis in neonates younger than 1 month includes aqueous crystalline penicillin G, 50,000 units/kg IV every 12 hours for 1 week, then every 8 hours for a total of 10–14 days. Infants older than 1 month receive aqueous crystalline penicillin G every 6 hours for 10–14 days. Serologic tests should be repeated until they become nonreactive. Persistent positive titers or a positive cerebrospinal fluid VDRL test result at 6 months should prompt retreatment.

> Contreras F, Pereda J. Congenital syphilis of the eye with lens involvement. *Arch Ophthalmol.* 1978;96:1052.
>
> Ingall D, Sanchez P. Syphilis. In: Remington JS, Klein JO, eds. *Infectious Diseases of the Fetus and Newborn Infant.* 5th ed. Philadelphia: Saunders; 2001.

Ophthalmia Neonatorum

Ophthalmia neonatorum refers to conjunctivitis occurring in the first month of life caused by a number of different agents, including bacterial, viral, and chemical ones. Widespread effective prophylaxis has diminished the morbidity of this problem to very low levels in industrialized countries, but ophthalmia neonatorum remains a significant source of ocular morbidity, blindness, and even death in medically underserved areas around the world.

Etiology

The infecting organism usually contaminates the infant through direct contact during passage through the birth canal. Infections are known to ascend to the uterus so that even infants delivered via cesarean section can be infected. This possibility is enhanced by prolonged rupture of membranes at the time of delivery.

Most Important Agents

Neisseria

The most serious form of ophthalmia neonatorum is caused by *Neisseria gonorrhoeae*. Onset is typically in the first 3–4 days of life but may be delayed for up to 3 weeks. Though some cases may present with mild conjunctival hyperemia and discharge, severe cases have marked chemosis, copious discharge, and possibly rapid corneal ulceration and perforation of the eye (Fig 17-4). Systemic infection can cause sepsis, meningitis, and arthritis.

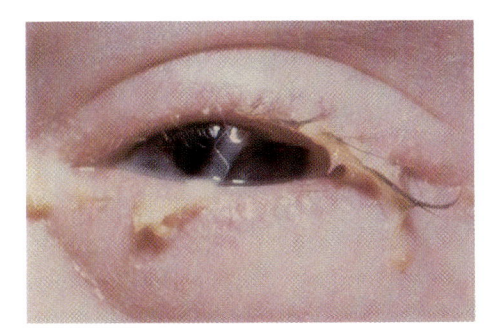

Figure 17-4 *Neisseria gonorrhoeae* conjunctivitis.

Diagnosis Gram's stain of the conjunctival exudate showing gram-negative intracellular diplococci allows a presumptive diagnosis of *N gonorrhoeae* infection, and treatment should be started immediately. Ophthalmia neonatorum from *Neisseria meningitidis* has been reported; the two *Neisseria* organisms cannot be differentiated by Gram's stain. Definitive diagnosis is based on culture of the conjunctival discharge. The specimen should be cultured on both selective (Thayer-Martin) and nonselective (chocolate agar) media and incubated at 37°C.

Treatment Treatment must be systemic. Increasing antibiotic resistance to traditionally effective antibiotics such as penicillin, tetracycline, and erythromycin has made treatment more difficult, but effective medications are available. Ceftriaxone given intravenously or intramuscularly daily for 1 week is highly effective. Penicillin (aqueous crystalline penicillin G) is effective for many susceptible strains.

Topical irrigation of the eyes can be helpful to mechanically débride large amounts of conjunctival discharge, but topical antibiotics, in the absence of corneal ulcer, provide no added benefit.

Chlamydia

Infection with *Chlamydia trachomatis* is the most common cause of ophthalmia neonatorum in the United States. The responsible agent (called *trachoma-inclusion conjunctivitis*, or *TRIC*) is an obligate intracellular organism. The infant comes into contact with the organism during passage through the birth canal of an infected mother, but like other organisms, the TRIC agent can ascend to the uterus and infect an infant delivered by cesarean section.

Onset of conjunctivitis in the infant usually occurs around 1 week of age, although onset may be earlier, especially in cases with premature rupture of membranes. Eye infection is characterized by usually mild swelling, hyperemia, and a papillary reaction with minimal to moderate discharge. Rare severe cases can be accompanied by more copious discharge and pseudomembrane formation. A follicular conjunctival reaction typical of adult inclusion conjunctivitis can occur after about 1 month of age.

Diagnosis Diagnosis can be made by culture from conjunctival scrapings. Several more rapid indirect laboratory tests are available, including enzyme-linked immunoassays and direct fluorescent antibody tests.

Treatment Chlamydial conjunctivitis is a self-limited disease, though it can last for a year or more in untreated cases. However, treatment is mandated in part because of the associated systemic involvement that can result in pneumonia or gastrointestinal infection. Treatment of the eye disease must be systemic; topical drops or ointment is superfluous.

The treatment of choice is oral erythromycin, 50 mg/kg per day in four divided doses for 10–14 days. As with other venereally transmitted diseases, public health authorities should be contacted to initiate evaluation and treatment of other maternal contacts.

Herpes simplex

Infection with HSV is a more rare form of ophthalmia neonatorum. It typically presents later than infection with *N gonorrhoeae* or *C trachomatis*, frequently in the second week of life. Please see the later discussion of herpes simplex conjunctivitis.

Chemical conjunctivitis

Chemical conjunctivitis refers to a mild, self-limited irritation and redness of the conjunctiva occurring in the first 24 hours after instillation of silver nitrate, a preparation used for prophylaxis of ophthalmia neonatorum. These symptoms can suggest the onset of conjunctivitis in the newborn, but it will improve spontaneously by the second day.

Prophylaxis for Ophthalmia Neonatorum

In 1880, Crede introduced the concept of widespread prophylaxis for gonorrheal ophthalmia neonatorum with 2% silver nitrate. It significantly reduced the incidence of gonorrheal conjunctivitis and is still used in many places today. This method is not effective against TRIC and therefore has been supplanted by agents effective against *Gonococcus* and TRIC, such as erythromycin and tetracycline ointments.

> Holland GN. Infectious diseases. In: Isenberg SJ, ed. *The Eye in Infancy*. 2nd ed. St Louis: Mosby; 1994:493–504.
>
> O'Hara MA. Ophthalmia neonatorum. *Pediatr Clin North Am*. 1993;40:715–725.

Conjunctivitis

Common causes of conjunctival inflammation, or *red eye*, in infants and children are listed in Table 17-1. The majority of cases of acute conjunctivitis in children are bacterial. About 20% of cases are caused by a virus. BCSC Section 8, *External Disease and Cornea*, discusses conjunctivitis in detail.

Common clinical findings in children with bacterial or viral conjunctivitis are burning, stinging, foreign body sensation, ocular discharge, and matting of the eyelids. Symptoms and signs may present unilaterally or bilaterally. The discharge, which can provide some diagnostic help, may be serous, mucopurulent, or purulent. Purulent discharge suggests a polymorphonuclear response to a bacterial infection, mucopurulence suggests a viral or chlamydial infection, and a serous or watery discharge suggests a viral or allergic reaction.

> Baum J, Barza M. The evolution of antibiotic therapy for bacterial conjunctivitis and keratitis: 1970–2000. *Cornea*. 2000;19:659–672.
>
> Feigin RD, Cherry JD, eds. *Textbook of Pediatric Infectious Disease*. 4th ed. Philadelphia: Saunders; 1998.
>
> Krachmer JH, Mannis MJ, Holland EJ, eds. *Cornea*. St Louis: Mosby; 1997.

Bacterial Conjunctivitis

The most common causes of bacterial conjunctivitis in school-age children are *Streptococcus pneumoniae*, some *Haemophilus* species, and *Moraxella*. The relative incidence of

Table 17-1 Causes of Conjunctival Inflammation in Children

> Infectious conjunctivitis
>   Bacterial
>   Viral
>   Chlamydial
>
> Blepharoconjunctivitis
>
> Allergic conjunctivitis
>
> Trauma
>
> Foreign body
>
> Drug, toxin, or chemical reaction
>
> Nasolacrimal duct obstruction
>
> Iritis
>
> Episcleritis or scleritis

infection from *Haemophilus* has dropped sharply in recent years since immunization for this genus has become widespread. In older children, cases present with unilateral or bilateral signs of conjunctival hyperemia, discharge, morning lid sealing, and perhaps foreign body sensation. In clinical practice, culture to identify the offending agent usually is not necessary. If untreated, symptoms will be self-limited but may last up to 2 weeks. A broad-spectrum topical ophthalmic drop or ointment should shorten the course to a few days. Usually effective medications include sulfacetamide, trimethoprim-polymyxin B, gentamicin or tobramycin, erythromycin ointment, or various newer fluoroquinolones.

More severe forms of bacterial conjunctivitis accompanied by copious discharge suggest infection with more virulent organisms, including *N gonorrhoeae, N meningitidis*, or various *Streptococcus, Staphylococcus,* or *Haemophilus* species. In such cases, calcium alginate swabs of the conjunctival surface should be obtained for Gram's stain and culture.

Although infection with *N gonorrhoeae* in children usually is associated with ophthalmia neonatorum from passage through an infected birth canal, older children who are sexually active or victims of sexual abuse can contract this infection.

For further discussion of diagnosis and treatment of gonorrheal conjunctivitis, see BCSC Section 8, *External Disease and Cornea.*

Viral Conjunctivitis

Most viral conjunctivitis is caused by adenovirus, a DNA virus that can cause a range of human disease including upper respiratory infection, gastroenteritis, and conjunctivitis. Some serotypes (types 18, 19, and 37) are associated with epidemic keratoconjunctivitis, others with pharyngoconjunctival fever (types 3 or 7), acute hemorrhagic conjunctivitis (types 11 or 21), or an acute follicular conjunctivitis (types 1, 2, 3, 4, 7, and 10).

Epidemic keratoconjunctivitis

Epidemic keratoconjunctivitis is a highly contagious conjunctivitis that tends to occur in epidemic outbreaks. This infection is an acute follicular conjunctivitis that is usually unilateral at onset and associated with preauricular lymphadenopathy. Initial complaints are foreign body sensation and periorbital pain. A diffuse superficial keratitis is followed by focal epithelial lesions that stain. After 11–15 days, subepithelial opacities begin to form under the focal epithelial infiltrates. The epithelial component fades by day 30, but the subepithelial opacities may linger for up to 2 years. In severe infections, particularly in infants, a conjunctival membrane and marked swelling of the eyelids occur and must be differentiated from orbital or preseptal cellulitis (discussed later under Orbital and Adnexal Infections).

The infection is easily transmitted and occurs in epidemic outbreaks. Infected children may need to be kept out of school or childcare for up to 2 weeks. Medical personnel who become infected should be excluded from ophthalmic examination areas for at least 2 weeks, and isolation areas should be designated for examination of patients known to have adenoviral infections.

Diagnosis is confirmed by isolation of the agent or increased antibody titer to the specific adenovirus type. The organism can be recovered from the eyes and throat for 2 weeks after onset, demonstrating that patients are infectious during this period. Complications include persistent subepithelial opacities and conjunctival scar formation. Treatment is supportive. Topical steroids administered three to four times daily may be used judiciously in severe cases causing visual compromise, but such agents may prolong the time to full recovery. Steroid use in adenovirus infections is seldom indicated in children.

Pharyngoconjunctival fever

Pharyngoconjunctival fever presents with conjunctival hyperemia and frequently with subconjunctival hemorrhage, edema, epiphora, and even lid swelling. Pharyngoconjunctival fever is accompanied by sore throat and fever. Within a few days, a follicular conjunctival reaction and preauricular adenopathy develop. Pharyngoconjunctival fever is caused by an adenovirus, usually type 3 or 7. Symptoms may last for 2 weeks or more. No topical or systemic treatment alters the course of the disease.

Herpes simplex conjunctivitis

HSV conjunctivitis can occur as a primary or secondary infection and typically presents with ocular redness, discomfort, foreign body sensation, or a combination thereof; a watery discharge; and preauricular adenopathy. HSV conjunctivitis is more commonly unilateral. Typical herpetic eye lid vesicles help identify the cause of the conjunctivitis, but they are not always present. Bulbar conjunctival ulceration, though rare, is highly suggestive of HSV infection.

Most cases of primary eye involvement are caused by HSV-1 and are associated with gingivostomatitis or recurrent orolabial infection. HSV-2 is associated with genital infection and is the more common cause of neonatal eye infections. Recurrent disease is characterized by dendritiform or geographic keratitis (Fig 17-5).

Treatment of pure conjunctival disease does not seem to alter the course of disease, although treatment is definitely indicated when the cornea is involved. Treatment includes topical drops of trifluridine 1%, nine drops per day, or vidarabine 3% ointment applied five times per day. For severe cases, oral acyclovir can be added, although this drug has

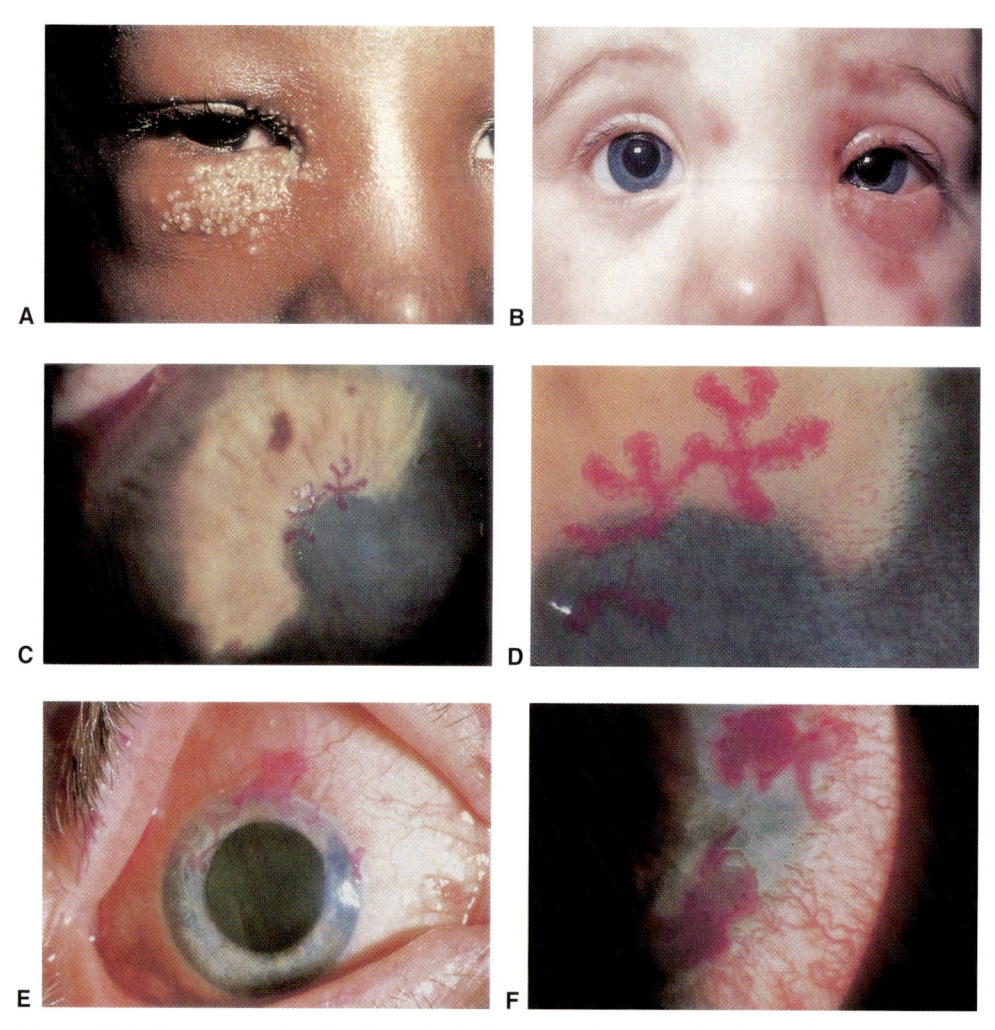

Figure 17-5 Herpes simplex. **A,** Vesicular lesions, right lower eyelid. **B,** Medial canthal distribution, left eye. **C** and **D,** Dendritic keratitis demonstrated by stain with rose bengal solution. **E** and **F,** Dendritic keratoconjunctivitis.

not been shown to be more efficacious for treatment of epithelial disease than topical treatment alone.

Corneal involvement can be treated with debridement of the infected area in addition to topical drops. See BCSC Section 8, *External Disease and Cornea,* for more discussion of the various forms of corneal disease and their treatment.

Herpes zoster

Children are seldom affected by herpes zoster, which rarely produces conjunctivitis. Vesicular lesions may erupt on the periorbital skin with subsequent ocular involvement (Fig 17-6).

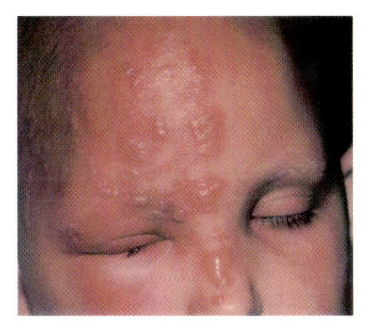

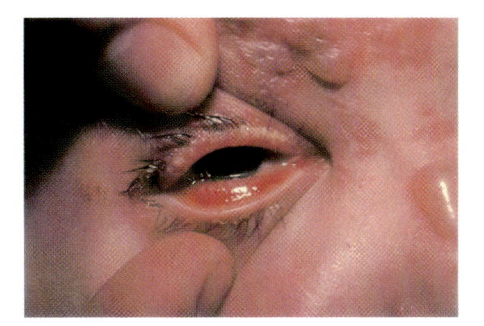

Figure 17-6 Herpes zoster.

Treatment includes steroids for the inflammation and for iritis, if present. Systemic antivirals (famciclovir, valacyclovir, acyclovir) can be used in infants and children with herpes zoster infection.

Infectious mononucleosis

Infectious mononucleosis is caused by Epstein-Barr virus. The disease usually occurs between ages 15 and 30 years and is benign and self-limited. Findings include fever, widespread lymphadenopathy, pharyngitis, hepatic involvement, and the presence of atypical lymphocytes and heterophil antibodies in the circulating blood. Conjunctivitis occurs in a very high percentage of cases. Treatment is supportive, including bed rest, antipyretics, analgesics, and cool compresses to the eyes.

Influenza virus

Acute conjunctivitis with superficial punctate or interstitial keratitis, chemosis, and secondary bacterial infection may be caused by influenza virus type A, B, or C. The clinical manifestations include headache, fever, malaise, myalgias, nasal congestion, nausea, cough, and pharyngitis. Treatment is supportive, with topical antibiotics to prevent secondary infection.

Mumps virus

Acute viremia may lead to ocular involvement. The conjunctival manifestations are chemosis, follicular or papillary conjunctivitis, hyperemia, and subconjunctival hemorrhages. Treatment is supportive, with topical antibiotics to prevent secondary bacterial infection.

Rubeola

Rubeola, an acute contagious febrile illness, primarily affects school-age children and is caused by a paramyxovirus. Clinical manifestations include maculopapular rash, keratoconjunctivitis, and inflammation of the respiratory tract. Treatment includes antipyretics, analgesics, and cool compresses on the eyelids.

Varicella (chickenpox)

Varicella is a contagious viral exanthem of childhood that causes fever and vesicular eruptions of skin and mucous membranes. The cause is varicella-zoster, a herpes family virus. Clinical manifestations include fever and characteristic skin lesions. Ocular involvement during primary childhood varicella is uncommon. Conjunctival vesicles or ulcerations and internal ophthalmoplegia can occur (Fig 17-7). The cornea may be involved with a dendritic ulcer, opacification, punctate epithelial keratitis, or interstitial keratitis.

Treatment is symptomatic. Topical steroids are contraindicated except for late non-ulcerative interstitial keratitis. Topical antibiotics may prevent secondary infection. Intravenous or oral acyclovir may be considered in the treatment of immunocompromised children with chickenpox but should be administered under the direction of an expert in pediatric infectious diseases.

Other Types of Conjunctivitis

Parinaud oculoglandular syndrome

Parinaud oculoglandular syndrome is a form of cat-scratch disease manifested as a unilateral granulomatous conjunctivitis associated with preauricular and submandibular adenopathy. The adenopathy can be very marked (Fig 17-8).

Cat-scratch disease is most commonly associated with a scratch from a young kitten, though a cat bite and perhaps even touching the eye with a hand that has been licked by an infected kitten can cause the disease. The etiologic agent, which is endemic in cats, has been identified as *Bartonella henselae*, a pleomorphic gram-negative bacillus.

Diagnosis is made on clinical grounds and supported by a compatible history of exposure to cats. An immunofluorescent assay directed at *B henselae* is available.

Treatment can be supportive in mild cases because the disease is self-limited and is not known to cause corneal complications. In more severe cases, oral ciprofloxacin, rifampin, trimethoprim-sulfamethoxazole, and erythromycin have been reported to be successful.

Other organisms that can cause similar disease are *Mycobacterium tuberculosis, Mycobacterium leprae, Francisella tularensis, Yersinia pseudotuberculosis, Treponema pallidum,* and *C trachomatis*.

> Grando D, Sullivan LJ, Flexman JP, et al. Bartonella henselae associated with Parinaud's oculoglandular syndrome. *Clin Infect Dis.* 1999;28:1156–1158.

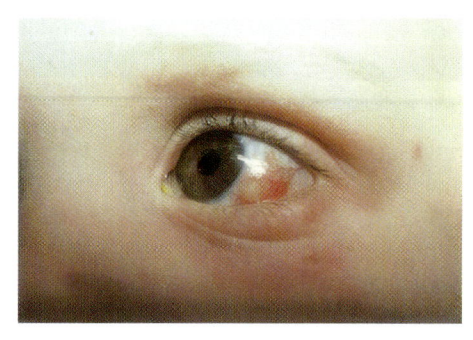

Figure 17-7 Varicella conjunctivitis, left eye.

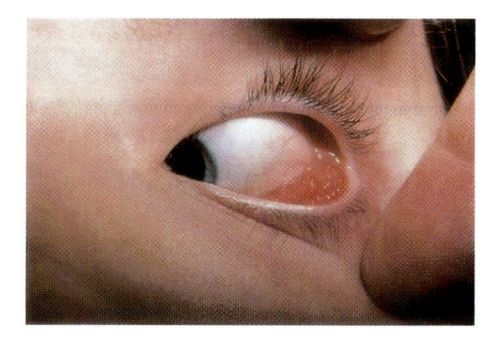

Figure 17-8 Parinaud oculoglandular syndrome, left eye.

Trachoma

Except in areas of the South and on Indian reservations, trachoma is uncommon in the United States. Most cases are mild. Clinical manifestations include acute purulent conjunctivitis, follicles, papillary hypertrophy, vascularization of the cornea, and progressive cicatricial changes of the cornea and conjunctiva. Diagnosis is made from corneal scrapings, which reveal cytoplasmic inclusion bodies. Expressed follicle material demonstrates large macrophages and lymphoblasts. Treatment includes topical or systemic sulfonamides (or both), erythromycin, and tetracyclines.

Orbital and Adnexal Infections

Orbital cellulitis and preseptal cellulitis are both usually more rapidly progressive and more severe in children than in adults. See also BCSC Section 7, *Orbit, Eyelids, and Lacrimal System*.

Preseptal Cellulitis

Preseptal cellulitis, a common infection in children, is an inflammatory process involving the tissues anterior to the orbital septum. Eyelid edema may extend into the eyebrow and forehead. The periorbital skin becomes taut and inflamed, and edema may appear on the contralateral eyelids. Proptosis is *not* a feature of preseptal cellulitis, and the globe remains uninflamed. Full ocular motility and absence of pain on eye movement help distinguish preseptal from orbital cellulitis.

Preseptal cellulitis can occur in one of three ways. Posttraumatic cellulitis occurs following puncture, laceration, or abrasion of the eyelid skin. In these cases, organisms found in the skin, such as *Staphylococcus aureus* or *Streptococcus pyogenes*, are the most common bacteria responsible for infection.

The second cause of preseptal cellulitis is severe conjunctivitis such as epidemic keratoconjunctivitis or skin infection such as impetigo or herpes-zoster infection.

The third mechanism for preseptal cellulitis tends to occur in young children and is secondary to upper respiratory or sinus infection or to unknown cause. Until the 1990s, *Haemophilus influenzae* was the most common causative agent. It could be recognized by a typical deep violaceous hue of the infected lids. *Haemophilus* preseptal cellulitis may still be seen in medically underserved regions, but the incidence has dropped markedly since widespread use of Hib vaccine began in the early 1990s. Now, *S pneumoniae* and other streptococcal infections and *S aureus* are the most common causes.

Children with nonsevere preseptal infections who are not systemically ill can be treated on an outpatient basis with oral antibiotics. Broad-spectrum drugs effective against the most common pathogens, such as cephalosporins or ampicillin–clavulanic acid combination, are usually effective.

If the child is younger than 1 year or has signs of systemic illness such as sepsis or meningeal involvement, hospitalization (for appropriate cultures, imaging of the sinuses and orbits, and intravenous antibiotics) is appropriate.

218 • Pediatric Ophthalmology and Strabismus

Orbital Cellulitis

Orbital cellulitis is an infection of the orbit that involves the tissues posterior to the orbital septum. Orbital cellulitis is commonly associated with ethmoid or frontal sinusitis and subperiosteal abscess and can follow penetrating injuries of the orbit. A retained foreign body can trigger orbital cellulitis months after the initial injury.

The etiologic agents most commonly responsible for orbital cellulitis vary with age. In general, children younger than 9 years have infections caused by a single aerobic pathogen. Children older than 9 years may have complex infections with multiple pathogens, both aerobic and anaerobic. *S aureus* and gram-negative bacilli are most common in the neonate. In older children and adults, *S aureus*, *S pyogenes*, *S pneumoniae*, and various anaerobic species are common pathogens. Gram-negative organisms are found primarily in immunosuppressed patients.

Diagnosis

Early signs and symptoms of orbital cellulitis include lethargy, fever, eyelid edema, rhinorrhea, headache, orbital pain, and tenderness on palpation. The nasal mucosa becomes hyperemic with a purulent nasal discharge. Increased venous congestion may cause elevated intraocular pressure. Proptosis and limited ocular rotations suggest orbital involvement. In general, children with orbital cellulitis appear much more ill than children of similar age with preseptal involvement only. It is crucial to distinguish orbital cellulitis from preseptal cellulitis because the former requires hospitalization with IV antibiotics. Paranasal sinusitis is the most common cause of bacterial orbital cellulitis (Fig 17-9). In children younger than 10 years, the ethmoid sinuses are most frequently involved. If orbital cellulitis is suspected, computed tomography is indicated to confirm orbital involvement, to document the presence and extent of sinusitis and subperiosteal abscess, and to rule out a foreign body in a patient with a history of trauma (Fig 17-10).

The differential diagnosis of orbital cellulitis includes inflammatory pseudotumor, benign orbital tumors such as lymphangioma and hemangioma, rhabdomyosarcoma or other malignant tumors, metastatic disease, and leukemia.

Complications of orbital cellulitis include cavernous sinus thrombosis or intracranial extension (subdural or brain abscesses, meningitis, periosteal abscess), which may result in death. Cavernous sinus thrombosis can be difficult to distinguish from simple orbital cellulitis. Paralysis of eye movement in cavernous sinus thrombosis is often out of proportion to the degree of proptosis. Pain on motion and tenderness to palpation are absent.

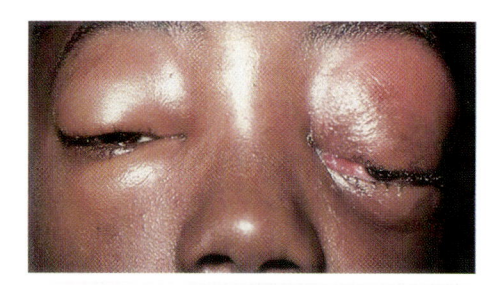

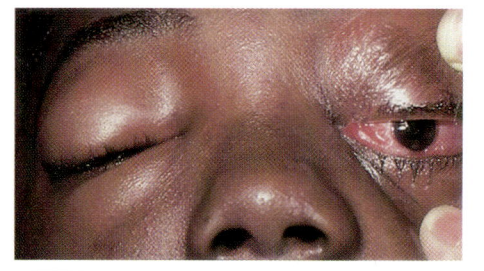

Figure 17-9 Orbital cellulitis secondary to pansinusitis.

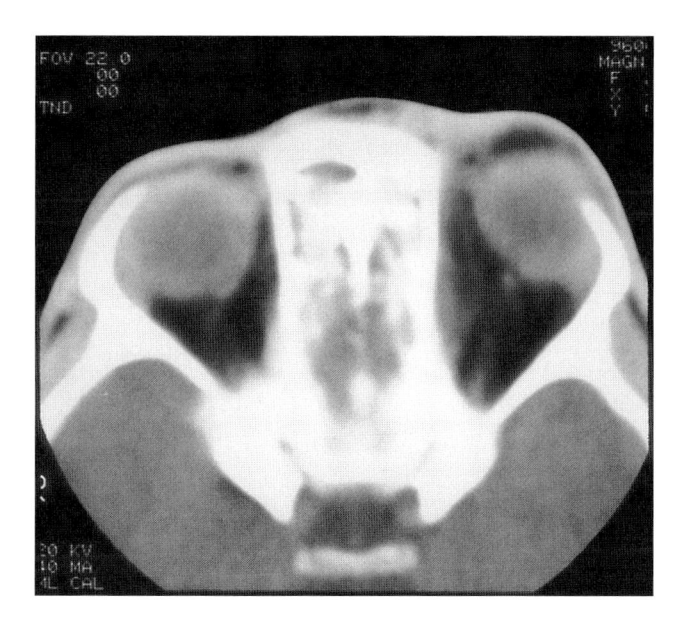

Figure 17-10 Axial CT showing a medial subperiosteal abscess of the left orbit associated with ethmoid sinusitis. *(Image courtesy of Mark S. Ruttum, MD.)*

Decreased sensation along the maxillary division of cranial nerve V (trigeminal) supports the diagnosis. Bilateral involvement is virtually diagnostic of cavernous sinus thrombosis.

Other complications of orbital cellulitis include corneal exposure with secondary ulcerative keratitis, neurotropic keratitis, secondary glaucoma, septic uveitis or retinitis, exudative retinal detachment, optic nerve edema, inflammatory neuritis, infectious neuritis, central retinal artery occlusion, and panophthalmitis.

Treatment

Orbital cellulitis in children is a serious disease that requires hospitalization and treatment with intravenous broad-spectrum antibiotics. Orbital computed tomography should be performed. If associated sinusitis is present, an otolaryngologist should be consulted. The patient should be followed closely for signs of visual compromise.

Choice of intravenous antibiotic should be based on the most likely pathogens until culture results from nasal, nasopharyngeal, or blood cultures are known. Nafcillin or oxacillin combined with cefuroxime or cefotaxime is a logical initial therapy for most patients. Vancomycin and chloramphenicol can be useful in patients with penicillin or cephalosporin allergy.

Emergency drainage of a subperiosteal abscess is indicated for a patient of any age with evidence of optic nerve compromise (decreasing vision, relative afferent pupillary defect) and an enlarging subperiosteal abscess. Even in the absence of optic nerve dysfunction, surgical drainage may be required for clinical deterioration despite 48 hours of intravenous antibiotics or to relieve significant discomfort.

Harris GJ. Subperiosteal abscess of the orbit: age as a factor in bacteriology and response to treatment. *Ophthalmology.* 1994;101:585–595.

Harris GJ. Subperiosteal abscess of the orbit: computed tomography and the clinical course. *Ophthal Plast Reconstr Surg.* 1996;12:1–8.

Related conditions

Maxillary osteomyelitis is a rare condition of early infancy. Infection spreads from the nose into the tooth buds with unilateral erythema and edema of the eyelids, cheek, and nose. Infection may spread and cause orbital cellulitis.

Fungal orbital cellulitis (mucormycosis) occurs most frequently in patients with ketoacidosis or severe immunosuppression. The infection causes thrombosing vasculitis with ischemic necrosis of involved tissue (Fig 17-11). Cranial nerves often are involved, and extension into the central nervous system is common. Smears and biopsy of the involved tissues reveal the fungal organisms. Treatment includes debridement of necrotic and infected tissue plus administration of amphotericin. Predisposing factors such as metabolic acidosis should be controlled.

Ocular Allergy

Allergic ocular disease is a common problem in children, often associated with asthma, allergic rhinitis, and atopic dermatitis. Marked itching and bilateral conjunctival inflammation of a chronic, recurrent, and possibly seasonal nature are hallmarks of external ocular disease of allergic origin. Other signs and symptoms may be nonspecific and include tearing, stinging, burning, and photophobia.

Three specific types of ocular allergy are discussed below: seasonal allergic conjunctivitis, vernal keratoconjunctivitis, and atopic keratoconjunctivitis. All have some element of type I hypersensitivity reaction caused by the interaction between an allergen and specific IgE antibodies on the surface of mast cells in the conjunctiva. This interaction results in the initiation of a cascade of biochemical events involved in mediation of the allergic response, including prostaglandins and leukotrienes. Among the mediators released as a result of these interactions is histamine. Histamine is known to cause much of the itching, vasodilation, and edema that is so characteristic of the ocular allergic response.

Seasonal Allergic Conjunctivitis

Seasonal allergic conjunctivitis is a common clinical entity, affecting approximately 40 million people living in the United States, including many children. As the name implies,

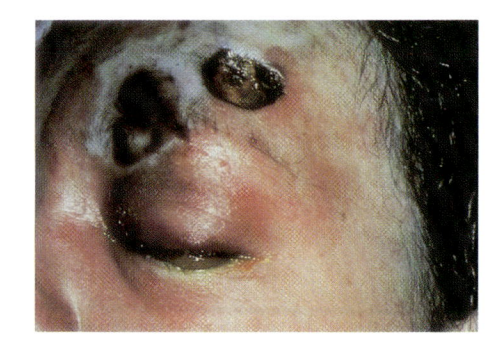

Figure 17-11 Mucormycosis, left orbit.

it is a seasonal affliction, occurring in the spring and fall and triggered by environmental contact with specific airborne allergens such as pollens from grasses, flowers, weeds, and trees. Conjunctival scrapings reveal eosinophils, a finding that is almost diagnostic of an allergic response. Patients typically present with reddened, watery eyes, boggy-appearing conjunctiva, and complaints of itchy eyes. Lower-lid ecchymoses termed *allergic shiners* are common.

Perennial allergic conjunctivitis is a related, though usually milder and less seasonal, form of type I hypersensitivity reaction to more ubiquitous household allergens, such as dust mites and dander from domestic pets.

Vernal Keratoconjunctivitis

Vernal keratoconjunctivitis shows evidence of a mast cell/lymphocyte-mediated allergic response. This condition most commonly affects males in the first two decades of life and, like seasonal allergic conjunctivitis, usually occurs in the spring and fall. It occurs in two forms, palpebral and bulbar, depending on which conjunctival surface is most affected.

The chief pathological findings include overgrowth of the subconjunctival tissues in the substantia propria. The tissue is infiltrated with lymphocytes, plasma cells, and eosinophils. With progression, large numbers of cells accumulate, forming nodules of tissue that project from the tarsal plate. New blood vessels are formed, producing giant papillae, the hallmark of this entity.

Clinically, the palpebral form of vernal keratoconjunctivitis preferentially affects the tarsal conjunctiva of the upper eyelid (Fig 17-12). Changes in the lower eyelid are rare and slight. In the early stages, the eye may be diffusely injected with little discharge and the conjunctiva appears milky. The most prominent features are photophobia and intense itching. There may be no progression beyond this stage. However, papillae may multiply, covering the tarsal area with a mosaic of flat papules. The conjunctiva is then covered with a milky veil.

The discharge is characteristically thick, ropy, and dirty white. It contains epithelial cells, leukocytes, and large numbers of eosinophils. Itching can be intense and accompanied by blepharospasm, foreign body sensation, and photophobia.

The limbal, or bulbar, form of vernal keratoconjunctivitis is also bilateral and seasonal, etiologically and pathogenically similar to the palpebral disease. Intense itching is

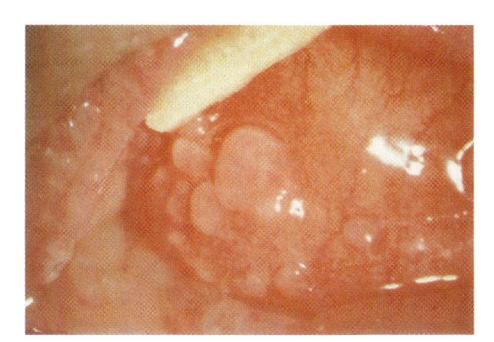

Figure 17-12 Palpebral vernal keratoconjunctivitis, upper eyelid.

the most constant clinical feature. The earliest changes are thickening and opacification of the conjunctiva at the limbus, usually most marked at the upper margin of the cornea. The discrete limbal nodules that appear in this thickened conjunctiva are gray, jellylike, elevated lumps with vascular cores. They may increase in number and become confluent. These nodules persist as long as the seasonal exacerbation of the disease lasts. A whitish center may occur in the raised lesion filled with eosinophils and epithelioid cells. The complex is called a *Trantas* or *Horner-Trantas dot.*

The cornea can become involved with punctate epithelial erosions, especially superiorly. Corneal involvement can progress to a large confluent area of epithelial defect, typically in the upper half of the cornea, called a *shield ulcer.* The ulcer is sterile and clinically looks like an ovoid corneal abrasion.

Atopic Keratoconjunctivitis

Atopic keratoconjunctivitis has elements of a variety of immune responses, including type I and cell-mediated response. This condition is relatively rare in children and tends to present in males from the late teens to the sixth decade of life. Atopic keratoconjunctivitis is not seasonal and occurs in atopic persons with a tendency to develop hypersensitivity reactions like atopic dermatitis, eczema, and asthma. Chronic inflammation of the eyelids is usually apparent. Unlike the case with vernal keratoconjunctivitis, the inferior palpebral conjunctiva is usually involved with papillae and scarring.

Other ocular involvement is common, including punctate corneal erosions and cataracts.

Treatment

Treatment of all allergic eye disorders is fundamentally similar to treatment of other allergy-related disorders. The most effective treatment is to remove the offending allergens from the patient's environment. Unfortunately, such attempts at removal frequently fall short of what is required to adequately alleviate the patient's symptoms.

Medical treatment can be systemic or topical. In general, oral medications—specifically, antihistamines aimed at ameliorating itching, swelling, and redness—are not very effective for ocular symptoms. The sedating effect of most drugs outweighs their therapeutic benefit for ocular allergy, although some recently introduced antihistamines induce less drowsiness than previous generations of these medications.

Topical eye drops are the preferred therapy for most patients. Therapeutic strategies are to stabilize mast cells, block H_1 receptors, or both. Available topical drops are listed in Table 17-2.

Cromolyn sodium, derived from khellin, a substance found in a Mediterranean plant, is the prototype mast cell stabilizer. Cromolyn acts by decreasing the release of granules containing inflammatory mediators from allergen-stimulated mast cells.

H_1-blocking antihistamines act by competitive inhibition of the H_1 sites responsible for the itching response and some of the vascular permeability and vasodilation reactions.

A topical nonsteroidal anti-inflammatory medication, ketorolac tromethamine (Acular), is also available.

Topical steroid drops used in pulsed doses can be effective in reducing allergic ocular symptoms, but patients using topical steroids, unlike those using other nonsteroidal

Table 17-2 Topical Drops for Treatment of Allergic Eye Disorders

Mast cell stabilizers
Cromolyn sodium (Crolom and Opticrom)
Lodoxamide tromethamine (Alomide)
Nedocromil sodium (Alocril)
Pemirolast potassium (Alamast)

H_1-receptor antagonists
Emedastine (Emadine)
Levocabastine hydrochloride (Livostin)

Drops with both mast cell stabilizer and H_1-blocking activity
Ketotifen fumarate (Zaditor)
Olopatadine hydrochloride (Patanol)

---

drops, must be closely monitored for steroid side effects, including glaucoma and cataracts.

> Bouchard C. The ocular immune response. In: Krachmer JH, Mannis MJ, Holland EJ, eds. *Cornea*. St Louis: Mosby; 1997.
>
> Dinowitz M, Rescigno R, Bielory L. Ocular allergic diseases: differential diagnosis, examination techniques, and testing. *Clin Allergy Immunol*. 2000;15:127–150.
>
> Heidemann DG. Atopic and vernal keratoconjunctivitis. In: *Focal Points: Clinical Modules for Ophthalmologists*. San Francisco: American Academy of Ophthalmology; 2001: vol 19, no 1.
>
> Mets MB, Noffke AS. Ocular infections of the external eye and cornea in children. In: *Focal Points: Clinical Modules for Ophthalmologists*. San Francisco: American Academy of Ophthalmology; 2002: vol 20, no 2.

Stevens-Johnson Syndrome (Erythema Multiforme)

Stevens-Johnson syndrome is an acute inflammatory polymorphic disease affecting skin and mucous membranes. All ages may be affected, and the incidence is equal in both sexes. This is a severe disease with a 5%–15% mortality rate. Ocular involvement, which occurs in as many as half of patients, varies from a mild mucopurulent conjunctivitis to severe perforating corneal ulcers. Blindness occasionally occurs in patients with a severe late-phase corneal complication, such as ulceration, vascularization, and perforation.

Stevens-Johnson syndrome has been associated with various bacterial, viral, mycotic, and protozoal infections. Vaccines, collagen diseases, and many drugs have also been implicated. The pathogenesis consists of angiitis leading to erythematous lesions that become edematous or bullous and darken, leaving concentric rings in a target shape. When bullae are present, they are subepidermal and without acantholysis.

Clinical manifestations range from mild to severe. A prodrome of chills is followed by pharyngitis, headache, tachypnea, and tachycardia. In several days, bullous mucosal lesions develop, especially in the oropharynx. These lesions rupture and ulcerate and become covered by gray-white membranes and a hemorrhagic crust.

Ocular involvement in Stevens-Johnson syndrome begins with edema, erythema, and encrustation of the eyelids. The palpebral conjunctiva becomes hyperemic, and distinct vesicles or bullae may occur. In many instances, a concomitant conjunctivitis appears that is characterized by watery discharge with mucoid strands (Fig 17-13). Secondary infection, most commonly with *Staphylococcus* species, may develop. In severe cases, a membranous or pseudomembranous conjunctivitis may result from coalescence of fibrin and necrotic cellular debris. Symblepharon formation may occur with severe pseudomembranous conjunctivitis. Primary corneal involvement and iritis are rare ocular manifestations of Stevens-Johnson syndrome.

Late ocular complications occur in about 20% of patients and include structural anomalies of eyelid position (ectropion and entropion), trichiasis, and symblepharon. Dry eye syndrome may also result from deficiencies in the tear film—either the aqueous layer from scarring of lacrimal duct orifices or, more commonly, the mucin layer from destruction of the conjunctival goblet cells.

Treatment

Early intervention is important in preventing the late ocular complications of Stevens-Johnson syndrome. Systemic therapy with corticosteroids is controversial. Antiviral treatment for cases associated with herpes simplex infection may be required. A discussion of systemic treatment is beyond the scope of this book. A dermatologist and pediatric infectious disease expert should be consulted.

Local measures should be instituted early in the course of the disease. Ocular lubrication with artificial tears and ointments (preferably preservative-free) should be applied regularly. Under topical anesthesia, the superior and inferior fornices should be inspected and débrided daily. A glass rod can be used for symblepharon lysis, but this may be ineffective. A symblepharon ring can be useful in severe cases in cooperative patients. Surveillance cultures for microbial infection should be taken as needed. See also BCSC Section 8, *External Disease and Cornea*.

> Wilkins J, Morrison L, White CR Jr. Oculocutaneous manifestations of the erythema multiforme/Stevens-Johnson syndrome/toxic epidermal necrolysis spectrum. *Dermatol Clin.* 1992;10:571–582.

Kawasaki Syndrome

Kawasaki syndrome, also known as *mucocutaneous lymph node syndrome*, is a febrile illness primarily affecting children younger than 5 years. The cause is unknown. The diagnostic criteria are an unexplainable fever lasting 5 or more days and at least four of the following:

- Bilateral conjunctival injection
- Mucous membrane changes of injected or fissured lips, injected pharynx, or "strawberry tongue"
- Extremity changes involving erythema of the palms or soles, edema of the hands or feet, or generalized or periungual desquamation
- Rash
- Cervical lymphadenopathy

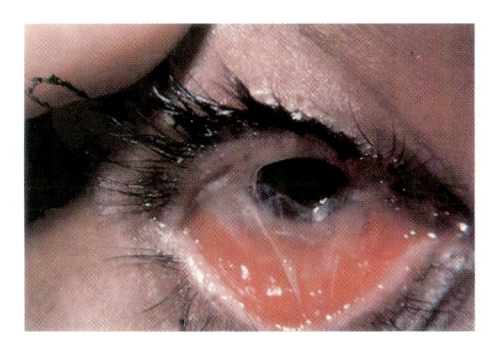

Figure 17-13 Stevens-Johnson syndrome. Early involvement of conjunctiva, right eye.

The most significant complication of Kawasaki syndrome is coronary artery aneurysm. Coronary artery evaluation by two-dimensional echocardiography is therefore indicated.

Anterior uveitis during the acute phase of the illness is common but generally self-limited. Conjunctival scarring can occur, and bilateral retinal ischemia has been observed histopathologically.

Treatment is mainly supportive, and aspirin is considered the drug of choice. Corticosteroid therapy is contraindicated because of its association with an increased rate of coronary artery aneurysm formation.

Blatt AN, Vogler L, Tychsen L. Incomplete presentations in a series of 37 children with Kawasaki disease: the role of the pediatric ophthalmologist. *J Pediatr Ophthalmol Strabismus.* 1996;33:114–119.

CHAPTER 18

The Lacrimal Drainage System

Tear fluid enters the lacrimal drainage system through the *puncta*, small (approximately 0.3 mm) round openings located in the upper and lower eyelids just nasal to the most medial of the meibomian gland orifices. The lower punctum is slightly more temporally located than the upper, and both are positioned so as to contact the surface of the eye. Each punctum continues as a *canaliculus* that runs vertically for 1–2 mm and then turns nasally toward the *lacrimal sac*, parallel to the eyelid margin. The canaliculi are lined with stratified squamous epithelium and surrounded by a layer of elastic tissue that permits considerable dilation. The tarsal plate does not extend into the portion of the eyelid containing the canaliculus, which consequently is easily torn. The upper and lower canaliculi join to form a very short *common canaliculus* before entering the lacrimal sac at *the valve of Rosenmüller*.

The lacrimal sac occupies the lacrimal fossa, which is formed by the lacrimal bone and the frontal process of the maxillary bone. The medial canthal ligament, which arises from the anterior lacrimal crest, lies in front of the upper portion of the sac. The epithelial lining of the sac is composed of a superficial columnar layer and a deeper layer of flattened cells as well as numerous mucus-secreting goblet cells. Similar epithelium lines the *nasolacrimal duct (NLD)*, which is the continuation of the sac, extending downward in a slightly lateral and posterior direction through a short bony canal to enter the lateral portion of the nose beneath the inferior turbinate at the *valve of Hasner*.

The lacrimal drainage passages arise embryologically from a solid epithelial cord formed by invagination of surface ectoderm, which canalizes toward the end of gestation. Persistence of a thin tissue membrane across the lower end of the duct at birth is very common.

Developmental Anomalies

Atresia of the Lacrimal Puncta

Atresia of the lacrimal puncta results from failure of the upper end of the developing lacrimal structures to canalize. Symptoms are typically limited to accumulation and overflow of clear tears; mucopurulence is not seen to the degree typical of an obstruction of the lacrimal duct. Often, only a thin epithelial punctal membrane obstructs a well-developed canalicular system. The site is easily identified in such cases, and perforating the membrane with a needle, followed by dilation, usually is curative. Other obstructions in the canalicular system cause symptoms similar to those of punctal atresia. More elaborate surgery may be required, ranging from an incisional punctoplasty combined with silicone intubation to conjunctivodacryocystorhinostomy in extreme cases.

Supernumerary Puncta

Supernumerary puncta occasionally occur nasal to the normal opening; they require no treatment.

Congenital Lacrimal Fistula

Congenital lacrimal fistula is an epithelial-lined tract extending from the common canaliculus or lacrimal sac to the skin surface of the lower eyelid, usually just inferonasal to the medial canthus. Discharge from the fistula often is associated with NLD obstruction and may cease to be a problem after the lower drainage system becomes patent. Persistence of bothersome symptoms necessitates surgical excision of the entire fistulous tract.

> Birchansky LD, Nerad JA, Kersten RC, et al. Management of congenital lacrimal sac fistula. *Arch Ophthalmol.* 1990;108:388–390.
> Cahill KV, Burns JA. Management of epiphora in the presence of congenital punctal and canalicular atresia. *Ophthal Plast Reconstr Surg.* 1991;7:167–172.
> Sevel D. Development and congenital abnormalities of the nasolacrimal apparatus. *J Pediatr Ophthalmol Strabismus.* 1982;18:13–19.

Dacryocele

Congenital dacryocele (sometimes called *mucocele, dacryocystocele,* or *amniotocele*) of the lacrimal sac is an uncommon condition, present at birth, in which cystic swelling accompanies obstruction of the lacrimal drainage system both above and below the sac. The lower blockage is usually membranous, similar to that responsible for the congenital NLD obstruction described below. Sometimes the upper part of the system is also obstructed anatomically, but often an unusually competent valve of Rosenmüller simply prevents reflux of accumulated fluid from the sac. Most authorities think the fluid originates as mucus secreted by the epithelium of the lacrimal sac, although lacrimal gland secretions and amniotic fluid have been suggested as alternatives. Involvement is occasionally bilateral.

Clinical Features

Dacryocele presents as a bluish swelling just below and nasal to the medial canthus. The appearance is distinctive, but there is the possibility of confusion with hemangioma, dermoid cyst, or encephalocele. Associated nasal mucocele (bulging of mucosa at the lower end of the NLD into the nasal cavity, which can be viewed with the nasal endoscope) can significantly compromise the airway. This finding also can be seen with NLD obstruction without a clinically apparent dacryocele. If the condition does not resolve spontaneously, infection with obvious local inflammatory changes usually develops within the first few weeks of life (Fig 18-1).

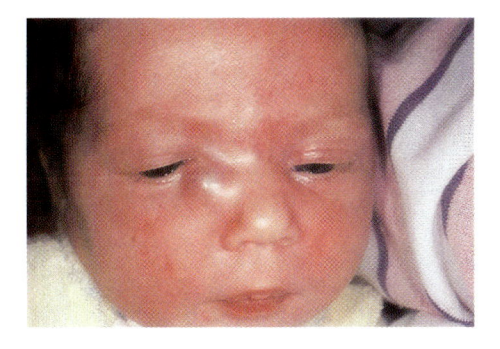

Figure 18-1 Congenital dacryocystocele, right eye, in a newborn girl. Note typical location and bluish discoloration of the overlying skin.

Management

A dacryocele sometimes can be decompressed by digital massage, which in combination with topical antibiotic administration may lead to resolution without complications. Lacrimal probing should be performed no later than 1 month after birth in persistent cases. Once dacryocystitis develops, systemic antibiotics are indicated, and prompt surgical decompression of the sac is usually necessary. This can be accomplished initially by passing a probe or lacrimal cannula through a canaliculus into the distended sac, but permanent and complete relief requires elimination of associated NLD obstruction. Any associated nasal mucocele can be marsupialized to facilitate drainage into the nose.

Probing the lower system can be difficult because of the considerable anatomical distortion that frequently accompanies dacryocele. Sometimes, intranasal surgery to marsupialize the bulging lower end of the duct is required. Incision and drainage of an infected dacryocele through the skin should be avoided because of the danger of creating a persistent fistulous tract.

> Paysse EA, Coats DK, Bernstein JM, et al. Management and complications of congenital dacryocele with concurrent intranasal mucocele. *J AAPOS*. 2000;4:46–53.

Nasolacrimal Duct Obstruction

Clinical Features

Obstruction of drainage below the lacrimal sac occurs in about 5% of full-term newborns. Usually, a thin mucosal membrane at the lower end of the NLD is the cause. Symptoms become manifest by age 1 month in 80%–90% of cases. Symptoms typically consist of epiphora and sticky mucoid or mucopurulent discharge that accumulates on the eyelid margins and lashes (Fig 18-2). The clinician can confirm the impatency of the drainage system by applying fluorescein solution to the tear film and noting significant retention after 5–10 minutes, with failure of dye to appear in the nose or pharynx after 10–15 minutes.

The severity of these manifestations may vary considerably from day to day. Digital pressure applied over the lacrimal sac often produces reflux of cloudy fluid through the punctum. Culture of the discharge typically indicates the presence of multiple strains of

Figure 18-2 Congenital nasolacrimal duct obstruction, right eye, in an infant boy. Note wetness and mucus accumulation, without evidence of inflammation.

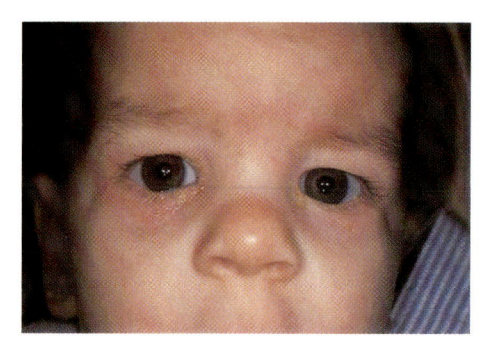

bacteria, but this step is not necessary for clinical management. Bilateral involvement is common.

The differential diagnosis of congenital NLD obstruction includes the following disorders:

- Punctal or canalicular atresia, which is ruled out by inspection
- Conjunctivitis
- Blepharitis, characterized by dry crusting on the eyelid margins
- Congenital glaucoma, in which epiphora caused by hypersecretion of tears is associated with nasal wetness and corneal enlargement or clouding, features that are absent from the clinical picture of lacrimal obstruction

Nonsurgical Management

Conservative management of congenital NLD obstruction includes lacrimal sac massage and administration of topical antibiotics. The antimicrobial agent should cover a broad spectrum of bacteria. Some clinicians prefer ointment because of its longer retention in the eye; others prefer drops, which are more likely to reach the sac.

Digital massage of the lacrimal sac and instillation of medication should be performed several times per day. Massage serves two purposes: it empties the sac, reducing opportunity for bacterial growth; and it applies hydrostatic pressure to the obstruction, which occasionally opens the duct and permanently relieves symptoms. To create sufficient pressure, it is necessary to compress the sac while initially occluding the canaliculi. The parent is instructed to place a finger above the medial canthus and then firmly press and slide downward along this side of the nose.

Congenital NLD obstruction resolves spontaneously with conservative management in a large majority of cases. Published series have shown clearing in 50%–90% of patients during the first 6 months of life. The probability that an affected 6-month-old will become asymptomatic by age 1 year is about 70%. The classic view has been that beyond age 1 year, the rate of spontaneous resolution is significantly reduced and the likelihood of permanent damage to the lacrimal drainage system from chronic repeated infections increases. More recent studies have shown that although extensive delay is not the treatment of choice, cases with membranous (ie, uncomplicated) obstruction presenting after the first year of life have success rates with simple probing comparable to those of younger infants. (See Chapter 14 of BCSC Section 7, *Orbit, Eyelids, and Lacrimal System*.)

> Kushner BJ. The management of nasolacrimal duct obstruction in children between 18 months and 4 years old. *J AAPOS*. 1998;2:57–60.

Surgical Management

Probing

The timing of surgery for congenital NLD obstruction is controversial. Early probing (before age 12 months) reduces the duration of bothersome symptoms, the burden of conservative management, and the potential for chronic infection. The procedure can be done in the office in the youngest patients, avoiding the risk of general anesthesia and the trouble and expense of even brief hospitalization. However, delaying probing until age 12 months or later may avoid surgery altogether in many cases. In the rest, probing in the operating room setting allows for increased control and provides the additional advantage of a better opportunity to evaluate and treat an obstructing inferior turbinate or an intranasal mucocele.

The surgical timing decision for a particular patient must be guided by the following factors:

- Severity of the child's symptoms
- The ophthalmologist's training, experience, and practice environment
- Availability of safe general anesthesia for pediatric patients
- Wishes and concerns of the family

The success rate of properly performed initial probing for congenital NLD obstruction exceeds 90% in infants up to 12 months old, and no convincing evidence has shown that delaying surgical treatment until age 12–15 months is harmful. Surgery performed after age 24 months fails to relieve symptoms with simple probing in as many as one third of cases. Two hypotheses have been proposed to explain this observation:

- Persistent obstruction of tear drainage with consequent infection and inflammation leads to scarring that progressively reduces the probability of successful probing over time.
- A small proportion of newborns with congenital NLD obstruction have anatomical variants that are unlikely to resolve spontaneously or be relieved by simple probing; as time passes and most other cases improve, this unchanging subgroup comes to account for an increasingly large fraction of the remaining affected population.

Before probing begins in an office setting, the unsedated infant is wrapped securely to immobilize the trunk and extremities as well as the head, and topical anesthetic is instilled. In the operating room, administration of inhalation agents by facial or laryngeal mask can provide adequate anesthesia, although some surgeons and anesthesiologists prefer to protect the airway with endotracheal intubation.

Before instruments are introduced, the lacrimal sac is emptied by digital compression, and the eyelid margins are cleansed of accumulated mucus. Observation of reflux from the puncta confirms patency of the canalicular system. The clinician initiates probing by dilating either the upper or the lower punctum. The risk of inadvertently causing significant damage to the canalicular system is said to be reduced by probing through the upper canaliculus, but the easier access afforded by the lower eyelid may outweigh this unproved advantage, particularly in the unanesthetized infant.

The instrument used for punctal dilation should have a slightly blunted tip and taper gradually up to a diameter of greater than 1 mm. (Some surgeons use the point of a large standard safety pin.) After the instrument is engaged in the punctal opening, it is immediately directed nasalward and advanced parallel to the eyelid margin while digital countertraction is applied to the eyelid. Holding constant pressure in this manner for 10–15 seconds usually suffices to dilate the punctum.

It is possible, before passing a probe through the NLD, to "hydrostatically" test the system by introducing a blunt-tipped irrigating cannula into the sac, directing it inferiorly and attempting to force a small amount of saline through the system from a syringe under moderate pressure. Reflux is prevented by compression of the canaliculi, but aspiration and laryngospasm are possible if fluid volume is excessive. This maneuver can confirm the presence of NLD obstruction and occasionally relieve it, either by the hydrostatic force of the irrigation or, if a longer-than-usual cannula is employed, by perforating the obstruction as a probe does.

If this preliminary maneuver is not successful, a Bowman probe judged to be of the appropriate size (usually No. 00, 0, or 1) can be advanced toward the sac along the canaliculus (Fig 18-3). If resistance is encountered (usually the result of kinking rather than anatomical obstruction in the canaliculus), the probe should be pulled back slightly and its direction modified until further advancement becomes possible. The probe should not be forced through the canalicular system. If this maneuver fails, passage through the other canaliculus should be tried.

Successful passage through the canalicular system is signaled by the feel of the probe tip against the nasal wall of the sac (bone under a thin layer of mucosa), which is distinctive. If a soft or spongy resistance is felt at the end of the canaliculus, the probe is probably caught at the valve of Rosenmüller. The probe should be gently maneuvered with the aid of countertraction on the eyelid and minimal force to get past this area.

When the surgeon is convinced that the nasal wall has been reached, the probe tip is held against the nasal wall of the sac and the probe is pivoted roughly 90°, directing it downward toward the floor of the nose, slightly rearward and temporally. The probe often must be subtly repositioned before it can be advanced smoothly. When there is distal membranous obstruction, as the probe slides through the NLD, a pop can be felt as the obstruction is overcome.

Sometimes, several minor barriers are overcome along the duct's course or a sense of constriction is felt throughout its length. Occasionally, despite repeated efforts to achieve smooth passage, grating resistance is felt, which may suggest that probing will be unsuccessful. (A precise description in the operative report of the feel of probe passage becomes valuable if later surgery is required.)

The distance traversed in probing from the punctum to the floor of the nasal cavity is approximately equal to the distance from the punctum to the external tip of the nose (<3 cm in a 1-year-old). The surgeon who fails to realize that the nasal floor has been

CHAPTER 18: The Lacrimal Drainage System • 233

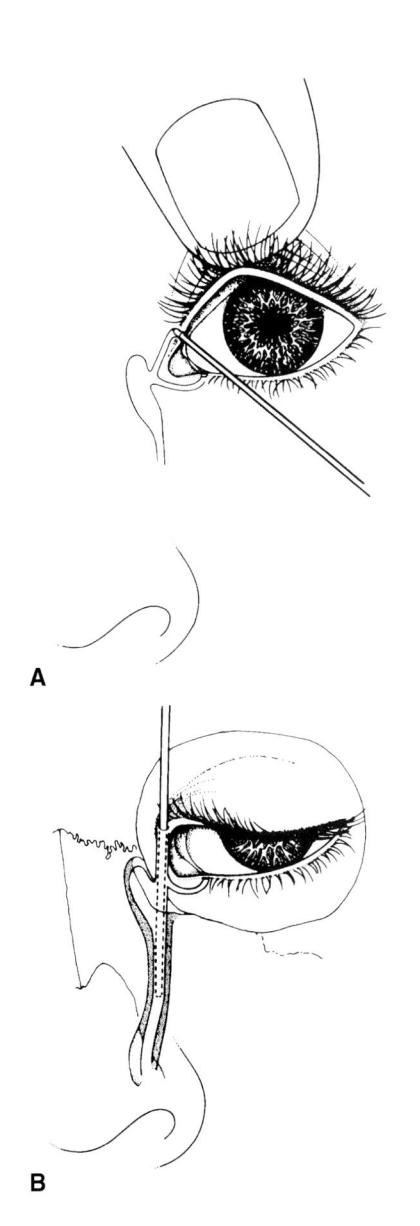

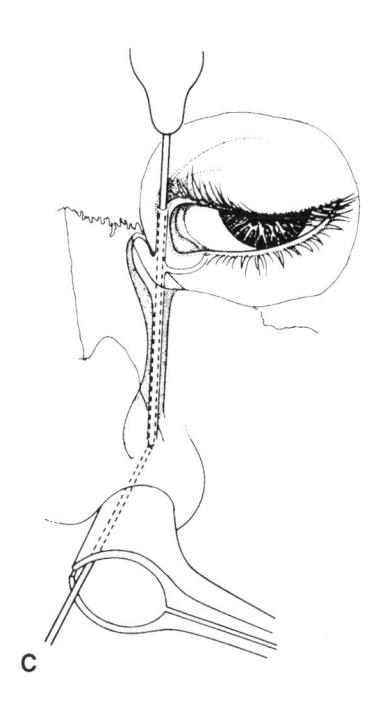

Figure 18-3 **A,** Introduction of probe tip through lacrimal punctum. **B,** Probe at completion of passage through canaliculus into lacrimal sac. **C,** Probe in transit through nasolacrimal duct. See text for detailed description of this surgical technique. *(Reproduced by permission from Calhoun JH, Nelson LB, Harley RD. Atlas of Pediatric Ophthalmic Surgery. Philadelphia: Saunders; 1987: 207–214.)*

reached can inadvertently push the probe through the palate into the oral cavity. To confirm emergence of the probe tip into the nose, a second probe is passed along the nasal floor close against the temporal wall underneath the inferior turbinate. The feel of metal on metal and the observed movement of the first probe as the second probe rubs directly against it confirms that the first probe is in the correct position. Alternatively, direct inspection with a nasal speculum and headlamp or with a special fiberoptic nasal endoscope can determine the precise position of the probe.

After probe withdrawal, irrigation through the drainage system should be possible with light pressure on the syringe; recovery of saline colored with fluorescein or methylene blue from the nose with a small suction catheter confirms patency.

Rarely, probing overcomes bony resistance. More often, the probe becomes misdirected into soft tissue or the maxillary sinus antrum. If either of these situations occur, the procedure should be aborted and reattempted on another occasion.

The most common undesired outcome of probing is passage into the nose along a route other than the true lacrimal drainage channel. Such *false passage* can result either from faulty manipulation of the probe or from anatomical variations that make it impossible for a straight instrument to follow the channel through its entire length. Intraoperative detection of false passage can be difficult or even impossible. Usually, the consequence of false passage is simply postoperative persistence or recurrence of symptoms, but occasionally damage to the tissue lining the canaliculus or NLD causes scarring that increases the difficulty of subsequent efforts to relieve drainage obstruction. Significant complications of probing are otherwise rare. Minor bleeding from the nose or into the tears sometimes occurs but requires no treatment.

Optional postoperative medications include antibiotic drops, corticosteroid drops, or both instilled in the eye two to four times per day for a period of several days or up to 2 weeks. Phenylephrine 1/8%; nose drops can be used concurrently for 2–3 days to promote tear flow by minimizing edema of the nasal mucosa. Because transient bacteremia can occur after probing, systemic antibiotic prophylaxis should be considered for the patient with congenital heart disease.

Resolution of symptoms is usually immediate and dramatic after probing, but the full effect of the procedure sometimes does not immediately become evident. Massage over the lacrimal sac should be continued for 1–2 weeks. Evaluation of the results is more accurate 1 week or more after discontinuing postoperative treatment. Recurrence after unsuccessful probing is nearly always obvious within 1 month. A postoperative office visit is not mandatory if the patient's family notifies the surgeon that the problem seems to have resolved. If the initial attempt to relieve congenital NLD obstruction with probing is substantially unsuccessful, it is appropriate to repeat the same procedure after an interval of a few weeks.

In some cases, epiphora still occurs occasionally, particularly outdoors in cold weather or in conjunction with an upper respiratory infection. This condition probably is attributable to a patent but narrow lacrimal drainage channel that is overwhelmed by mild hypersecretion or becomes occluded when the nasal mucosa swells. A similar clinical picture is occasionally encountered in an infant or young child without a prior history of complete obstruction. Usually, no treatment is required. Spontaneous improvement is likely over time.

Infracture of the inferior turbinate

Some surgeons routinely perform infracture of the inferior turbinate as an addition to the initial probing irrespective of the nature of the obstruction because of possible interference with tear flow if the turbinate encroaches on the distal opening of the lacrimal duct. Most surgeons reserve this procedure for when firm resistance is felt as the advancing probe approaches the lowest portion of the bony nasolacrimal canal or for subsequent procedures after initial probing fails.

Infracture is accomplished by placing a small periosteal elevator beneath the turbinate or by grasping it with a hemostat, then rotating the instrument to force the turbinate inward until its core fractures, without disrupting the overlying soft tissue. The value of this widely practiced maneuver is debatable in merely membranous obstructions.

Balloon catheter dilation

In recent years, dilation of a lacrimal drainage system that appears to be blocked by scarring or constriction rather than by a distal membrane, by means of an inflatable balloon carried on a probe (similar to coronary angioplasty), has become popular. Some observers think that the method increases the success rate of delayed treatment but is applicable at any age. Although the original proponents of this procedure have advocated prolonged pre- and posttreatment use of systemic antibiotics and corticosteroids, most ophthalmologists do not employ these measures.

> Gunton KB, Chung CW, Schnall BM, et al. Comparison of balloon dacryocystoplasty to probing as the primary treatment of congenital nasolacrimal duct obstruction. *J AAPOS.* 2001;5:139–142.
>
> Hutcheson KA, Drack AV, Lambert SR. Balloon dilatation for treatment of resistant nasolacrimal duct obstruction. *J AAPOS.* 1997;1:241–244.

Intubation

Silicone intubation of the lacrimal system is usually recommended when one or more simple probings have failed. In the most commonly employed technique, the silicone tubing is swedged onto a thin probe whose end is modified with a bulbed tip. Once passed into the nose, the probe tip is engaged with a specially configured hook and withdrawn from the nares. Both the upper and lower eyelids are intubated, leaving a small loop of silicone tubing between the puncta. A variety of measures are employed to secure the ends of the tubing in the nose, such as placing knots in the tubing, passing the tubing through a bolster, or suturing the tubes to the lateral nasal wall to prevent retrograde entry into the NLD. Additional modifications, such as placement of suture material in the lumen of the tube to allow the cut ends to be smoothly tied together, have been made.

An alternative method involves intubation via one canaliculus only. The supposed advantages of this method, which employs the Monoka tube, are ease of insertion and removal of the tube and its easily achieved fixation in the intended location once passed. Acceptance of this technique has been limited by the prominent rate of corneal complications. No approach offers the ideal combination of ease of placement and removal along with high resistance to accidental displacement.

Ideally, the silicone tubing should be left in place for 3–6 months to maximize the probability of a patent lacrimal drainage system after the tubing has been removed, but shorter periods of intubation can be successful. Occasionally, the tubing becomes dislodged and protrudes excessively out of the nose or the puncta. Such situations warrant attempts to reposition the tubing. A tube laterally displaced at the puncta sometimes can be repositioned by rethreading, although it usually must be removed. Ophthalmic ointment on the tubing may facilitate this maneuver.

If the tubing protrudes out of the nose, a cotton-tipped applicator or forceps can be used to replace the tubing. Repositioning can be facilitated by having the child sniff. The parents should be cautioned about the possibility of punctal lacerations. Early removal is necessary in these cases.

The technique chosen for tube removal depends on the age of the patient, how the tubing was secured, and its position (in place or partially dislodged). If the ends were secured with a very small knot, the tubing can be removed by cutting and retracting through the punctum. A more cumbersome closure in the nose often requires anesthesia because the tube will have to be removed from the nose.

> Pashby RC, Crawford JS. Lacrimal apparatus: treatment of obstruction of the lacrimal passages. In: Crawford JS, Morin JD. *The Eye in Childhood.* New York: Grune & Stratton; 1983:183–190.
>
> Pe MRL, Langford JD, Linberg JV, et al. Ritleng intubation system for treatment of congenital nasolacrimal duct obstruction. *Arch Ophthalmol.* 1998;116:387–391.

Dacryocystorhinostomy

Dacryocystorhinostomy may be necessary when intubation cannot be accomplished or when significant symptoms recur after tubing is removed. BCSC Section 7, *Orbit, Eyelids, and Lacrimal System,* discusses dacryocystorhinostomy and the other procedures covered in this chapter.

> Gardiner JA, Forte V, Pashby RC, et al. The role of nasal endoscopy in repeat pediatric nasolacrimal duct probings. *J AAPOS.* 2001;5:148–152.

CHAPTER 19

Diseases of the Cornea and Anterior Segment

This chapter focuses on corneal and anterior segment problems that begin in infancy and childhood. To understand how developmental anomalies affect the cornea and anterior segment, it is helpful to review the embryology of these regions of the eye.

Embryology of the Cornea and Anterior Segment

The lens vesicle separates from the surface ectoderm by the sixth week of gestation. The optic cup, which arises from neural ectoderm, has reached the periphery of the lens by this time, and a triangular mass of undifferentiated neural crest cells overrides the rim of the cup and surrounds the anterior periphery of the lens. Three waves of tissue move forward between the surface ectoderm and the lens. The first of these layers differentiates into the primordial corneal endothelium by the eighth week and subsequently produces Descemet's membrane. The second wave of tissue produces the stroma of the cornea, and the third wave gives rise to the pupillary membrane and the iris stroma. The pigment epithelial layer of the iris develops in later months from neural ectoderm.

By the beginning of the fifth fetal month, a complete endothelial lining overlies the primitive anterior chamber, creating a closed cavity. In addition, the iris insertion is now well anterior to the neural crest tissue destined to become the trabecular meshwork. The endothelial lining undergoes fenestration in the final weeks of gestation and the first weeks after birth. The iris insertion also repositions posteriorly to gradually uncover the developing trabecular meshwork. This repositioning, or posterior sliding, probably occurs secondary to differential growth rates and is not merely the result of a cleavage or an atrophy of tissue. At birth, the iris insertion has normally reached the level of the scleral spur. Posterior migration of the iris normally continues for about the first year of life.

A spectrum of anterior segment dysgenesis syndromes can result from abnormalities of neural crest cell migration, proliferation, or differentiation. A developmental arrest late in gestation can result in retention of primordial endothelium and incomplete posterior iris migration. BCSC Section 2, *Fundamentals and Principles of Ophthalmology*, discusses these issues in greater detail with illustrations in Part II, Embryology.

Congenital Corneal Anomalies

Abnormalities of Corneal Size and Shape

The normal horizontal corneal diameter in the newborn is 9.5–10.5 mm. The average 12 mm adult corneal diameter is reached by age 2 years. Abnormalities of corneal size and shape in childhood include simple megalocornea, keratoglobus, keratoconus, and microcornea. (See also the discussion of congenital anomalies in BCSC Section 8, *External Disease and Cornea*.)

Megalocornea

If the horizontal diameter is greater than 13 mm (or 12 mm in the newborn), megalocornea is present. The most common type of megalocornea is *anterior megalophthalmos*, which is X-linked recessive and bilateral. In this condition, the normal-sized lens is too small for the enlarged ciliary ring, which may result in subluxation. The iris is hypoplastic with defects visible by transillumination, and the pupil is often ectopic. There is a greatly increased risk of glaucoma. *Simple megalocornea* is a rare condition in which both corneas exceed 13 mm in horizontal diameter but associated abnormalities are absent. This condition must be differentiated from congenital glaucoma.

Keratoglobus

In keratoglobus, the cornea is thinner than normal and arcs high over the iris, creating a deeper than normal anterior chamber. Spontaneous breaks in Descemet's membrane may produce acute corneal edema, and the cornea is easily ruptured by minor blunt trauma. Patients with keratoglobus should be advised to wear protective lenses indefinitely. This rare autosomal recessive disorder can be part of the *Ehlers-Danlos type VI syndrome*, which is characterized by generalized thinning and anterior bulging of the cornea accompanied by hyperextensible joints, blue sclera, and gradually progressive neurosensory hearing loss.

Keratoconus

In keratoconus, the central or paracentral cornea undergoes progressive thinning and bulging, so that the cornea takes on the shape of a cone. The disease can present and progress during the adolescent years. Keratoconus is associated with Down syndrome, other conditions with mental retardation, and atopic disease. There is a hereditary component in some families.

Microcornea

Microcornea is present if the corneal diameter is smaller than 10 mm (or smaller than 9 mm in the newborn) (Fig 19-1). Microcornea may follow a pattern of autosomal dominant inheritance, particularly as part of the oculodentodigital dysplasia syndrome, or may appear sporadically. Microcornea may be accompanied by many other abnormalities of the eye, including cataracts, colobomas, high myopia, or persistent hyperplastic primary vitreous. Microcornea can be seen in nanophthalmos, in which the entire eye is smaller than normal without other major structural abnormalities.

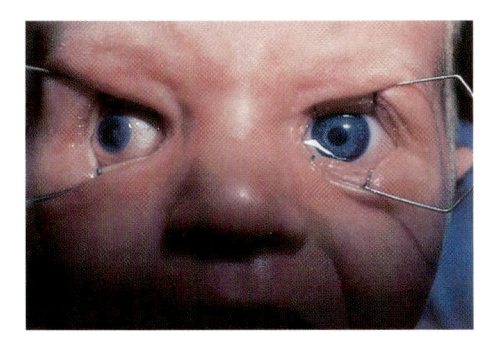

Figure 19-1 Microcornea, right eye.

Anterior Segment Dysgenesis: Peripheral Developmental Abnormalities

The spectrum of developmental anomalies known as *anterior segment dysgenesis* is sometimes called *mesenchymal dysgenesis* and was previously known as *anterior chamber cleavage syndrome* or *mesectodermal dysgenesis*.

> Wilson ME. Congenital iris ectropion and a new classification for anterior segment dysgenesis. *J Pediatr Ophthalmol Strabismus*. 1990;27:48–55.

Posterior embryotoxon

Posterior embryotoxon is seen as a central thickening and displacement of Schwalbe's line. Posterior embryotoxon is visible with the slit lamp as an irregular white line just concentric with and anterior to the limbus (Fig 19-2). Gonioscopically, the condition appears as a continuous or broken ridge protruding into the anterior chamber. Posterior embryotoxon often has pigmented spots on the internal surface of this ridge. This anomaly is also called a *prominent Schwalbe's ring*. It is most often associated with Axenfeld-Rieger syndrome but is also found in arteriohepatic dysplasia (Alagille syndrome) and may be an isolated finding in 15% of normal patients.

> Nischal KK, Hingorani M, Bentley CR, et al. Ocular ultrasound in Alagille syndrome: a new sign. *Ophthalmology*. 1997;104:79–85.

Axenfeld-Rieger syndrome

Axenfeld-Rieger syndrome represents a spectrum of developmental disorders characterized by an anteriorly displaced Schwalbe's line (posterior embryotoxon) with attached iris strands, iris hypoplasia, and anterior chamber dysgenesis leading to glaucoma in childhood or adulthood in 50% of cases (Figs 19-3, 19-4, 19-5). The conditions previously called *Axenfeld anomaly*, *Rieger anomaly*, and *Rieger syndrome* often have overlapping findings and are now considered a single entity known as *Axenfeld-Rieger syndrome*. With the identification of causative genes for these disorders, nomenclature has become even more complex. There are cases in which the same ocular appearance is caused by different genes, and others in which very different ocular presentations, which would have previously been confidently classified as *Peters anomaly* versus *Rieger anomaly* versus *primary glaucoma*, for example, are caused by the same mutated gene.

In Axenfeld-Rieger syndrome, a glassy, smooth, cryptless iris surface and a high iris insertion are present, sometimes accompanied by iris transillumination. Iris hypoplasia

240 • Pediatric Ophthalmology and Strabismus

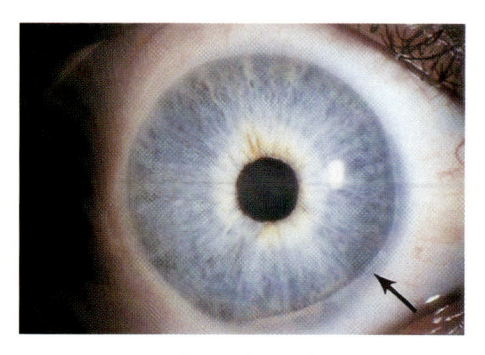

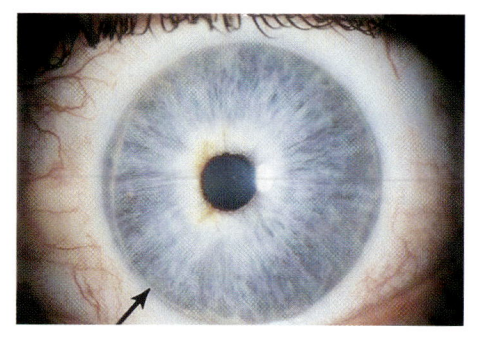

Figure 19-2 Posterior embryotoxon *(arrows)*, bilateral, in Axenfeld-Rieger syndrome.

Figure 19-3 Gonioscopic view in Axenfeld-Rieger syndrome.

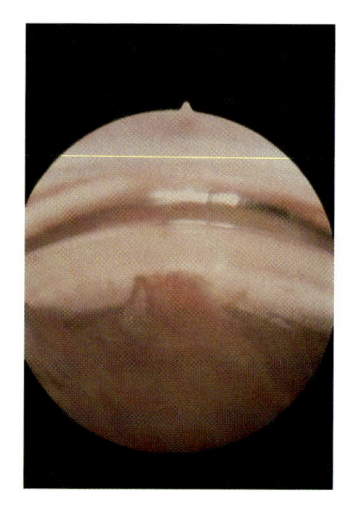

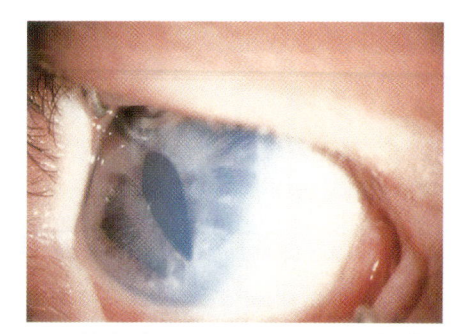

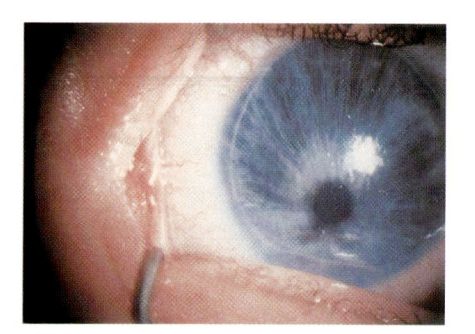

Figure 19-4 Axenfeld-Rieger syndrome, bilateral.

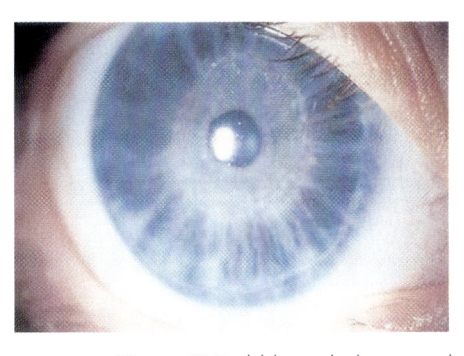

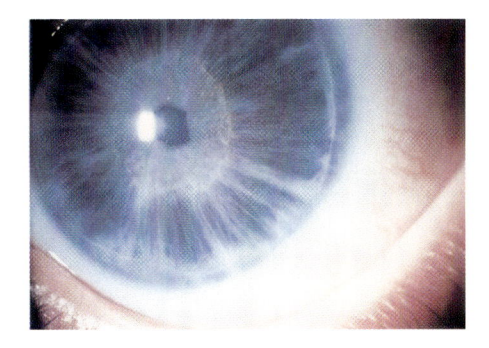

Figure 19-5 Iridogoniodysgenesis, bilateral. *(Courtesy of Jane D. Kivlin, MD.)*

can range from mild stromal thinning to marked atrophy with hole formation, corectopia, and ectropion uveae. Megalocornea or microcornea can occur. Glaucoma develops in 50% of cases. Developmental defects of the teeth and facial bones may be associated. Redundant periumbilical skin, hypospadias, and anomalies in the region of the pituitary gland have also been reported. Autosomal dominant inheritance is most common. Mutations in the *RIEG1/PITX2* gene have been identified. Patients with mutations of *PITX2* have been reported with phenotypes of aniridia, Peters anomaly, Rieger anomaly, and Axenfeld anomaly. The nonocular findings are actually more consistent and should be sought with any of these ocular phenotypes. Mutations in the forkhead transcription factor gene *FKHL7* also cause Axenfeld-Rieger syndrome as well as autosomal dominant iris hypoplasia, juvenile glaucoma, and primary congenital glaucoma. These genes are also important in craniofacial, dental, umbilical, cardiac, and pituitary development.

Nishimura DY, Swiderski RE, Alward WL, et al. The forkhead transcription factor gene FKHL7 is responsible for glaucoma phenotypes which map to 6p25. *Nat Genet.* 1998;19:140–147.

Perveen R, Lloyd IC, Clayton-Smith J, et al. Phenotypic variability and asymmetry of Rieger syndrome associated with PITX2 mutations. *Invest Ophthalmol Vis Sci.* 2000;41:2456–2460.

Traboulsi EI. Ocular malformations and developmental genes. *J AAPOS.* 1998;2:317–323.

Walter MA, Mirzayans F, Mears AJ, et al. Autosomal-dominant iridogoniodysgenesis and Axenfeld-Rieger syndrome are genetically distinct. *Ophthalmology.* 1996;103:1907–1915.

Anterior Segment Dysgenesis: Central Developmental Abnormalities

With central developmental abnormalities, the basic finding is a localized loss or attenuation of the corneal endothelium or Descemet's membrane, which is usually associated with an overlying stromal and epithelial opacity.

Posterior corneal depression (central posterior keratoconus)

Posterior corneal depression, a discrete posterior corneal indentation, is best detected with a retinoscope or direct ophthalmoscope that reveals an abnormal red reflex. This condition can also be diagnosed with the slit lamp by moving the beam across the defect to discern increased convexity of the posterior corneal surface. Sometimes, pigment deposits appear on the border of the posterior defect. The anterior curvature of the cornea is normal. This defect usually causes irregular astigmatism and can result in amblyopia if the refractive error is not corrected.

Peters anomaly

Peters anomaly consists of a posterior corneal defect with stromal opacity and often adherent iris strands. In many cases, the stromal opacity decreases with time. In some cases, lysis of adherent iris strands may improve corneal clarity. The size and density of the opacity can range from a faint stromal opacity to a dense opaque central leukoma. In extreme cases, the central leukoma may be vascularized and protrude above the level of the cornea. The strands from the iris to the borders of this defect vary in number and density. A more severe variety of this condition involves adherence of the lens to the cornea at the site of the central defect (Fig 19-6). Peters anomaly is the end result of many defects, including the genetic Axenfeld-Rieger syndrome and nongenetic conditions such as congenital rubella.

Bilateral Peters anomaly is often associated with a syndrome. When associated with microphthalmia and reddish linear skin lesions, Peters anomaly may be part of a syndrome that includes life-threatening cardiac arrhythmias. Bilateral cases warrant complete genetic and systemic workup. Unilateral cases are usually isolated.

> Doward W, Perveen R, Lloyd IC, et al. A mutation in the RIEG1 gene associated with Peters' anomaly. *J Med Genet.* 1999;36:152–155.
> Hanson IM, Fletcher JM, Jordan T, et al. Mutations at the PAX6 locus are found in heterogeneous anterior segment malformations including Peters' anomaly. *Nat Genet.* 1994;6: 168–173.
> Mulet M, Caldwell D. Corneal abnormalities. In: Wright KW, ed. *Pediatric Ophthalmology and Strabismus.* St Louis: Mosby; 1995;321–348.
> Traboulsi EI, Maumenee IH. Peters' anomaly and associated congenital malformations. *Arch Ophthalmol.* 1992;110:1739–1742.

Infantile Corneal Opacities

Peters anomaly has already been discussed. Table 19-1 lists the other possibilities to be considered in a differential diagnosis.

Sclerocornea

In sclerocornea, a congenital condition, the cornea is opaque and resembles the sclera, making the limbus indistinct. The central cornea is clearer than the periphery in nearly all cases. Severe cases show no increased corneal curvature and no apparent scleral sulcus. Sclerocornea is often associated with other ocular or systemic abnormalities.

Tears, breaks, or ruptures of Descemet's membrane

Injuries to Descemet's membrane may be caused by forceps trauma to the eye during a difficult delivery. Rupture of Descemet's membrane leads to stromal and sometimes epithelial edema. Other signs of trauma are frequently apparent on the child. In most cases, the stromal and epithelial edema regresses, but the edges of the broken Descemet's membrane persist indefinitely and can be seen as ridges protruding slightly from the posterior

CHAPTER 19: Diseases of the Cornea and Anterior Segment • 243

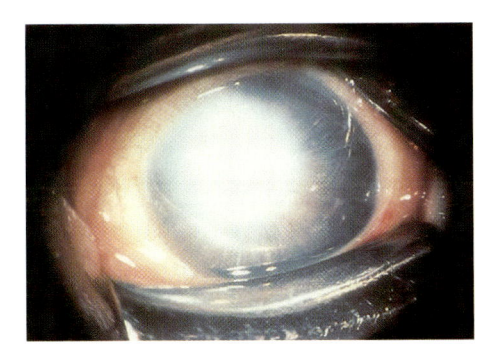

Figure 19-6 Peters anomaly, left eye.

Table 19-1 **Differential Diagnosis of Infantile Corneal Opacities**

Entity	Location and Description of Opacity	Other Signs	Method of Diagnosis
Sclerocornea	Peripheral opacity, clearest centrally; unilateral or bilateral	Flat cornea	Inspection
Forceps injury	Central opacity; unilateral	Breaks in Descemet's membrane	History
Mucopolysaccharidosis, mucolipidosis	Diffuse opacity; bilateral	Smooth epithelium	Conjunctival biopsy; biochemical testing
Posterior corneal defects	Central opacity; unilateral or bilateral	Iris adherence to cornea; posterior keratoconus	Inspection
Congenital hereditary endothelial dystrophy (CHED)	Diffuse opacity; bilateral	Thickened cornea	Inspection
Dermoid	Temporal opacity; unilateral; raised; hair on surface; keratinized	Associated with Goldenhar syndrome	Inspection
Infantile glaucoma	Diffuse opacity; unilateral or bilateral	Enlarged cornea; breaks in Descemet's membrane	Elevated intraocular pressure
Congenital hereditary stromal dystrophy (CHSD)	Diffuse opacity; bilateral	Stromal opacities, normal thickness, normal epithelium	Autosomal dominant; examine family members

corneal surface. Severe amblyopia may result from the corneal opacity. The high astigmatism induced by the trauma can cause severe amblyopia even if the cornea clears quickly. Aggressive optical correction and patching can reverse the amblyopia.

Mucopolysaccharidosis and mucolipidosis

The varied systemic findings and ultrastructural abnormalities of the lysosomal disorders mucopolysaccharidosis and mucolipidosis are beyond the scope of this discussion (see Chapter 29, Table 24-1; BCSC Section 8, *External Disease and Cornea;* and BCSC Section 12, *Retina and Vitreous*). However, corneal clouding and haziness may be present in early life in at least two of these conditions: in *mucopolysaccharidosis IH*, or *Hurler syndrome*, corneal clouding occurs by age 6 months (Fig 19-7); in *mucopolysaccharidosis IS*, or *Scheie syndrome*, corneal clouding occurs by age 12–24 months. In *mucolipidosis IV*, corneal clouding has been reported as early as age 6 weeks. Enzymatic and DNA analyses usually can identify the metabolic defect. Conjunctival biopsies show abnormal cytoplasmic inclusions on electron microscopy.

Congenital hereditary endothelial dystrophy (CHED)

CHED is an uncommon corneal dystrophy with onset at birth or shortly thereafter. The cornea is diffusely and uniformly edematous secondary to a defect of the corneal endothelium and Descemet's membrane. The edema involves both the stroma and epithelium. The hallmark of CHED is increased corneal thickness. The appearance of the cornea is similar to that in congenital glaucoma but without increased corneal diameter and elevated intraocular pressure. CHED can be inherited in an autosomal dominant or autosomal recessive manner. The dominant and recessive forms are caused by different genes. The dominant form maps to the same genetic locus as posterior polymorphous dystrophy on pericentromeric chromosome 20. The autosomal recessive form maps to another locus on chromosome 20.

> Hand CK, Harmon DL, Kennedy SM, et al. Localization of the gene for autosomal recessive congenital hereditary endothelial dystrophy (CHED2) to chromosome 20 by homozygosity mapping. *Genomics.* 1999;61:1–4.

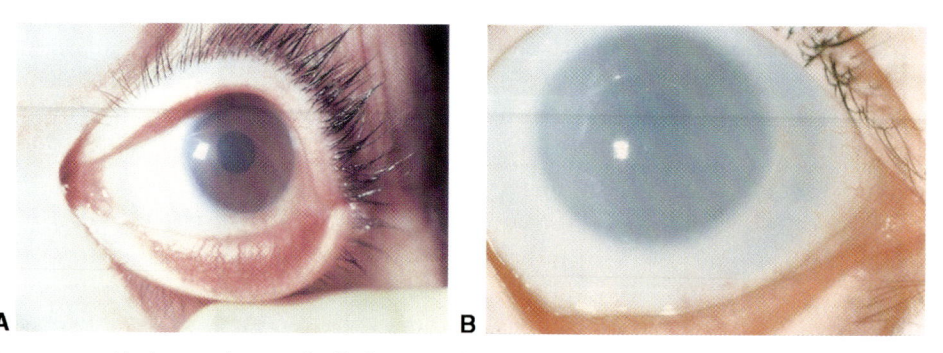

Figure 19-7 Hurler syndrome. **A,** Early corneal clouding. **B,** Late corneal clouding. *(Courtesy of Jane D. Kivlin, MD.)*

Dermoids

A corneal dermoid is a hamartoma composed of fibrofatty tissue covered by keratinized epithelium. Dermoids sometimes contain hair follicles, sebaceous glands, and sweat glands. Dermoids can range up to 8–10 mm in diameter and usually straddle the limbus. Dermoids may extend into the corneal stroma and adjacent sclera but seldom occupy the full thickness of either cornea or sclera. Most dermoids are on the inferior temporal limbus. Many dermoids produce a lipoid infiltration of the corneal stroma at their leading edge.

Limbal dermoids are often seen with Goldenhar syndrome (see Chapter 28). They are sometimes continuous with subconjunctival lipodermoids that involve the upper outer quadrant of the eye and extend into the orbit under the lateral aspect of the upper eyelid. Large dermoids can cover the visual axis; small dermoids can produce astigmatism with secondary amblyopia. Surgical excision may result in scarring and astigmatism, which can also lead to amblyopia.

Congenital or infantile glaucoma

Glaucoma in an infant can make the cornea hazy, cloudy, opaque, enlarged, or any combination thereof. Chapter 21 discusses pediatric glaucoma in more detail.

Congenital hereditary stromal dystrophy

Congenital hereditary stromal dystrophy is a very rare congenital stationary opacification of the cornea transmitted in an autosomal dominant manner. Flaky or feathery clouding of the stroma, which is of normal thickness, is covered by a smooth, normal epithelium. These features are in contrast with CHED, which has a thickened stroma and epithelial edema.

Treatment

The treatment of congenital corneal opacities is difficult and often visually unrewarding. If bilateral dense opacities are present, keratoplasty should be considered for one eye as soon as possible. If the opacity is unilateral, the decision is more difficult. Keratoplasty should be undertaken only if the family and the physicians involved in the care of the child are prepared for the tremendous commitment of time and effort needed to combat the corneal graft rejection that often occurs in children as well as the amblyopia. The team should include ophthalmologists skilled in the management of pediatric corneal surgery, pediatric glaucoma, amblyopia, and strabismus. Contact lens expertise is important for fitting infants with small eyes and large refractive errors. Examinations under anesthesia are required, and infectious keratitis may occur. Social service support is often needed.

Although there is ample evidence that deprivation amblyopia must be reversed before the age of 3 months to achieve excellent vision, it may be appropriate to delay corneal transplantation until the child is older in some cases of Peters anomaly. Some studies have found better final vision in patients treated at about the age of 1 year as opposed to age 3 months because older children showed less rejection and ultimately a clearer cornea. Very few patients in either group achieved good vision, however.

Systemic Diseases With Corneal Manifestations in Childhood

The mucopolysaccharidoses are discussed above. All of the mucopolysaccharidoses except mucopolysaccharidosis II (Hunter syndrome) may involve deposits in the cornea leading to some degree of clinical corneal clouding (see Fig 19-7).

Cystinosis

Cystinosis, a metabolic disease characterized by elevated levels of cystine within the cell, is rare. French Canada has the highest incidence in the world. Cystine crystals are deposited in various places throughout the body. In the infantile form of the disease, the major presenting symptoms are failure to thrive, rickets, and progressive renal failure, collectively called *Fanconi syndrome*. The ocular findings are pathognomonic. Iridescent elongated corneal crystals appear at approximately 1 year of age, first in the peripheral part of the cornea and the anterior part of the stroma. These crystals are also present in the uvea and can be seen with the slit lamp on the surface of the iris (Fig 19-8). Severe photophobia can make a slit-lamp examination almost impossible without anesthesia. Cystine can be found in conjunctival biopsy specimens. Oral cysteamine has been shown to help the systemic problems but not the corneal crystal deposition. Topical cysteamine drops must be applied every 1–2 hours, have an unpleasant odor, and are difficult to obtain but can markedly reduce crystal deposition in the cornea.

> Graf M, Grote A, Wagner F. [Cysteamine eyedrops for treatment of corneal cysteine deposits in infantile cystinosis.] *Klin Monatsbl Augenheilkd.* 1992;201:48–50.
> Kaiser-Kupfer MI, Fujikawa L, Kuwabara T, et al. Removal of corneal crystals by topical cysteamine in nephropathic cystinosis. *N Engl J Med.* 1987;316:775–779.
> Richler M, Milot J, Quigley M, et al. Ocular manifestations of nephropathic cystinosis. The French-Canadian experience in a genetically homogeneous population. *Arch Ophthalmol.* 1991;109:359–362.

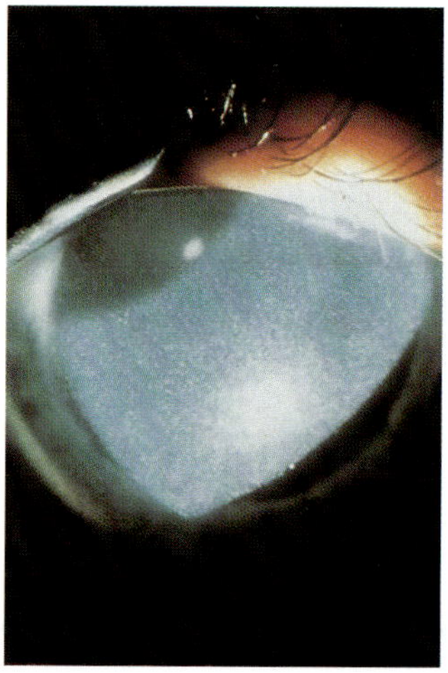

Figure 19-8 Cystinosis with corneal involvement.

Hepatolenticular degeneration (Wilson disease)

Hepatolenticular degeneration, an autosomal recessive inborn error of metabolism, results in excess copper deposition in the liver, kidney, and basal ganglia of the brain, leading to cirrhosis, renal tubular damage, and a Parkinson-like defect of motor function. The characteristic copper-colored Kayser-Fleischer ring is limited to Descemet's membrane and is thus separated from the limbus. The ring may be several millimeters in width. The initial deposits are in the corneal periphery at 12 and 6 o'clock. This arc of deposits spreads, eventually encircling the entire cornea. The ring resolves with treatment. Because it can develop fairly late, laboratory tests for serum copper and ceruloplasmin are better than an eye examination for early diagnosis.

Congenital syphilis

Interstitial keratitis may occur in the first decade of life secondary to congenital syphilis. The keratitis presents as rapidly progressive corneal edema followed by abnormal vascularization in the deep stroma adjacent to Descemet's membrane. Intense vascularization may give the cornea a salmon-pink color—hence the term *salmon patch*. Blood flow through these vessels gradually ceases over several weeks to several months, leaving empty "ghost" vessels in the corneal stroma (Fig 19-9). Immune-mediated iritis, arthritis, and hearing loss may also develop and recur even after treatment.

Familial dysautonomia (Riley-Day syndrome)

Familial dysautonomia, a complex autosomal recessive condition, occurs largely in children of eastern European Jewish (Ashkenazi) descent. It is characterized by autonomic dysfunction, relative insensitivity to pain, temperature instability, and absence of the fungiform papillae of the tongue. Exposure keratitis and corneal ulcers with secondary opacification are a frequent problem because of the abnormal lacrimation and decreased corneal sensitivity. Preventive measures include supplemental tears and tarsorrhaphies. The gene has been mapped to chromosome 9q.

   Blumenfeld A, Slaugenhaupt SA, Liebert CB, et al. Precise genetic mapping and haplotype analysis for the familial dysautonomia gene on human chromosome 9q31. *Am J Hum Genet.* 1999;64:1110–1118.
   Mulet M, Caldwell D. Corneal abnormalities. In: Wright KW, ed. *Pediatric Ophthalmology and Strabismus.* St Louis: Mosby; 1995:321–348.

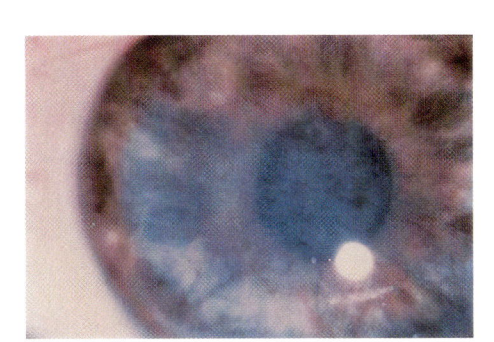

Figure 19-9 Interstitial keratitis secondary to congenital syphilis.

CHAPTER 20

Iris Abnormalities

Aniridia

Aniridia is a panocular, bilateral disorder. The term *aniridia* is a misnomer because at least a rudimentary iris is always present. Variations range from almost total absence to only mild hypoplasia of the iris. In addition to iris involvement, foveal and optic nerve hypoplasia are present, resulting in a congenital sensory nystagmus and leading to reduced visual acuity, usually 20/100 or worse. Cataracts, glaucoma, and corneal opacification often develop later in childhood, and these conditions may lead to progressive deterioration of visual acuity.

The typical presentation of aniridia is an infant with nystagmus who appears to have absent irides or dilated, unresponsive pupils. Photophobia may also be present. Examination findings commonly include small anterior polar cataracts with attached persistent pupillary membrane strands (Fig 20-1).

A defect in the *PAX6* gene on chromosome 11p13 is the cause of aniridia, which can be sporadic or familial. The familial form is autosomal dominant with complete penetrance but variable expressivity. There are reports of autosomal dominant pedigrees in which patients have severe glaucoma but normal maculas and good central vision. Two thirds of all aniridic children have affected parents. The *PAX6* gene is the master control gene for eye morphogenesis. This gene is probably involved in the complex inductive interactions between the optic cup, surface ectoderm, and neural crest during formation of the iris and other ocular structures. Inadequate gene dosage may thus lead to global impairment of morphogenesis. Parts II (Embryology) and III (Genetics) of BCSC Section 2, *Fundamentals and Principles of Ophthalmology*, discuss aniridia.

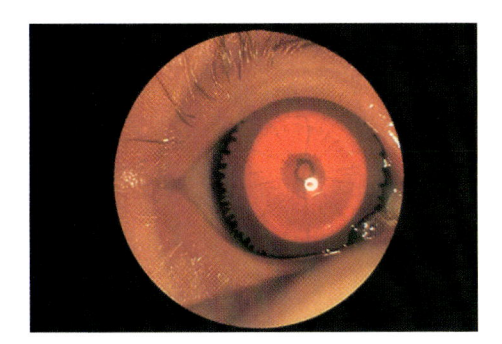

Figure 20-1 Aniridia in an infant. Both the ciliary processes and the edge of the lens are visible. Also present are persistent pupillary membrane fibers and a small central anterior polar cataract.

Sporadic aniridia is associated with *Wilms tumor (nephroblastoma)* in as many as one third of cases. When associated with aniridia, Wilms tumor is diagnosed before patients reach age 5 in 80% of cases. The combination of aniridia and Wilms tumor represents a contiguous gene syndrome in which the adjacent *PAX6* and Wilms tumor *(Wt1)* genes are both deleted. Some deletions create the WAGR complex of Wilms tumor, aniridia, genitourinary malformations, and mental retardation. All children with sporadic aniridia should undergo chromosomal analysis for the Wilms tumor gene defect. Positive results necessitate consultation with an oncologist along with repeated abdominal ultrasonographic and clinical examinations. Patients with familial aniridia are rarely at risk for Wilms tumor.

> Drechsler M, Meijers-Heijboer EJ, Schneider S, et al. Molecular analysis of aniridia patients for deletions involving the Wilms' tumor gene. *Hum Genet.* 1994;94:331–338.
>
> Hanson IM, Fletcher JM, Jordan T, et al. Mutations at the PAX6 locus in aniridia. *Hum Mol Genet.* 1994;2:915–920.
>
> Ivanov I, Shuper A, Shohat M, et al. Aniridia: recent achievements in paediatric practice. *Eur J Pediatr.* 1995;154:795–800.

Coloboma of the Iris

Iris colobomas are classified as *typical* if they occur in the inferonasal quadrant and can thus be explained by failure of the embryonic fissure to close in the fifth week of gestation. With a typical iris coloboma, the pupil is shaped like a light bulb, keyhole, or inverted teardrop (Fig 20-2). Typical colobomas may involve the ciliary body, choroid, retina, and optic nerve. These colobomas are part of a continuum that extends to microphthalmos and anophthalmos. Nystagmus may be present if both optic nerves or both maculas are involved. Isolated colobomatous microphthalmia may be inherited as an autosomal dominant trait in about 20% of cases. Parents of an affected child may have small previously undetected chorioretinal or iris defects in an inferonasal location, so careful examination of family members is indicated.

Atypical iris colobomas occur in areas other than the inferonasal quadrant and are not associated with more posterior uveal colobomas. These colobomas probably result from fibrovascular remnants of the anterior hyaloid system and pupillary membrane.

Figure 20-2 Typical iris coloboma, right eye.

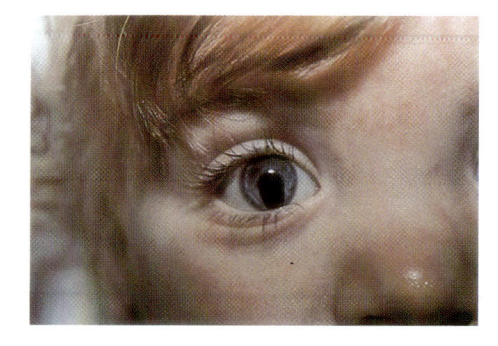

Any child with a coloboma and at least one other organ system abnormality should undergo karyotype analysis with extended banding. Although iris colobomas can be associated with almost any chromosomal abnormality, the most common associations are:

- Triploidy, especially trisomy 13 (cat's eye syndrome) or 18
- 4p– Wolf-Hirschhorn syndrome
- 11q–
- 18r (ring)
- 13r
- Klinefelter syndrome
- Turner syndrome (rarely)

In addition, many well-characterized syndromes are associated with uveal colobomas. These syndromes include:

- CHARGE association (ocular *c*oloboma, *h*eart defects, choanal *a*tresia, mental *r*etardation, and *g*enitourinary and *e*ar anomalies), which accounts for about 15% of cases
- Lenz microphthalmos syndrome
- Goltz focal dermal hypoplasia
- Basal cell nevus syndrome
- Meckel syndrome
- Warburg syndrome
- Aicardi syndrome
- Rubinstein-Taybi syndrome
- Linear sebaceous nevus syndrome
- Goldenhar syndrome

Mets MB, Erzurum SA. Uveal tract in infants. In: Isenberg SJ, ed. *The Eye in Infancy*. 2nd ed. St Louis: Mosby; 1994:308–317.

Pagon RA. Ocular coloboma [review]. *Surv Ophthalmol*. 1981;25:223–236.

Wilson ME, O'Neil JW. Pediatric iris abnormalities. In: Wright KW, ed. *Pediatric Ophthalmology and Strabismus*. St Louis: Mosby; 1995:349–365.

Iris Nodules

Lisch Nodules

Lisch nodules are neural crest hamartomas commonly associated with *neurofibromatosis type 1*. These nodules are raised and usually tan in color but can vary significantly in appearance (Fig 20-3). The prevalence of Lisch nodules in neurofibromatosis type 1 increases with age, being approximately 10 times the patient's age (up to 9 years) (Fig 20-4). (See also Chapter 27.) For example, by age 8 years, Lisch nodules are present in approximately 80% of patients.

Figure 20-3 Lisch nodules in neurofibromatosis type 1.

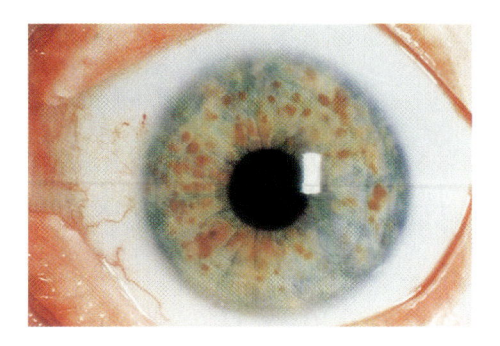

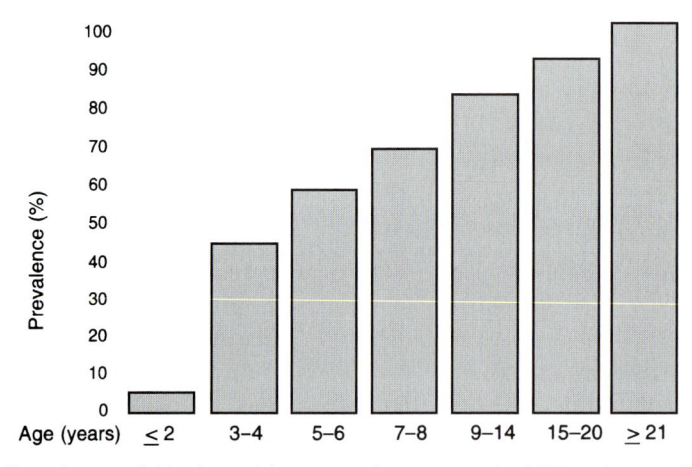

Figure 20-4 Prevalence of Lisch nodules according to age in 167 patients with neurofibromatosis type 1. *(Modified from Lubs ML, Bauer MS, Formas ME, et al. Lisch nodules in neurofibromatosis type 1. N Engl J Med. 1991;324:1264–1266.)*

Juvenile Xanthogranuloma

Juvenile xanthogranuloma is primarily a cutaneous disorder with a predilection for the head and face. Vascular iris lesions may occur as discrete yellowish or reddish nodules or as diffuse infiltration causing heterochromia. Spontaneous hyphema can occur. (See also Chapter 25.)

Primary Iris Cysts

Cysts of Iris Pigment Epithelium

Spontaneous cysts of the iris pigment epithelium result from a separation of the two layers of epithelium anywhere between the pupil and ciliary body (Fig 20-5). Clinically, these cysts tend to be stable and rarely cause ocular complications. They are usually not diagnosed until the teenage years.

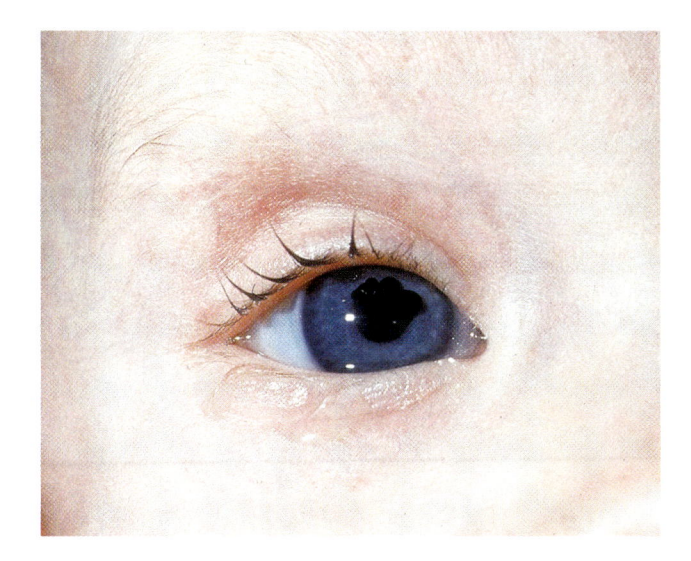

Figure 20-5 Cysts of the pigmented epithelium of the iris.

Central (Pupillary) Cysts

Pigment epithelial cysts at the pupillary border are sometimes hereditary. They are usually diagnosed in infancy. They may enlarge slowly but generally remain asymptomatic and rarely require treatment. Rupture of these cysts can result in *iris flocculi*. Potent cholinesterase-inhibiting eyedrops may produce similar pupillary cysts, especially in young phakic persons. Discontinuation of the drug or concomitant administration of phenylephrine generally results in improvement.

Cysts of Iris Stroma

Primary iris stromal cysts are often diagnosed in infancy. They are most likely caused by sequestration of epithelium during embryologic development. The epithelium-lined stromal cysts usually contain goblet cells, and they may enlarge, causing obstruction of the visual axis, glaucoma, corneal decompensation, or iritis from cyst leakage. Numerous treatment modalities have been described, including cyst aspiration and photocoagulation or photodisruption, but the sudden release of cystic contents may result in transient iritis and glaucoma. Because of inherent complications or frequent cyst recurrences with other methods, surgical excision may be the preferred treatment method. Iris stromal cysts account for about 16% of childhood iris cysts.

Secondary Iris Cysts

Secondary iris cysts have been reported in childhood after trauma and associated with tumor or iris nevus.

> Shields JA, Shields CL, Lois N, et al. Iris cysts in children: classification, incidence, and management. The 1998 Torrence A Makley Jr Lecture. *Br J Ophthalmol* 1999;83:334–338.

Sidoti PA, Valencia M, Chen N, et al. Echographic evaluation of primary cysts of the iris pigment epithelium. *Am J Ophthalmol.* 1995;120:161–167.

Brushfield Spots (Wofflin Nodules)

Focal areas of iris stromal hyperplasia surrounded by relative hypoplasia occur in up to 90% of patients with Down syndrome, in whom these areas are known as *Brushfield spots.* These are hypopigmented spots. Essentially identical areas, known as *Wofflin nodules,* occur in 24% of patients who do not have Down syndrome. Neither condition is pathological.

Heterochromia Iridis

The differential diagnosis of pediatric heterochromia iridis is extensive. Causes can be classified on the basis of whether the condition is congenital or acquired and whether the affected eye is hypopigmented or hyperpigmented (Fig 20-6; Table 20-1). Trauma,

Figure 20-6 Heterochromia iridis. The left iris has become darker after developing a traumatic cataract. *(Photograph courtesy of John W. Simon, MD.)*

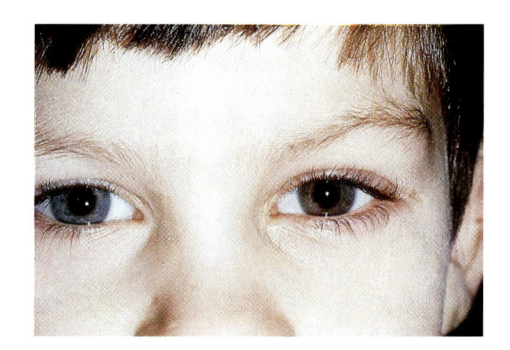

Table 20-1 Pediatric Heterochromia Iridis

Hypochromic heterochromia
  Horner syndrome (congenital or early in life)
  Incontinentia pigmenti (rare)
  Fuchs heterochromia
  Waardenburg-Klein syndrome
  Nonpigmented tumors
  Hypomelanosis of Ito

Hyperchromic heterochromia
  Oculodermal melanocytosis (associated with glaucoma in nonwhite adults)
  Pigmented tumors
  Siderosis
  Iris ectropion syndrome
  Extensive rubeosis

(Modified from Roy FH. *Ocular Differential Diagnosis.* 3rd ed. Philadelphia: Lea & Febiger; 1984.)

chronic iridocyclitis, and intraocular surgery are important causes of acquired hyperpigmented heterochromia in children. Whether congenital or acquired, hypopigmented heterochromia, if associated with a more miotic pupil on the ipsilateral side, should prompt a workup for Horner syndrome. This may be related to a benign entity, such as shoulder dystocia at birth, or a life-threatening one, such as neuroblastoma along the sympathetic chain.

Persistent Pupillary Membranes

Persistent pupillary membranes are the most common developmental abnormality of the iris. They are present in about 95% of newborns, and trace remnants are common in older children and adults. Persistent pupillary membranes are rarely of any visual significance. However, if especially prominent, they can adhere to the anterior lens capsule, causing a small anterior polar cataract. They may also be associated with various other anterior segment abnormalities (Fig 20-7). See the discussion of posterior synechiae at the end of this chapter.

Abnormalities in the Size, Shape, or Location of the Pupil

Congenital Miosis

Congenital miosis, or *microcoria*, may represent an absence or malformation of the dilator pupillae muscle. Congenital miosis can also occur secondary to contracture of fibrous material on the pupil margin from remnants of the tunica vasculosa lentis or neural crest cell anomalies. The condition may be unilateral or bilateral and sporadic or hereditary. Severe cases require surgical pupilloplasty.

The pupil diameter rarely exceeds 2 mm, is often eccentric, and reacts poorly to mydriatic drops. Some patients with eccentric microcoria also have lens subluxation and are therefore part of the spectrum of ectopia lentis et pupillae. Congenital miosis may be associated with microcornea, megalocornea, iris atrophy, iris transillumination, myopia, and glaucoma. Congenital miosis can also be seen with congenital rubella syndrome and hereditary ataxia and in 20% of patients with Lowe oculocerebrorenal syndrome.

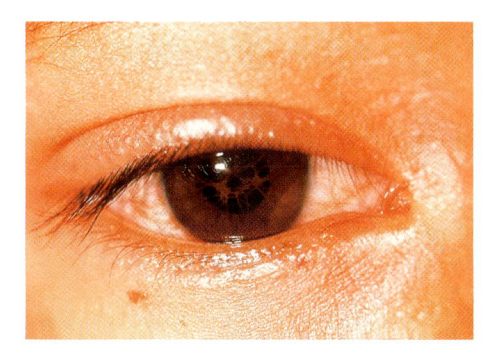

Figure 20-7 Persistent pupillary membrane. Uncorrected visual acuity is 20/40.

Toulemont PJ, Urvoy M, Coscas G, et al. Association of congenital microcoria with myopia and glaucoma. A study of 23 patients with congenital microcoria. *Ophthalmology.* 1995; 102:193–198.

Congenital Mydriasis

Congenitally dilated and fixed pupils with normal-appearing irides have been reported under the names *familial iridoplegia* and *congenital bilateral mydriasis.* Iris sphincter trauma, pharmacologic mydriasis, or acquired neurologic disease affecting the parasympathetic innervation to the pupil must also be considered. Many cases of congenital mydriasis may fall within the aniridia spectrum, especially if the central iris structures from the collarette to the pupillary sphincter are absent.

Dyscoria

The term *dyscoria* refers to an abnormality of the shape of the pupil and is usually reserved for congenital malformations. Acquired inflammatory conditions can lead to posterior synechiae, which can also produce a misshapen pupil. Colobomatous iris defects that produce a dyscoric pupil are discussed above. Iris hypoplasia, especially if sectorial, can produce dyscoria as well as corectopia (see below). Slitlike pupils have been described in the Axenfeld-Rieger syndrome (see Chapter 19, Fig 19-4), in ectopia lentis et pupillae (see following discussion of corectopia), and rarely as an isolated condition with normal visual acuity.

Corectopia

Corectopia refers to displacement of the pupil. Normally, the pupil is situated about 0.5 mm inferonasally from the center of the iris. Minor deviations up to 1 mm are usually cosmetically insignificant and should probably not be considered abnormal. Sector iris hypoplasia or other colobomatous lesions can lead to corectopia, and isolated noncolobomatous autosomal dominant corectopia has also been reported. More commonly, however, corectopia is associated with lens subluxation, and this combination is called *ectopia lentis et pupillae.* The condition is almost always bilateral, with the pupils and lenses displaced in opposite directions.

The pupils may be oval or slit-shaped, and they often dilate poorly. Iris transillumination may occur, and microspherophakia has been reported.

Progressive corectopia can be associated with the Axenfeld-Rieger spectrum as well as iridocorneal endothelial (ICE) syndrome.

Polycoria and Pseudopolycoria

True polycoria, which must by definition include a sphincter mechanism in each pupil, is very rare. The vast majority of accessory iris openings can be classified as *pseudopolycoria.* These iris holes may be congenital or may develop in response to progressive corectopia and iris hypoplasia in Axenfeld-Rieger syndrome or ICE syndrome (Fig 20-8). Pseudopolycoria can also result from trauma or surgery.

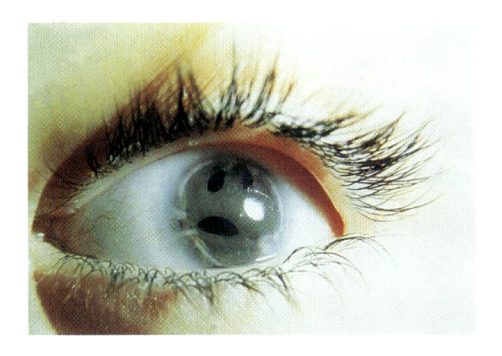

Figure 20-8 Pseudopolycoria that is secondary to Axenfeld-Rieger syndrome. *(Photograph courtesy of John W. Simon, MD.)*

Congenital Iris Ectropion

Ectropion of the posterior pigment epithelium onto the anterior surface of the iris is called *ectropion uveae* in much of the literature. This term is a misnomer because the iris posterior epithelium is derived from neural ectoderm and is not considered part of the uvea. This iris ectropion can occur as an acquired tractional abnormality, often associated with rubeosis iridis, or as a congenital nonprogressive abnormality. The combination of unilateral congenital iris ectropion; a glassy smooth, cryptless iris surface; a high iris insertion; dysgenesis of the drainage angle; and glaucoma has been called *congenital iris ectropion syndrome* (Fig 20-9). In some cases, congenital iris ectropion has been associated with neurofibromatosis and has been reported more rarely with facial hemihypertrophy and Prader-Willi syndrome.

> Wilson ME. Congenital iris ectropion and a new classification for anterior segment dysgenesis. *J Pediatr Ophthalmol Strabismus.* 1990;27:48–55.

Iris Transillumination

In albinism, iris transillumination results from the absence of pigmentation in the posterior epithelial layers. Iris hypoplasia can also lead to iris transillumination, especially as part of Axenfeld-Rieger or ICE syndrome. Iris transillumination has also been reported

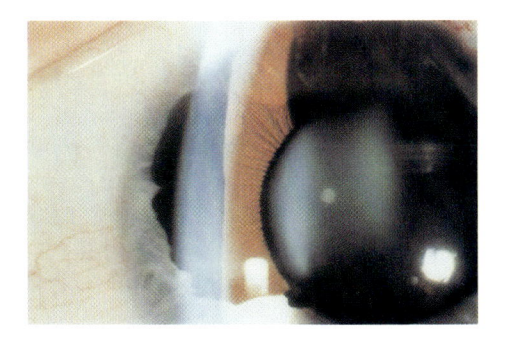

Figure 20-9 Congenital iris ectropion syndrome. A glassy-smooth, cryptless iris surface is present along with marked ectropion of the posterior pigmented epithelium onto the anterior iris surface.

in Marfan syndrome, ectopia lentis et pupillae, and microcoria. Patchy areas of transillumination can also be seen after trauma, surgery, or uveitis.

Posterior Synechiae

Congenital adhesions between the iris margin and lens capsule may occur in association with cataracts, aniridia, intrauterine inflammation, or other developmental abnormalities. These adhesions can also be isolated, benign remnants of the tunica vasculosa lentis. Acquired posterior synechiae secondary to iridocyclitis occur more frequently. In pediatric sarcoidosis, inflammatory iris nodules (Koeppe or Busacca) may be associated with posterior synechiae.

CHAPTER 21

Pediatric Glaucomas

Pediatric glaucomas constitute a heterogeneous group of diseases, which may result from an intrinsic disease or structural abnormality of the aqueous outflow pathways *(primary glaucoma)* or from abnormalities affecting other regions of the eye *(secondary glaucoma)*. A variety of systemic abnormalities are also associated with pediatric glaucoma.

Primary Congenital Glaucoma

Primary congenital open-angle glaucoma is also commonly called *congenital*, or *infantile*, *glaucoma*. Primary congenital glaucoma occurs in about 1 out of 10,000 births and results in blindness in 2%–15% of cases. Visual acuity is worse than 20/50 in at least 50% of cases. This condition is bilateral in about two thirds of patients and occurs more frequently in males (65%) than in females (35%). No specific racial or geographic prevalence has been identified.

Although diagnosis is made in only 25% of affected infants at birth, disease onset occurs within the first year of life in more than 80% of cases. If this disease presents later in childhood (after about age 3–4 years), it is considered *primary juvenile open-angle glaucoma*, a disease that appears to have a different genetic origin (see below) and often responds to therapy classically used for adult open-angle glaucoma (see BCSC Section 10, *Glaucoma*).

> Buckley EG. Primary congenital open angle glaucoma. In: Epstein DL, Allingham RR, Schuman JS, eds. *Chandler and Grant's Glaucoma*. 4th ed. Baltimore: Williams & Wilkins; 1997:598–608.
>
> deLuise VP, Anderson DR. Primary infantile glaucoma (congenital glaucoma). *Surv Ophthalmol.* 1983;28:1–19.

Genetics

Most cases of primary congenital glaucoma occur sporadically, but an autosomal recessive form with variable penetrance has been identified. A major locus for recessively inherited primary congenital glaucoma (GLC3 gene) has recently been identified on the short arm of chromosome 2 (2p21). The association of congenital glaucoma with abnormalities of other chromosomes has previously been reported in the regions of 6p21, 6p25, 11p, and 11q. Autosomal dominant juvenile-onset primary open-angle glaucoma has been mapped to the long arm of chromosome 1.

When no family history of congenital glaucoma exists, the chance of an affected parent having an affected child is approximately 5%. If the first child is affected, the risk of a second child being affected is still approximately 5%, rising to approximately 25% per subsequent offspring if two siblings are affected. Primary congenital glaucoma does not appear to be associated with adult primary open-angle glaucoma; the incidence of steroid-induced intraocular pressure (IOP) elevation is no higher in parents of affected children than in controls.

> Broughton WL, Fine BS, Zimmerman LE. Congenital glaucoma associated with a chromosomal defect. A histologic study. *Arch Ophthalmol.* 1981;99:481–486.
>
> Sarfarazi M, Akarsu AN, Hossain A, et al. Assignment of a locus (GLC3A) for primary congenital glaucoma (buphthalmos) to 2p21 and evidence for genetic heterogeneity. *Genomics.* 1995;30:171–177.

Pathophysiology

The basic pathological defect in primary congenital glaucoma remains obscure. Although Barkan originally proposed a thin imperforate membrane that covered the anterior chamber angle and blocked aqueous outflow, the site of obstruction is now thought to be the trabecular meshwork itself. This disease may represent a developmental arrest of anterior chamber tissue derived from neural crest cells during the late embryologic period.

> Anderson DR. The development of the trabecular meshwork and its abnormality in primary infantile glaucoma. *Trans Am Ophthalmol Soc.* 1981;79:458–485.
>
> Beck AD, Lynch MG. Pediatric glaucoma. In: *Focal Points: Clinical Modules for Ophthalmologists.* San Francisco: American Academy of Ophthalmology; 1997: vol XV, no 5.
>
> Walton DS. Primary congenital open angle glaucoma: a study of the anterior segment abnormalities. *Trans Am Ophthalmol Soc.* 1981;77:746–768.

Clinical Manifestations and Diagnosis

Primary congenital glaucoma usually presents in the neonatal or infantile period with a combination of signs and symptoms. *Epiphora, photophobia,* and *blepharospasm* constitute the classic "clinical triad" of primary congenital glaucoma. Other symptoms include clouding and enlargement of the cornea (Fig 21-1).

Corneal edema results from elevated IOP and may be gradual or sudden in onset. Corneal edema is often the presenting sign in infants younger than 3 months. Microcystic edema initially involves the corneal epithelium but later extends also to the stroma, often accompanied by one or more curvilinear breaks in Descemet's membrane *(Haab striae).* Although edema may resolve with IOP reduction, a scar will remain permanently at the site of Haab striae. Photophobia, epiphora, and blepharospasm result from the glare and epithelial abnormalities associated with corneal edema and opacification.

Corneal enlargement occurs with gradual stretching of the cornea as a result of elevated IOP and often appears in slightly older infants up to about 2–3 years of age. The normal newborn has a horizontal corneal diameter of 9.5–10.5 mm; a diameter of greater than 11.5 mm is suggestive of glaucoma. By age 1 year, normal corneal diameter

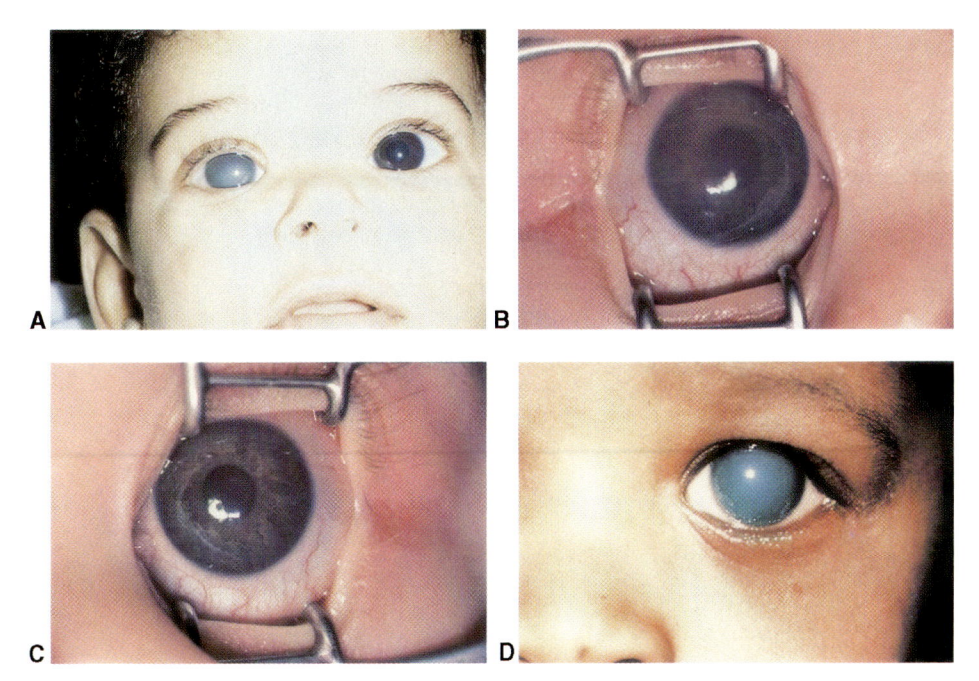

Figure 21-1 A, Congenital glaucoma, right eye. **B,** Right cornea larger and hazy. **C,** Left cornea clear. **D,** Late congenital glaucoma, left eye.

is 10–11.5 mm; a diameter greater than 12.5 mm suggests abnormality. Glaucoma should be suspected in any child with a corneal diameter greater than 13 mm.

The signs and symptoms described for primary congenital glaucoma can also occur in infants with other primary developmental and secondary glaucomas as a nonspecific result of expansion of the infant eye when faced with high IOP. Nonglaucomatous conditions may also cause some of the signs and the symptoms seen in primary congenital glaucoma (Table 21-1) (see also BCSC Section 10, *Glaucoma*).

Diagnostic examination

A full ophthalmic examination of every child suspected of glaucoma is imperative. Vision is often poorer in the affected eye in unilateral cases and may be poor in both eyes when glaucoma is bilateral. The child's ability to fix and follow and the presence of nystagmus should also be noted. *Refraction*, when possible, often reveals myopia or astigmatism (or both) from eye enlargement and corneal irregularity.

Corneal inspection The cornea should be examined for size, possible edema, and Haab striae. A penlight, millimeter ruler, direct ophthalmoscope, and retinoscope are useful. Inspection can often reveal even a half-millimeter difference in corneal diameter between the eyes. Haab striae are often seen well against the red reflex after pupil dilation (Fig 21-2).

Table 21-1 Differential Diagnosis of Signs in Primary Congenital Glaucoma

Conditions sharing signs of epiphora and red eye
Conjunctivitis
Congenital nasolacrimal duct obstruction
Corneal epithelial defect/abrasion
Ocular inflammation (uveitis, trauma)

Conditions sharing signs of corneal edema or opacification
Corneal dystrophy
  Congenital hereditary endothelial dystrophy
  Posterior polymorphous dystrophy
Obstetric birth trauma with Descemet's tears
Storage disease
  Mucopolysaccharidoses
  Cystinosis
Congenital anomalies
  Sclerocornea
  Peters anomaly
Keratitis
  Maternal rubella keratitis
  Herpetic
  Phlyctenular
Idiopathic (diagnosis of exclusion only)

Conditions sharing sign of corneal enlargement
Axial myopia
Megalocornea

Conditions sharing sign of optic nerve cupping (real or apparent)
Physiologic optic nerve cupping
Optic nerve coloboma
Optic atrophy
Optic nerve hypoplasia
Optic nerve malformation

(Reproduced with modification from Buckley EG. Primary congenital open angle glaucoma. In: Epstein DL, Allingham RR, Schuman JS, eds. *Chandler and Grant's Glaucoma*. 4th ed. Baltimore: Williams & Wilkins; 1997:598–608.)

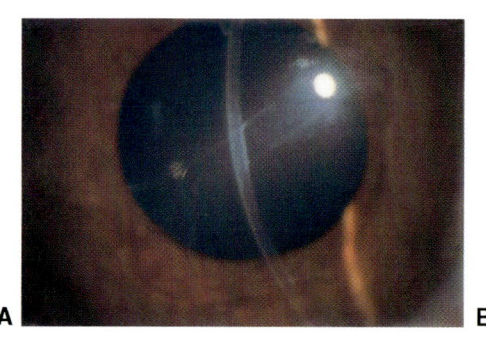

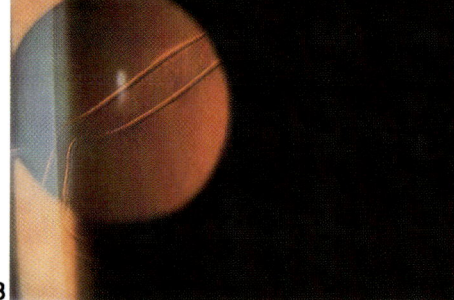

Figure 21-2 **A,** Breaks in Descemet's membrane (Haab striae), right eye. **B,** Retroillumination, same eye.

Tonometry and intraocular pressure IOP is best measured using topical anesthesia in a cooperative child because IOP may be falsely elevated in a struggling child and unpredictably altered (usually lowered) when systemic sedatives and anesthetics are administered. A useful technique is to bring the child in slightly hungry and then bottle feed at the time of pressure measurement. The Perkins applanation tonometer and the Tono-Pen are useful in infants and young children, and Goldmann applanation readings can frequently be achieved in older children.

In primary congenital glaucoma, unanesthetized IOP commonly ranges between 30 and 40 mm Hg, and it is usually greater than 20 mm Hg even under anesthesia.

The normal IOP in infants and young children is lower than that of normal adults; mean IOP is between 10 and 12 mm Hg in newborn infants and reaches approximately 14 mm Hg by age 7–8 years. Asymmetrical IOP readings in a quiet or anesthetized child should also raise suspicion of glaucoma in the eye with the higher IOP. Conscious sedation with chloral hydrate (50 mg/kg PO or PR, up to 1000 mg maximum dose) allows IOP readings that are minimally altered from those in an awake state. Conscious sedation should be performed with close monitoring of the child's vital signs and oxygenation by pulse oximetry.

Anterior segment examination After tonometry has been attempted, the portable slit lamp allows detailed inspection of the anterior segments. An abnormally deep anterior chamber and relative peripheral iris stromal hypoplasia are characteristic of primary congenital glaucoma.

Gonioscopy provides important information regarding the mechanism of glaucoma. It is best performed using a Koeppe contact lens and portable slit lamp or loupes. Often, a preliminary examination can be performed on a quiet infant in the office, with more detailed assessment possible in the operating room under anesthesia. Figure 21-3 gives examples of gonioscopic photographs of adult patients. The anterior chamber angle of a *normal* infant differs from that of an adult in the following ways:

- The trabecular meshwork is more lightly pigmented
- Schwalbe's line is often less distinct
- The uveal meshwork is translucent so that the junction between scleral spur and ciliary body band is often not well seen

In congenital glaucoma, the iris often shows an insertion more anterior than that of the normal angle, and the translucency of the uveal meshwork is altered, making ciliary body band, trabecular meshwork, and scleral spur indistinct. (The membrane described by Barkan may indeed be these translucent uveal meshwork cells.) The scalloped border of the iris pigmented epithelium is often unusually prominent, especially when peripheral iris stromal hypoplasia is present. In contrast, the open angle usually appears normal in juvenile open-angle glaucoma.

Optic nerve examination The optic nerve, when visible, usually shows an increased cup/disc ratio, which can improve with successful treatment and lowering of IOP. The pattern of generalized enlargement of the optic cup seen in very young patients with glaucoma has been attributed to stretching of the optic canal and backward bowing of the lamina

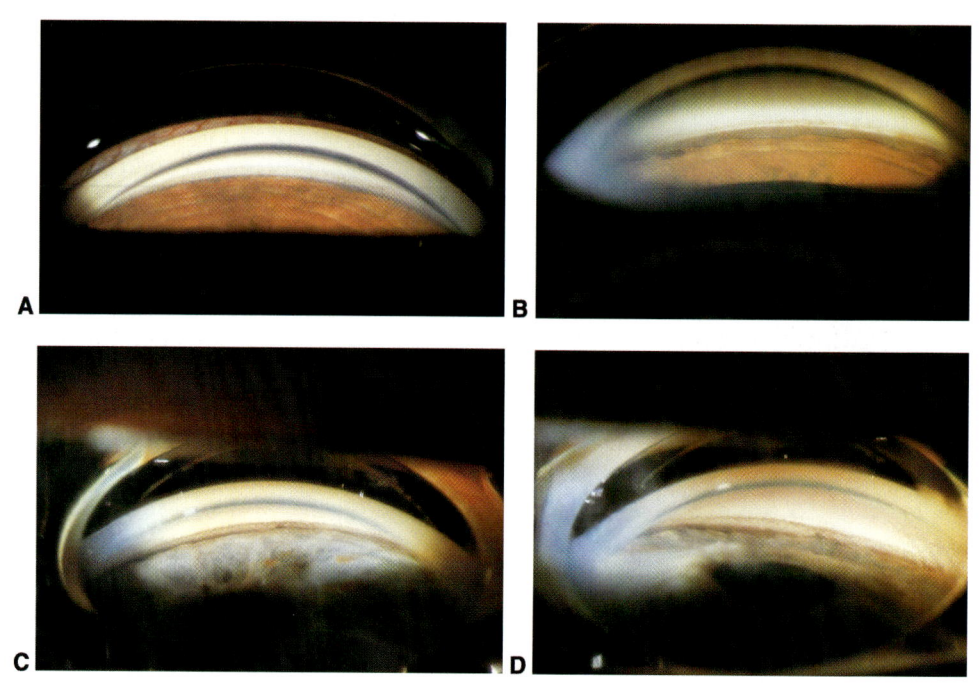

Figure 21-3 Gonioscopy in adults. **A,** Normal open angle. Gonioscopic photograph shows trace pigmentation of the posterior trabecular meshwork and normal insertion of the iris into a narrow ciliary body band. The Goldmann lens was used. **B,** Normal open angle. This gonioscopic view using the Goldmann lens shows mild pigmentation of the posterior trabecular meshwork. A wide ciliary body band with posterior insertion of the iris can also be seen. **C,** Narrow angle. This gonioscopic view using the Zeiss lens without indentation shows pigment in inferior angle but poor visualization of angle anatomy. **D,** Same angle as shown in **C.** Gonioscopy with a Zeiss lens with indentation shows peripheral anterior synechiae in the posterior trabecular meshwork. Pigment deposits on Schwalbe's line can also be seen. *(Photographs courtesy of Elizabeth A. Hodapp, MD.)*

cribrosa, which can be reversible (Fig 21-4). In most cases of primary congenital glaucoma, the cup/disc ratio exceeds 0.3; in contrast, 97% of normal newborn eyes show a cup/disc ratio of less than 0.3. Cup/disc asymmetry between two eyes of an infant is also suspicious for glaucoma on the more cupped side.

> Buckley EG. Primary congenital open angle glaucoma. In: Epstein DL, Allingham RR, Schuman JS, eds. *Chandler and Grant's Glaucoma.* 4th ed. Baltimore: Williams & Wilkins; 1997:598–608.
>
> Shaffer RN, Weiss DI. *Congenital and Pediatric Glaucomas.* St Louis: Mosby; 1970.

Natural History

In almost all cases of untreated primary congenital glaucoma, the disease progresses and leads to blindness. The cornea becomes irreversibly opacified and may vascularize. It may continue to enlarge through the first 2–3 years of life, reaching a diameter up to 16–17 mm. As the entire eye enlarges, pseudoproptosis and an "ox eye" appearance, called *buphthalmos,* may result. Scleral thinning and myopic fundus changes may occur, and

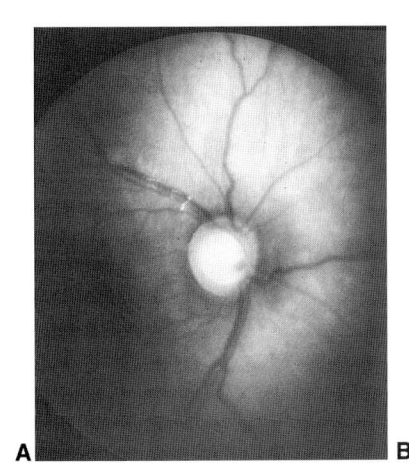

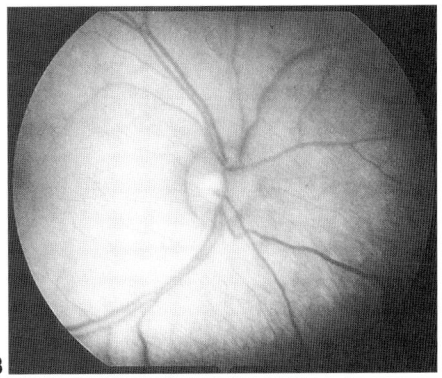

Figure 21-4 Optic nerve changes after treatment for congenital glaucoma. **A,** Preoperative enlarged optic disc cup. **B,** Resolution of disc cupping after pressure is reduced by goniotomy. *(Photographs courtesy of Sharon Freedman, MD.)*

spontaneous lens dislocation can result. Optic nerve cupping also increases and may finally lead to complete blindness.

Other Primary Developmental and Secondary Pediatric Glaucomas

Primary Developmental Glaucomas

In addition to primary congenital open-angle glaucoma, other primary developmental glaucomas can present at birth or shortly after. The ophthalmologist and pediatrician should carefully examine the newborn or infant with glaucoma to uncover associated ocular and systemic abnormalities. Examples of associated systemic abnormalities include:

- Congenital rubella
- Oculocerebrorenal (Lowe) syndrome
- Sturge-Weber syndrome (nevus flammeus, or port-wine stain, of the face on the affected side)
- Neurofibromatosis
- Homocystinuria

Infantile glaucoma can present with the following ocular abnormalities:

- Aniridia
- Axenfeld-Rieger syndrome
- Congenital iris ectropion
- Peters anomaly
- Sclerocornea

- Posterior polymorphous dystrophy
- Congenital hereditary endothelial dystrophy

See BCSC Section 10, *Glaucoma*.

Treatment of infants with primary developmental glaucomas should usually follow the same guidelines as those for primary congenital glaucoma (see Treatment, below). In some cases (eg, aniridia and Axenfeld-Rieger syndrome), secondary glaucoma may also occur later in childhood, and treatment again resembles that for other secondary glaucomas in childhood.

Secondary Glaucoma

Secondary glaucomas in children may result from trauma, inflammation, or uveitis (eg, juvenile rheumatoid arthritis). Aphakic glaucoma after congenital cataract surgery, secondary angle-closure glaucoma in cases of cicatricial retinopathy of prematurity, and glaucoma associated with childhood intraocular neoplasm (eg, retinoblastoma, juvenile xanthogranuloma, and medulloepithelioma) are secondary glaucomas specific to children. Less commonly, secondary glaucoma can result from some of the same causes as in adults, such as steroid use. In general, secondary glaucoma in children is managed as it is managed in adults. Eyes with angle closure usually require peripheral iridectomy or lensectomy; with other secondary glaucomas, medical therapy is attempted first.

Aphakic glaucoma deserves special comment. Acute or subacute angle closure with iris bombé is rare; although it usually occurs soon after surgery, onset can be delayed by a year or more. Treatment consists of surgical iridectomy, often with goniosynechialysis and anterior vitrectomy. The incidence of the more common open-angle glaucoma after removal of congenital cataracts varies from 15% to 30%, with a mean time to onset of 5 years after surgery. The risk of glaucoma seems higher in infants who undergo surgery prior to age 1 year, in those whose initial corneal diameter exceeds 10 mm, and in those with persistent hyperplastic primary vitreous. Children who are aphakic are at lifelong risk for glaucoma and need regular careful examination (including IOP evaluation).

> Egbert JE, Wright MM, Dahlhauser KF, et al. A prospective study of ocular hypertension and glaucoma after pediatric cataract surgery. *Ophthalmology*. 1995;102:1098–1101.
>
> Hoskins HD Jr, Shaffer RN, Hetherington J. Anatomical classification of the developmental glaucomas. *Arch Ophthalmol*. 1984;102:1331–1336.
>
> Walton DS. Unusual pediatric glaucomas. In: Epstein DL, Allingham RR, Schuman JS, eds. *Chandler and Grant's Glaucoma*. 4th ed. Baltimore: Williams & Wilkins; 1997:623–638.

Treatment

Although it is true that juvenile open-angle glaucoma and most secondary glaucomas of childhood are managed in much the same way as similar conditions in adults, differences in approach do exist. Management of adult glaucoma is more likely to delay surgery until medical options have been pursued.

Surgical Therapy

Surgical intervention is the treatment of choice for primary congenital glaucoma and most of the other primary developmental glaucomas presenting in infancy and early childhood. BCSC Section 10, *Glaucoma*, also covers the procedures discussed in this chapter.

Angle surgery is the preferred initial surgical intervention in these cases. *Goniotomy*, in which the trabecular meshwork is incised under direct gonioscopic visualization, is often preferred when the cornea is clear; *trabeculotomy*, which uses an external approach to identify, cannulate, and then connect Schlemm's canal with the anterior chamber by tearing through the poorly functioning trabecular meshwork, is preferable in cases of poor visualization of the angle. A modification of this technique uses a 6–0 Prolene suture to cannulate and open Schlemm's canal for its entire 360° circumference in one surgery.

Usually, at least two angle surgeries are performed prior to proceeding with an additional surgical modality. IOP is controlled with one or two angle surgeries in approximately 80% of infants with primary congenital glaucoma presenting from 3 months to 1 year of age. If angle surgery is unsuccessful and medical therapy (see below) is inadequate to control IOP and glaucoma, additional options include trabeculectomy with antifibrotic therapy (eg, mitomycin), glaucoma implant procedures, or cycloablative procedures.

Trabeculectomy with the use of mitomycin-C is successful in approximately 50%–95% of children. The reported success rate may vary tremendously with characteristics of the patient and the eye. Patients younger than 1 year and those who are aphakic often do not fare as well. The long-term risk of bleb leaks and endophthalmitis seem to be particularly high with mitomycin-augmented trabeculectomy in children.

The reported success rate of glaucoma *implant surgery* with the Molteno, Baerveldt, and Ahmed implants has varied between 54% and approximately 80%–85%. Although most of these children must remain on adjunctive topical medical therapy to control IOP after surgery, their blebs are thicker and may be less prone to leaking and infection than those of mitomycin-augmented trabeculectomy.

Cycloablation via the Nd:YAG laser, the diode laser, or cyclocryotherapy is generally reserved for extremely resistant cases or those not amenable to the intraocular surgeries noted above. These techniques decrease ciliary body production of aqueous humor. Cyclocryotherapy (freeze treatment to the ciliary body through the sclera) has a reported success rate of about 33%. Repeat applications are the rule, and the risk of phthisis and blindness is significant (approximately 10%). Transscleral laser cycloablation with the Nd:YAG or the diode laser has also been used in refractory cases. Short-term success is about 50% with a retreatment rate of about 70% with either laser. The recent success rate of endoscopic cycloablation using the diode laser in pediatric cases has been 50%. The endoscopic route also may require less retreatment than the transscleral routes.

Medical Therapy

The menu of glaucoma medications continues to expand. See also BCSC Section 10, *Glaucoma*.

Carbonic anhydrase inhibitors have been used for many years as aqueous suppressants in children, and they may be quite effective. Acetazolamide (Diamox), the most commonly used agent, is effective at oral doses of 10–20 mg/kg/day divided into three or four doses. Care must be taken to watch for weight loss, lethargy, or metabolic acidosis, although many children tolerate this medication well.

The topical carbonic anhydrase inhibitor dorzolamide (Trusopt) is available as a 2.0% solution. Preliminary studies using dorzolamide three times a day indicate that this drug is effective in many cases, although it produces a smaller reduction in IOP (<15%) than does full-dose oral acetazolamide in the same child (~20%). A second topical carbonic anhydrase inhibitor, brinzolamide (Azopt), has shown effects similar to those of dorzolamide in some children.

Topical beta-blocker therapy has been used in children since 1978, and it often lowers IOP about 20%. The major risks of this therapy are respiratory distress caused by apnea or bronchospasm and bradycardia, which occurs mostly in very tiny infants and in children with a history of bronchospasm. Timolol (or its equivalent) or betaxolol (Betoptic S) should be used at 0.25% strength twice a day for initial therapy. The parent should be instructed how to perform nasolacrimal occlusion with these drugs. The gel-forming preparations of timolol (Timoptic XE) seem effective in some children but should be avoided in eyes with aphakic contact lenses.

Miotic therapy is rarely effective in cases of primary congenital glaucoma, perhaps because of the high iris insertion in these cases. Long-acting or slow-release miotics such as pilocarpine (Pilopine gel and Ocusert) or echothiophate (Phospholine Iodide—for aphakic patients) can be helpful, particularly in cases of juvenile open-angle glaucoma and some secondary childhood glaucomas.

Adrenergic agents such as epinephrine or dipivefrin (Propine) are not usually effective in children, particularly when a nonselective beta blocker is already in use. The α_2-adrenergic agonist apraclonidine (Iopidine) has been useful when short-term IOP reduction is essential, but this drug shows a high incidence of tachyphylaxis and allergy in young children. The α_2-adrenergic antagonist brimonidine (Alphagan) effectively reduces IOP in some cases of pediatric glaucoma, but this agent can produce severe systemic side effects in infants and small children (among them lethargy, hypotonia, hypothermia, and serious CNS depression).

The *prostaglandin derivative* latanoprost (Xalatan) has recently become available at a strength of 0.005% for use at bedtime. Early experience shows an excellent systemic safety profile but varied IOP reduction with this medication in pediatric patients with glaucoma. Among pediatric patients, those with juvenile open-angle glaucoma are the most likely to respond to latanoprost.

> Freedman SF. Medical and surgical treatments for childhood glaucomas. In: Epstein DL, Allingham RR, Schuman JS, eds. *Chandler and Grant's Glaucoma*. 4th ed. Baltimore: Williams & Wilkins; 1997:609–622.
>
> Freedman SF, Buckley EG. Goniotomy and trabeculectomy. In: Buckley EG, Freedman SF, Shields MB, eds. *Atlas of Ophthalmic Surgery*. St Louis: Mosby; 1995. *Strabismus and Glaucoma;* vol 3.

Prognosis and Follow-Up

If primary congenital glaucoma presents at birth, the prognosis for IOP control and visual preservation is poor, with at least half of these eyes becoming legally blind. With a corneal diameter greater than 14 mm at diagnosis, the visual prognosis is similarly poor. Up to 80%–90% of cases in the "favorable prognostic group" (onset, 3–12 months) can be controlled with angle surgery. The remaining 10%–20% of these cases, and many of the remaining cases of primary and secondary glaucomas, often present a lifelong challenge.

Visual loss in childhood glaucoma is multifactorial. Visual loss may result not only from corneal scarring and opacification or optic nerve damage but also from significant myopic astigmatism and associated anisometropic and strabismic amblyopia, especially in unilateral cases. Myopia results from axial enlargement of the eye in the setting of high IOP; astigmatism often results from unequal expansion of the anterior segment, corneal scarring and opacification, or dislocation of the lens. Careful assessment of vision, refraction, and amblyopia therapy are needed to optimize visual function in these children.

All cases of childhood glaucoma require diligent follow-up, which should also be performed when glaucoma is suspected but cannot yet be confirmed. After any given surgical intervention or change in medical therapy, control of IOP should be assessed within 1–2 weeks. The status of the cornea in terms of its size and clarity, the appearance of the optic nerve, and the refractive error can all often provide clues regarding improved IOP control. If IOP cannot be determined in the office, examination may require sedation with chloral hydrate or occasionally anesthesia. The IOP should be considered not as an isolated finding but rather in conjunction with other features of the examination. If the IOP is less than 20 mm Hg under anesthesia but clinical evidence shows persistent corneal edema or enlargement, progressive optic nerve cupping, or myopic progression, further intervention should be pursued despite the IOP reading. By contrast, IOP of about 20 mm Hg in a young child who shows evidence of clinical improvement may be followed carefully in the short term without any other intervention.

Careful repeated follow-up of all parameters associated with glaucoma in children is the only way to ensure disease control and optimal preservation of visual function. Even those children apparently "cured" after angle surgery can experience relapse years later with elevated IOP and subsequent visual loss. Although helpful in following disease progression in older children, visual fields are rarely useful in children younger than 6–8 years. Optic nerve photographs should be taken whenever possible, and these can be helpful for comparison during later examinations. As discussed above, refractive error and corneal size and clarity are also helpful to follow as evidence of ocular stability over time. Serial axial length measurement may be followed as well, but it is no more reliable than corneal diameter measurement.

CHAPTER 22

Childhood Cataracts and Other Pediatric Lens Disorders

Abnormalities of the pediatric lens include those of opacification (cataract), shape, size, location, and development; such abnormalities constitute a significant source of visual impairment in children (Table 22-1). The incidence is approximately 6 per 10,000 infants. Abnormalities of the pediatric lens are associated with diseases of the central nervous system, urinary tract, skeletal system, and skin. Pediatric lens abnormalities must be treated promptly to avoid lifelong visual loss. BCSC Section 11, *Lens and Cataract*, also covers conditions and procedures discussed in this chapter.

Structural or Positional Lens Abnormalities

Congenital aphakia
Absence of the lens at birth is rare. This condition is usually associated with a markedly abnormal eye.

Table 22-1 **Congenital Lens Abnormalities**

Opacification	Shape
Lamellar	Lenticonus
Speckled	Lentiglobus
Membranous	Spherophakia
Pulverulent	Coloboma
Polar	
Zonular	**Location**
Subcapsular	Subluxed
Nuclear	Luxed
Total	
	Developmental
Size	Persistent hyperplastic primary vitreous
Microspherophakia	Mittendorf dot
Disciform	

Spherophakia

A lens that is spherical and smaller than a normal lens is called *spherophakic*. This condition is usually bilateral. The lens may dislocate, causing secondary glaucoma (Fig 22-1).

Coloboma

A lens coloboma (a misnomer) involves flattening or notching of the lens periphery (Fig 22-2). A coloboma can be associated with a defect in the iris, optic nerve, or retina and is due to the abnormal closure of the embryonic fissure. The coloboma is usually located inferonasally, and zonular fibers are typically absent in the colobomatous area, resulting in a flattening of the lens at that location without any dislocation. In significant colobomatous defects, lens dislocations occur superiorly and temporally. Most colobomatous lenses do not worsen progressively.

Posterior lenticonus/lentiglobus

Posterior lenticonus/lentiglobus (Fig 22-3) describes a group of lens abnormalities due to a central ectasia of the lens surface; such abnormalities can develop into opacification. Over 90% of lenticonus cases are unilateral. Initially, the change in lens architecture

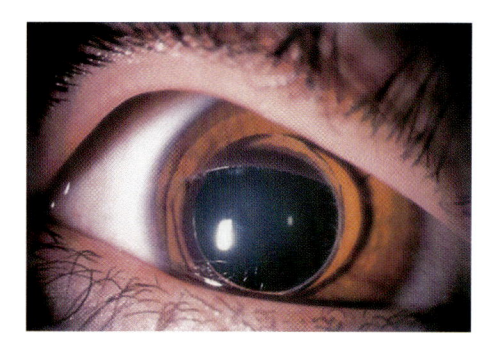

Figure 22-1 Spherophakia with lens dislocation into anterior chamber, left eye.

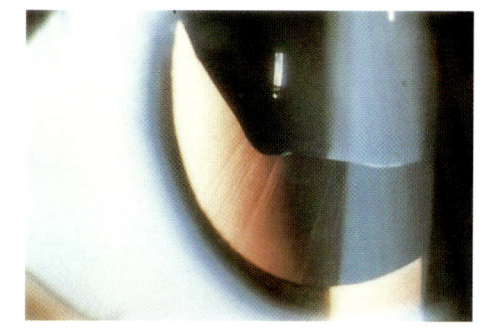

Figure 22-2 Lens equator flattening (with dislocation), which may be referred to as *lens coloboma*.

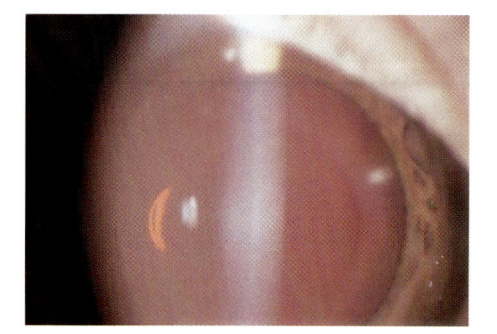

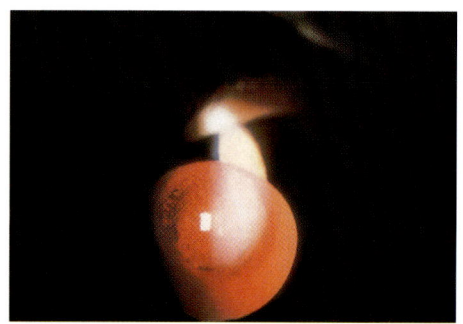

Figure 22-3 Posterior lenticonus.

results in myopia and irregular astigmatism. Over time, the distorted posterior lens cortex becomes opacified and occasionally ruptures, resulting in total lens opacification. Because opacification does not usually occur until age 4 or 5, the postsurgical prognosis for vision is generally good. Anterior lenticonus may be associated with nerve deafness and nephritis (Alport syndrome).

Dislocated Lenses in Children

When the lens is not in its normal anatomical position, it is said to be *dislocated, subluxed, subluxated, luxed, luxated,* or *ectopic.* Luxed or luxated lenses are completely detached from the ciliary body and are either loose in the posterior chamber or vitreous or can prolapse to the anterior chamber. The amount of dislocation can vary from only slight displacement with minimal iridodonesis to severe displacement with the edge of the lens totally out of the pupillary margin. Lens dislocation is often associated with multisystem disease or an inborn error of metabolism (Table 22-2). Lens dislocation can occur with trauma, although this is not common and usually involves a significant injury to the eye. Spontaneous lens dislocation has been reported in aniridia and rarely with exfoliation syndrome and buphthalmos (secondary to congenital glaucoma).

Simple ectopia lentis

Simple ectopia lentis is usually bilateral and symmetrical with upward and temporal lens displacement. Autosomal dominant inheritance is most common. The onset may be congenital or can occur between the ages of 20 and 65 years. Glaucoma is common in the late-onset type.

Ectopia lentis et pupillae

Also known as *ectopia of the lens and pupil,* this condition is a rare autosomal recessive condition. It is manifested by bilateral displacement of the pupil, usually inferotem-

Table 22-2 **Subluxed Lenses**

Systemic Conditions
Marfan syndrome
Homocystinuria
Weill-Marchesani syndrome
Hyperlysinemia
Sulfite oxidase deficiency
Syphilis
Ehlers-Danlos syndrome

Ocular Conditions
Aniridia
Iris coloboma
Trauma
Hereditary ectopic lentis
Congenital glaucoma

porally, with lens dislocation in the opposite direction (Fig 22-4). Patients have microspherophakia, miosis, and poor pupillary dilation with mydriatics. This condition is thought to be due to a defect in neuroectodermal tissue development because the pigmented layers of the iris, zonules, and iris dilator are all involved. Some family members may have only subluxation without the pupillary displacement. The condition is nonprogressive.

Marfan syndrome

Marfan syndrome is the systemic disease most commonly associated with dislocated lenses. The syndrome consists of abnormalities of the cardiovascular, musculoskeletal, and ocular systems. It is inherited as an autosomal dominant trait, but family history is negative in 15% of cases. Marfan syndrome is caused by mutations in the fibrillin gene on chromosome 15. These patients are characteristically tall with long limbs and fingers (arachnodactyly); loose, flexible joints; scoliosis; and chest deformities. Cardiovascular abnormalities are a source of significant mortality and manifest as enlargement of the aortic root, dilatation of a descending aorta, dissecting aneurysm, and floppy mitral valve. The life expectancy of patients with Marfan syndrome is about half that of the normal population. Ocular abnormalities occur in over 80% of patients, with lens dislocation being the most common. In approximately 75% of cases, the lens is upwardly dislocated (Fig 22-5). Typically, the zonules that are visible are intact and unbroken, in contradistinction to the broken zonules seen in homocystinuria. Examination of the iris may reveal transillumination defects that are more marked near the iris base. The pupil is small and dilates poorly. The axial length is increased, and the patients are usually myopic. Retinal detachment often occurs spontaneously in the second and third decades of life.

Homocystinuria

Homocystinuria is a rare autosomal recessive condition caused by an abnormality in the enzyme cystathionine β-synthase. This abnormality causes homocystine to accumulate in the plasma and to be excreted in the urine. Homocystinuria occurs in approximately 1 in 100,000 births.

The clinical manifestations of homocystinuria vary markedly and affect the eye, skeletal system, central nervous system, and vascular system. Most of the abnormalities develop after birth and become progressively worse with age. Ocular findings consist mainly

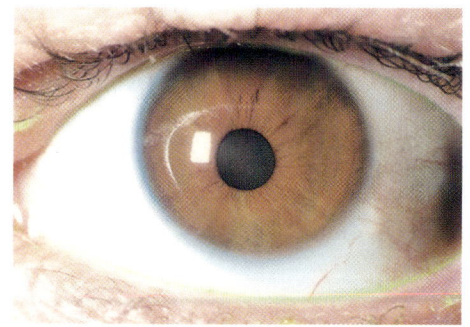

Figure 22-4 Ectopia lentis et pupillae, left eye.

CHAPTER 22: Childhood Cataracts and Other Pediatric Lens Disorders • 275

of dislocated lenses (normally downward), a condition that typically occurs between the ages of 3 and 10 years. The lenses may dislocate into the anterior chamber, a finding suggestive of homocystinuria (Fig 22-6).

Systemically, vascular complications are common and secondary to thrombotic disease, which affects large or medium-sized arteries and veins anywhere in the body. Partial or complete vascular obstruction is present in various organs, and hypertension, cardiac murmurs, and cardiomegaly are common. Anesthesia holds a higher risk for patients with homocystinuria because of thromboembolic phenomena. These patients are usually

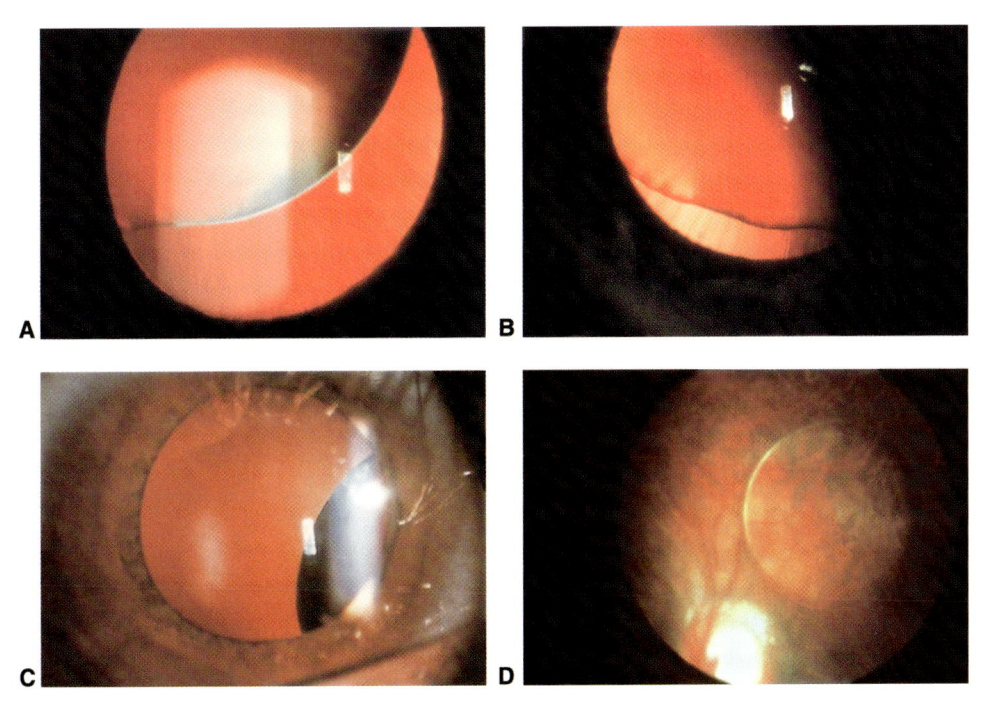

Figure 22-5 Marfan syndrome. **A** and **B,** Superotemporal displacement of lenses, bilateral. **C,** Inferonasal displacement, right eye. **D,** Lens dislocation into vitreous, left eye.

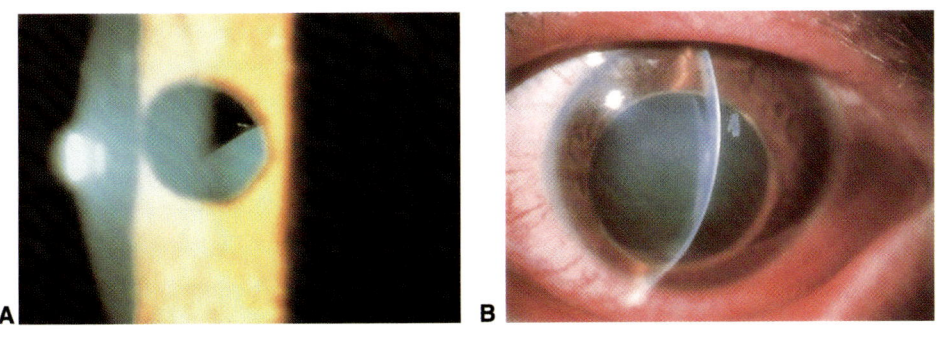

Figure 22-6 Homocystinuria. **A,** Inferonasal lens dislocation, right eye. **B,** Lens may dislocate into anterior chamber with acute pupillary-block glaucoma (same patient).

tall with osteoporosis, scoliosis, and chest deformities. Central nervous system abnormalities occur in approximately 50% of patients, with mental retardation and seizures being the most common.

Diagnosis is confirmed by detecting disulfides, including homocystine, in the urine. The medical management of homocystinuria is directed toward normalizing the biochemical abnormality. Dietary management (low methionine and high cystine) has been attempted, and coenzyme supplements (pyridoxine or vitamin B_6) are effective in about 50% of cases.

Weill-Marchesani syndrome

Patients with Weill-Marchesani syndrome characteristically are short with short fingers and limbs, and they can be thought of as clinical opposites of patients with Marfan syndrome. Inheritance can be autosomal dominant or recessive. The lenses are also small and nearly round *(microspherophakia)*. With time, the lens dislocates anteriorly and pupillary block glaucoma may occur. Because of this, prophylactic laser peripheral iridectomy is recommended.

> Jensen AD, Cross HE, Paton D. Ocular complications in the Weill-Marchesani syndrome. *Am J Ophthalmol.* 1974;77:261–269.

Hyperlysinemia

Hyperlysinemia is the result of a definciency of lysine α-ketoglutarate reductase and has been found in mentally retarded patients, some of whom have had dislocated lenses. However, the same biochemical abnormality and enzyme deficiency have been found in normal persons identified through newborn screening. The association between hyperlysinemia and dislocated lenses is not clearly documented.

Sulfite oxidase deficiency

Sulfite oxidase deficiency is a very rare hereditary disorder of sulfur metabolism manifested by severe neurologic disorders and ectopia lentis. The enzyme deficiency interferes with conversion of sulfite to sulphate, resulting in increased urine secretion of sulfite. The diagnosis can be confirmed by the absence of sulfite oxidase activity in skin fibroblasts. Neurologic abnormalities include infantile hemiplegia, choreoathetosis, and seizures. Irreversible brain damage and death usually occur by age 5.

> Halpert M, BenEzra D. Surgery of the hereditary subluxated lens in children. *Ophthalmology.* 1996;103:681–686.
>
> Maumenee IH. The eye in the Marfan syndrome. *Trans Am Ophthalmol Soc.* 1981;79:684–733.

Treatment

Optical correction

Optical correction of the refractive error caused by lens dislocation is often difficult. Depending on the extent of the dislocation, the patient may see better with a myopic astigmatic correction or an aphakic correction. With very mild subluxation, the patient may be only myopic and corrected visual function may be good. More severe amounts of dislocation cause optical distortion because the patient is looking through the far peripheral part of the lens. Because the resultant myopic astigmatism is difficult to accurately measure by retinoscopy, or automated refractometry, visual acuity using the aphakic correction may be superior. Pre- and postdilation refractions are often helpful in deciding on the best choice. If satisfactory visual function cannot be obtained, or if visual function is worsening over time, lens removal should be considered.

Surgery

Subluxed lenses can be removed either from the anterior segment through a limbal incision or through the pars plana. In most circumstances, complete lensectomy is indicated. Postoperative visual rehabilitation can be achieved using contact lenses or glasses, and postoperative visual results are quite good. The use of sutured intraocular lenses, lens capsular bag expanders, or other types of lens supporting maneuvers has undergone limited testing in children. Caution should be exercised in patients with Marfan syndrome because there is an increased risk of retinal detachment, which may occur years after surgery.

> Plager DA, Parks MM, Helveston EM, et al. Surgical treatment of subluxed lenses in children. *Ophthalmology.* 1992;99:1018–1023.

Pediatric Cataracts

Congenital cataracts are responsible for nearly 10% of all visual loss in children worldwide (Fig 22-7). It is estimated that 1 in 250 newborns has some form of cataract. Cataracts can be inherited, most commonly as a result of an autosomal dominant pattern, but X-linked and autosomal recessive types have been reported. Cataract development has been linked to chromosome 1, 2, 16, and 17 (Table 22-3). Chromosomal disorders such as trisomy 13, 18, and 21 have been associated with lens opacities. Trauma is also a known cause of cataracts and should be investigated in children who present with other signs suggesting child abuse (see Chapter 30). The cause of the vast majority of cataracts is unknown. A large number of systemic and metabolic disorders can result in cataract formation (Table 22-4; Fig 22-8). The visual significance of cataracts depends on the age

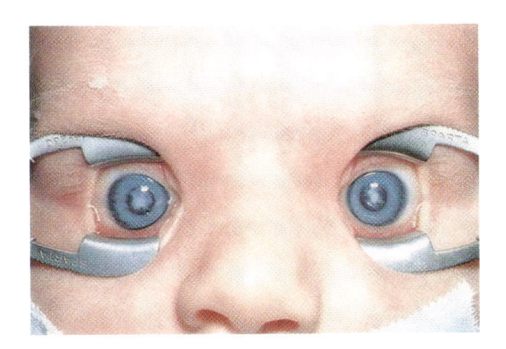

Figure 22-7 Bilateral congenital cataracts.

Table 22-3 Hereditary Factors in Pediatric Cataracts

Mendelian inheritance
Autosomal dominant chromosome
  1
  2
  16
  17
Autosomal recessive
X-linked
  Nance-Horan syndrome

Chromosomal disorders
Trisomy
  21 (Down syndrome)
  13–15
  18 (Edward syndrome)
  10q
  20p
Turner syndrome
Translocation
  3:4
  2:14
  2:16
Cri du chat syndrome

of onset, location, and morphology. These parameters provide important clues to the cause and visual prognosis.

Onset

In general, the younger the child is at diagnosis, the greater the potential impact on vision. Cataracts present at birth are the most serious because the visual system is not fully developed and because vision will be lost irreversibly if the visual axis is not cleared by 6–8 weeks of life. Unilateral opacities are more likely to cause permanent visual loss than bilateral opacities because of the competition between eyes (amblyopia). The development of nystagmus is a poor prognostic sign in terms of visual development. If the opacity occurs later in infancy or early childhood, the prognosis is improved for normal visual function, but prompt removal is still necessary, especially in unilateral cases. Even traumatic cataracts occurring at age 4 or 5 can result in significant permanent visual loss (<20/200) if not treated promptly.

Location

The more posterior and central the cataract, the greater the effect on vision. This is because of the optical characteristics of the lens. A small central posterior subcapsular opacity decreases vision more than a larger opacity located in the pericentral mid cortex. A small anterior polar cataract is rarely visually significant.

Table 22-4 Etiology of Pediatric Cataracts

Bilateral cataracts
  Idiopathic
  Hereditary cataracts (autosomal dominant most common,
    also autosomal recessive or X-linked)
  Genetic and metabolic diseases
    Down syndrome
    Hallermann-Streiff syndrome
    Lowe syndrome
    Galactosemia
    Marfan syndrome
    Trisomy 13–15
    Hypoglycemia
    Alport syndrome
    Myotonic dystrophy
    Fabry disease
    Hypoparathyroidism
    Conradi syndrome
  Maternal infection
    Rubella
    Cytomegalovirus
    Varicella
    Syphilis
    Toxoplasmosis
  Ocular anomalies
    Aniridia
    Anterior segment dysgenesis syndrome
  Toxic
    Corticosteroids
    Radiation (may also be unilateral)

Unilateral cataracts
  Idiopathic
  Ocular anomalies
    Persistent hyperplastic primary vitreous (PHPV)
    Anterior segment dysgenesis
    Posterior lenticonus
    Posterior pole tumors
  Traumatic (rule out child abuse)
  Rubella
  Masked bilateral cataract

Morphologic Types of Cataracts

Polar cataracts

Polar cataracts are opacities involving the subcapsular cortex or capsule in the polar regions of the lens. These cataracts are usually small (<3 mm), white, and located in the center of the lens capsule (Fig 22-9). Polar cataracts are thought to arise from abnormal separation of the lens vesicle during embryonic lens development. They can be inherited as an autosomal dominant trait. Although these cataracts are mostly visually insignificant, a small percentage can progress and may require surgery.

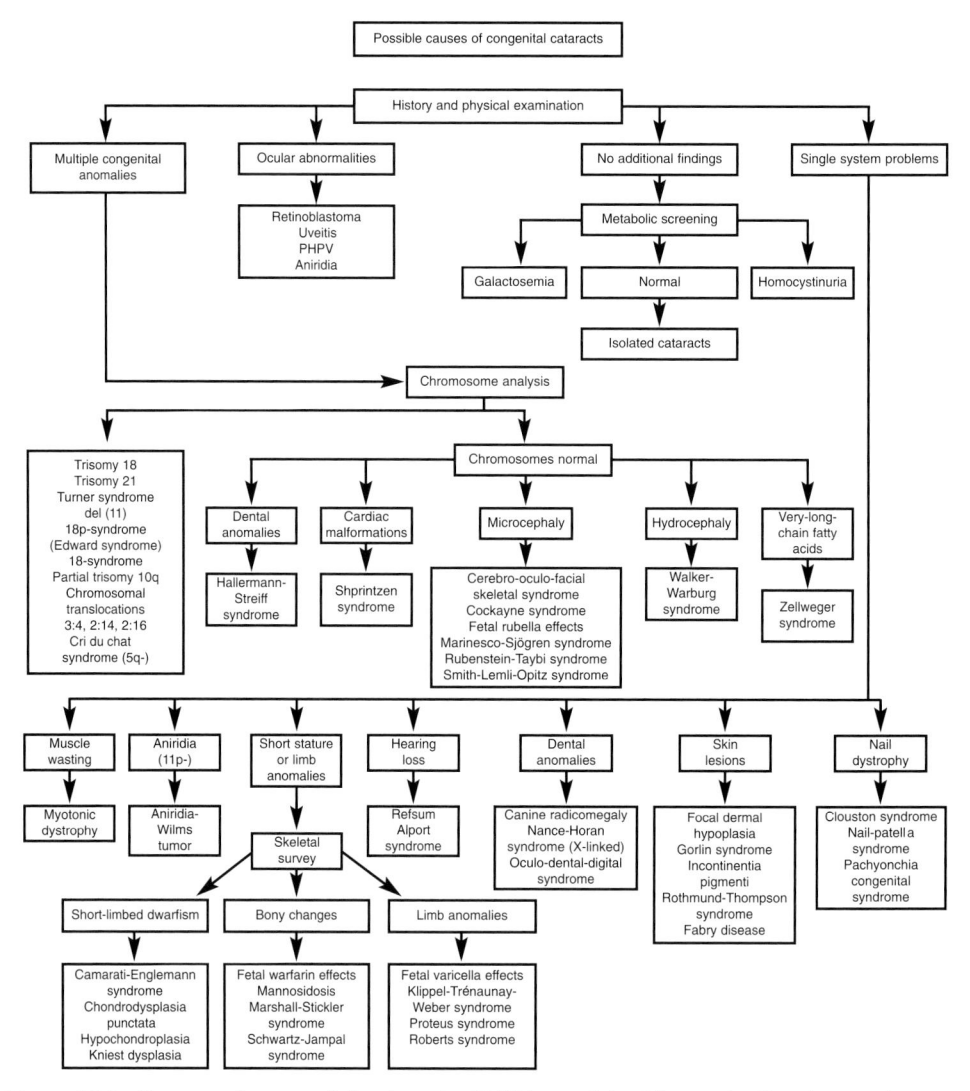

Figure 22-8 Causes of congenital cataracts. PHPV, persistent hyperplastic primary vitreous. *(Adapted from Buckley EG. Pediatric cataracts. In: Parrish R, ed. Bascom Palmer Eye Institute's Atlas of Ophthalmology. Philadelphia: Current Medicine; 2000.)*

Lamellar cataracts

Lamellar cataracts are characterized by layers of opacification peripheral to the Y-sutures with a clear nucleus (Fig 22-10). These cataracts are generally bilateral, 5 mm or more in diameter, and of varying density; they are found in normal-sized eyes. These cataracts are often inherited, and they are considered acquired and progressive rather than truly congenital. Some affected children have visually insignificant cataracts and do not require surgery or require it late, even if the cataract appears dense. Visual prognosis is very good.

Nuclear cataracts

Nuclear cataracts are typically congenital, dense axial opacities of 3 mm or more (Fig 22-11). They are frequently associated with mild to moderate microphthalmos and inherited as autosomal dominant traits. Visual results are generally only fair if surgery is performed early and poor if surgery is performed late.

Posterior lenticonus/lentiglobus

Posterior lenticonus/lentiglobus presents as a posterior lens opacity associated with bulging of the posterior lens capsule (Fig 22-12). Although frequently mistaken for a con-

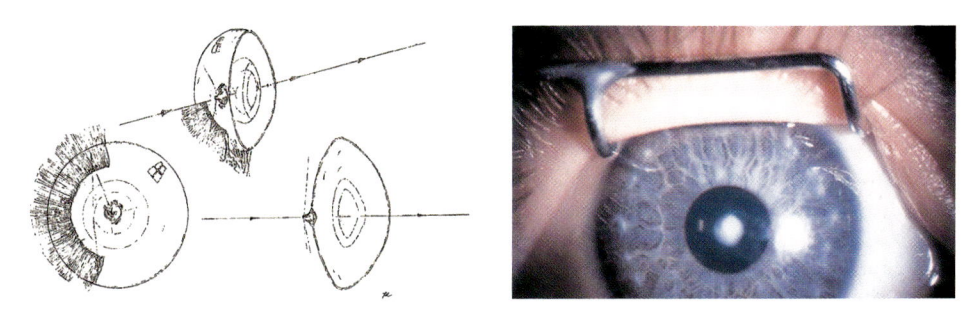

Figure 22-9 Anterior polar cataract. *(Illustration courtesy of Alan Y. Chow, MD.)*

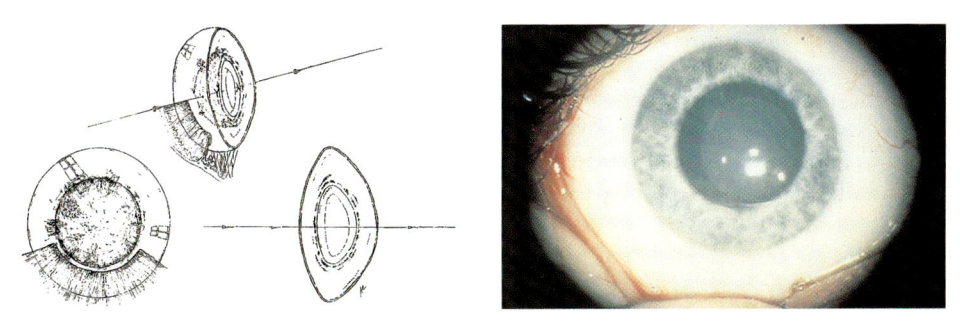

Figure 22-10 Lamellar cataract. Note that in photograph on the right, the opacity surrounds the nucleus and is outside the Y-sutures. *(Illustration courtesy of Alan Y. Chow, MD.)*

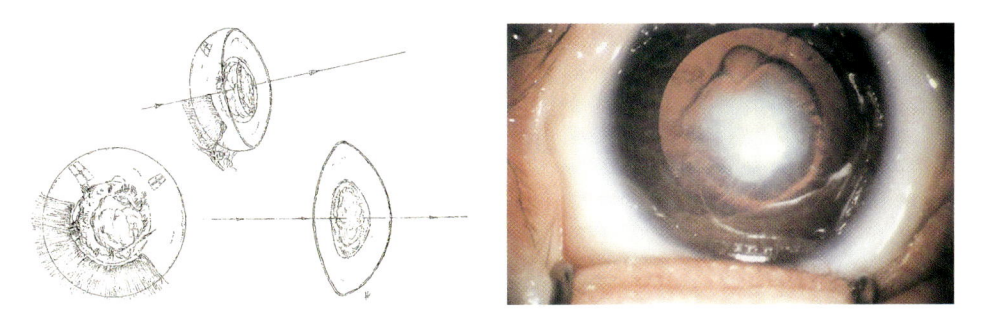

Figure 22-11 Nuclear cataract. *(Illustration courtesy of Alan Y. Chow, MD.)*

282 • Pediatric Ophthalmology and Strabismus

genital cataract, this opacity is usually acquired in infancy and is slowly progressive. The eyes are of normal size, and visual results are excellent with surgery.

Persistent hyperplastic primary vitreous (persistent fetal vasculature)

Persistent hyperplastic primary vitreous (Fig 22-13) is caused by failure of the primitive hyaloid vascular system to regress. Clinically, there is a retrolenticular fibrovascular membrane, which may be accompanied by a fibrovascular stalk extending from the posterior lens capsule to the optic disc. The vascular membrane can extend to involve the ciliary processes. Frequently, the lens is pushed forward by the membrane and glaucoma may develop. The eyes are usually mildly microphthalmic. Visual prognosis depends on the amount of microphthalmos and the extent of involvement of the posterior pole with fibrovascular proliferation.

Evaluation

All newborns deserve screening eye examinations, which should include an evaluation of the red reflexes and ophthalmoscopy. Examination of the red reflex can reveal even minute opacities. Detailed evaluation of the normally symmetrical red reflexes is easily

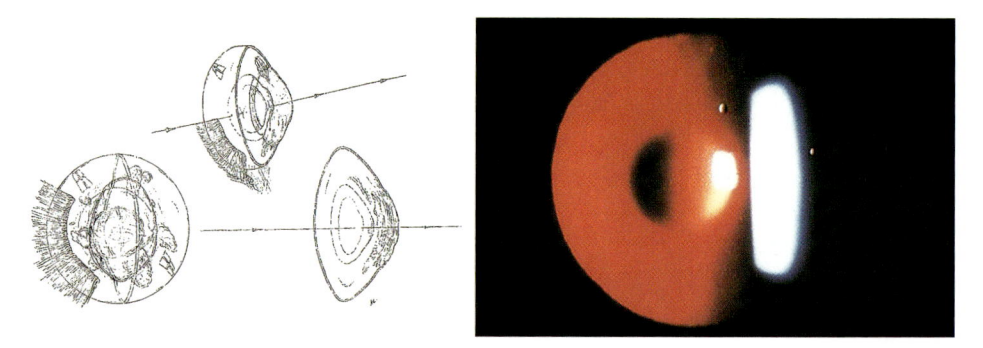

Figure 22-12 Posterior lenticonus/lentiglobus. *(Illustration courtesy of Alan Y. Chow, MD.)*

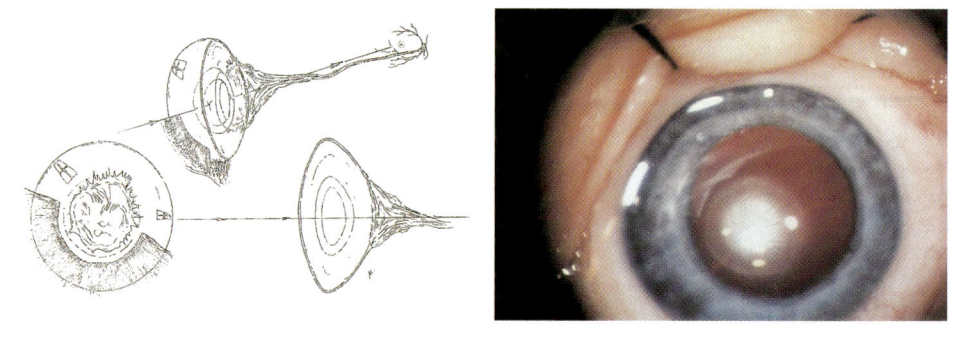

Figure 22-13 Persistent hyperplastic primary vitreous, also known as *persistent fetal vasculature*. Note that in the photograph on the right, the ciliary processes are pulled centrally and are visible inside the pupillary border. *(Illustration courtesy of Alan Y. Chow, MD.)*

accomplished in a darkened room by shining a bright direct ophthalmoscope into both eyes simultaneously. This test, which is called the *illumination test, red reflex test,* or *Brückner test,* can easily be used for routine ocular screening by nurses, pediatricians, and family practitioners. Retinoscopy through the child's undilated pupil is helpful for estimating potential vision in an eye harboring a cataract. Any central opacity or surrounding cortical distortion greater than 3 mm can be assumed to be visually significant.

History

A detailed history concerning the age of onset of visual signs and symptoms or ocular status on previous eye examinations can be helpful in assessing visual prognosis after treatment.

Visual Function

Visual function can be assessed by history, observation of the fixation and following reflex, behavioral testing, and electrophysiologic examination. Infants with complete bilateral congenital cataracts usually demonstrate decreased visual interest and experience delayed development. Ocular fixation and following movements may be decreased or absent. Strabismus is sometimes a presenting sign, especially in children with unilateral cataracts. Nystagmus results from early visual deprivation and signals that vision may be poor even after treatment.

Anterior Segment Evaluation

Slit-lamp examination clarifies the morphology of the cataract and may help determine, along with associated findings, the cause and prognosis (Table 22-5). Associated abnormalities of the cornea, iris, and pupil should be noted. A portable handheld slit lamp is especially helpful for examining infants and young children. Glaucoma should be ruled out because cataracts and glaucoma are associated with congenital rubella and Lowe syndrome.

Table 22-5 Congenital Cataracts: Cataract Appearance

Cataract Morphology	Diagnosis	Other Possible Findings
Spokelike	Fabry syndrome	+ Urine sediment
	Mannosidosis	Hepatosplenomegaly
Vacuoles	Diabetes	Blood glucose level increased
Multicolor flecks	Hypoparathyroidism	Serum calcium
	Myotonic dystrophy	Characteristic facial features, tonic "grip"
Green "sunflower"	Wilson disease	Kayser-Fleischer corneal ring
Thin disciform	Lowe syndrome	Hypotonia
Lamellar	Galactosemia	RBC enzymes
	Hypoglycemia	Blood glucose level decreased

RBC = red blood cell

Funduscopic Examination

An attempt should be made to visualize the retina, fovea, and optic disc to estimate the visual potential for the eye. When the cataract completely obstructs the visual axis, B-scan ultrasonography may be used to rule out potential retinal and vitreous pathology. This is especially important in patients with dense bilateral cataracts because these eyes could be harboring retinoblastoma.

Workup

In some cases, the cause of the cataract is obvious and costly laboratory tests are not warranted. A positive family history of childhood cataract or evidence of a minor opacity of the same type in one parent can confirm a diagnosis of hereditary congenital cataract. Unilateral infantile cataracts are generally not metabolic or genetic in origin, and therefore laboratory tests are not helpful. With bilateral cortical or lamellar cataracts, the laboratory can provide valuable information for diagnosis and management, particularly in Lowe syndrome and galactosemia (Fig 22-14). Table 22-6 summarizes the medical evaluation of congenital cataracts.

Surgery

Lensectomy (No Intraocular Lens)

In children in whom contact lenses or spectacles are the preferred means of aphakic optical correction, lensectomy is performed through a small limbal or pars plana incision via a vitreous-cutting instrument or a manual aspirating device. Irrigation can be provided by an integrated infusion sleeve or by a separate cannula for bimanual surgery (Fig 22-15A). Lens cortex and nucleus are generally soft, and ultrasonic phacoemulsification is not required (Fig 22-15B). Tough, fibrotic plaques are best handled by increasing vitrectomy port size, increasing suction, and reducing cutting speed or by manually removing the plaques with intraocular scissors and forceps. A large round anterior capsulectomy is easily performed either before or (preferably) after complete cortical removal.

Figure 22-14 Galactosemia, late.

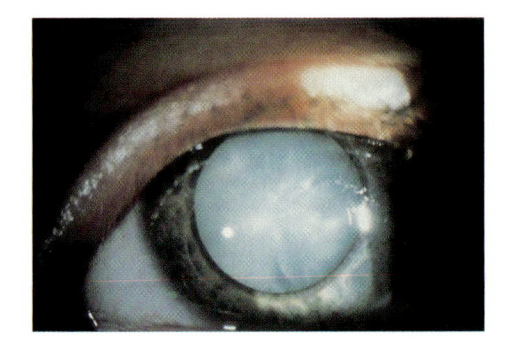

Table 22-6 Evaluation of Pediatric Cataracts

    Family history (autosomal dominant or X-linked)
    Pediatric physical examination
    Ocular examination including
      Corneal diameter
      Iris configuration
      Anterior chamber depth
      Lens position
      Cataract morphology
      Posterior segment
        Rule out posterior mass
        Rule out retinal detachment
        Rule out optic nerve stalk to lens
      Intraocular pressure
    Laboratory studies
      Bilateral cataracts
        Urine for reducing substance after milk feeding
        TORCH titer and VDRL
        Optional: Urine for amino acids, blood for calcium and
          phosphorus, red-cell galactokinase level
      Unilateral cataract
        TORCH titer

Because posterior capsule opacification occurs rapidly, a controlled moderate posterior capsulectomy and anterior vitrectomy should be performed at the time of surgery (Fig 22-15C). This technique allows for rapid, permanent establishment of a clear visual access for retinoscopy and prompt fitting and monitoring of aphakic optical correction, which is important in the age group subject to amblyopia. Sufficient peripheral posterior capsular remnants should be left, if possible, to facilitate secondary posterior chamber IOL implantation at a later date.

Postoperative optical rehabilitation

The choice of optical device for correction of aphakia depends on various factors. Aphakic spectacles are the safest method available and can be easily changed to accommodate the refractive shifts that occur with growth. These spectacles are not practical in monocular aphakia because of induced aniseikonia. Until the child can use a bifocal lens, the power selected should make the child slightly myopic when wearing the glasses. Contact lenses are the most popular method and are excellent for monocular cases. The power change for lenses is relatively easy, and some lenses can be worn 24 hours a day. Unfortunately, contact lenses are easily displaced by eye rubbing and can be expensive to replace. In addition, spectacle correction is necessary if a clear image is desired for both distance and near functions. Contact lenses also pose a risk of recurring infections and corneal ulcers.

Figure 22-15 A, Unlike cataractous adult lenses, the pediatric lens is soft and can easily be aspirated through a small port. This avoids the large corneal or limbal opening required for extracapsular extraction or phacoemulsification. A two-port closed system technique with an infusion source and a separate aspiration instrument or vitrector is ideal and allows the instrument to be switched from one side to the other, thereby facilitating cortical removal. An anterior capsule opening can be created with a vitrector. **B,** Both nucleus and surrounding cortex are aspirated. Complete cortical removal is important because remaining pediatric lens fibers will quickly proliferate, causing opacification and adhesions. **C,** After lens removal a large posterior capsulectomy and limited anterior vitrectomy are necessary to minimize the development of recurrent pupillary membranes, iris capsular adhesions, and posterior membranes. A small rim of capsule should be left to support possible secondary intraocular lens implants in the future. *(Photographs courtesy of Edward G. Buckley, MD.)*

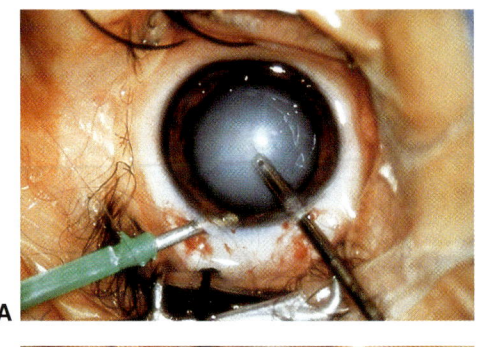

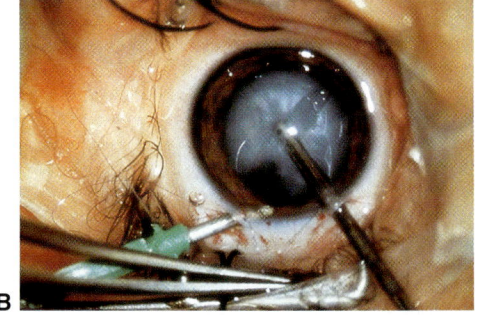

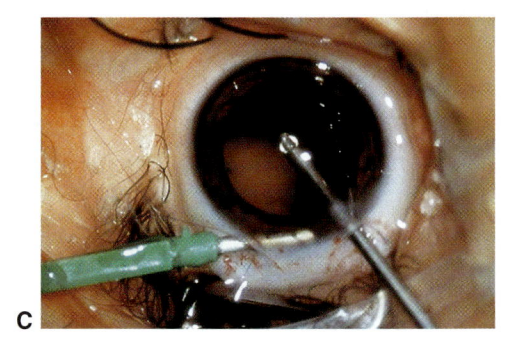

Intraocular Lens Implant

When an implant is to be used, the main adjustment in childhood cataract surgery involves the management of the anterior and posterior capsules. A controlled opening in the anterior capsule (by capsulorrhexis, or by "vitrectorrhexis," with a vitreous-cutting instrument) is important to help ensure in-the-bag placement of the posterior chamber IOL. Capsular fixation of the implant is thought to be far superior to sulcus fixation in terms of safety and stability of the lens. The posterior capsule can be left intact if it is clear at the end of the procedure and if the child is considered cooperative for Nd:YAG laser capsulotomy (generally, the child should be at least 4 years old). Alternatively, the posterior capsule can be opened primarily in conjunction with a limited anterior vitrectomy prior to IOL placement. Some surgeons prefer to close the anterior wound after IOL placement and perform posterior capsulotomy through a pars plana approach (Fig 22-16).

CHAPTER 22: Childhood Cataracts and Other Pediatric Lens Disorders • 287

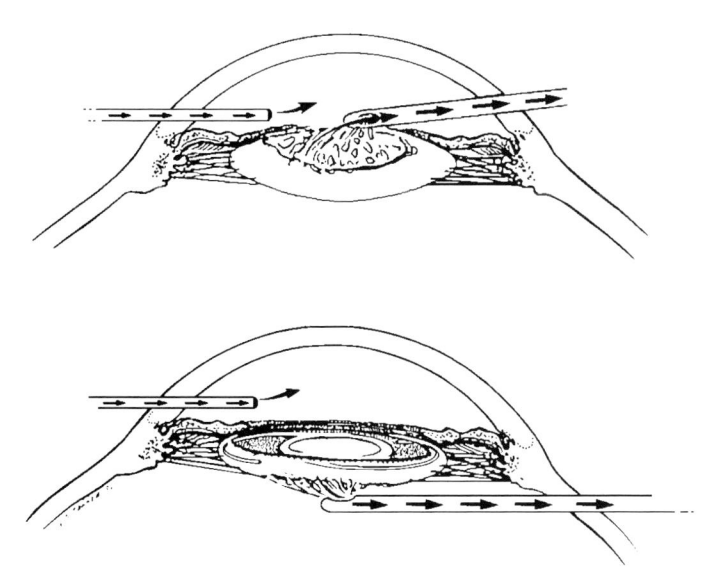

Figure 22-16 The posterior capsule can be removed primarily either (1) before the lens implantation from an anterior approach or (2) after lens implantation in one of two ways, anteriorly from the limbus or posteriorly via the pars plana. The pars plana approach has the advantage that the intraocular lens is implanted with an intact posterior capsule. The technique involves maintaining an anterior chamber infusion source, which helps bow the posterior capsule backward. A pars plana incision made approximately 2 mm from the limbus is performed. The vitrector is set at a low-cut suction rate and the capsule is opened in the center and enlarged to approximately 4 mm. *(Illustrations courtesy of Edward G. Buckley, MD.)*

IOL power selection

Because the child's eye continues to elongate until the age of 11, the selection of an appropriate IOL power is complicated. Studies have shown that the refractive error of aphakic children undergoes a myopic shift of 7–8 D from age 1 to age 10. Thus, if a child is made emmetropic at age 1, refraction at age 10 would be expected to be about -8.00 D. Therefore, lens implantation requires a compromise that accounts for the age of the child and the target refraction at the time of surgery. Most surgeons implant IOLs with powers that will be required in adulthood, allowing the child to grow into the power selection of the lens. Thus, the child is undercorrected and will require hyperopic spectacles of decreasing powers until the teenage years. Other surgeons strive for emmetropia at the time of lens implantation, especially in unilateral situations, to avoid anisometropia and facilitate development of binocular function. These children become progressively more myopic with time and eventually require a secondary procedure in order to eliminate the increasing anisometropia.

Enyedi L, Peterseim M, Freedman SF, et al. Refractive changes in pediatric patients with pseudophakia. *Am J Ophthalmol.* 1998;126:772–781.

IOL lens material

The most popular type of material used in pediatric lens implants is PMMA; experience is longest with this material, and it has been shown to be safe and predictable in this population. Recently, foldable acrylic lenses have gained acceptance and seem to be equally well tolerated. Silicone lenses have not been well studied in children.

Postoperative Care

Medical therapy

Intensive therapy with topical corticosteroids is advisable after childhood cataract surgery because of significant postoperative inflammation. Some clinicians advocate a short course of oral corticosteroids, particularly if a posterior chamber IOL has been implanted. Mydriasis should be maintained for at least several weeks with atropine or cyclopentolate therapy.

Amblyopia management

Amblyopia therapy, if necessary, should begin as soon as possible after surgery. For patients left aphakic, corrective lenses—contact lenses for unilateral or bilateral aphakia, spectacles for bilateral aphakia—can be dispensed as early as 1 week after surgery. Patching of the better eye is frequently indicated in cases of unilateral cataracts or asymmetrical bilateral cataracts. The amount of patching should be titrated to the degree of amblyopia and the age of the child. Part-time occlusion in the neonatal period may allow stimulation of binocular vision and may help to prevent associated strabismus.

Complications

In children, complications after lens extraction are different than in adults. Retinal detachments, macular edema, and corneal abnormalities are rare in children. The incidence of postoperative infections and bleeding are similar in adults and in children. Glaucoma associated with pediatric aphakia may develop many years after lens extraction but has been reported to occur in up to 25% of patients. The recent increase in the use of IOLs may reduce this incidence.

Visual Outcome After Cataract Extraction

Good visual outcome after cataract surgery depends on many factors, including the timing of surgery, optical correction, and treatment of amblyopia. Visual acuity is best in patients who undergo surgery before age 2 months and who comply with amblyopia treatment. Early surgery by itself does not ensure good outcome. Optimal visual acuity requires careful postoperative management to avoid amblyopia. Conversely, even when congenital cataracts are detected late (after age 4 months), cataract removal combined with a strong postoperative visual rehabilitation program can achieve good vision in some eyes (Fig 22-17).

In general, children with bilateral aphakia do much better than children with monocular aphakia, and both experience worse visual outcomes than adults. This poor outcome is undoubtedly due to the effect of aphakia on the developing visual system. Patients

CHAPTER 22: Childhood Cataracts and Other Pediatric Lens Disorders • 289

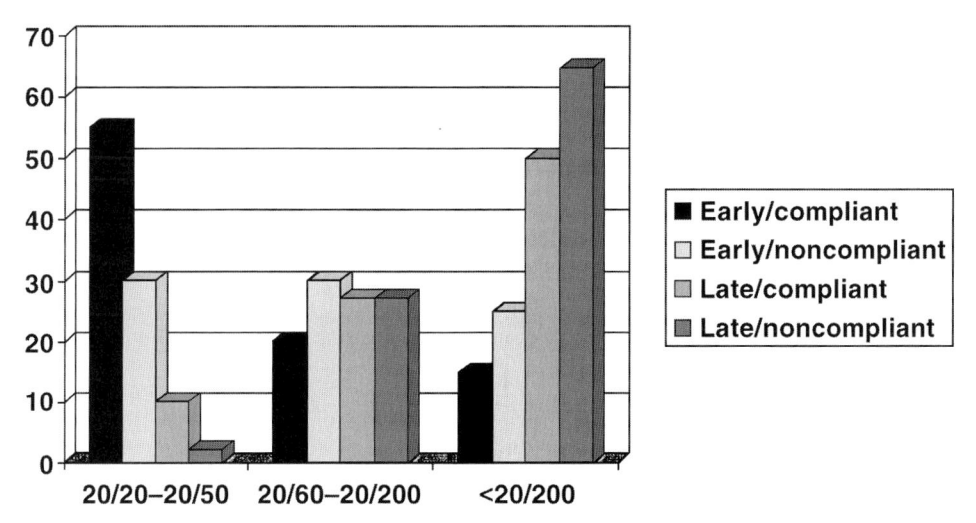

Figure 22-17 Visual outcomes in monocular dense congenital cataracts. Good visual outcome after cataract surgery depends on many factors, including the timing of surgery, optical correction, and treatment of amblyopia. The best visual acuity occurs in patients who undergo early surgery before age 2 months and comply with amblyopia treatment. Conversely, even when cataracts are detected late (after age 4 months), cataract removal combined with a strong postoperative visual rehabilitation program can achieve good vision in some eyes. *(From Seaber JH, Buckley EG. Functional outcome of monocular and binocular congenital cataract. Part 1: visual acuity. Am Orthoptic J. 1997;47:29–38.)*

with monocular aphakia have the added difficulty of interocular competition, which invariably results in better vision in the phakic eye. The data comparing contact lenses with IOLs indicate slightly better results with IOLs; however, selection biases may explain this finding.

Birch EE, Stager DR. The critical period for surgical treatment of dense congenital unilateral cataract. *Invest Ophthalmol Vis Sci.* 1996;37:1532–1538.

Buckley EG. Pediatric lens surgery. In: Parrish R, ed. *Bascom Palmer Eye Institute's Atlas of Ophthalmology*. Philadelphia: Current Medicine; 2000.

Ruttum MS. Childhood cataracts. In: *Focal Points: Clinical Modules for Ophthalmologists*. San Francisco: American Academy of Ophthalmology; 1996: vol 14, no 1.

Seaber JH, Buckley EG. Functional outcome of monocular and binocular congenital cataract. Part 1: visual acuity. *Am Orthoptic J.* 1997;47:29–38.

Wilson ME. Management of aphakia in childhood. In: *Focal Points: Clinical Modules for Ophthalmologists*. San Francisco: American Academy of Ophthalmology; 1999: vol 17, no 1.

CHAPTER 23

Uveitis in the Pediatric Age Group

Uveitis in the pediatric age group is relatively uncommon, occurring at an annual rate of 6/100,000 and accounting for only 2%–8% of the total cases of uveitis. Nevertheless, uveitis in children can present unique challenges to the physician. Children may not verbalize symptoms until disease is advanced. Therapeutic options may be limited by potential side effects, the need for general anesthesia, or poor compliance with self-administered medications. In addition, the rates of corticosteroid-induced glaucoma, cataract, and band keratopathy are increased in children. Finally, the risk of amblyopia is unique to children.

Classification

As in adults, uveitis in children can be classified by a number of methods, including anatomical location (anterior, posterior, intermediate, or panuveitis); pathology (granulomatous, nongranulomatous); course (acute, chronic, recurrent); or cause (traumatic, autoimmune, infectious, masquerade syndromes, idiopathic). Anatomical location can be helpful in determining cause (Table 23-1). A specific cause is found in 50%–65% of pediatric cases. Traditionally, posterior uveitis has been thought to account for 40%–50% of uveitis cases in children, anterior uveitis 30%–40%, intermediate uveitis about 20%, and panuveitis less than 10%. Toxoplasmosis is the most commonly identified infectious cause, and juvenile rheumatoid arthritis (JRA) is the most commonly identified cause overall. In a recently studied population, JRA accounted for over 40% of childhood uveitis cases.

Clinical Features

Children with uveitis may present in a number of ways. Although pain, redness, and photophobia are common in acute anterior uveitis, these symptoms are often absent in patients with chronic uveitis such as that associated with JRA, who may present with decreased vision secondary to cataract or band keratopathy. Clinical features of uveitis and mechanisms of inflammation are well described in BCSC Section 9, *Intraocular Inflammation and Uveitis,* Chapter 6. For the differential diagnosis of uveitis, see Table 23-1.

Table 23-1 Differential Diagnosis of Uveitis

Anterior uveitis
  Juvenile rheumatoid arthritis
  Trauma
  Sarcoidosis
  Disease related to HLA-B27
  Herpetic disease
  Sympathetic ophthalmia
  Syphilis
  Lyme disease
  Fuchs heterochromic iridocyclitis
  Kawasaki syndrome
  Acute interstitial nephritis, viral syndromes
  Unknown cause

Intermediate uveitis
  Pars planitis
  Sarcoidosis
  Tuberculosis
  Toxocariasis
  Lyme disease
  Unknown cause

Posterior uveitis
  Toxoplasmosis
  Ocular histoplasmosis
  Herpetic disease
  Syphilis
  Sympathetic ophthalmia
  Lyme disease
  Unknown cause

Panuveitis
  Sarcoidosis
  Vogt-Koyanagi-Harada syndrome
  Behçet syndrome
  Unknown cause

Cunningham ET Jr. Diagnosis and management of anterior uveitis. In: *Focal Points: Clinical Modules for Ophthalmologists*. San Francisco: American Academy of Ophthalmology; 2002: vol 20, no 1.

Dunn JP. Uveitis in children. In: *Focal Points: Clinical Modules for Ophthalmologists*. San Francisco: American Academy of Ophthalmology; 1995: vol 13, no 4.

Tugal-Tutkun I, Havrlikova K, Power WJ, et al. Changing patterns of uveitis in childhood. *Ophthalmology*. 1996;103:375–383.

Anterior Uveitis

In approximately 50% of children presenting with anterior uveitis, the cause cannot be determined. Many ophthalmologists prefer to postpone workup of anterior uveitis unless it is chronic, recurrent, or unresponsive to initial therapy.

Juvenile Rheumatoid Arthritis

JRA is the most common cause of anterior uveitis in children. JRA comprises a group of diseases characterized by chronic synovitis associated with a number of extraarticular manifestations. Three broad clinical groups are recognized today:

- Pauciarticular disease
- Polyarticular disease
- Systemic disease (Still disease)

These three classes of JRA differ in many features, including the likelihood of iridocyclitis. Characteristics of these groups are listed in Table 23-2. (See also Chapter 7 of BCSC Section 9, *Intraocular Inflammation and Uveitis*.)

The prevalence of JRA in North America and Europe is 64–113 per 100,000 children. An estimated 240,000 children in the United States have JRA, and 190,000 are at risk for JRA-associated iridocyclitis. Onset may occur at any time during childhood but is rare before the second year of life. JRA is a major cause of long-term illness and disability in children.

JRA is characterized by chronic nonsuppurative synovial inflammation. Increased secretion of joint fluid causes joint effusions. With continued synovitis, the articular cartilage and other joint structures are destroyed. Bone deformity then occurs.

Iridocyclitis is most frequently associated with the pauciarticular form of JRA. At particular risk for anterior uveitis are girls with early onset of pauciarticular JRA (ie, onset at age 2–3 years), positive antinuclear antibody test results, and negative rheumatoid factor. Approximately 25% of patients in this group develop anterior uveitis. Patients with polyarticular disease are at lower risk for iridocyclitis. In children with the systemic form of JRA, iridocyclitis is rare.

Diagnosis

The cause of rheumatoid arthritis and the mechanism of anterior uveitis remain unknown. Correlation between the course of arthritis and uveitis may be weak, although 90% of patients with JRA who develop uveitis do so within 7 years of the onset of arthritis. Occasionally, uveitis is diagnosed before the onset of joint symptoms. No strong correlation among JRA, iridocyclitis, and human leukocyte antigen (HLA) haplotypes, including HLA-B27, has been found.

The uveitis associated with JRA is usually asymptomatic and chronic. Such uveitis is characterized by anterior chamber cells and flare. Prolonged inflammation may lead to posterior synechiae, band keratopathy, cataract, hypotony, and glaucoma (Fig 23-1).

Table 23-2 Subgroups of Juvenile Rheumatoid Arthritis

Type of Onset	% of JRA Patients	Number of Joints Affected	% With Uveitis
Pauciarticular	50	≤4	20–30
Polyarticular	30	>4	2–5
Systemic	20	Variable	1–2

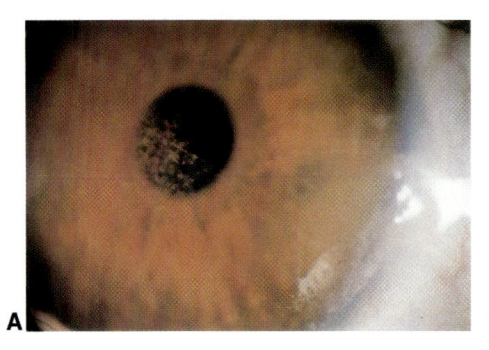

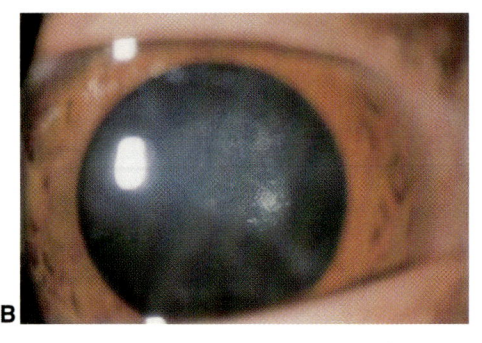

Figure 23-1 Juvenile rheumatoid arthritis. **A,** Early band keratopathy: note presence of calcium deposits in superficial cornea. **B,** Early cataract formation: note posterior subcapsular location of opacity.

Vitritis and macular edema occur infrequently. Visual loss in JRA may be associated with multiple factors, including amblyopia in susceptible patients.

The differential diagnosis of arthritis and uveitis in children includes sarcoidosis, Lyme disease, psoriatic arthritis, juvenile Reiter syndrome, and inflammatory bowel disease. In addition, boys with pauciarticular arthritis who are positive for HLA-B27 may be at increased risk for anterior uveitis, although this uveitis is generally more acute than in JRA. Some of these boys develop ankylosing spondylitis in later life.

Management

The combination of topical corticosteroid and mydriatic therapy is the mainstay of treatment for children with JRA-associated uveitis. The goals of treatment are to decrease the number of anterior chamber cells and prevent the formation of posterior synechiae; chronic flare is less responsive to corticosteroid therapy and does not require treatment in the absence of cells. Periocular injections of depot corticosteroids may be useful in patients who show poor compliance for topical corticosteroid therapy or in whom topical therapy is ineffective. Short courses of oral corticosteroids may be used, but long-term use should be avoided because of significant side effects in young children.

Nonsteroidal anti-inflammatory drugs (NSAIDs) may allow a reduction in the dose of corticosteroids required to treat chronic uveitis. Naproxen and tolmetin are the NSAIDs most commonly used in children.

Systemic immunosuppressive therapy may be recommended for patients who have persistent inflammation despite aggressive treatment with corticosteroids and NSAIDs. Methotrexate, azathioprine, chlorambucil, cyclophosphamide, and cyclosporine may be used under the guidance of a rheumatologist experienced in the use of these agents.

Surgery for cataracts and severe band keratopathy may be necessary for children with severe uveitis. Cataract surgery should be performed only in eyes that have been quiet for several months. Aggressive postoperative anti-inflammatory therapy is required. Severe band keratopathy may require chelation therapy with ethylenediaminetetraacetic acid after debridement of the epithelium. Chelation may be performed for decreased vision, for pain associated with recurrent erosions, or to improve the appearance of the eye.

Routine screening for uveitis in children with JRA is important because of the insidious nature of the intraocular inflammation. An eye examination schedule for children with JRA developed by the Sections on Rheumatology and Ophthalmology of the American Academy of Pediatrics is shown in Table 23-3.

>American Academy of Pediatrics Section on Rheumatology and Section on Ophthalmology. Guidelines for ophthalmic examinations in children with juvenile rheumatoid arthritis. *Pediatrics.* 1993;92:295–296.
>Ceisler EJ, Foster CS. Juvenile rheumatoid arthritis and uveitis: minimizing the blinding complications. *Int Ophthalmol Clin.* 1996;36:91–107.
>Nussenblatt RB, Whitcup SM, Palestine AG. *Uveitis: Fundamentals and Clinical Practice.* 2nd ed. St Louis: Mosby; 1996:270–273.

Trauma

Traumatic iritis is generally a self-limited disease that is characterized by pain and photophobia occurring hours to days after a blunt injury to the eye. Typical findings include ciliary flush and anterior chamber cells and flare. Intraocular pressure may be abnormally high or low. Penetrating injuries to the eye can result in retained intraocular foreign bodies, infectious endophthalmitis, and sympathetic ophthalmia.

Treatment includes topical steroids and cycloplegic agents for mild cases. Intravitreal antibiotic administration, vitreoretinal surgery, or both may be indicated in cases of retained intraocular foreign body or endophthalmitis.

Sarcoidosis

Sarcoidosis is a multisystem granulomatous disease of unknown cause. It is relatively uncommon in children. The majority of cases of childhood sarcoidosis occur in the southeastern and south central United States. The disease is 10–17 times more common in African Americans than in Caucasians. There is no clear gender predominance.

Sarcoidosis in children has two distinct forms. Older children usually present with a multisystem disease similar to the adult manifestation, with frequent lymphadenopathy and pulmonary involvement as well as generalized signs and symptoms such as fever and malaise. In contrast, early-onset childhood sarcoidosis is a unique form of the disease characterized by the triad of rash, uveitis, and arthritis presenting before age 4 years. This variant can be difficult to distinguish from JRA.

Ocular involvement is common in childhood sarcoidosis. Visual symptoms include pain, blurred vision, and photophobia. Anterior uveitis is the most common manifestation, occurring in about 90% of cases of early-onset sarcoidosis (compared with 20%–30% of cases of later-onset disease). Conjunctival granulomas are also common. Band keratopathy, cataracts, and glaucoma may occur. Multifocal chorioretinal granulomas, with or without disc edema and vitritis, have also been documented. Orbital infiltration may occur. Eyelid, lacrimal gland, and scleral involvement are uncommon in children.

No laboratory test is diagnostic of sarcoidosis. The chest radiograph appears abnormal in at least 60% of patients. Laboratory testing may reveal an elevated erythrocyte sedimentation rate. Anemia, leukopenia, and eosinophilia are common. Angiotensin-converting enzyme is elevated in up to 80% of patients with late-onset sarcoidosis.

Table 23-3 Examination Schedule for Children With JRA Without Known Iridocyclitis

JRA Subtype	Age at Onset <7 years	Age at Onset ≥7 years
Pauciarticular		
Positive ANA		
Less than 4 years', duration	Every 3–4 months	Every 6 months
4–7 years' duration	Every 6 months	Annually
More than 7 years' duration	Annually	Annually
Negative ANA		
Less than 4 years' duration	Every 6 months	Every 6 months
4–7 years' duration	Every 6 months	Annually
More than 7 years' duration	Annually	Annually
Polyarticular		
Positive ANA		
Less than 4 years' duration	Every 3–4 months	Every 6 months
4–7 years' duration	Every 6 months	Annually
More than 7 years' duration	Annually	Annually
Negative ANA		
Less than 4 years' duration	Every 6 months	Every 6 months
4–7 years' duration	Every 6 months	Annually
More than 7 years' duration	Annually	Annually
Systemic	Annually, regardless of duration	Annually, regardless of duration

(Adapted from American Academy of Pediatrics, Sections on Rheumatology and Ophthalmology. Guidelines for Ophathalmic Examinations in Children with Juvenile Rheumatoid Arthritis. *Pediatrics.* 1993; 92:295–296.)

Hypercalcemia, hypercalciuria, or both may be found. The diagnosis of sarcoidosis is confirmed by demonstration of a typical noncaseating granuloma on a biopsy specimen, usually from the skin or conjunctiva.

Sarcoid uveitis is usually treated with topical steroids and cycloplegic agents. Systemic administration and local injections of steroids are generally reserved for more severe cases. Methotrexate given orally in low doses is effective and safe and has steroid-sparing properties. The natural history of sarcoidosis in children is not well established. The disease is usually chronic, although spontaneous recovery is possible. Patients with early-onset disease may experience a chronic progressive course.

> Hoover DL, Khan JA, Giangiacomo J. Pediatric ocular sarcoidosis. *Surv Ophthalmol.* 1986;30:215–228.
>
> Shetty AK, Gedilia A. Sarcoidosis: a pediatric perspective. *Clin Pediatr.* 1998;37:707–717.

Diseases Related to HLA-B27

This group of disorders includes ankylosing spondylitis, Reiter syndrome, inflammatory bowel disease, and psoriatic arthritis. In most series of childhood uveitis, diseases related to HLA-B27 account for less than 1% of cases; however, in one series, such diseases accounted for 16% of cases of anterior uveitis. See BCSC Section 9, *Intraocular Inflammation and Uveitis,* for a discussion of these disorders.

Herpetic Iridocyclitis

Acute anterior uveitis is often associated with herpetic viral disease, usually as keratouveitis secondary to corneal disease but occasionally as an isolated finding. Both herpes simplex and varicella-zoster have been infrequently observed as causes of anterior uveitis in children. These disorders are discussed extensively in BCSC Section 8, *External Disease and Cornea*, and Section 9, *Intraocular Inflammation and Uveitis*, as well as later in this chapter.

Sympathetic Ophthalmia

Sympathetic ophthalmia is a bilateral granulomatous panuveitis that occurs after injury or surgery to one eye followed by a latent period with development of uveitis in the fellow eye (called the *sympathizing eye*). The incidence of sympathetic ophthalmia has diminished significantly since the advent of improved wound closure techniques and perhaps because severely damaged eyes tend to be removed early.

Sympathetic ophthalmia is more common after penetrating trauma than after planned ophthalmic procedures. The cause is unknown but may involve an autoimmune response to one of the proteins associated with the retina, uveal tract, or both. See also BCSC Section 9, *Intraocular Inflammation and Uveitis*.

Syphilis

Syphilis is a systemic communicable infection characterized by periods of clinical activity followed by prolonged latency. Acquired syphilis requires contact between an infective lesion and a break in the skin or mucosa. *Treponema pallidum*, the spirochete responsible for syphilis, can cross the placenta, and congenital syphilis is contracted from the mother, whose infection is usually latent.

Congenital infection characteristically presents with a salt-and-pepper chorioretinitis affecting both eyes. The fundus examination may also reveal optic nerve pallor. Anterior uveitis and interstitial keratitis may be present. See Chapter 17 for a more extensive discussion of this disorder.

Other Causes

Anterior uveitis may also be associated with Kawasaki syndrome, acute interstitial nephritis, HLA-B27–positive syndromes, and Fuchs heterochromic iridocyclitis.

Intermediate Uveitis (Pars Planitis)

The term *intermediate uveitis*, which is a diagnosis based on the anatomical location of inflammation, is preferred by the International Committee on Uveitis Nomenclature. It replaces the terms *peripheral uveitis* and *chronic cyclitis*. Pars planitis is now considered a type of intermediate uveitis in which a white opacity *(snowbank)* occurs over the peripheral retina and pars plana. Pars planitis is the most common type of intermediate uveitis, accounting for approximately 85%–90% of cases. The distinction between pars planitis and intermediate uveitis is not always clear in common usage, and the two terms are often used interchangeably. Intermediate uveitis accounts for 5%–15% of all cases of uveitis and about 25% of uveitis in the pediatric age group. The cause is most often unknown.

Snowbank formation in the region of the pars plana is made up of mononuclear cells, hyperplastic nonpigmented ciliary epithelial cells, and an occasional fibroblastlike cell (Fig 23-2). Fibroglial proliferation is present at the vitreous base, drawing the peripheral retina into the snowbank. The retinal veins are sheathed with lymphocytes.

Intermediate uveitis has a gradual onset, and the course may be mild in as many as 50% of patients. About 75% of patients have bilateral involvement. Initially, a peripheral perivasculitis usually occurs along with small exudates adjacent to the inflamed peripheral retinal vessels. These exudates enter the vitreous, giving rise to floaters in the field of vision. In addition, the patient may note blurring of distance vision and difficulties with accommodation. The anterior chamber has a minimal response, but the retrolenticular space and anterior vitreous are filled with freely moving cells. Exudate is seen in the region of the pars plana inferiorly. With time, the vitreous exudate extends nasally, temporally, and posteriorly. Cystoid macular edema, optic nerve inflammation, posterior subcapsular cataract, glaucoma, exudative retinal detachment, and even phthisis bulbi may develop.

Diagnosis

The diagnosis is made clinically. Because of the high incidence of bilaterality in intermediate uveitis, unilateral inflammation should cause the clinician to consider sarcoidosis, toxocariasis, peripheral toxoplasmosis, or a retained intraocular foreign body.

Treatment

Topical administration or periocular injection of corticosteroids may improve intermediate uveitis considerably. Because the disorder is chronic with recurrences and remissions, treatment should be reserved for patients with a moderate decrease in visual acuity, macular edema, or increased vitreous debris. About 10% of cases follow a self-limited course; 60% follow a prolonged course without exacerbations; and 30% follow a chronic, smoldering course with exacerbations. If treatment with topical and sub-Tenon's injection of corticosteroids every 2–6 weeks does not result in improvement, systemic corticosteroids may be used.

Figure 23-2 Intermediate uveitis with inferior snowbank formation, right eye.

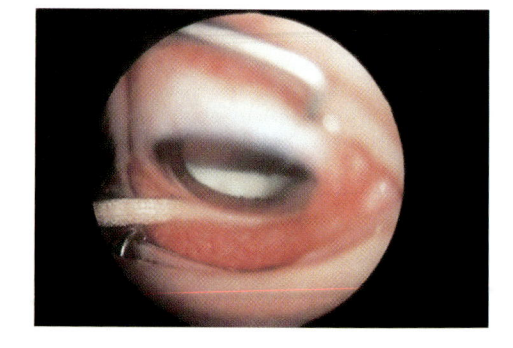

Immunosuppressive agents are considered if systemic steroids are inadequate or if posterior subcapsular cataracts begin to form. Transscleral diathermy and cryotherapy have also been applied. Vitrectomy may be indicated in severe cases.

Hooper PL. Pars planitis. In: *Focal Points: Clinical Modules for Ophthalmologists.* San Francisco: American Academy of Ophthalmology; 1993: vol 11, no 11.

Posterior Uveitis

More than 50% of pediatric cases of uveitis involve posterior inflammation. No etiologic agent or disease is documented in about one third of these cases.

Toxoplasmosis

Toxoplasmosis is the most common cause of posterior uveitis in children, accounting for 30%–50% of cases. The *Toxoplasma* organisms described in Chapter 17 have been identified only in the retina, where they have a predilection for the nerve fiber layer. The organisms survive best in the tissues of the central nervous system, particularly the brain and retina. Ocular toxoplasmosis may be asymptomatic and sometimes goes unrecognized.

The initial symptoms are floaters and blurred or reduced vision. Anterior chamber cells and flare may be present. Vitreous cells and opacities are seen. Yellow, slightly raised, indistinct lesions are seen in the retina but may be obscured by dense vitreous inflammation that gives rise to the characteristic appearance of a headlight in the fog. An exudative focal retinitis involves the anterior layers of the retina. With time, these affected areas usually heal, leaving atrophied areas with pronounced pigmentation around their edges.

The disease may run a course of 6 months before healing occurs. Recurrence may first be noted in *satellite lesions.* Recurrence often brings about severe anterior uveitis with mutton fat keratic precipitates, marked anterior chamber cell and flare formation, iris nodules, and posterior synechial development. Papilledema, vitreous precipitates, and glaucoma can all result from toxoplasmosis infection of the eye.

The diagnosis of toxoplasmosis is based on clinical manifestations and laboratory tests and is described in Chapter 17. The standard treatment for ocular toxoplasmosis is combination therapy with pyrimethamine and sulfadiazine. Corticosteroid therapy may also be considered in conjunction with antibiotics. Drug treatment schedules for children vary. Because of significant systemic side effects from the medications, the patient's pediatric or infectious disease specialist should participate in management. Cryotherapy, photocoagulation, and vitrectomy have also been attempted. The prognosis depends on the patient's immune status, age, and sex; the location of the lesion; and the virulence of the organisms themselves.

Mets MB, Holfels E, Boyer KM, et al. Eye manifestations of congenital toxoplasmosis. *Am J Ophthalmol.* 1996;122:309–324.

Ocular Histoplasmosis

Ocular histoplasmosis is a fungal infection that is benign and asymptomatic most of the time. It is uncommon in children. Ocular histoplasmosis has several classic clinical manifestations, including disseminated choroiditis with scattered areas of retinal pigment epithelium atrophy *(histo spots)*, maculopathy, peripapillary pigment changes, and a clear vitreous. The presence of cells in the vitreous dictates reconsideration of the diagnosis. See Chapter 17 for a more extensive discussion of the diagnosis and management of this disorder.

Toxocariasis

The nematode larvae of a common intestinal parasite of dogs *(Toxocara canis)* or cats *(Toxocara cati)* cause toxocariasis. Children contract the disease by ingesting the ova from dirt contaminated by dog or cat feces. Infection may also result from eating improperly cleaned foods such as lettuce or carrots. Ingested ova produce larvae in the human intestine that invade the intestinal walls, penetrate the blood vessels and lymphatic system, and proceed to the liver, lung, and eyes. The exact incidence is unknown.

Organisms from the cat have not been identified in the human eye; therefore, the dog is considered a more likely source of infection for children. *Toxocara* may have a predilection for the retina. As the larvae move through the retinal tissues, they leave tracks and can cause hemorrhage, necrosis, and inflammation. The pathological lesion is an eosinophilic granuloma consisting of fibrin, lymphocytes, epithelioid cells, giant cells, and numerous eosinophils.

The average age of the child infected with ocular *Toxocara* is 7–8 years, ranging from 2 to 9 years. Children with this disease present with chronic unilateral uveitis and a marked vitreous opacification that overlies a primary eosinophilic granuloma. Exudative retinal detachment, posterior synechiae, and a cyclitic membrane may be present. The *Toxocara* granuloma is white, dome-shaped, and confined principally to the retina. Overlying vitreal inflammation may occur, and ocular toxocariasis can present as chronic endophthalmitis or a peripheral granuloma.

Diagnosis is based on clinical findings and specific laboratory tests. An enzyme-linked immunosorbent assay specific for *Toxocara* has been developed. Eosinophils may be elevated in peripheral blood and found on aqueous cytologic examination. Calcification is rare in this lesion, in contrast with retinoblastoma.

Active inflammation can be managed with topical, periocular, or systemic corticosteroids. Because inflammation from *Toxocara* infection usually begins after the larvae die, corticosteroids are the drug of choice despite the fact that thiabendazole has been proven effective against living *Toxocara* organisms. Destruction of the larvae is not sufficient because an inflammatory response from the destruction can itself cause ocular damage. However, it may be desirable to kill the larvae if they appear to be moving toward the macula. In the presence of a cataract or cyclitic membrane, pars plana vitrectomy and lensectomy may be indicated.

The prognosis depends on the form and location of the infection. Chronic endophthalmitis usually compromises vision in the eye. Peripheral granulomas cause distortion of the macula with loss of central vision, but the globe can usually be preserved (Fig 23-3).

Other Causes

Posterior uveitis can also be caused by herpes simplex, syphilis, sympathetic ophthalmia, Vogt-Koyanagi-Harada syndrome, Behçet syndrome, and *Candida albicans* (see BCSC Section 9, *Intraocular Inflammation and Uveitis*). When posterior uveitis is associated with significant anterior chamber inflammation, it is designated *panuveitis*.

Masquerade Syndromes

Other conditions can simulate uveitis in the pediatric age group. These *masquerade syndromes* are listed together with their diagnostic features in Table 23-4. The evaluation of uveitis in the pediatric age group should include assessment of the patient by a pediatrician, which may include testing for rheumatic and gastrointestinal disorders, tuberculin skin testing, FTA-ABS, serum protein electrophoresis, chest radiography, sacroiliac radiography (when indicated), and general health. The clinician should also obtain ocular ultrasound images and radiographs to rule out foreign body or tumor. Laboratory tests for various types of uveitis are listed in Table 23-5.

> Forster DJ, Rao NA. Uveitis in children. In: Wright KW, ed. *Pediatric Ophthalmology and Strabismus*. St Louis: Mosby; 1995:409–430.

Treatment of Uveitis in Children

The goal of uveitis treatment in children is to suppress inflammation in order to prevent the complications of cataract, glaucoma, cystoid macular edema, retinal detachment, band keratopathy, and amblyopia.

Medical Treatment

Infectious causes should be treated appropriately as described above. For noninfectious disease, mild anterior segment inflammation is treated with topical corticosteroid and mydriatic/cycloplegic agents. Because topical corticosteroids do not penetrate well into the vitreous or posterior segment, posterior sub-Tenon injections of a corticosteroid may be useful in treating older children with intermediate uveitis. The use of oral corticosteroids and immunosuppressants should be limited to cases in which the benefit clearly outweighs the risk, and these agents are best used in conjunction with the patient's pediatrician or rheumatologist.

Complications of medical therapy

Glaucoma and cataract formation are two of the most serious side effects of corticosteroid therapy. In general, the most potent corticosteroids are those most likely to produce an increase in intraocular pressure. Periocular injections of depot corticosteroids can produce elevations in intraocular pressure weeks to months after injection. Children appear

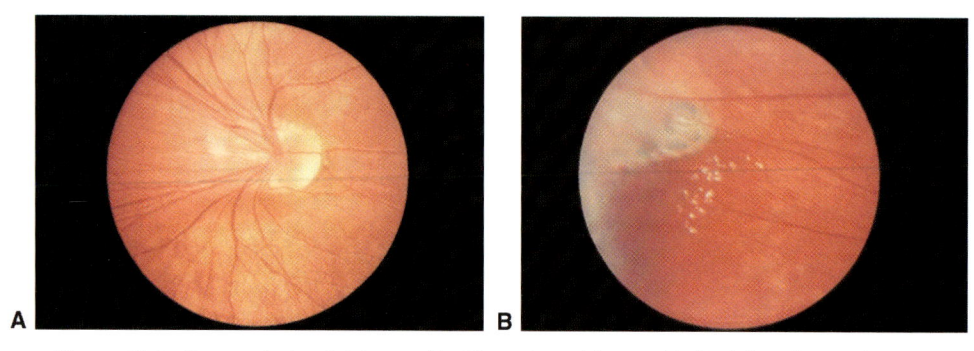

Figure 23-3 Toxocariasis, right eye. **A,** Distortion of fovea. **B,** Peripheral granuloma.

Table 23-4 **Masquerade Syndromes**

Disease	Age (Years)	Signs of Inflammation	Diagnostic Studies
Anterior segment			
Retinoblastoma	<15	Flare, cells, pseudohypopyon	Ultrasound; CT
Leukemia	<15	Flare, cells, heterochromia	Bone marrow, peripheral blood smear
Intraocular foreign body	Any age	Flare, cells	X-ray, ultrasound
Malignant melanoma	Any age	Flare, cells	Fluorescein angiography, ultrasound
Juvenile xanthogranuloma	<15	Flare, cells, hyphema	Examination of skin, iris biopsy
Peripheral retinal detachment	Any age	Flare, cells	Ophthalmoscopy
Posterior segment			
Retinitis pigmentosa	Any age	Cells in vitreous	ERG, EOG, visual fields
Reticulum cell sarcoma	15+	Vitreous exudate, retinal hemorrhage or exudates, retinal pigment epithelium infiltrates	Cytology study of aqueous and vitreous
Lymphoma	15+	Retinal hemorrhage or exudates, vitreous cells	Node biopsy, bone marrow, physical examination
Retinoblastoma	<15	Vitreous cells, retinal exudates	Ultrasound, CT
Malignant melanoma	15+	Vitreous cell	Fluorescein angiography, ultrasound
Multiple sclerosis	15+	Periphlebitis	Neurologic examination

CT, computed tomography; ERG, electroretinogram; EOG, electro-oculogram.

Table 23-5 Laboratory Tests for Various Types of Uveitis

Anterior
  Complete blood count (to rule out leukemia)
  Antinuclear antibody (to subtype JRA)
  Serum lysozyme (to rule out sarcoidosis)
  Serum protein electrophoresis (to look for alpha$_2$ globulin fraction in sarcoidosis)
  FTA-ABS (to rule out syphilis)
  HLA-B27 (to rule out ankylosing spondylitis and Reiter syndrome)
  PCR, ELISA, IFA, for Lyme disease
  Tuberculin skin test, chest x-ray (to rule out sarcoidosis and tuberculosis)
  GI series (if ulcerative colitis or regional enteritis [Crohn disease] is suspected)
  Angiotensin-converting enzyme (ACE)

Intermediate
  Serum lysozyme (to rule out sarcoidosis)
  FTA-ABS (to rule out syphilis)
  Chest x-ray (to rule out sarcoidosis or tuberculosis)
  Tuberculin skin test
  PCR, ELISA for toxocariasis
  Angiotensin-converting enzyme

Posterior
  PCR, ELISA for toxoplasmosis
  PCR, ELISA for toxocariasis
  Serum lysozyme (to rule out sarcoidosis)
  FTA-ABS (to rule out syphilis)
  PCR, blood cultures, viral cultures, or antibody levels if cytomegalovirus, herpes simplex (especially in a newborn), or rubella is suspected
  PCR, ELISA, IFA, for Lyme disease
  Angiotensin-converting enzyme

---

to develop posterior subcortical cataracts following oral corticosteroid therapy sooner and at lower doses than is the case with adults, but these cataracts may be reversible after cessation of treatment.

Other risks of long-term systemic corticosteroid use in children include retardation of skeletal maturation and growth, osteoporosis and bone fractures, cushingoid appearance, peptic ulcers, myopathy, hypertension, altered mental status, pseudotumor cerebri, and increased mortality from infection. Patients may also require increased doses of corticosteroids during times of stress to avoid an addisonian crisis.

Cytotoxic therapy carries a risk of sterility, bone marrow depression, cancer, and infection.

Surgical Treatment

Band keratopathy can often be alleviated by removal of corneal epithelium followed by chelation with ethylenediaminetetraacetic acid. Several treatments may be needed.

Cataract surgery in patients with uveitis can be complicated by hypotony, glaucoma, synechiae formation, cystoid macular edema, and retinal detachment. In patients with JRA, a combined lensectomy/vitrectomy appears to give better results than cataract extraction alone. Uveitis must be aggressively treated so that it is under control both before and after surgery. IOL implantation in children with uveitis is highly controversial.

Glaucoma surgery may become necessary in children with uveitis. Conventional filtering surgery has a low success rate. The role of setons and antimetabolites in the pediatric population is under investigation. Cyclotherapy is rarely successful in the long term.

BenEzra D, Cohen E. Cataract surgery in children with chronic uveitis. *Ophthalmology.* 2000;107:1255–1260.

CHAPTER 24

Vitreous and Retinal Diseases and Disorders

Vitreous and retinal disorders in children are uncommon. Many of these conditions are associated with an underlying systemic disorder. A careful family history, a history of growth and development, and any details about other sensory or health problems should be part of the evaluation of these children.

> Drack AV, Stone EM. Patterns of retinal disease in children. In: Wright KW, ed. *Pediatric Ophthalmology and Strabismus.* St Louis: Mosby; 1995:563–580.

Leukocoria

The term *leukocoria* means "white pupil." Depending on the lesion, the pupil may appear normal in room light but have no red reflex on ophthalmoscopy. The differential diagnosis of leukocoria includes:

- Retinoblastoma
- Persistent hyperplastic primary vitreous, also known as *persistent fetal vasculature*
- Retinopathy of prematurity—stage 5 with total retinal detachment and fibrous membrane
- Cataract
- Chorioretinal colobomas
- Uveitis
- Toxocariasis
- Congenital retinal folds
- Coats disease
- Vitreous hemorrhage
- Retinal dysplasia
- Other tumors (eg, hamartomas, choroidal hemangiomas, diktyomas)

The major retinal causes are discussed in this chapter with the exception of retinoblastoma, which is covered in Chapter 26. See also BCSC Section 12, *Retina and Vitreous*, for more information about these conditions.

Persistent Hyperplastic Primary Vitreous

Persistent hyperplastic primary vitreous (PHPV) is usually a congenital, nonhereditary malformation of the eye that is unilateral and not associated with systemic defects. Bilateral cases may be a harbinger of other systemic or neurologic abnormalities. The term *persistent fetal vasculature* is more accurate but has not yet supplanted the widespread *PHPV*. The spectrum of severity is broad. Mild cases feature eyes with prominent hyaloid vessel remnants, large Mittendorf dots, and Bergmeister papillae. At the other end of the spectrum are microphthalmic eyes with progressive shallowing of the anterior chamber and angle-closure glaucoma from fibrovascular invasion of the lens through a defect in the posterior lens capsule. Peripheral and posterior central retinal detachments may also occur in these more severely involved eyes. The hyaloid artery may be replaced by a thick fibrous stalk. The ciliary processes may be elongated and visible through the dilated pupil, and prominent radial vessels are often noted on the iris surface (Fig 24-1). The retrolental plaque is usually most dense centrally, and it may contain cartilage as well as fibrovascular tissue. Eccentric plaques may also occur.

The natural history of the more severely affected untreated eyes is usually one of relentless, progressive cataract formation with concomitant shallowing of the anterior chamber, eventually resulting in angle-closure glaucoma. Retinal detachment, intraocular hemorrhage, and angle-closure glaucoma are the most severe complications in PHPV. The hemorrhages presumably originate in the fibrovascular membrane in the retrolental space. Affected eyes are almost always smaller than the normal fellow eye, although this finding may be apparent only by ultrasonography or careful caliper measurement of the corneal diameters. It is important to document microphthalmos because retinoblastoma is rarely found in microphthalmic eyes, and retinoblastoma may be part of the initial differential diagnosis. The presence of a cataract is also evidence against the diagnosis of retinoblastoma, although lens opacities may develop in advanced cases.

Many eyes with PHPV can be saved by early cataract surgery combined with membrane excision. In cases with minimal posterior involvement, it is even possible to obtain some degree of central vision if early surgical intervention is followed by aggressive contact lens wear combined with carefully monitored patching of the uninvolved eye. The visual prognosis depends on the degree of retinal involvement.

Various surgical approaches to the management of PHPV have been proposed. In most cases, the retrolenticular tissues can be cauterized and removed by vitreous-cutting instruments. Both limbal and pars plicata/pars plana approaches have been successfully employed. If the macula and optic nerve appear normal postoperatively, a vigorous effort should be made to optically correct aphakia and to patch as would be done with a unilateral cataract.

> Goldberg MF. Persistent fetal vasculature (PFV): an integrated interpretation of signs and symptoms associated with persistent hyperplastic primary vitreous (PHPV). *Am J Ophthalmol.* 1997;124:587–626.
>
> Haddad R, Font RL, Reeser F. Persistent hyperplastic primary vitreous. A clinicopathologic study of 62 cases and review of the literature. *Surv Ophthalmol.* 1978;23:123–134.
>
> Karr DJ, Scott WE. Visual acuity results following treatment of persistent hyperplastic primary vitreous. *Arch Ophthalmol.* 1986;104:662–667.

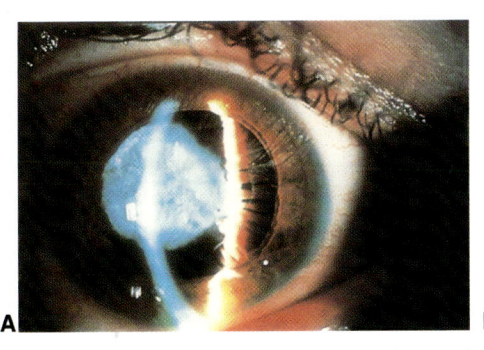

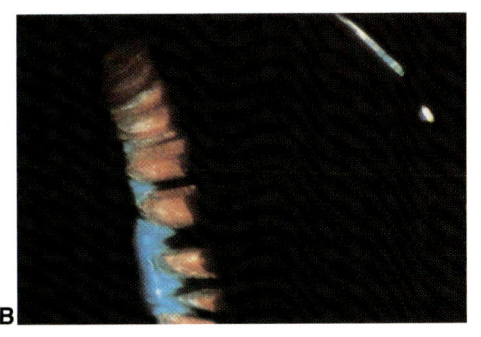

Figure 24-1 Persistent hyperplastic primary vitreous (also called *persistent fetal vasculature*). **A,** Elongated ciliary processes are adherent to lens. Note the dense fibrous plaque on the lens. **B,** Close-up of ciliary processes dragged into the pupillary axis.

> Wright KW, Christensen LE, Noguchi BA. Results of late surgery for presumed congenital cataracts. *Am J Ophthalmol.* 1992;114:409–415.

Retinopathy of Prematurity

Retinopathy of prematurity (ROP) is the current designation for what was previously called *retrolental fibroplasia*. ROP includes the acute disease seen in the nursery and the cicatricial disease seen later.

Normally, retinal vascular development begins during week 16 of gestation. Mesenchymal tissue containing spindle cells is the source of retinal vessels. The mesenchyme grows centrifugally from the optic disc, reaching the nasal ora serrata in the eighth month of gestation and the temporal ora serrata up to 1–2 months later. Premature birth may trigger the onset of ROP, in which normal retinal vascular development is altered and abnormal neovascularization occurs. The pathological process may stop or reverse itself at any point, or the disease may eventually progress to fibroglial proliferation and lead to vitreoretinal traction and retinal detachment.

ROP is rare in infants with a birth weight greater than 2000 g. Premature infants weighing less than 1500 g at birth are at risk for serious visual sequelae from ROP, and the risk increases as gestational age and birth weight decrease. In the multicenter trial of cryotherapy for ROP (CRYO-ROP Study), 37% of infants weighing less than 750 g developed severe (stage 3, see below) ROP, whereas only 21.9% of those weighing 750–999 g and 8.5% of those weighing 1000–1250 g did so.

Administration of supplemental oxygen to the newborn has been implicated as the cause of ROP; however, extremely premature infants vary highly in severity of and susceptibility to ROP, suggesting that factors other than hyperoxia play a role in the etiology of this disease. Currently, birth weight is a greater predictor of ROP than is oxygen exposure. ROP, or a disease process similar to it, has also been reported in infants who did not receive supplemental oxygen. Oxygen monitoring is considered the standard of care in the intensive care nursery. Oxygen deprivation can cause loss of life or of neurologic function, limiting how significantly oxygen administration can be cut back in these very ill infants.

Factors other than oxygen have been studied as well. Several studies have examined vitamin E (α-tocopherol) as a preventive treatment, with conflicting results. Intraventricular hemorrhage, necrotizing enterocolitis, and death have been associated with high-dose IV vitamin E use. Vitamin E is usually administered to achieve physiologic levels. The possibility of premature exposure to light as a factor has also been raised but was recently refuted in a multicenter trial. Reduction of light in the nursery to allow for better rest is a national trend in the United States.

The ultimate prevention of ROP would be prevention of premature birth itself. Good early prenatal care can greatly affect the incidence of premature birth. The cost of prenatal efforts pales in comparison with the measures that may be necessitated by the lack of this care.

Gestational age and birth weight are inversely correlated with the development of ROP. The amount of time in oxygen therapy is a strong correlate, but the level of oxygenation is a weaker correlate. Other characteristics that correlate with the development of ROP are multiple births and transfer after birth to a hospital with a neonatal intensive care unit. Severe ROP is also more prevalent in white newborns, especially males.

Among infants who develop ROP, certain diseases are common, particularly various forms of respiratory distress syndrome, including hyaline membrane disease, pulmonary interstitial emphysema, pneumothorax, and bronchopulmonary dysplasia. Other disease entities observed include patent ductus arteriosus, apnea and bradycardia, intracranial hemorrhage, suspected sepsis, anemia, and jaundice.

Classification

The 1984 international classification of ROP describes the disease by stage, zone, and extent. It has functioned very well in the CRYO-ROP study and will probably be the standard classification for many years (Table 24-1; Figs 24-2 through 24-6). BCSC Section 12, *Retina and Vitreous*, discusses this classification in detail. *Plus disease* refers to arteriolar tortuosity and venous engorgement of the posterior pole.

Management

Fundus examination of the premature infant must be performed with extreme care; these infants are fragile, and the examination is stressful. The recommended solution to be used in the examination is Cyclomydril (0.2% cyclopentolate and 1.0% phenylephrine). Phenylephrine 10% (Neo-Synephrine) should never be used because of its potential to cause hypertension. Concentrations of cyclopentolate greater than 0.5% should be avoided as well because of induced feeding intolerance. If an examination must be postponed, the postponement and medical reason should be documented in the patient's chart.

It has been recommended that the initial fundus examination for infants weighing less than 1500 g take place 5–6 weeks after birth, and if no ROP is apparent, the examination should be repeated 1–2 weeks later (Table 24-2). Screening fundus examinations are no longer needed when the retina is fully vascularized.

The screening clinician is initially looking for ROP and retinal vessel development. Regardless of the presence or absence of ROP, if the normal retinal vessels do not extend past zone I on early examinations, the chance that treatment will be needed becomes

Table 24-1 International Classification of Acute Stages of Retinopathy of Prematurity

Location—Zones II and III are based on convention rather than strict anatomy (Fig 24-7)

   Zone I (posterior pole)—Circle with radius of 30°, twice disc-macula distance

   Zone II—From edge of zone I to point tangential to nasal ora serrata and around to area near the temporal equator

   Zone III—Residual crescent anterior to zone II

Extent—Specified as hours of the clock as observer looks at each eye

Staging the disease

   Stage 1—Demarcation line (see Fig 24-2)

   Stage 2—Ridge, ± small tufts of fibrovascular proliferation (popcorns) (see Fig 24-3)

   Stage 3—Ridge with extraretinal fibrovascular proliferation (see Fig 24-4)
- Mild fibrovascular proliferation
- Moderate fibrovascular proliferation
- Severe fibrovascular proliferation

   Stage 4—Subtotal retinal detachment (see Fig 24-5)
   A. Extrafoveal
   B. Retinal detachment including fovea

   Stage 5—Total retinal detachment

   Funnel: Anterior   Posterior
                Open   Open
                Narrow   Narrow

Plus disease—Plus (+) is added when vasular shunting is so marked that the veins are enlarged and the arteries tortuous in the posterior pole (see Fig 24-6).

(Modified from the Committee for Classification of Retinopathy of Prematurity: An international classification of retinopathy of prematurity. *Arch Ophthalmol.* 1984;102:1130–1134.

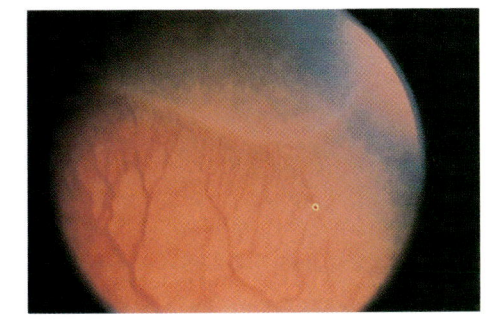

Figure 24-2 Late stage 1 ROP. Demarcation line has no height. *(Reprinted courtesy of Oregon Health Sciences University Ophthalmic Photography Department.)*

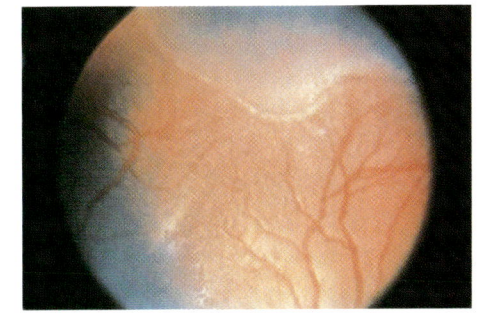

Figure 24-3 Early stage 2 ROP. Demarcation height and width, creating a ridge. *(Reprinted courtesy of Oregon Health Sciences University Ophthalmic Photography Department and CRYO-ROP Cooperative Group.)*

310 • Pediatric Ophthalmology and Strabismus

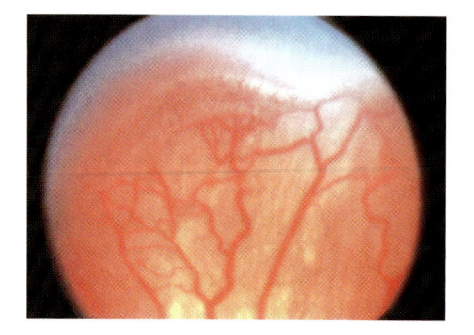

Figure 24-4 Stage 3 ROP. Ridge with extraretinal fibrovascular proliferation (top right shows stage 2). *(Reprinted by permission from Arch Ophthalmol. 1984;102:1132. ©1988 American Medical Association.)*

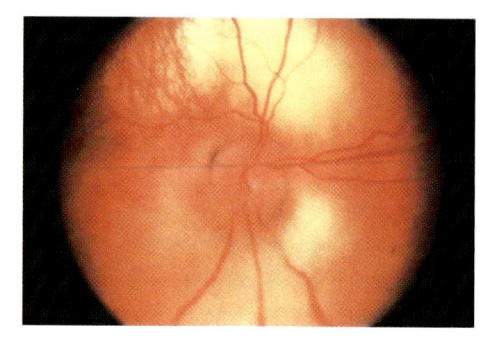

Figure 24-5 Stage 4 ROP. Subtotal retinal detachment. *(Reprinted by permission from Arch Ophthalmol. 1984;102:1134. ©1988 American Medical Association.)*

Figure 24-6 Classic plus disease.

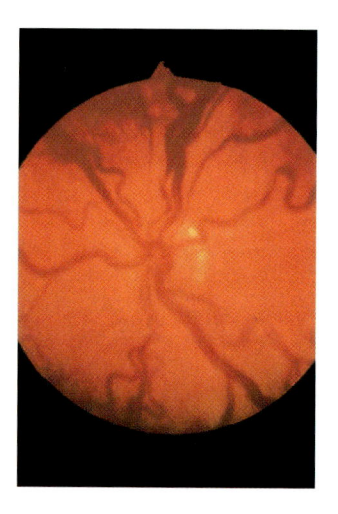

much higher. In infants less than 1000 g at birth who are not vascularized beyond zone I, weekly examinations may be advisable even if no ROP is present. Such infants are predisposed to rush disease, in which plus disease and retinal detachment develop rapidly, without intervening stages. On follow-up examinations, the patient is observed for development of ROP, spontaneous resolution of ROP, or progression to threshold disease. *Threshold disease* is stage 3+ ROP in zone I or II, involving at least five contiguous clock-hour sectors or at least eight interrupted clock-hour sectors (see Table 24-2, Fig 24-7). The iris vessels can become visibly congested just prior to the development of threshold disease (Fig 24-8).

The CRYO-ROP study has shown that 6% of infants with a birth weight less than 1251 g will develop threshold disease and that 45% of these will have vision of 20/200 or worse at age 3½ years if not treated. If cryotherapy is applied to the avascular areas of retina in these eyes, only 26% of these patients will have vision of 20/200 or worse at age

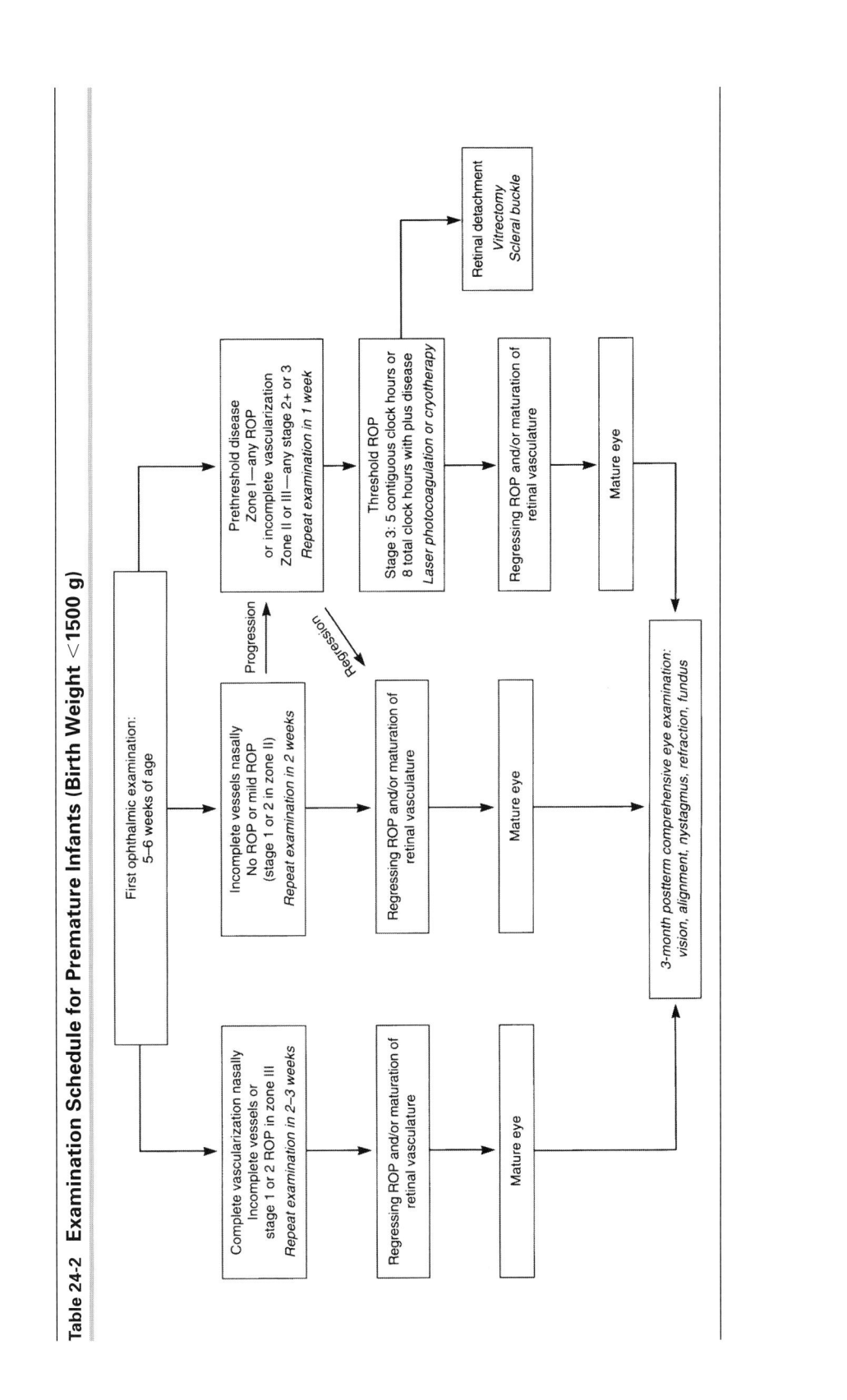

Table 24-2 Examination Schedule for Premature Infants (Birth Weight <1500 g)

```
                        First ophthalmic examination:
                              5–6 weeks of age
          ┌──────────────────────┬──────────────────────┐
          ▼                      ▼                      ▼
  Complete vascularization  Incomplete vessels     Prethreshold disease
  nasally                   nasally                Zone I—any ROP
  Incomplete vessels or     No ROP or mild ROP     or incomplete vascularization
  stage 1 or 2 ROP in       (stage 1 or 2 in       Zone II or III—any stage 2+ or 3
  zone III                  zone II)               Repeat examination in 1 week
  Repeat examination in     Repeat examination
  2–3 weeks                 in 2 weeks
          │                      │   ▲  │                │
          │                      │   │Progression        │
          │                      │   │  │Regression      │
          ▼                      ▼   │  ▼                ▼
  Regressing ROP and/or     Regressing ROP and/or    Threshold ROP
  maturation of retinal     maturation of retinal    Stage 3: 5 contiguous clock hours or
  vasculature               vasculature              8 total clock hours with plus disease
                                                     Laser photocoagulation or cryotherapy
          │                      │                        │
          ▼                      ▼                        ▼
      Mature eye             Mature eye           Regressing ROP and/or maturation of
                                                  retinal vasculature
                                                          │
                                                          ▼
                                                      Mature eye ────► Retinal detachment
                                                                       Vitrectomy
                                                                       Scleral buckle
          │                      │                        │
          └──────────────────────┼────────────────────────┘
                                 ▼
                   3-month postterm comprehensive eye examination:
                   vision, alignment, nystagmus, refraction, fundus
```

312 • Pediatric Ophthalmology and Strabismus

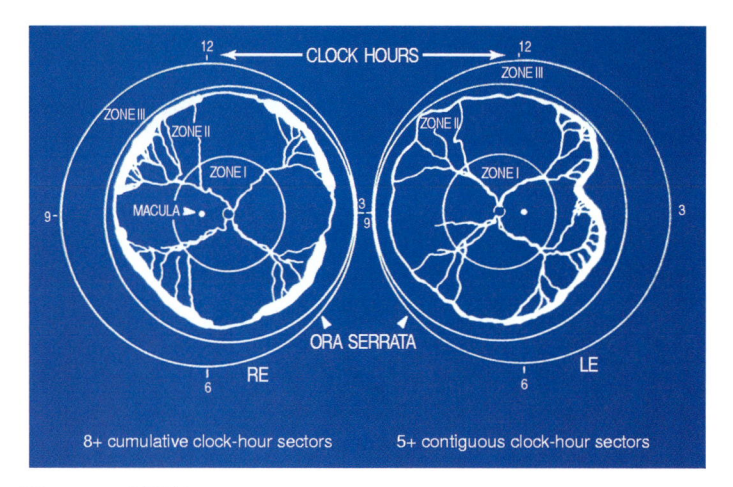

Figure 24-7 Diagram of ROP zones. *(Reprinted by permission from* Arch Ophthalmol. *1988;106:472. © 1988 American Medical Association.)*

Figure 24-8 Congested iris vessels associated with stage 3+ ROP.

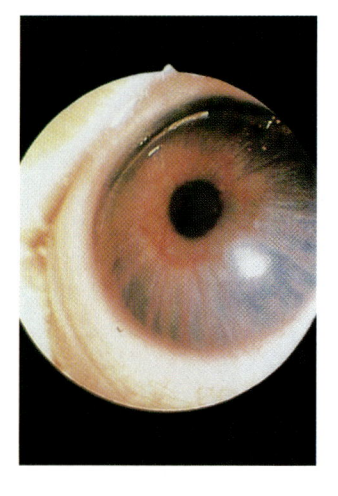

3½ years (Fig 24-9). Therefore, cryotherapy reduces severe vision loss by about half. The study showed that at age 5½ years, treated eyes were still much less likely to have very poor vision. However, more of the untreated eyes with quantifiable vision had vision of 20/40 or better than did the treated eyes. Longer-term follow-up studies are necessary to see whether this trend persists, particularly after the patients go through teenage years, a common time for secondary retinal detachments in severe ROP. Mild constriction of visual field has been measured in treated eyes; the benefit of preserved acuity outweighs this disadvantage.

The median age at which eyes reached threshold disease in the CRYO-ROP study was 36.9 weeks post conception; 90% of cases reached threshold between 33.6 and 42 weeks post conception. This age can coincide with the age at which the patient is transferred to another facility or discharged to home. If a child has worsening ROP at this

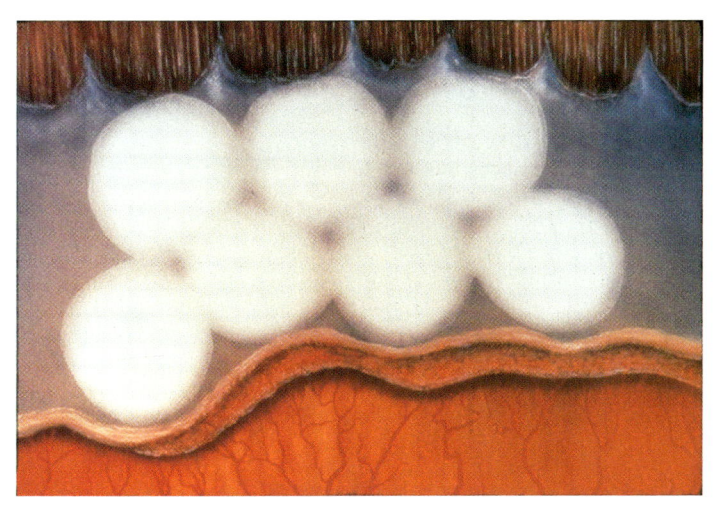

Figure 24-9 Cryotherapy as a row at ora serrata extending posteriorly to anterior edge of ridge. *(Reprinted by permission from* Arch Ophthalmol. *1988;106:474. © 1988 American Medical Association.)*

age, the discharge plans should include consideration of follow-up and treatment possibilities. Follow-up examinations should be performed according to the schedule presented in Table 24-2.

Laser photocoagulation is a newer treatment modality that has been as effective as cryotherapy in halting threshold disease in several series. The major advantages of laser over cryotherapy are:

- Greater facility in reaching more posterior locations
- Less trauma to ocular tissues
- Less discomfort to the patient
- Less ultimate myopia in some studies

Laser is not without complications, however. Laser causes an intense inflammatory response in some eyes. For this reason, a postoperative regimen of topical steroids and cycloplegia is imperative for the first week. Hyphema and cataract may also occur. Such cataracts are often accompanied by hypotony, and many infants lose the eye.

Although ROP regresses in most cases, sequelae of advanced disease (stage 3) can include both peripheral and posterior retinal changes. Therefore, a child who has had ROP requires periodic ophthalmic examinations beyond the newborn period to reach maximum visual function. Vitreoretinal traction may cause retinal detachment in the first or second decade of life. Retinal folds and dragging of the macula can also occur, causing visual impairment (Fig 24-10). Amblyopia may be present as a result of high myopia, macular dragging, or strabismus. Pseudostrabismus caused by dragging of the macula can occur, often giving the appearance of an exotropia as a result of a large positive angle kappa (Fig 24-11). These children need particular attention to their development and education because they are often multiply handicapped beyond their visual problems.

When laser or cryotherapy has not prevented the progression of ROP to stage 4 or retinal detachment, scleral buckling and vitrectomy are also used. The outcome continues

314 • Pediatric Ophthalmology and Strabismus

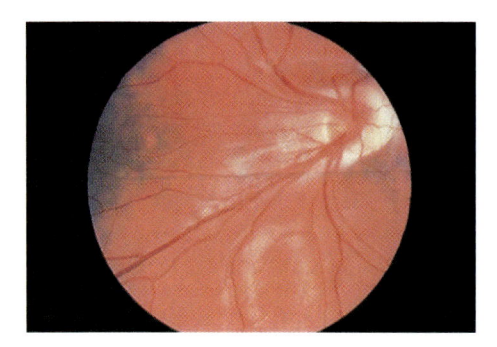

Figure 24-10 Posterior pole traction/dragging, a sequela of ROP, right eye. Central acuity is usually diminished in such eyes.

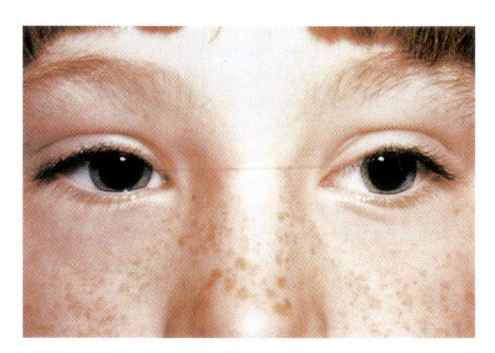

Figure 24-11 Pseudoexotropia in a fixating left eye in ROP. Patient has a positive angle kappa as a result of macular dragging.

to be poor. Anatomical reattachment is achieved in only about 60% of eyes, and a much smaller number recover some vision. Even with laser and cryotherapy treatment, several hundred babies are blinded by this disease in the United States yearly.

Other late changes associated with stage 5 ROP include microphthalmos, cataract, glaucoma, and phthisis bulbi. Glaucoma is caused by peripheral anterior synechiae and angle closure resulting from forward movement of the lens–iris diaphragm. Such eyes are often blind but may be preserved by cycloplegic agents, steroids, lensectomy, and iridectomy. In seeing eyes, progressive myopia may indicate progression of lens movement and rounding and may be a harbinger of angle closure. In blind eyes, enucleation is sometimes necessary for pain relief.

See the end of this chapter for the joint statement on ROP screening approved by the American Academy of Pediatrics, the American Association for Pediatric Ophthalmology and Strabismus, and the American Academy of Ophthalmology.

> Cryotherapy for Retinopathy of Prematurity Cooperative Group. Multicenter trial of cryotherapy for retinopathy of prematurity: Snellen visual acuity and structural outcome at 5 1 years after randomization. *Arch Ophthalmol.* 1996;114:417–424.
>
> Palmer EA. Retinopathy of prematurity. In: *Focal Points: Clinical Modules for Ophthalmologists.* San Francisco: American Academy of Ophthalmology; 1993: vol 11, no 3.
>
> Quinn GE, Young TL. Retinopathy of prematurity. In: *Focal Points: Clinical Modules for Ophthalmologists.* San Francisco: American Academy of Ophthalmology; 2001: vol 19, no 11.
>
> Reynolds JD, Hardy RJ, Kennedy KA, et al. Lack of efficacy of light reduction in preventing retinopathy of prematurity. Light Reduction in Retinopathy of Prematurity (LIGHT-ROP) Cooperative Group. *N Engl J Med.* 1998;338:1572–1576.

Coats Disease

Coats disease is an important mimicker of retinoblastoma. The definition of this condition has been narrowed, and Coats disease is now understood to mean the presence of abnormal retinal vessels with a fundus picture showing yellow subretinal exudates. The term *telangiectasia* is frequently used to indicate these anomalous grapelike clusters of vessels. The macular area is a favored site for exudation. Once the fovea is detached and the subretinal exudate becomes organized, the prognosis for restoration of central vision is poor. See also BCSC Section 12, *Retina and Vitreous*.

In the juvenile form of Coats disease, males are affected more frequently than females. This condition is usually, but not always, unilateral. The typical age at diagnosis is 8–10 years, but the disease has also been observed in infants (Fig 24-12). The most widely held theory is that the subretinal exudation originates from the leaking anomalous vessels. Hence, the diagnosis of Coats disease requires the presence of the abnormal retinal vessels, which occasionally are small and difficult to find. Fluorescein angioscopy and angiography may be helpful in demonstrating leakage from the telangiectatic vessels and in assessing the effectiveness of therapy.

The differential diagnosis includes angiomatosis retinae, retinoblastoma, PHPV, ROP, toxocariasis, metastatic retinitis, familial exudative vitreoretinopathy, massive retinal fibrosis, Eales disease, sickle cell retinopathy, leukemia, anemia, and cavernous retinal hemangioma.

Treatment is directed at obliterating the abnormal vessels and includes cryotherapy or laser photocoagulation. The disease is stopped when the leaking vessels are destroyed. Eyes with progressive disease develop exudative retinal detachments and subretinal fibrosis. Scleral buckling may be used on eyes with retinal detachments. Some eyes develop intractable glaucoma.

In one study, 22 untreated patients were followed for an average of 5 years. The ocular disease progressed in about half of patients, remaining stable in the other half. Ridley and coworkers (1982) reported on 43 eyes, of which 29 were treated. Of the treated group, 8 (27.5%) deteriorated, 15 (52%) stabilized, and 6 (20.5%) improved. Aggressive treatment of the abnormal vessels and prolonged follow-up were recommended.

Hereditary Retinal Disease

Nystagmus is the most definitive presenting sign of a hereditary retinal disorder in the preverbal child. The onset of nystagmus typically occurs between 8 and 12 weeks of age. Poor visual function can also be the presenting abnormality in a young child, and school-age children with retinal disease often fail a vision screening. Workup requires a complete

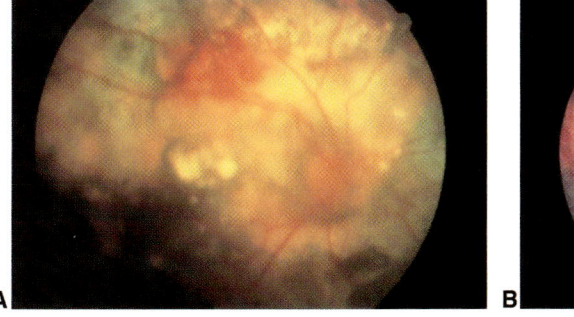

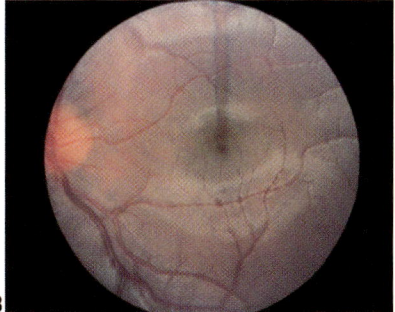

Figure 24-12 Coats disease. **A,** Affected right eye. Note extensive subretinal exudate and exudative retinal detachment. **B,** Normal left eye.

ophthalmologic examination and an electroretinogram (ERG). Older children can be examined further with an electro-oculogram (EOG), color vision testing, visual fields, and dark adaptation testing.

Table 24-3 outlines the causes of nystagmus in the first 3 months of life. Optic nerve disorders, infectious diseases, and congenital motor nystagmus are discussed elsewhere in this book (see Chapters 12, 17, and 25). Hereditary retinal diseases with onset late in childhood are much like adult hereditary retinal diseases and are thoroughly covered in BCSC Section 12, *Retina and Vitreous*.

Leber Congenital Amaurosis

Leber congenital amaurosis is an autosomal recessive disorder that affects both rods and cones. It presents with decreased vision during the first year of life, usually manifesting as nystagmus beginning in the second or third month. Vision ranges from 20/200 to bare light perception in most patients. Hyperopic refraction and sluggish pupillary responses are characteristic findings, although some patients are myopic. Ophthalmoscopic appearance varies highly, ranging from a normal appearance, particularly in infancy, to one resembling classic retinitis pigmentosa with bone spicules, attenuation of arterioles, and disc pallor. Other reported fundus findings include irregularity of the retinal pigment epithelium, extensive chorioretinal atrophy, macular coloboma, white dots (similar to

Table 24-3 Causes of Nystagmus in First 3 Months of Life

Primary sensory retinal abnormality
  Leber congenital amaurosis
  Achromatopsia
  Blue-cone monochromatism
  Congenital stationary night blindness (X-linked and autosomal recessive)

Vitreoretinal abnormality
  Norrie disease
  Familial exudative vitreoretinopathy

Foveal hypoplasia
  Associated with albinism
  Associated with aniridia
  Isolated

Optic nerve disorder
  Optic nerve hypoplasia
  Optic nerve coloboma
  Optic atrophy

Infectious disease
  Congenital toxoplasmosis
  Cytomegalovirus
  Rubella
  Syphilis

Congenital motor nystagmus

Generalized central nervous system disorder
  Aicardi syndrome
  Others

retinitis punctata albescens), marbleized retinal appearance, and disc edema (Fig 24-13). Additional ocular abnormalities include oculodigital reflex (eye poking), cataracts, keratoconus, and keratoglobus. The incidence of neurologic and renal disorders is significant in these patients. See Familial Oculorenal Syndromes, later in this chapter.

Given such variability, the diagnosis of Leber congenital amaurosis cannot be based on fundus appearance alone and requires an ERG. However, electroretinography can be technically difficult to perform in infants, and there is a maturation of the response. Thus, an ERG can appear highly abnormal in an infant who will later develop a more normal response. It is often advisable either to delay the ERG until age 6 months or to repeat the ERG after this time.

The characteristic clinical picture in this disorder is of an infant in the first 6 months of life presenting with nystagmus and an ERG that is nearly or essentially flat. Histologic examination shows diffuse absence of photoreceptors. No treatment is available. Leber congenital amaurosis is genetically heterogeneous. Mutations of the photoreceptor-specific guanylate cyclase gene *(RETGC1)*, the *RPE65* gene, and the *CRX* gene account for about 27% of cases. Other genes are being sought. Patients with *RETGC1* mutations may experience a more stable course than those with *RPE65* mutations.

Both *Refsum disease* (infantile phytanic acid storage disease) and *Bassen-Kornzweig syndrome* (abetalipoproteinemia) have been reported to present as Leber congenital amaurosis. Because these are potentially treatable metabolic disorders (via reduction of phytanic acid intake and vitamin A and E therapy, respectively), it is recommended that the evaluation of a new patient with findings of Leber congenital amaurosis include a complete blood lipid profile, inspection of peripheral smear for acanthocytes (Bassen-Kornzweig syndrome), and measurement of serum phytanic acid levels.

Lambert SR, Taylor D, Kriss A. The infant with nystagmus, normal appearing fundi, but an abnormal ERG. *Surv Ophthalmol.* 1989;34:173–186.

Perrault I, Rozet JM, Gerber S, et al. Leber congenital amaurosis. *Mol Genet Metab.* 1999;68:200–208.

Achromatopsia

Achromatopsia can be difficult to distinguish initially from Leber congenital amaurosis, but infants with achromatopsia develop better visual functioning and less photophobia over time. Complete achromatopsia, or *rod monochromatism*, is a stationary autosomal

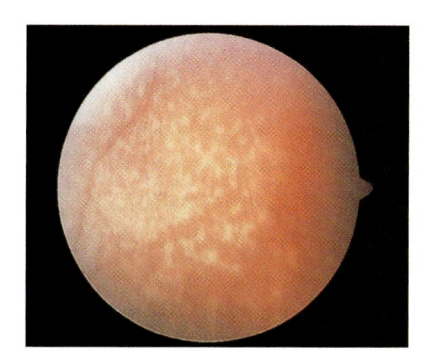

Figure 24-13 Leber congenital amaurosis, marbleized fundus type.

recessive disorder in which patients have no color vision, poor central vision, nystagmus, and photophobia. The photophobia is actually a desire to avoid bright light rather than true pain or discomfort, and photophobia may be manifested by squinting or rapid fluttering of the eyelids in normal indoor illumination. It may not appear until several months of age.

Retinal examination is usually normal, with the possible exception of a decreased or absent foveal reflex. Color vision testing results are markedly abnormal, as is the ERG, which shows extinguished photopic responses. Dark glasses or red glasses that exclude short wavelengths may help. Autosomal recessive achromatopsia is associated with mutations of the *CNGA3* gene on chromosome 2. This encodes the α-subunit of the cone cyclic nucleotide–gated cation channel, which generates the light-evoked electrical responses of the cones. In the Pingelapese islanders of Micronesia, mutations have been found in the *CNBG3* gene on chromosome 8. This gene encodes the β-subunit of the cone cyclic nucleotide–gated cation channel. Incomplete autosomal recessive forms of achromatopsia occur less often.

> Pokorny J, Smith VC, Pinckers AJ, et al. Classification of complete and incomplete autosomal recessive achromatopsia. *Graefes Arch Clin Exp Ophthalmol.* 1982;219:121–130.
>
> Sundin OH, Yang JM, Li Y, et al. Genetic basis of total colour blindness among the Pingelapese islanders. *Nat Genet.* 2000;25:289–293.

Blue-Cone Monochromatism

Blue-cone monochromatism is an X-linked cone disorder that may present with nystagmus in the first few months of life. These patients are less severely affected clinically than those with complete achromatopsia. Vision may decline slowly over time. Patients have a characteristic color vision abnormality and visual acuity ranging from 20/60 to 20/200. Fundus examination appears essentially normal. Although the short-wavelength (blue) cones are functioning, the photopic ERG is essentially extinguished. Mutations in the red and green pigment gene array at Xq28 are responsible.

> Ladekjaer-Mikkelsen AS, Rosenberg T, Jorgensen AL. A new mechanism in blue cone monochromatism. *Hum Genet.* 1996;98:403–408.

Congenital Stationary Night Blindness

The following classification scheme for congenital stationary night blindness (CSNB) was proposed by Carr (1974). Forms with normal fundi are:

- Autosomal dominant
- Autosomal recessive
- X-linked

Forms with abnormal fundi are:

- Oguchi disease: yellow sheen after light exposure that disappears following dark adaptation
- Fundus albipunctatus: yellow-white dots, normal vessels

Both autosomal recessive and X-linked forms of CSNB can present in early infancy with nystagmus and normal fundi. These forms are often also associated with myopia and decreased acuity in the range of 20/200. The retina appears normal, although the optic nerve may show some temporal pallor. The ERG shows two characteristic patterns; in both, the scotopic b-wave amplitude is greatly reduced. Dark adaptation is abnormal in all patients. Infants with CSNB may have a flat ERG until approximately 6 months of age, when it converts to the classic negative configuration. Other forms of CSNB are discussed in BCSC Section 12, *Retina and Vitreous*.

Carr RE. Congenital stationary night blindness. *Trans Am Ophthalmol Soc.* 1974;72:448–487.

Foveal Hypoplasia

Foveal hypoplasia, or incomplete development of the fovea, is another cause of nystagmus in early infancy. This condition is most often associated with albinism or aniridia but may also be an isolated finding. The ophthalmoscopic appearance is of a decreased or absent foveal reflex with varying degrees of hypoplasia of the macula itself (patients with complete achromatopsia also show decreased foveal reflex). The ERG appears normal in these cases. Foveal hypoplasia can be familial and may be related to a defect in the *PAX6* gene.

Aicardi Syndrome

Aicardi syndrome is a disorder characterized by round or oval, widespread, depigmented chorioretinal lesions (Fig 24-14). Optic nerve head colobomas and microphthalmos also occur. CT reveals agenesis of the corpus callosum. Affected patients have infantile spasms and severe mental retardation. Aicardi syndrome is an X-linked dominant disorder, lethal in males.

Carney SH, Brodsky MC, Good WV, et al. Aicardi syndrome: more than meets the eye. *Surv Ophthalmol.* 1993;37:419–424.

Menezes AV, MacGregor DL, Buncic JR. Aicardi syndrome: natural history and possible predictors of severity. *Pediatr Neurol.* 1994;11:313–318.

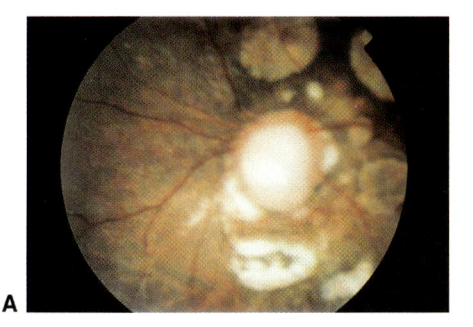

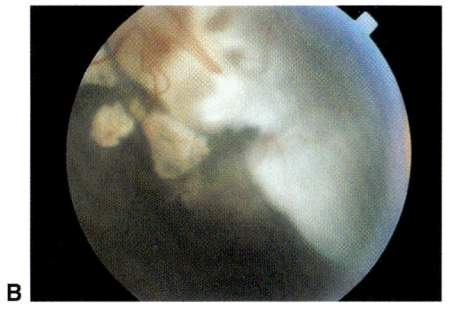

Figure 24-14 Aicardi syndrome. **A,** Fundus photograph showing disc and adjacent chorioretinal lacunae. **B,** Peripheral view of same patient showing large chorioretinal lacuna.

Hereditary Macular Dystrophies

The macula can be involved in a hereditary disorder in three possible ways:
- The macula may appear abnormal secondary to a hereditary systemic disease (eg, the cherry-red spot seen in generalized gangliosidosis).
- The macula may be involved in a generalized primary retinal disorder, as in some cases of Leber congenital amaurosis. Tests of overall retinal function such as the ERG reveal abnormal results in this situation.
- The macula alone may be affected by a hereditary disorder such as Stargardt disease, Best vitelliform dystrophy, and familial drusen.

Stargardt Disease

Stargardt disease (juvenile macular degeneration) is the most common hereditary macular dystrophy. It is a bilateral, symmetrical, progressive condition in which acuity levels off at approximately 20/200. Vision typically begins to deteriorate between ages 8 and 15 years. The fundus appears normal early in the course of the disease, even when some vision has been lost. The first ophthalmoscopic changes observed are loss of foveal reflex, followed by development of a characteristic bull's-eye lesion. Yellow flecks in the posterior pole are characteristic, but they are not required for the diagnosis (Fig 24-15). Eventually, the macula may acquire an atrophic appearance, with a peculiar light-reflecting quality that has been described as beaten bronze. The lesion then enlarges and deepens and may finally show choroidal atrophy with prominent choroidal vessels at its base. The dark choroid sign on fluorescein angiography is distinctive but not always present. Progressive cone–rod dystrophy may present like Stargardt disease in children but has a much worse prognosis, often resulting in very little vision. Repeat ERG and acuity measurements over the first year are recommended before a definitive diagnosis is made.

Fundus flavimaculatus

When more retinal flecks develop in the periphery and evidence suggests generalized retinal involvement, the condition has been called fundus flavimaculatus (Fig 24-16). ERG abnormalities are usually very mild in Stargardt disease and more significant in

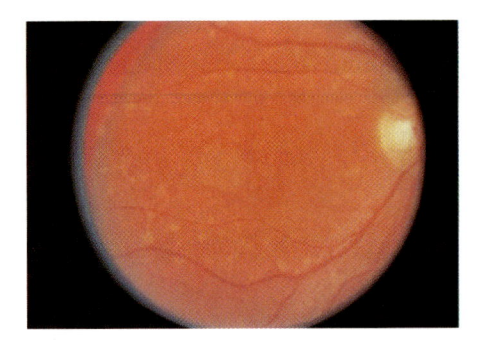

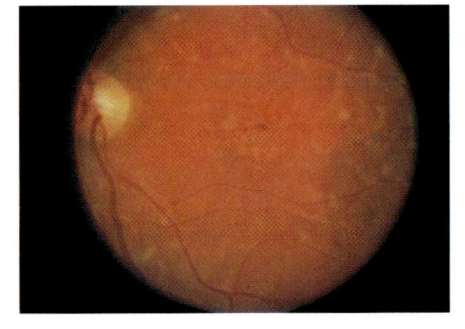

Figure 24-15 Stargardt disease, bilateral. Note atrophic, beaten-metal appearance of macula. Early in the disease, usually at presentation, the macula appears normal.

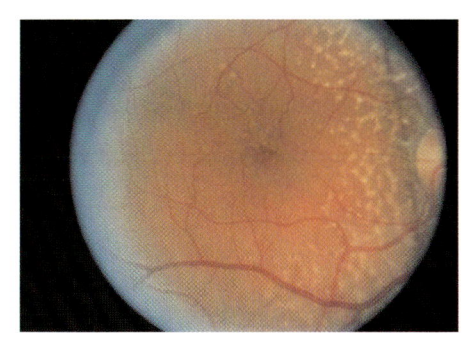

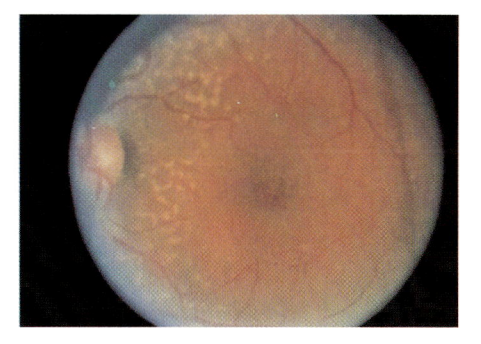

Figure 24-16 Fundus flavimaculatus. Note pisciform yellowish flecks.

fundus flavimaculatus. Many authors now group the two entities together as Stargardt disease/fundus flavimaculatus because of reports of families in which both forms exist in different members with the same genetic mutations. Both disorders also map to the same genetic locus. Stargardt disease is caused by mutations in the retina-specific ATP binding transporter gene (ABCR). Interestingly, this gene is expressed in rods, not cones, although clinically Stargardt disease manifests primarily in the cones.

> Rozet JM, Gerber S, Ghazi I, et al. Mutations of the retinal specific ATP binding transporter gene (ABCR) in a single family segregating both autosomal recessive retinitis pigmentosa and Stargardt disease: evidence of clinical heterogeneity at this locus. *J Med Genet.* 1999;36:447–451.

Best Vitelliform Dystrophy

The retina may at first appear normal in Best vitelliform dystrophy even though the EOG appears abnormal (Fig 24-17). The vitelliform stage begins between 4 and 10 years of age and is seen as a yellow-orange cystlike structure, usually in the macula, although the lesion may occur elsewhere and can occasionally be multiple. It is usually 1.5–5.0 disc diameters in size. The *sunny-side up* appearance is associated with good central vision. With time, the cystic material may become granular, giving rise to the *scrambled egg* stage. Central vision usually remains good.

The contents of the retinal pigment epithelial cyst may rupture and become partially resorbed, and pseudohypopyon may form with liquefaction of the cystic contents. Eventually, atrophy of the macula ensues. There may be subretinal neovascularization and serous detachment of the retinal pigment epithelium, and subretinal hemorrhage may occur. Most patients see surprisingly well for many years; eventually, however, central vision often deteriorates to 20/100 or worse.

The EOG appears abnormal in all affected patients and in carriers. This disorder is one of the few in which the EOG appears abnormal and the ERG appears normal. Carriers can be identified by the presence of an abnormal-appearing EOG in the absence of morphologic abnormalities. The condition is autosomal dominant and is caused by mutations in the vitelliform macular dystrophy gene *(VMD2)*, also called *bestrophin*, on chromosome 11.

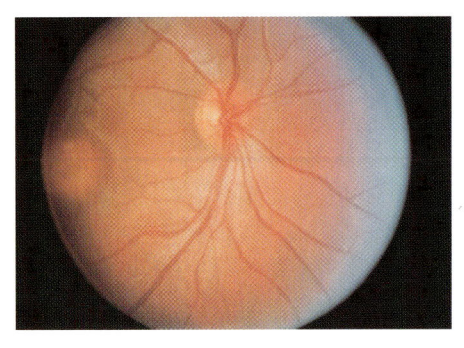

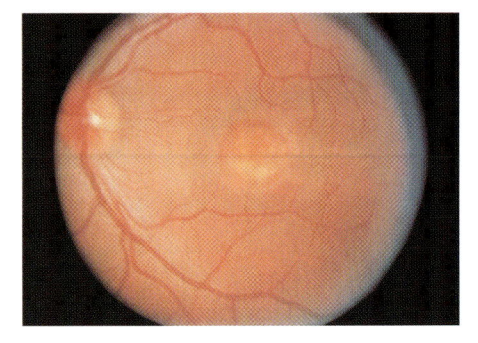

Figure 24-17 Best vitelliform dystrophy, bilateral. Even with pronounced vitelliform maculopathy as seen here, vision may be nearly normal.

Petrukhin K, Koisti MJ, Bakall B, et al. Identification of the gene responsible for Best macular dystrophy. *Nat Genet.* 1998;19:241–247.

Familial Drusen

In this dominantly transmitted disorder, drusen appear on Bruch's membrane. Decreased central acuity is rare before age 40, but macular drusen are occasionally seen in children. The drusen are small, yellow-white, and round or oval. They are similar to the lesions of fundus albipunctatus except that familial drusen tend to form grapelike clusters. Complications in adult life include macular edema, hemorrhage, and macular degenerations of various types following subretinal neovascularization.

Hereditary Vitreoretinopathies

The vitreoretinopathies include a broad range of disease entities. The ones discussed here characteristically present in childhood.

Juvenile Retinoschisis

Foveal retinoschisis is present in almost all cases of juvenile retinoschisis. About 50% of patients have peripheral retinoschisis in addition to foveal involvement. The retinoschisis occurs in the nerve fiber layer. The fovea has a star-shaped or spokelike configuration; vitreous veils or strands are common (Fig 24-18); and vitreal syneresis is prominent. Visual acuity varies extremely but may gradually deteriorate to the finger-counting range. Complications include vitreous hemorrhages and retinal detachments. The ERG shows a reduction of the scotopic b-wave with preservation of the a-wave; the EOG appears normal. The condition is usually transmitted as an X-linked trait.

Stickler Syndrome

Stickler syndrome is an autosomal dominant disease characterized by progressive arthropathy, high myopia, retinal detachment, degenerative joint changes, epiphyseal dysplasia, flat midface, progressive hearing loss, and heart defects. A single family can show

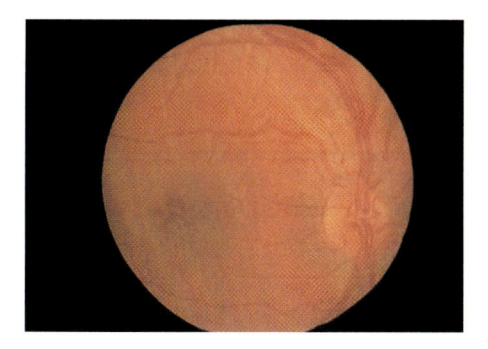

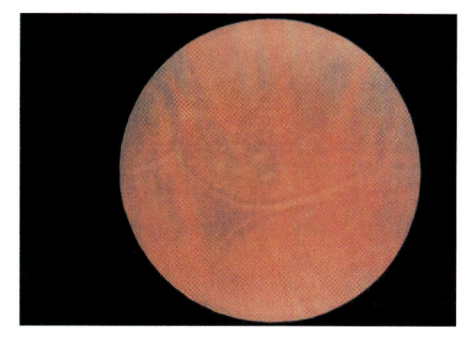

Figure 24-18 Juvenile retinoschisis. Central (macular) and peripheral schisis may be present.

great variability in expression of the syndrome, and individuals may manifest only a few of the characteristic findings. In many families, a defect in the type II procollagen gene has been found. Type II collagen is the major structural component of secondary vitreous.

A significant percentage of patients with Stickler syndrome also have the Pierre Robin sequence of cleft palate, small mandible, and backward displacement of the tongue. These patients can be detected in infancy because of their vulnerability to serious respiratory and feeding problems, but others with only ophthalmic defects may go unrecognized until later in childhood. The ophthalmic manifestations are not only frequent but also extremely severe and vision-threatening. Myopia, usually of a high degree, is the most common finding, and it is often associated with a radial type of lattice retinal degeneration with pigment clumping around the retinal vessels. There is a high incidence of retinal detachment with large retinal breaks and proliferative vitreoretinopathy. Angle anomalies, ectopia lentis, cataracts, ptosis, and strabismus are less frequently associated. The incidence of vitreous loss during cataract surgery is high, as is the rate of subsequent retinal detachments. When possible, retinal folds and breaks should be treated before cataract extraction.

Early diagnosis may aid in preventing some of the severe complications of the ocular pathology and allow treatment of mild joint involvement. Although the arthropathy may not be symptomatic initially, these children often show radiographic abnormalities of long bones and joints.

> Snead MP, Payne SJ, Barton DE, et al. Stickler syndrome: correlation between vitreoretinal phenotypes and linkage to COL 2A1. *Eye*. 1994;8:609–614.
>
> Vandenberg P. Molecular basis of heritable connective tissue disease. *Biochem Med Metab Biol*. 1993;49:1–12.

Familial Exudative Vitreoretinopathy

Both vitreous traction and posterior vitreous detachment are present in familial exudative vitreoretinopathy (also known as *FEVR*). The peripheral retina shows lack of vascularization and white areas with and without pressure. Thick peripheral exudates develop both in and under the retina. The combined effect of exudates and vitreous membranes results in retinal traction and subsequent retinal break. Early signs include decreased vision from retinal detachment and cataract. Family members can show marked variation of severity, from minimal straightening of vessels and peripheral nonperfusion to total retinal detachment. Differential diagnosis includes ROP and Coats disease.

The disease is usually autosomal dominant as a result of a mutation of the *FEVR1* locus on chromosome 11. X-linked transmission has also been reported in families with a defect in the same gene that causes Norrie disease and primary retinal dysplasia. Cryopexy, photocoagulation, retinal detachment surgery, vitrectomy, and cataract surgery have all been used to manage this disorder.

> Shastry BS, Hejtmancik JF, Trese MT. Identification of novel missense mutations in the Norrie disease gene associated with one X-linked and four sporadic cases of familial exudative vitreoretinopathy. *Hum Mutat.* 1997;9:396–401.

Norrie Disease

Norrie disease is an X-linked disorder that is characterized by bilateral congenital blindness associated with varying degrees of hearing impairment and mental retardation. Affected boys are typically born blind, although the external ocular appearance may initially be normal. During the first few days or weeks of life, a yellowish retinal detachment appears bilaterally, followed by a whiter mass behind the clear lens. Over time, the lenses, and later the cornea, opacify; phthisis bulbi may ensue by the age of 10 years or earlier. Before the end stage is reached, the retina shows dysplasia histopathologically. DNA testing is possible for genetic counseling.

> Mintz-Hittner HA, Ferrell RE, Sims KB, et al. Peripheral retinopathy in offspring of carriers of Norrie disease gene mutations. Possible transplacental effect of abnormal Norrin. *Ophthalmology.* 1996;103:2128–2134.

Goldmann-Favre Vitreoretinal Dystrophy

Goldmann-Favre vitreoretinal dystrophy consists of vitreous strands and veils as well as foveal and peripheral retinoschisis. The peripheral retina shows changes similar to those seen in retinitis pigmentosa, including optic nerve pallor and attenuation of the retinal vessels. The pigmentary disturbance tends to be in a nummular, rather than a bone spicule, configuration; in some cases, little pigment is seen. Decreased central acuity and night blindness are prominent early findings in the second decade of life, and complicated cataracts subsequently develop. Inheritance is autosomal recessive.

> Brown DM, Weingeist TA. Disorders of the vitreous and the vitreoretinal interface. In: Wright KW, ed. *Pediatric Ophthalmology and Strabismus.* St Louis: Mosby; 1995:467–476.

Systemic Diseases and Disorders With Retinal Manifestations

Diabetes Mellitus

Type 1, or *insulin-dependent, diabetes mellitus* was formerly called *juvenile-onset diabetes mellitus.* The prevalence of retinopathy in this condition is directly proportional to the duration of diabetes after puberty. Retinopathy rarely occurs less than 3 years after the onset of diabetes mellitus. Fundus photography or angiography reveals that about 50%

of patients have nonproliferative (background) retinopathy after 7 years, although only half of these cases can be recognized by direct ophthalmoscopy. The prevalence of retinopathy increases to approximately 90% in patients who have had type 1 diabetes for 15 years or more. Proliferative diabetic retinopathy is rare in pediatric cases and is not covered in this section. For further discussion see BCSC Section 12, *Retina and Vitreous*.

A variety of nonproliferative changes may occur in the pediatric age group. These changes are thought to result from obstruction of retinal capillaries and abnormal capillary permeability. Microaneurysms are the first ophthalmoscopic sign; they may be followed by retinal hemorrhages, areas of retinal nonperfusion, cotton-wool spots, hard exudates, intraretinal microvascular abnormalities, and venous dilatation. A rapid rise of blood glucose may produce myopia, and sudden reduction of blood glucose can induce hyperopia. Several weeks may be required before acuity returns to normal.

True diabetic cataracts are uncommon, occurring most often in patients with poorly controlled disease. Such cataracts resemble a snowstorm affecting the anterior and posterior cortices of young patients. Diabetic cataracts are caused by collection of sorbitol within the lens. Sorbitol concentration increases the lens osmolarity, leading to lens swelling and leakage of intralenticular contents. Such cataracts may require surgery.

Management

Specific treatment is not indicated for nonproliferative retinopathy in children. A schedule of ophthalmic examinations proposed by the American Academy of Pediatrics includes an initial discussion between the parents and the endocrinologist regarding ocular complications and the need for surveillance; this discussion should take place within the first year after diagnosis of type 1 diabetes mellitus. An initial eye examination should be performed at age 9 if the glucose is poorly controlled or 3 years after puberty if glucose is well controlled, with annual follow-up examinations. (See the statement, Screening Examination of Premature Infants for Retinopathy of Prematurity, at the end of this chapter.)

Leukemia

Ocular abnormalities occur in patients with acute lymphoblastic, acute myelogenous, and acute monocytic leukemia. Retinopathy appears less often in children than in adults. Two series describe a poorer prognosis for children with ocular manifestations. Histopathologically, the choroid is the most frequently affected ocular tissue, but choroidal involvement is usually not apparent clinically. Indirect ophthalmoscopy sometimes reveals mildly pale fundus areas, but choroidal involvement is more accurately detected ultrasonically.

The most common eye findings are retinal hemorrhages, especially flame-shaped lesions in the nerve fiber layer (Fig 24-19). They involve the posterior fundus and can have some correlation with other aspects of the disease such as anemia, thrombocytopenia, or coagulation abnormalities. At times, these retinal hemorrhages have white centers similar to the hemorrhages described in pernicious anemia, subacute bacterial endocarditis, scurvy, and septicemia. These hemorrhages can also resemble those associated with intracranial hemorrhages and trauma in infants in that the white centers are fibrin thrombi. However, collections of leukocytes have also been found on histopathologic

326 • Pediatric Ophthalmology and Strabismus

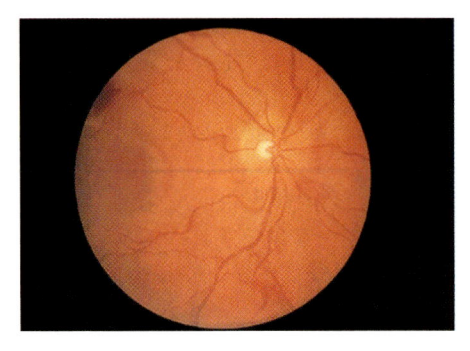

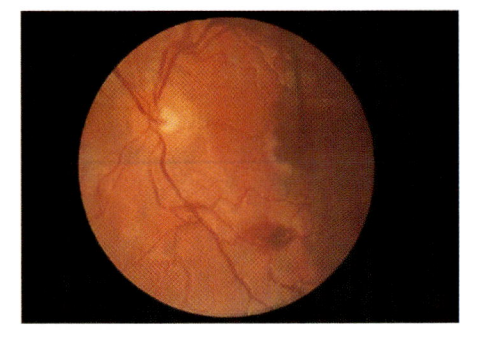

Figure 24-19 Retinal hemorrhages in bilateral leukemia.

examination. Other forms of retinal involvement include localized perivascular infiltrations, microinfarction, and discrete tumor infiltrations.

Optic nerve involvement is visible if the disc is infiltrated by leukemic cells (Fig 24-20). Translucent swelling of the disc obscures the normal landmarks; with florid involvement, only a white mass is visible in the region of the disc. If the nerve is involved centrally, a papilledema-like fundus picture ensues; such retrolaminar optic nerve involvement results in the loss of central vision. Therefore, a leukemic child with papilledema and a loss of central vision should be considered to have this complication. Early optic nerve involvement in leukemia constitutes a medical emergency because permanent loss of central vision is imminent. Such patients should undergo radiation therapy as soon as possible. However, patients receiving cancer chemotherapy may be abnormally sensitive to radiation therapy; blinding optic nerve atrophy has been reported in these patients.

Leukemic infiltrates in the anterior segment may lead to heterochromia iridis, a change in the architecture of the iris; frank iris infiltrates; spontaneous hyphemas; leukemic cells in the anterior chamber; and hypopyon. Keratic precipitates may be seen, and some affected eyes develop glaucoma from tumor cells clogging the trabecular meshwork. Other possible glaucoma mechanisms include posterior synechiae formation, seclusion of the pupil, and pupillary block. Anterior chamber paracentesis for cytologic studies may be diagnostic in cases involving the anterior segment. Topical steroids and local irradiation are effective for anterior segment complications.

Leukemic involvement of the iris may be confused with juvenile xanthogranuloma. Methods for distinguishing between these two eye disorders of children include the following:

- Biopsy of skin lesions of juvenile xanthogranuloma
- Peripheral blood analysis
- Bone marrow biopsy
- Anterior chamber taps for cytologic studies

Leukemic infiltration of the orbit is relatively uncommon and is more characteristic of acute myelogenous leukemia. Orbital involvement may be difficult to distinguish from bacterial or fungal orbital cellulitis. Leukemic orbital infiltration may be best managed

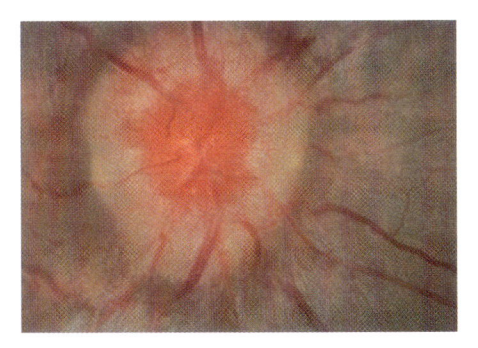

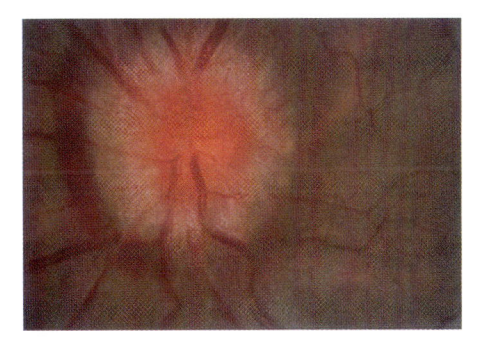

CHAPTER 24: Vitreous and Retinal Diseases and Disorders • 327

Figure 24-20 Leukemic infiltration of optic nerves, bilateral.

by radiation therapy. Ocular involvement is highly correlated with central nervous system involvement when the cerebrospinal fluid contains abnormal cells.

> Kaikov Y. Optic nerve head infiltration in acute leukemia in children: an indication for emergency optic nerve radiation therapy. *Med Pediatr Oncol.* 1996;26:101–104.
> Ohkoshi K, Tsiaras WG. Prognostic importance of ophthalmic manifestations in childhood leukaemia. *Br J Ophthalmol.* 1992;76:651–655.

Albinism

Albinism is a group of various conditions that involve the melanin system of the skin, eye, or both (Table 24-4; see also BCSC Section 12, *Retina and Vitreous*). The most common forms are *oculocutaneous albinism* (both tyrosinase positive and negative) and *X-linked ocular albinism.* The primary morbidity for most forms of albinism is ocular, so the ophthalmologist may be the physician who educates the family about heredity and skin protection from the sun.

The major ophthalmologic findings in albinism are iris transillumination from decreased pigmentation, foveal aplasia or hypoplasia, and a characteristic deficit of pigment in the retina, especially peripheral to the posterior pole (Fig 24-21). Nystagmus, light sensitivity, high refractive errors, and reduced central acuity are often present, and visual acuity ranges from 20/40 to 20/200. If a child has significant foveal hypoplasia, nystagmus will begin at 2–3 months of life. The severity of the visual defect tends to be proportionate to the degree of hypopigmentation. An abnormally large number of crossed fibers appear in the optic chiasm of patients and animals with albinism, precluding stereopsis and normal representation of space in the central nervous system. Asymmetrical visually evoked cortical potentials reflect this abnormality.

All forms of albinism are heritable, and genetic counseling is important. Unlike other recessive disorders, the defective genes responsible for albinism are fairly common, so parents of the patients are usually not related. Different ethnic groups show large variations in incidence. Africans and African Americans have a much higher incidence than Caucasians but frequently have incomplete forms. Defects in the *P* gene are commonly the cause of albinism in people of African descent; mutations of the tyrosinase gene are more common in Caucasians. Albinism resulting from *P* gene mutations presents as nystagmus in a child with pigment but who is more lightly pigmented than expected for

Table 24-4 Albinism

Disease	Ocular Manifestations	Systemic Manifestations	Inheritance
OCA1A (tyrosinase-negative)	Iris is thin, pale blue; characteristic orange reflex from the iris occurs because of marked transillumination defect; prominent choroidal vessels with poorly defined fovea; nystagmus; head-nodding; frequently myopic astigmatism and strabismus; vision 20/100–20/200; marked photophobia	White hair throughout life; tyrosinase absent, serum tyrosine levels normal; stage I and II melanosomes only; increased susceptibility to skin neoplasia	Autosomal recessive, chromosome 11q14–21; tyrosinase gene
OCA1B (with pigment)	At birth complete albinism with blue, translucent irides and albinotic fundal reflex; nystagmus and photophobia; increasing pigmentation with age	White hair and skin at birth; increasing pigmentation with yellow-red hair and light normal skin that tans; biochemically, intermediate reaction between tyrosinase positive and negative; stage III pheomelanosomes	Autosomal recessive; allelic with OCA1A; tyrosinase gene
OCA2 (tyrosinase-positive)	Eye color blue, yellow, or brown (age and race dependent); pigment cartwheel effect at pupil and limbus; red reflex minimal to absent in dark-skinned adults; moderate to severe nystagmus; photophobia; moderately severe visual defect; 20/80–20/100	Hair and skin color white at birth, darkening slightly by 2 years; melanosomes to early stage III polyphagosomes; hair bulbs develop pigmentation upon incubation in tyrosine; increased susceptibility to skin neoplasia; hyperkeratoses and freckling in exposed areas of skin	Autosomal recessive, chromosome 15q11.2–q12; P gene
Hermansky-Pudlak syndrome	Eye color blue-gray to brown (age and race dependent); iris normal to cartwheel effect; red reflex present in light-skinned individuals; mild to severe nystagmus and photophobia; slight to moderate decrease in visual acuity; high frequency in Puerto Rico	Platelet bleeding disorder, pulmonary fibrosis; hair color variable, white to dark red-brown; cream-colored skin; melanosis on exposed skin; pigmented nevi and freckles; susceptibility to skin neoplasia; serum tyrosine levels normal to decreased; platelet defect; ceroid storage, cytoplasmic bodies	Autosomal recessive, chromosome 10q2; HPS1 gene ADTB3A gene
OCA3 (Brown)	Blue to brown irides; transillumination of irides; retinal hypopigmentation; nystagmus; strabismus	Skin and hair light brown; freckles present; areas of hypopigmentation	Autosomal recessive, TRP-1 gene
Oculocerebral hypopigmentation (Cross syndrome)	Gray-blue eye color; cataracts; microphthalmos; nystagmus; blindness	White to light blond hair; white to pink skin; pigmented nevi; freckles; scanty melanosomes, stage III, some stage IV; oligophrenia; gingival fibromatosis; athetosis; urinary tract abnormalities	Autosomal recessive

Ocular	*X-linked form:* Marked deficiency of pigment in iris and choroid; nystagmus and myopic astigmatism; in blacks, may be limited to nystagmus, foveal hypoplasia, and tessellated fundus; mosaic pigment pattern in fundi *Autosomal recessive form:* Ocular signs as above, females as severely affected as males, and obligate heterozygotes have normal fundi	Normal pigmentation elsewhere; occasional hypopigmented cutaneous macules; giant melanosomes in normal skin; patients appear more lightly pigmented than their relatives May be the same as brown albinism	X-linked recessive, Xp22.3; *OA1* gene Autosomal recessive
Chédiak-Higashi syndrome	Partial albinism; diminished uveal and retinal pigmentation with photophobia and nystagmus On histologic examination: papilledema; lymphocytic infiltration of the optic nerve; leukocytes containing the typical metachromatic inclusion granules in the limbal area, iris, and choroid	Early death from recurrent infections; silver tinge to hair; neutropenia with tendency toward lymphocytosis, anemia, and thrombocytopenia, hepatosplenomegaly, lymphadenopathy; leukemia, lymphoma	Autosomal recessive, chromosome 1q42–43; *LYST* gene
Temperature sensitive (OCA1TS)	Similar to findings for OCA1A	White hair on warmer parts of body including scalp, darker hair on extremities	Autosomal recessive, allelic with OCA1A form due to a temperature-sensitive tyrosinase
OCA1MP (minimal pigment)	Vision 20/50–20/200; some iris pigment develops; foveal hypoplasia and nystagmus	Minimal hair and skin pigment; low tyrosinase levels	Autosomal recessive
With deafness	Typical ocular changes	Typical albinism with nerve deafness	X-linked recessive
Dominant oculocutaneous	Fine diffuse pattern of depigmentation on irides	Hypomelanism of skin, hair	Autosomal dominant, very rare

(Adapted and updated from Nelson LB, Calhoun JH, Harley RD, eds. *Pediatric Ophthalmology*. 3rd ed. Philadelphia: Saunders; 1991.)

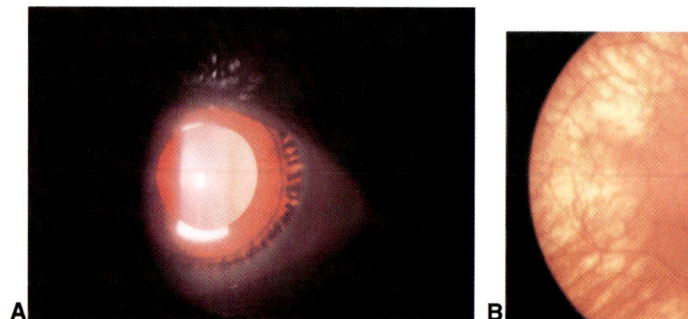

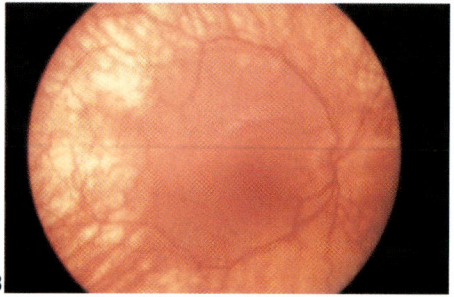

Figure 24-21 A, Transillumination of iris in albinism, right eye. **B,** Fundus in albinism, right eye, demonstrating complete lack of pigment and macular agenesis. In some incomplete forms of albinism, transillumination defects may be difficult to detect and retinal pigment may appear nearly normal, but the foveal reflex is absent.

ethnicity and other family members. Because pigment is present, motor nystagmus is a common misdiagnosis. The pigment such patients possess, however, does not protect against ultraviolet damage, and skin cancer is common unless sunscreen and skin protection are used starting in childhood. All children with nystagmus should undergo a careful examination that looks for iris transillumination defects and macular hypoplasia, which are diagnostic, before motor nystagmus is diagnosed.

Most children with albinism can attend regular schools with some assistance, but few see well enough to obtain a regular driver's license. Treatment is nonspecific and includes refraction, tinted glasses, and low-vision aids for older patients. When either Chédiak-Higashi albinism syndrome (with susceptibility to infections) or Hermansky-Pudlak syndrome (bleeding diathesis, more common in people of Puerto Rican descent) is suspected, hematologic consultation is advised because of the lethal nature of these forms of albinism.

> Creel D, Witkop CJ Jr, King RA. Asymmetric visually evoked potential in human albinos: evidence for visual system anomalies. *Invest Ophthalmol.* 1974;13:430–440.
>
> Kerr R, Stevens G, Manga P, et al. Identification of P gene mutations in individuals with oculocutaneous albinism in sub-Saharan Africa. *Hum Mutat.* 2000;15:166–172.
>
> Oetting WS, Summers CG, King RA. Albinism and the associated ocular defects. *Metab Pediatr Syst Ophthalmol.* 1994;17:5–9.

Familial Oculorenal Syndromes

Oculorenal syndromes include *Lowe (oculocerebral) syndrome.* This X-linked recessive disorder with renal defects presents in the first year of life, producing aminoaciduria, metabolic acidosis, proteinuria, hematuria, granular casts in the urine, and rickets. Affected children are mentally retarded, hypotonic, and areflexic. The biochemical defect is in a phosphatase important in Golgi complex vesicular transport. No specific treatment exists.

The most common eye defect is cataract. The lenses are small, thick, and opaque and may demonstrate posterior lenticonus. Congenital glaucoma may be present. Surgery is often difficult, with recurrent cyclitic membranes and recalcitrant glaucoma. Mothers of affected children may have punctate snowflake opacities within the lens cortex.

Lavin CW, McKeown CA. The oculocerebrorenal syndrome of Lowe. *Int Ophthalmol Clin.* 1993;33:179–191.

Alport syndrome is usually transmitted as an X-linked disorder but is autosomal recessive in approximately 10% of cases. It is a disorder of basement membranes that produces progressive renal failure, deafness, anterior lenticonus, cataract of the crystalline lens, and fleck retinopathy. Hematuria begins in childhood. Proteinuria and renal casts develop, with hypertension and kidney failure occurring late in the course of the disease. Mutations in collagen genes on the X chromosome or chromosome 2 are responsible for this disorder.

Colville D, Savige J, Morfis M, et al. Ocular manifestations of autosomal recessive Alport syndrome. *Ophthalmic Genet.* 1997;18:119–128.

Familial renal-retinal dystrophy is an autosomal recessive inherited condition characterized by interstitial nephritis and pigmentary retinal degeneration. Polyuria, polydipsia, and progressive azotemia are the rule. The eye signs and symptoms are characteristic of retinitis pigmentosa. Some patients who present early in life appear similar to those with Leber congenital amaurosis.

Clarke MP, Sullivan TJ, Francis C, et al. Senior-Loken syndrome. Case reports of two siblings and association with sensorineural deafness. *Br J Ophthalmol.* 1992;76:171–172.
Warady BA, Cibis G, Alon V, et al. Senior-Loken syndrome: revisited. *Pediatrics.* 1994;94:111–112.

Ocular findings in chronic renal disease are often those of hypertensive retinopathy. Diffuse retinal and disc edema are common. Nonrhegmatogenous bullous retinal detachments, usually involving the inferior retina, may occur. Calcium salts may be deposited in the cornea and conjunctiva. Punctate stippling of the lens capsule occurs in many patients with chronic renal disease, and dense lens opacities develop in some patients. Steroid-induced glaucoma and cataract may follow transplantation. Cytomegalic inclusion retinitis and *Candida* retinitis may develop following renal transplantation.

Cherry-Red Spot

The appearance of a cherry-red spot in the macula is caused by loss of transparency of the perifoveal retina due to edema or deposition of abnormal materials in the retinal ganglion cells. Ophthalmologists are often consulted to determine whether a cherry-red spot is present because such a spot may confirm the diagnosis of a number of disorders, especially some of the storage diseases. The most common causes of a cherry-red spot are:

- Tay-Sachs disease (GM_2 gangliosidosis type I)
- Sandhoff disease (GM_2 gangliosidosis type II)
- Niemann-Pick disease
- Sialidosis

- Farber lipogranulomatosis
- Metachromatic leukodystrophy
- GM$_1$ gangliosidosis
- Central retinal artery occlusion
- Trauma (retinal edema)

The cherry-red spot of storage diseases may disappear over time, so an absent spot should not be used to rule out a diagnosis, especially in older children. Even so, the presence of a cherry-red spot may be diagnostic. More detailed descriptions of the major storage diseases associated with cherry-red spot follow.

Gangliosidoses

In *GM$_1$ type I gangliosidosis,* all three β-galactosidase isoenzymes (hexosaminidase A, B, and C) are absent. This severe disease often occurs with congenital edema and hepatosplenomegaly. A cherry-red spot is present in 50% of patients. Acuity is greatly diminished, and pendular nystagmus is present. Tortuous conjunctival vessels with saccular microaneurysms, optic atrophy, occasional corneal clouding, papilledema, and high myopia may be present. Other features of this disease include psychomotor retardation, hypotonia, Hurler-like facial features, kyphosis, and congestive heart failure. Affected children usually die by age 2 years.

In *GM$_1$ type II gangliosidosis (Derry disease),* β-galactosidase isoenzymes B and C are lacking. There is no cherry-red spot, but nystagmus, esotropia, pigmentary retinopathy, and optic atrophy have been observed. The first sign is locomotor ataxia followed by progressive psychomotor deterioration and seizures. Affected children are decerebrate and rigid by the end of their second year of life. Death occurs between the ages of 3 and 10.

GM$_2$ type I gangliosidosis (Tay-Sachs disease) is caused by a deficiency in isoenzyme hexosaminidase A. A foveal cherry-red spot is characteristic by age 6 months, and vision is reduced by age 12–18 months. The pathological finding is the white ring resulting from accumulation of storage material in the ganglion cells around the normally pigmented macula. Nystagmus, optic atrophy, and narrowing of the retinal vessels develop. As the ganglion cells of the retina die, the cherry-red spot can disappear. Affected children become apathetic, hypotonic, and abnormally sensitive to sound. Seizures and progressive neurologic deterioration ensue, and patients usually die by age 24–30 months.

This disease is the most common of the gangliosidoses. It used to occur most often in persons of eastern European Jewish (Ashkenazi) descent. An effective genetic screening and counseling program in that population has reduced the number of cases of Tay-Sachs disease by 90% in the United States. Other groups such as French Canadians can also be affected more often than the general population. The heterozygous condition can be identified so that carriers can be counseled, and the homozygous state can be diagnosed in utero by amniocentesis.

In *GM$_2$ type II gangliosidosis (Sandhoff disease),* hexosaminidase A and B are absent. Ocular findings include decreased visual acuity, strabismus, inconspicuous corneal clouding, a prominent cherry-red spot, and normal-appearing optic nerves. This disorder has an ocular and systemic course similar to that of Tay-Sachs disease. Hepatosplenomegaly is not a conspicuous feature. Most affected children die as a result of progressive psychomotor deterioration by the age of 2–12 years.

In *GM₂ type III gangliosidosis (Bernheimer-Seitelberger disease)*, hexosaminidase A is partially deficient. The eye findings include late-onset visual loss, optic atrophy, and pigmentary retinopathy. No cherry-red spot appears. The disorder begins in early childhood with progressive psychomotor retardation, locomotor ataxia, speech loss, and spasticity. This disease leads to death before the age of 15 years.

The causative genes for many of the gangliosidoses are known, and carrier detection and treatment strategies are evolving.

Many other subtypes of gangliosidoses, with differing genetic defects, occur. Most present later in life with motor problems, and few have cherry-red spots.

> Chavany C, Jendoubi M. Biology and potential strategies for the treatment of GM2 gangliosidoses. *Mol Med Today.* 1998;4:158–165.
>
> Kivlin JD, Sanborn GE, Myers GG. The cherry red spot in Tay-Sachs and other storage diseases. *Ann Neurol.* 1985;17:356–360.

SCREENING EXAMINATION OF PREMATURE INFANTS FOR RETINOPATHY OF PREMATURITY

A Joint Statement of the American Academy of Pediatrics, Section on Ophthalmology; The American Association for Pediatric Ophthalmology and Strabismus; and the American Academy of Ophthalmology

Retinopathy of prematurity (ROP) is a retinal disorder of low birth weight premature infants potentially leading to blindness in a small but significant percentage of those infants. The results of the Multicenter Trial of Cryotherapy for Retinopathy of Prematurity Cooperative Group indicated that treament is associated with a 41% decrease in the occurrence of posterior retinal traction folds or detachments and a 19% to 24% decrease in the incidence of blindness when evaluated 5 years later.[1-3] Because of the sequential nature of the progression of ROP, the proven benefits of cryotherapy and, more recently, the acceptance of at least equivalent therapeutic benefit of laser therapy for the same indications,[4-7] standards of practice now demand carefully timed retinal examination of at-risk infants by an ophthalmologist experienced in the examination of preterm infants for ROP to minimize the risk of visual loss by those infants.

This statement outlines the principles on which a screening program to detect ROP in infants at risk might be based. The goal of an effective screening program must be to identify the relatively few preterm infants who require treatment for ROP from among the much larger number born each year while minimizing the number of stressful examinations required for these sick infants. Any screening program designed to implement an evolving standard of care has inherent defects, such as overreferral or underreferral, and cannot, by its very nature, duplicate the precision and rigor of a scientifically based clinical trial. With that in mind and on the basis of information published thus far, the sponsoring organizations of this statement suggest the following guidelines for the United States:

1. Infants with a birth weight of less than 1500 g or with a gestational age of 28 weeks or less, as well as selected infants between 1500 and 2000 g with an unstable

clinical course who are believed to be at high risk by their attending pediatrician or neonatologist, should have at least two fundus examinations performed after pupillary dilation using binocular indirect ophthalmoscopy to detect ROP. One examination is sufficient only if it unequivocally shows the retina to be fully vascularized bilaterally.

2. Examination for ROP should be performed by an ophthalmologist with sufficient regular experience and knowledge in the examination of preterm infants for ROP to identify the location and sequential retinal changes in this disorder using binocular indirect opthalmoscopy. The location and sequential retinal changes, if any, should be recorded using the *International Classification of Retinopathy of Prematurity.*[8]

3. The first examination should normally be performed between 4 and 6 weeks of chronologic (postnatal) age or, alternatively, within the 31st to 33rd week of postconceptional or postmenstrual age (gestational age at birth plus chronologic age), whichever is later, as determined by the infant's attending pediatrician or neonatologist. If using the postconceptional age guideline, examinations are generally not needed in the first 4 weeks after birth. The timing of the initial screening examination may be adjusted appropriately on the basis of other reliable data, such as local incidence and onset of ROP or the presence of other recognized risk factors.[8,9] The initial screening examination and subsequent examinations should be timed to permit sufficient time for treament, including any extra time required for transfer to another facility for treatment, if necessary. Treatment should be accomplished within 72 hours of determination of the presence of threshold 1 ROP to minimize the risk of retinal detachment before treatment.

4. Scheduling of follow-up examinations at the recommendation of the examining ophthalmologist is best determined by the finding at the first examination using the *International Classification of Retinopathy of Prematurity*. For example, if the retinal vasculature is immature and extends into zone II but no retinopathy is present, follow-up examination should be planned at approximately 2- to 3-week intervals until normal vascularization proceeds to zone III (ie, in the nasal periphery, there is no retinopathy and normal vessels are present within 1 disk diameter of the ora serrata).

5. Once an infant has been determined on first examination to be at risk for ROP, the following schedule is suggested:

    A. Infants with ROP that may soon progress to threshold ROP should be examined at least weekly. These include:

    1. Any infant with ROP less than threshold in zone I
    2. Infants with ROP in zone II, including:

        a. those with stage 3 ROP without plus disease (defined as posterior pole dilation and tortuosity of the retinal vessels);
        b. those with stage 2 ROP with plus disease; and
        c. those with stage 3 ROP with plus disease not yet extensive enough to justify ablative surgery.

B. Infants with less severe ROP in zone II should be examined at 2-week intervals. Those without ROP but with incomplete vascularization in zone I should be seen at 1- to 2-week intervals until retinal vascularization has reached zone III or until threshold conditions are reached.

C. If the retinal vascularization is incomplete in zone II but no ROP is detected, follow-up examination should be planned at approximately 2- to 3-week intervals until vascularization proceeds tinto zone III.

D. Retinas with incomplete vascularization only in zone III usually mature completely; ROP in zone III normally regresses (involutes) without adverse consequences. However, the finding or normal vascularization in zone III is unusual in the initial examination of very low gestational age infants. In cases in which zone III vascular maturation seems to be present on initial examination of very low birth weight infants, this finding should be verified by at least 1 repeat examination within 2 to 3 weeks.

6. Infants reaching threshold 1 disease (stage 3 ROP in zone I or II in 5 or more continuous clock hours or 8 cumulative clock hours [30° sectors] with plus disease [posterior retinal vessel dilation and tortuosity]) should receive ablative therapy for at least 1 eye within 72 hours of diagnosis, generally before the onset of retinal detachment. Stage 3 ROP with vascularization in zone I or borderline zone I to II may appear different from purely zone II stage 3 disease in that proliferation may appear flat, only appearing to be significantly elevated when it has become extremely severe. In view of this difficulty in distinguishing between stages 2 and 3 in posterior regions, infants with suspected stage 3 ROP in zone I or border zone I to II with plus disease should be examined especially carefully to determine if they meet the threshold criteria noted above.

7. Parents of infants with ROP should be informed of the nature and possible consequences of this disorder throughout the infant's hospital stay, beginning at the time of first diagnosis and continuing on an ongoing basis with updates on its progression during hospitalization.

8. Responsibility for examination and follow-up of infants at risk for ROP must be carefully defined by each neonatal intensive care unit. Unit-specific criteria for examination for ROP should be established for each neonatal intensive care unit by consultation and agreement between neonatology and ophthalmology services. These criteria should be recorded and should automatically trigger scheduled ophthalmology examinations. If hospital discharge or transfer to another neonatal unit or hospital is contemplated before retinal maturation into zone III has taken place, the availability of appropriate follow-up ophthalmologic examination must be ensured, and specific arrangement for that examination must be made before such discharge or transfer occurs. The transferring primary physician should have the responsibility of communicating orally and in writing what eye examinations are needed and their required timing to the infant's new primary physician. The new primary physician should ascertain the current ocular examination status of the infant from the record and through communication with the transferring physician so that any necessary examinations by an ophthalmologist with regular

experience and knowledge of the examination of preterm infants for ROP can be arranged promptly at the receiving facility. If responsibility for arranging follow-up after discharge is delegated to the parents, it must be clearly understood by the parents that blindness is a possible outcome, that there is a critical time window to be met if treatment is to be successful, and that timely follow-up examination is essential to successful treatment; this information should be transmitted to the parents orally and in writing. If such arrangements for follow-up after transfer or discharge cannot be made, the infant should not be transferred or discharged.

These recommendations replace the previous American Academy of Pediatrics statement on ROP,[10] are evolving, and may be modified as additional ROP risk factors, treatment, and long-term outcomes are known.

RETINOPATHY OF PREMATURITY SUBCOMMITTEE, 1997–2001
  Walter M. Fierson, MD, Chairperson
  Earl A. Palmer, MD
  Robert A. Petersen, MD
  Dale L. Phelps, MD
  Richard A. Saunders, MD
SECTION ON OPHTHALMOLOGY, 2000–2001
  Gary T. Denslow, MD, MPH, Chairperson
  Jay Bernstein, MD
  Edward G. Buckley, MD
  Allan M. Eisenbaum, MD
  George S. Ellis, Jr, MD
  Howard L. Freedman, MD
  Steven J. Lichtenstein, MD
CONSULTANT
  Harold P. Koller, MD, Immediate Past Chairperson
STAFF
  Stephanie Mucha
AMERICAN ASSOCIATION FOR PEDIATRIC OPHTHALMOLOGY AND
    STRABISMUS
AMERICAN ACADEMY OF OPHTHALMOLOGY

References

1. Cryotherapy for Retinopathy of Prematurity Cooperative Group. Multicenter trial of cryotherapy retinopathy of prematurity; preliminary results. *Arch Ophthalmol.* 1988;106:471–479.
2. Cryotherapy for Retinopathy of Prematurity Cooperative Group. Multicenter trial of cryotherapy retinopathy of prematurity; 3½ year outcome–structure and function. *Arch Ophthalmol.* 1993;111:339–344.
3. Cryotherapy for Retinopathy of Prematurity Cooperative Group. Multicenter trial of cryotherapy retinopathy of prematurity; Snellen visual acuity and structural outcome at 5½ years after randomization. *Arch Ophthalmol.* 1996;114:417–424.

4. McNamara JA, Tasman W, Brown GC, Federman JL. Laser photocoagulation for stage 3+ retinopathy of prematurity. *Ophthalmology.* 1991;98:576–580.
5. Hunter DG, Repka MX. Diode laser photocoagulation for threshold retinopathy of prematurity. A randomized study. *Ophthalmology.* 1991;100:238–244.
6. Laser ROP STudy Group. Laser therapy for retinopathy of prematurity. *Arch Ophthalmol.* 1994;112:154–156.
7. Iverson DA, Trese MT, Orgel IK, Williams GA. Laser photocoagulation for threshold retinopathy of prematurity. *Arch Ophthalmol.* 1992;109:1342–1343.
8. Committee for the Classification of Retinopathy of Prematurity. An international classification of retinopathy of prematurity. *Arch Ophthalmol.* 1984;102:1130–1134.
9. Hussain N, Clive J, Bhandari V. Current incidence of retinopathy of prematurity, 1989–1997. *Pediatrics.* 199;104(3). Available at: URL:http://www.pediatrics.org/cgi/content/full/104/3/e26.
10. American Academy of Pediatrics, American Academy of Ophthalmology, American Association for Pediatric Ophthalmology and Strabismus. screening exmination of premature infants for retinopathy of prematurity. *Pediatrics.* 1997;100:273. *Ophthalmology.* 1997;104:888–889.

Related Readings

Hutchinson AK, Saunders RA, O'Neil JW, et al. Timing of initial screening examination in retinopathy of prematurity. *Arch Ophthalmology.* 1998;116:608–612.

Palmer EA, Flynn JT, Hardy RH, et al. Incidence and early course of retinopathy of prematurity. *Ophthalmology.* 1991;98:1628–1640.

The recommendations in this statement do not indicate an exclusive course of treatment or serve as a standard of medical care. Variations, taking into account individual circumstances, may be appropriate.

©2001 by the American Academy of Pediatrics. No part of this statement may be reproduced in any form or by any means without written permission from the American Academy of Pediatrics except for one copy for personal use.

CHAPTER 25

Optic Disc Abnormalities

Developmental Anomalies

Morning glory disc anomaly

A striking congenital abnormality of the optic disc and surrounding retina, morning glory disc anomaly is due to either an abnormal closure of the embryonic fissure or abnormal development of the distal optic stalk at its junction with the primitive optic vesicle. Clinically, the anomaly appears as a funnel-shaped excavation of the posterior fundus that incorporates the optic disc. The surrounding retinal pigment epithelium is elevated, with an increased number of blood vessels looping at the edges of the disc (Fig 25-1). A central core of white glial tissue occupies the position of the normal cup. This tissue may have contractile elements, and the optic cup can actually be seen to open and close with some periodicity. Visual acuity can range anywhere from 20/20 to no light perception but in general is approximately 20/100 to 20/200. Serous retinal detachments can occur in approximately one third of affected patients, but the source of the subretinal fluid is unknown. Morning glory disc anomaly has been associated with basal encephalocele in patients with midfacial anomalies.

Coloboma of the optic nerve

Coloboma of the optic nerve may be part of a complete chorioretinal coloboma that involves the entire embryonic fissure, or the coloboma may involve only the proximal portion of the fissure, causing a deformity of the optic disc alone. Mild optic disc colobomas resemble deep physiologic cupping and may be confused with glaucomatous damage. More extensive disorders appear as an enlargement of the peripapillary area with a

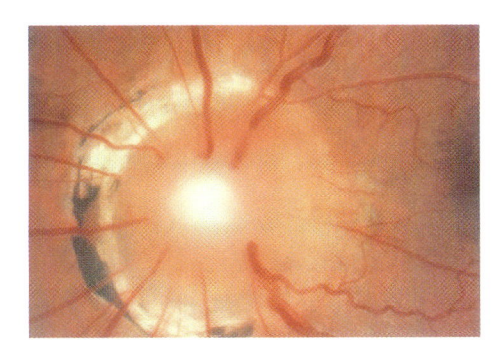

Figure 25-1 Morning glory disc anomaly, left eye.

deep central excavation lined by a glistening white tissue, with blood vessels crossing over the edge of this deep cavity (Fig 25-2). The defects usually extend inferonasally and are often associated with retinal coloboma in the periphery. Nonrhegmatogenous retinal detachments may occur. This condition may be unilateral or bilateral and can be very asymmetrical. Visual acuity may be mildly or severely decreased and is difficult to predict from the optic disc appearance. Ocular colobomas may also be accompanied by multiple systemic abnormalities (CHARGE association: *c*oloboma, *h*eart, *c*hoanal *a*tresia, mental *r*etardation, *g*enitourinary abnormalities, and *e*ar abnormalities—see Chapter 20.)

Brodsky MC. Congenital optic disk anomalies. *Surv Ophthalmol.* 1994;39:89–112.

Myelinated (medullated) retinal nerve fibers

Normal myelination starts at the lateral geniculate ganglion and stops at the lamina cribrosa. Occasionally, some of the fibers in the retina acquire a myelin sheath. Clinically, this appears as a white superficial retinal area with frayed and feathered edges that tends to follow the same orientation as the normal retinal nerve fibers (Fig 25-3). Retinal vessels that pass within the superficial layer of the nerve fibers are obscured. The myelinated fibers may occur as a single spot or in several noncontiguous isolated patches. The most common location is along the disc margin. Visual loss can occur if the macula is involved or from an associated anisometropic amblyopia due to unilateral high myopia. In these cases, the macula can also be hypoplastic. Treatment for amblyopia should be attempted but may be unsuccessful because of the macular pathology. Absolute scotomas occur in the visual field that corresponds to the area of the myelination.

Tilted disc syndrome (Fuchs coloboma)

In tilted disc syndrome, the superior pole of the optic disc appears elevated and the inferior nasal disc is posteriorly displaced, resulting in an oval-appearing optic disc with an obliquely oriented long axis (Fig 25-4). This condition is often accompanied by a scleral crescent located inferiorly or inferonasally, situs inversus (a nasal detour of the temporal retinal vessels as they emerge from the disc before turning back temporally), and posterior ectasia of the inferior nasal fundus.

Because of the fundus abnormality, affected patients have myopic astigmatism with the plus axis oriented parallel to the ectasia. Patients may demonstrate a bitemporal

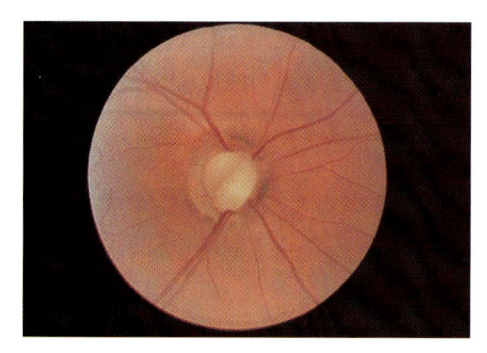

Figure 25-2 Optic nerve coloboma, right eye.

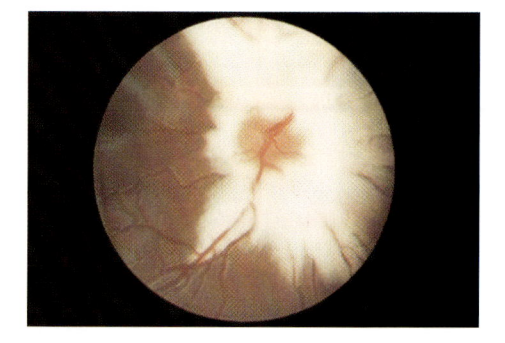

Figure 25-3 Myelinated nerve fibers of optic nerve and retina, right eye.

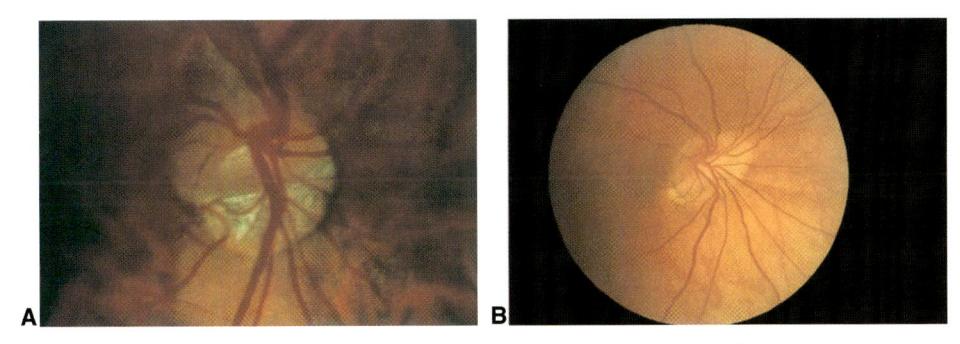

Figure 25-4 Tilted disc syndrome. **A,** Right eye. **B,** Left eye.

hemianopia, which is typically incomplete and preferentially involves the superior quadrants. The hemianopia can usually be distinguished from a chiasmal lesion because the defect does not respect the vertical midline. Large and small isopters are fairly normal; medium-sized isopters are severely constricted. Appropriate refractive correction often results in elimination of the visual field defect. Tilted discs, myopic astigmatism, bilateral decreased vision, and visual difficulty at night should suggest the possibility of X-linked congenital stationary night blindness (see Chapter 24).

Apple DJ, Rabb MF, Walsh PM. Congenital anomalies of the optic disc. *Surv Ophthalmol.* 1982;27:3–41.

Bergmeister papillae (persistent hyaloid artery)

Bergmeister papillae results when the hyaloid artery is not resorbed before birth. The entire artery may remain as a fine thread or cord extending from the optic disc to the lens and can be associated with persistent hyperplastic primary vitreous. The hyaloid artery may be patent and contain blood where it was attached to the posterior lens capsule. In mild cases, the attachment to the posterior lens capsule is located inferonasally (Mittendorfs dot) and is usually visually insignificant. When all that remains of the hyaloid artery is glial tissue on the disc in association with avascular prepapillary veils and epipapillary membranes, the term *Bergmeister's papillae* is used.

Megalopapilla

Megalopapilla features an abnormally large optic disc diameter and is often associated with an increased cup/disc ratio that can be confused with normal-tension glaucoma. Visual acuity is usually normal or slightly decreased, and visual fields may demonstrate a slightly enlarged blind spot. Rarely, megalopapilla has been associated with optic nerve glioma. The condition can be unilateral or bilateral, and the cause is unknown.

Optic nerve hypoplasia

Histologically, optic nerve hypoplasia is characterized by a decreased number of optic nerve axons of otherwise normal architecture. Clinically, the disc is pale and smaller than normal. This condition can be unilateral or bilateral and is often asymmetrical. It may be associated with a yellow to white ring around the disc *(double ring sign)* (Fig 25-5). Because the size of the surrounding ring often corresponds to the normal disc diameter, careful observation is necessary to avoid mistaking the entire hypoplastic disc/ring com-

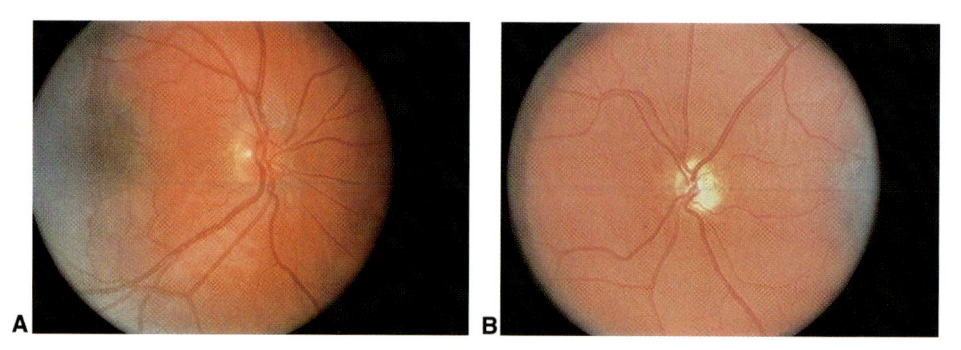

Figure 25-5 Optic nerve hypoplasia. **A,** Normal right optic nerve. **B,** Hypoplastic left optic nerve.

plex for a normal-sized disc. The vascular pattern is also abnormal and can be associated with too few or too many disc vessels. Retinal vascular tortuosity is common.

Visual acuity ranges from normal to light perception, and visual field defects are invariably present. Visual acuity is related to the integrity of the macular fibers and often does not correlate with the overall size of the disc. Because patients with optic nerve hypoplasia also have strabismus, unilateral visual loss may result from amblyopia and may respond to patching therapy.

The cause of optic nerve hypoplasia is multifactorial. Usually, this condition results from an insult in the first trimester as the optic nerves are developing. Any intrauterine damage to the visual pathway can result in optic nerve hypoplasia. Segmental hypoplasia occurs in some children of mothers with insulin-dependent diabetes.

Optic nerve hypoplasia has been associated with midline central nervous system anomalies consisting of absence of the septum pellucidum and agenesis of the corpus callosum. Septo-optic dysplasia *(de Morsier syndrome)* is occasionally accompanied by manifestations of hypothalamic and pituitary dysfunction, such as growth hormone deficiency, neonatal hypoglycemia, diabetes insipidus, panhypopituitarism, hyperprolactinemia, and hypothyroidism.

MRI is preferred for evaluating central nervous system abnormalities in patients with optic nerve hypoplasia. These abnormalities include small intracranial optic nerves, absent septum pellucidum, agenesis of the corpus callosum, and cerebral hemisphere abnormalities such as schizencephaly, leukomalacia, or encephalomalacia. Absence of the septum pellucidum or agenesis of the corpus callosum is not detectable by clinical evaluation. Neurodevelopmental defects, when present, are usually the result of associated cerebral hemispheric abnormalities.

During MRI, special attention should be directed to the pituitary infundibulum, where ectopia of the posterior pituitary may be found. Posterior pituitary ectopia appears on MRI as an absence of the pituitary infundibulum with an abnormal bright spot at the upper infundibulum area. This abnormality is present in approximately 15% of patients and suggests posterior pituitary hormone deficiency, requiring further endocrinologic workup.

The laboratory evaluation of patients with optic nerve hypoplasia is directed by their clinical appearance and MRI findings. A history of neonatal jaundice suggests hypothyroidism; neonatal hypoglycemia or seizures indicates possible panhypopituitarism. A T_4 level should be obtained in infants with optic nerve hypoplasia to rule out hypothyroidism. Because of the difficulty of measuring normal growth hormone levels, these values should not be assessed unless growth is retarded or MRI shows evidence of posterior pituitary ectopia. Patients with optic nerve hypoplasia and diabetes insipidus can have significant problems with thermal regulation and must be monitored carefully during febrile illnesses.

> Coston G, Murphree AL. Hypothalamic-pituitary function in children with optic nerve hypoplasia. *Am J Dis Child.* 1995;139:249–254.
>
> Hoyt WF, Kaplan SL, Grumbach MM, et al. Septo-optic dysplasia and pituitary dwarfism. *Lancet.* 1970;1:893–894.

Optic nerve aplasia
Optic nerve aplasia is rare. There are no optic nerve or retinal blood vessels, making the choroidal pattern clearly visible.

Optic pits or holes
The developmental defects of optic pits or holes can be considered similar to colobomas. Pits usually appear in the inferotemporal quadrant or central portion of the disc. A pit may be shallow or very deep, and it is usually unilateral and often covered with a gray veil of tissue. Optic pits have been associated with serous retinal detachments occurring mainly during the second and third decades of life (Fig 25-6).

Peripapillary staphyloma
Peripapillary staphyloma is a posterior bulging of the sclera in which the optic disc occupies the bottom of the bowl. The disc may be normal but is surrounded by stretched choroid, thereby exposing the white sclera encircling the disc. Visual acuity is usually poor.

Optic Atrophy

Optic atrophy in children usually results from anterior visual pathway disease (Table 25-1) such as inflammation (optic neuritis), hereditary optic atrophy, perinatal disease,

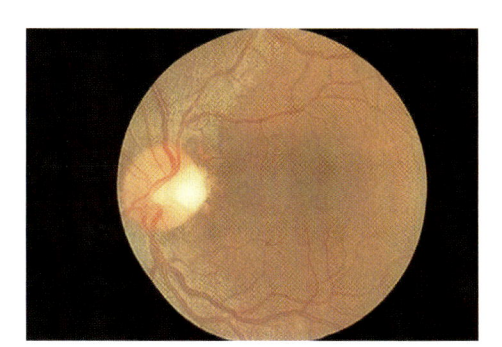

Figure 25-6 Temporal optic nerve pit with serous retinal detachment, left eye.

Table 25-1 **Causes of Acquired Optic Atrophy in Childhood**

> Craniopharyngioma
> Optic nerve/chiasmal glioma
> Retinal degenerative disease
> Hydrocephalus
> Optic neuritis
> Postpapilledema
> Hereditary

hydrocephalus, and optic nerve tumors. The workup should include neuroimaging in all cases of uncertain cause (negative family history, normal neurologic examination results) because a tumor or hydrocephalus is present in over 40% of these cases.

Hereditary Optic Atrophy

Bilateral slow loss of central vision in childhood may be due to hereditary optic atrophy. This condition usually begins before the age of 10 years with mild visual loss, ranging from 20/40 to 20/100. Visual fields show central or cecocentral scotomata with normal peripheral isopters. Color vision testing is diagnostic, revealing generalized dyschromatopsia. Clinically, the optic disc shows temporal pallor with an area of triangular excavation. Inheritance is usually autosomal dominant but can be recessive, and family pedigrees are hard to elicit. Long-term prognosis is good, with visual function rarely reduced to the 20/200 level.

A rare recessive optic atrophy can occur with severe bilateral visual loss before the age of 5. Nystagmus is present in approximately half of these patients. Funduscopic examination reveals a pale optic disc with vascular attenuation of the type characteristically seen in retinal degeneration. ERG results are normal, however.

Behr optic atrophy

A hereditary disorder, Behr optic atrophy occurs mainly in males, with onset in childhood. This condition is associated with increased deep tendon reflexes, cerebellar ataxia, bladder dysfunction, mental retardation, hypotonia of the extremities, and external ophthalmoplegia.

Leber hereditary optic neuropathy (LHON)

A maternally inherited (mitochondrial) disease, LHON is characterized by acute or subacute bilateral loss of central vision, acquired red–green dyschromatopsia, and central or cecocentral scotomata in otherwise healthy patients (usually males) in their second to fourth decade of life. Progressive atrophy results in a flat, pale disc with dense central scotoma. Clinically, this disorder presents as a low-grade optic neuritis with circumpapillary telangiectasia, pseudoedema of the disc, and absence of fluorescein staining. Pallor of the entire disc indistinguishable from primary atrophy generally develops within a few weeks after onset of visual disturbance. Final visual acuity is rarely better than 20/200. Associated neurologic abnormalities may include paraplegia, dementia, deafness, migraines, vertigo, spasticity, and a cardiac preexcitation arrhythmia *(Wolff-Parkinson-White)* syndrome.

LHON is transmitted by female carriers and involves the mitochondrial DNA (mtDNA). Primary mtDNA point mutations have been located at nucleotide positions 11778, 3460, and 14484. Molecular genetic analysis of mtDNA from leukocytes is currently available, and the finding of a primary mutation is pathognomonic for the disease. No effective treatment exists.

Optic Neuritis

Optic neuritis in childhood frequently presents after systemic infections such as measles, mumps, chickenpox, and viral illnesses (Fig 25-7). It can also be associated with immunizations. Visual loss can be severe and is often bilateral. In over half of affected children, the history suggests central nervous system involvement including headache, nausea, vomiting, lethargy, or malaise. Disc swelling, when present, can be extensive and may result in a macular star formation (*Leber idiopathic stellate neuroretinitis;* Fig 25-8).

The cause of this postinfectious form of viral optic neuritis is unknown. It has been speculated that a presumed autoimmune process, triggered by previous viral infection, may result in a demyelinative injury. Spontaneous recovery can occur, but visual function can be dramatically improved with intravenous corticosteroid treatment.

The relationship between optic neuritis and the development of multiple sclerosis, which is common in adults, is less clear in children. A small subset of children with optic neuritis eventually develop signs and symptoms consistent with multiple sclerosis within 1 year. Most of the neurologic deficits are minor, but disability can be severe. BCSC Section 5, *Neuro-Ophthalmology*, discusses the relationship between optic neuritis and multiple sclerosis at length.

> Steinlin MI, Blaser SI, MacGregor DL, et al. Eye problems in children with multiple sclerosis. *Pediatr Neurol.* 1995;12:207–212.

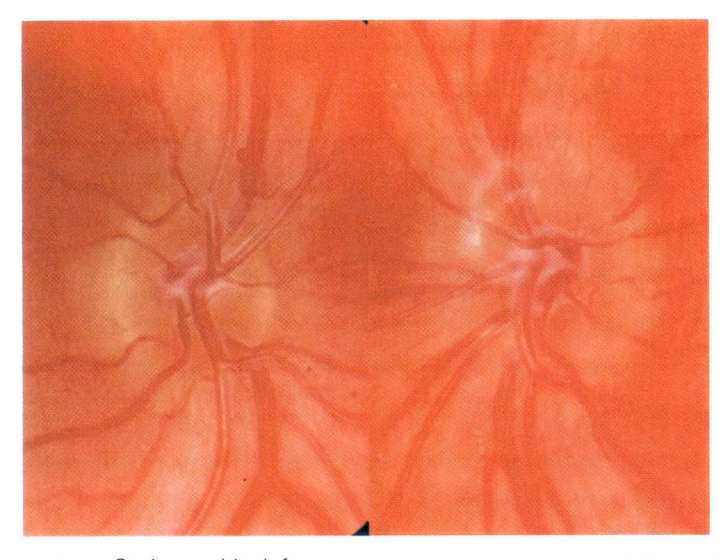

Figure 25-7 Optic neuritis, left eye. *(Photograph courtesy of Edward G. Buckley, MD.)*

Figure 25-8 Leber idiopathic stellate neuroretinitis.

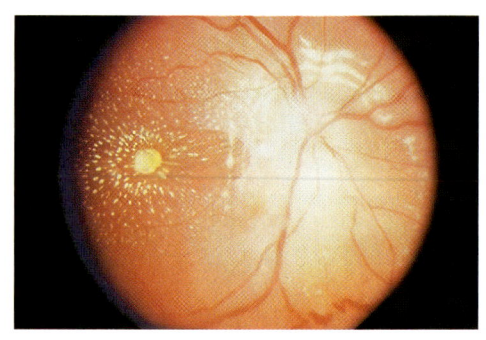

Papilledema

Increased intracranial pressure in children can be caused by hydrocephalus, a mass lesion, or pseudotumor cerebri. A full evaluation, including neuroimaging and lumbar puncture, is indicated. In infants, increased intracranial pressure results in firmness and distension of the open fontanelles. Significantly elevated pressure is usually accompanied by nausea, vomiting, and headaches. The older child may experience transient visual obscurations. Esotropia and diplopia may result from injury to the sixth nerve, which usually resolves once intracranial pressure is reduced.

Pseudotumor Cerebri

A benign condition, pseudotumor cerebri consists of increased intracranial pressure of unknown cause and duration. The presenting symptoms are headache and visual loss. Pseudotumor cerebri can occur in children of any age and has been associated with viral infections, drug use (tetracycline, corticosteroids, vitamin A, and nalidixic acid), thyroid medications, and venous sinus thrombosis. Often the cause is not determined. Ocular examination reveals excellent visual acuity with marked swelling of both optic nerves. The patient should be monitored closely for signs of visual loss and worsening headaches. Medical treatments include acetazolamide and corticosteroids. Repeated lumbar punctures have been used to control intracranial pressure, and optic nerve sheath fenestration has been shown to reduce the incidence of visual loss. Severe cases require lumbar or ventricular shunts. The visual prognosis is excellent: spontaneous resolution occurs in most cases within 12–18 months.

Pseudopapilledema

Pseudopapilledema refers to any elevated anomaly of the optic disc that resembles papilledema (Table 25-2). Disc anomalies that are frequently confused with papilledema in children include drusen, hyperopia, and prominent glial tissue. Pseudopapilledema can be differentiated from true papilledema by the absence of associated venous dilation and retinal hemorrhages or exudates and by the lack of any systemic findings that are usually associated with increased intracranial pressure.

Table 25-2 Conditions Associated With Pediatric Optic Disc Swelling

Papillitis
Optic neuritis (postinfectious)
Toxoplasmosis
Lyme disease
Bartonella infection
Neuroretinitis
Leber hereditary optic neuropathy
Toxocara infection of disc
Papilledema
  Intracranial mass
  Pseudotumor cerebri
    Dural sinus thrombosis
  Hypertension
  Cranial synostosis
  Hydrocephalus
    Chiari malformation
    Aqueductal stenosis
    Dandy-Walker syndrome
    Infection
Astrocytoma of optic disc (tuberous sclerosis)
Optic disc drusen
Hyperopia
Glial veils
Leukemia infiltrate

Drusen

Interpapillary *drusen*, which are the most common cause of pseudopapilledema in children, can appear within the first or second decade of life (Fig 25-9). Drusen are frequently inherited, and examination of the parents is helpful when drusen are suspected in children.

Clinically, the elevated disc does not obscure the retinal arterioles lying anteriorly and often has an irregular border suggesting the presence of drusen beneath the surface. There is no pallor, dilatation of the papillary network, exudates, or hemorrhages. When drusen are not buried, they appear as shiny refractile bodies visible on the surface with a gray-yellow translucent appearance. Visual defects are frequently associated; lower nasal field defects are most common. However, central defects, arcuate scotoma, and concentric narrowing can also occur. These defects can be slowly progressive, and central visual acuity is rarely affected.

Although most patients with drusen can be identified by simple funduscopic evaluation, occasionally it is difficult to tell for certain that drusen are responsible for the swollen disc appearance. B-scan ultrasonography can be helpful in this situation. This technique permits detection of bright objects in the end of the optic nerve. CT can also detect these particles.

    Arnold AC. Differential diagnosis of optic disc edema. In: *Focal Points: Clinical Modules for Ophthalmologists.* San Francisco: American Academy of Ophthalmology; 1999: vol 17, no 2.

348 • Pediatric Ophthalmology and Strabismus

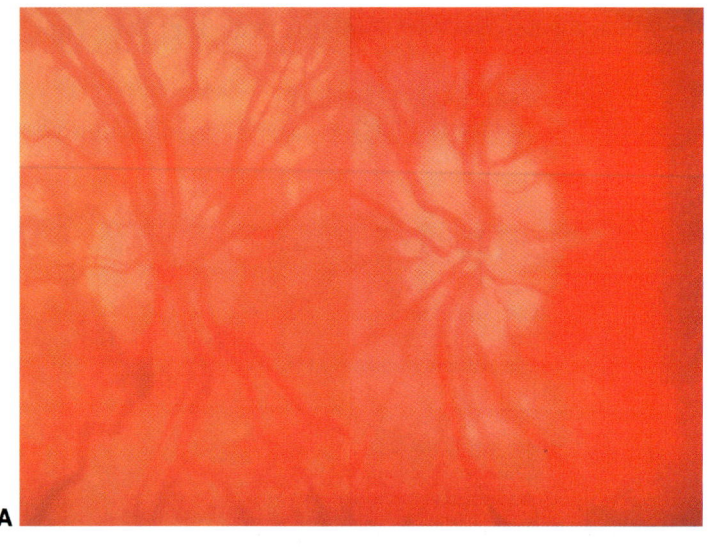

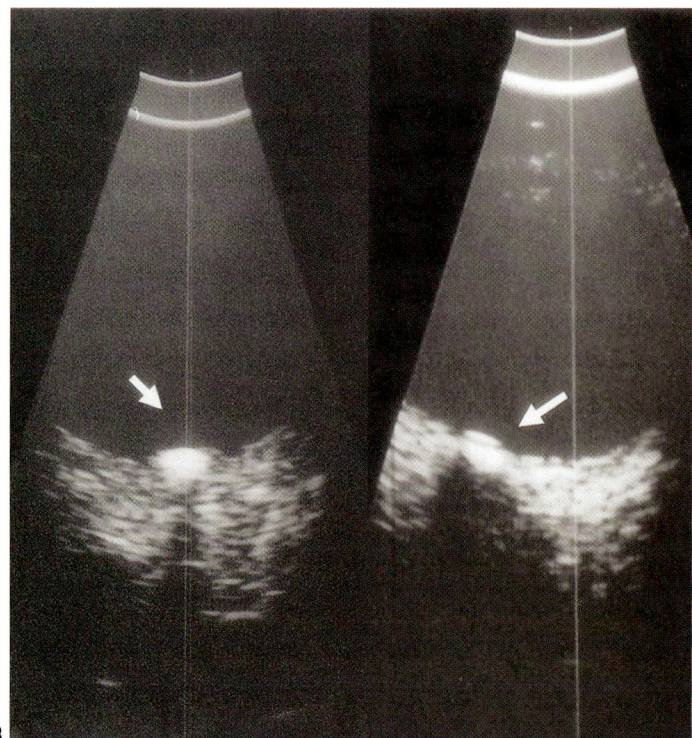

Figure 25-9 **A,** Optic nerve drusen, right eye. **B,** Ultrasound image of bright spot in nerve *(arrows)* consistent with drusen. *(Photographs courtesy of Edward G. Buckley, MD.)*

CHAPTER 26

Ocular Tumors in Childhood

Ocular and orbital tumors, both benign and malignant, occur relatively frequently in infants and children. Benign masses are much more common than malignant tumors in the orbital region. *Hamartomas*, defined as focal overgrowths of mature cells identical to those normally found at the site of origin but lacking normal tissue architecture and organization, also occur frequently.

Many tumors of childhood show variable qualities and are sometimes difficult to categorize. The overall incidence of ophthalmic malignancy is greater during the first 5 years of life than during any subsequent age interval until the sixth decade of life. Compared with other forms of childhood cancer, however, tumors with significant ocular involvement are uncommon, accounting for only about 4% of the total. See also BCSC Section 4, *Ophthalmic Pathology and Intraocular Tumors*.

Differential Diagnosis

The diagnosis of space-occupying lesions in the orbit is a particular challenge for the ophthalmologist because their clinical manifestations are relatively limited in variety and nonspecific:

- Proptosis or other displacement of the globe
- Swelling or discoloration of the eyelids
- Palpable subcutaneous mass
- Ptosis
- Strabismus

This list constitutes the presenting signs of most orbital tumors as well as numerous other disorders (Table 26-1).

The problem of differential diagnosis in childhood is compounded by the fact that, in young patients, both benign and malignant tumors often enlarge very rapidly, making them difficult to distinguish from one another, from infectious and inflammatory disorders such as orbital cellulitis, and from the effects of trauma, which occurs with high frequency and often without a reliable history. Furthermore, mild to moderate proptosis can be difficult to detect in an uncooperative child with associated eyelid swelling.

Typical presentations of the common benign orbital and periorbital masses in infants and children (capillary hemangioma, dermoid cyst) are sufficiently distinctive to permit confident clinical diagnosis in a large majority of cases. A malignant process should be

Table 26-1 Differential Diagnosis of Proptosis in Childhood

Malignant neoplastic
  Rhabdomyosarcoma
  Other primary sarcoma
  Metastatic neuroblastoma
  Extraocular retinoblastoma
  Other secondary tumor
  Leukemic infiltration
  Burkitt lymphoma
  Malignant histiocytosis

Benign proliferative
  Capillary hemangioma
  Lymphangioma
  Optic glioma
  Meningioma
  Fibrous dysplasia
  Ossifying fibroma
  Juvenile fibromatosis
  Eosinophilic granuloma

Infectious/inflammatory
  Cellulitis
  Sinus mucocele
  Echinococcal cyst
  Idiopathic pseudotumor

Traumatic
  Hematoma
  Foreign body
  Carotid cavernous fistula
  Encephalocele

Endocrine/metabolic
  Graves disease
  Osteopetrosis
  Infantile cortical hyperostosis

Developmental
  Infantile glaucoma
  Axial high myopia
  Craniofacial dysostosis
  Encephalocele
  Colobomatous cyst
  Dermoid cyst
  Teratoma

suspected when proptosis and eyelid swelling suggestive of cellulitis are *not* accompanied by warmth of the overlying skin, or when periorbital ecchymosis or hematoma develops in the absence of an unequivocal trauma history.

The current widespread availability of high-quality imaging permits orbital masses to be noninvasively differentiated with confidence in most cases. For initial diagnostic evaluation of the orbit, CT has advantages over MRI because of CT's high sensitivity to disturbances of bony architecture, its avoidance of interference from the high MRI signal intensity of orbital fat, and the greater ease of its use (although sedation is still generally required for young children). Dermoid cysts, teratomas, colobomatous cysts, and encephaloceles have highly distinctive appearances on CT, as do the blood-filled cavities found in acutely deteriorated lymphangiomas. The superior ability of MRI to differentiate various tissue types makes it a valuable adjunctive study in many cases, and its lack of radiation exposure is an advantage when repeated imaging is required. In experienced hands, ultrasonography may also provide important diagnostic information about the orbit.

Definitive diagnosis still often requires biopsy. A pediatric oncologist should be consulted and an appropriate metastatic workup should be completed before resorting to orbital surgery; sometimes, other more easily accessible sites can be used as tissue sources.

Pseudoproptosis can result from a mismatch between the volume of the globe and the capacity of the orbit. Examples include the elongation of the eyeball from infantile glaucoma or high myopia and the shallowness of the orbit in craniofacial syndromes with midfacial hypoplasia (sometimes called *exorbitism*). Confusion with orbital space-occupying lesions is unlikely to be a problem in such cases.

Musarella MA, Chan HSL, Gallie BL. Malignant pediatric ocular tumors: a sixty-year review from the Hospital for Sick Children. *Ophthalmol Clin North Am.* 1990;3:177–193.

Nicholson DH, Green WR. *Pediatric Ocular Tumors.* New York: Masson; 1981.

Orbital Tumors

A wide variety of space-occupying lesions can develop in the region of the orbit during childhood. Several of the most important pediatric malignancies show a predilection for orbital involvement. Benign adnexal masses are common and, in many cases, constitute a threat to vision. BCSC Section 7, *Orbit, Eyelids, and Lacrimal System*, and Section 4, *Ophthalmic Pathology and Intraocular Tumors*, also discuss and illustrate orbital tumors.

Meldrum ML. Pediatric orbital tumors. *Ophthalmol Clin North Am.* 1999;12:279–292.

Shields JA. *Diagnosis and Management of Orbital Tumors.* Philadelphia: Saunders; 1989.

Primary Malignant Neoplasms

Malignant diseases of the orbit include primary tumors arising from orbital tissue elements, secondary growth of solid tumors originating elsewhere in the body (metastasis), and abnormally proliferating cells of the hematopoietic or lymphoreticular systems. A large majority of primary malignant tumors of the orbit in childhood are sarcomas. Tumors of epithelial origin (eg, carcinoma of the lacrimal gland) are extremely rare.

Rhabdomyosarcoma

The most common primary pediatric orbital malignancy is rhabdomyosarcoma. The incidence of this disease (which is found in about 5% of orbital biopsies from children and adolescents) exceeds that of all other sarcomas combined. The orbit is the origin of 10% of rhabdomyosarcomas; an additional 25% develop elsewhere in the head and neck, occasionally involving the orbit secondarily. The average age of onset is about 5–7 years. Roughly 5% of cases manifest before age 1 year; 90% have occurred before age 16 years.

Proptosis is the usual presenting sign of orbital rhabdomyosarcoma and can develop rapidly (over a few days). Ptosis and strabismus are also common signs (Fig 26-1). The tumor can also arise as a localized mass in the eyelid or conjunctiva. CT or MRI demonstrates an irregular but well-circumscribed mass of uniform density.

A biopsy is required for confirmation of the diagnosis whenever rhabdomyosarcoma is suspected. The most common histopathologic type is *embryonal,* which shows few cells containing characteristic cross-striations. Second in frequency is the prognostically unfavorable *alveolar* pattern, showing poorly differentiated tumor cells compartmentalized by orderly connective tissue septa. The *botryoid* (grapelike) or well-differentiated *pleomorphic* tumors are rarely found in the orbit. The *botryoid* type may originate from conjunctiva.

Small encapsulated or otherwise well-localized rhabdomyosarcomas should be totally excised when possible. For larger or more extensive tumors, chemotherapy and radiation are now the mainstays of treatment; exenteration of the orbit is seldom indicated. Primary orbital rhabdomyosarcoma has the best prognosis of any site, with a long-term survival rate of nearly 90% in a large multicenter study.

> Wharam M, Beltangady M, Hays D, et al. Localized orbital rhabdomyosarcoma. An interim report of the Intergroup Rhabdomyosarcoma Study Committee. *Ophthalmology.* 1987; 94:251–254.

Other sarcomas

Osteosarcoma, chondrosarcoma, and *fibrosarcoma* can also develop in the orbit during childhood. The risk of these tumors increases in children with a history of heritable retinoblastoma, particularly when external-beam radiation treatment has been given.

Metastatic Tumors

In contrast with adults, children with secondary ocular malignancy are much more likely to show involvement of the orbit than the globe.

Neuroblastoma

One of the most common childhood cancers is neuroblastoma, the most frequent source of orbital metastasis. It usually originates in either the adrenal gland or the sympathetic ganglion chain in the retroperitoneum or mediastinum. Approximately 20% of all pa-

Figure 26-1 Rhabdomyosarcoma in a 4-year-old boy presenting with right upper eyelid ptosis of 3 weeks' duration and a palpable subcutaneous mass.

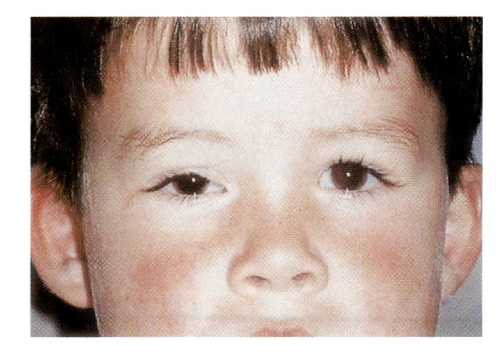

tients with neuroblastoma show clinical evidence of ocular involvement, which is sometimes the initial manifestation of the tumor.

Unilateral or bilateral proptosis and lid ecchymosis are the classic presentations of metastatic neuroblastoma (Fig 26-2). Patients may also have eyelid swelling, ocular motility disturbances, ptosis, and Horner syndrome caused by a thoracic tumor (Fig 26-3). *Opsoclonus*, characterized by rapid, multidirectional saccadic eye movements, is a unique paraneoplastic syndrome that is not related to orbital involvement and is associated with a good prognosis. Other signs and symptoms may include abdominal fullness and pain, venous obstructions and edema, hypertension caused by renal vascular compromise, and bone pain. Incisional biopsy showing small round blue cells confirms the diagnosis. Urinalysis for catecholamines is positive in 90%–95% of cases.

The mean age at diagnosis of patients with orbital neuroblastoma metastasis is about 2 years. Even with intensive treatment including radiation and chemotherapy, only about 10%–25% of affected patients survive. The prognosis for disseminated neuroblastoma is considerably better in infants under age 1 year than in older children.

Nonorbital neuroblastoma has a relatively good prognosis. In a recent series, long-term survival was documented in 11 of 14 cases of neuroblastoma with Horner syndrome and in all cases of opsoclonus.

Ewing sarcoma

Ewing sarcoma is a tumor composed of small round cells that usually originates in the long bones of the extremities or the axial skeleton. Ewing sarcoma is the second most frequent solid tumor source of orbital metastasis. Contemporary treatment regimens involving surgery, radiation, and chemotherapy permit long-term survival in many cases with disseminated disease.

Wilms tumor

One of the most common childhood cancers, Wilms tumor rarely metastasizes from the kidney to the orbit.

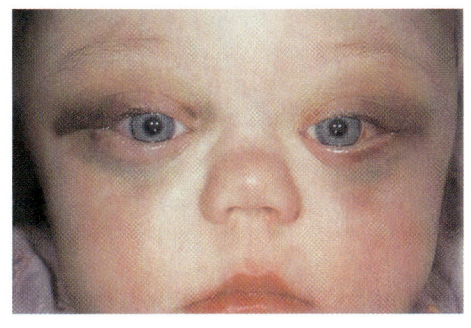

Figure 26-2 Bilateral orbital metastasis of neuroblastoma, presenting with periorbital ecchymosis in a 2-year-old girl.

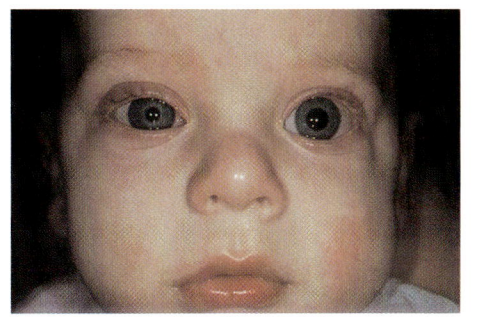

Figure 26-3 Right Horner syndrome, the presenting sign of localized intrathoracic neuroblastoma in a 6-month-old boy.

Leukemia

By far the most common malignancy of childhood, leukemia is acute in 95% of cases, more often lymphocytic than myelocytic. Aside from retinal hemorrhage, orbital infiltration (causing proptosis, eyelid swelling, and ecchymosis) is leukemia's most frequent clinically evident ocular manifestation, occurring in 1%–2% of patients. Infiltration of the optic nerve by leukemic cells may cause optic disc edema and loss of vision, requiring prompt treatment with low-dose radiation.

Granulocytic sarcoma, or *chloroma* (in reference to the greenish color of involved tissue), is a localized accumulation of leukemic cells in the orbit more characteristic of myelocytic than of lymphocytic disease in childhood. This lesion typically develops several months before leukemia becomes hematologically evident.

> Davis JL, Parke DW II, Font RL. Granulocytic sarcoma of the orbit. A clinicopathologic study. *Ophthalmology.* 1985;92:1758–1762.

Lymphoma

In contrast with adult disease, lymphoma in children very rarely involves the orbit. Burkitt lymphoma, endemic to east Africa and uncommon in North America, is the most likely form to involve the orbit.

Histiocytosis X (Langerhans cell histiocytosis)

Histiocytosis X is the collective term for a group of disorders involving abnormal proliferation of histiocytes, often within bone. More specifically, the cells are of the dendritic type, which are considered to be immune accessory or antigen-processing and -presenting cells as opposed to phagocytic cells. *Eosinophilic granuloma*, the most localized and benign form of histiocytosis, produces bone lesions that involve the orbit, skull, ribs, and long bones in childhood or adolescence. Symptoms may include proptosis, ptosis, and periorbital swelling, and localized pain and tenderness are relatively common. Radiography and CT characteristically demonstrate sharply demarcated osteolytic lesions without surrounding sclerosis (Fig 26-4). Treatment consists of observation of isolated asymptomatic lesions, excision of painful and easily accessible lesions, systemic corticosteroid administration, or low-dose radiation; all modalities have a high rate of success.

Hand-Schüller-Christian disease is a more disseminated and aggressive form of histiocytosis X that is likely to produce proptosis from involvement of the bony orbit in childhood. Diabetes insipidus is common. Chemotherapy is often required, but prognosis

Figure 26-4 Axial CT image showing eosinophilic granuloma with partial destruction of the right posterior lateral orbital wall in a 15-year-old boy, who presented with retrobulbar pain and mild edema and erythema of the right upper eyelid.

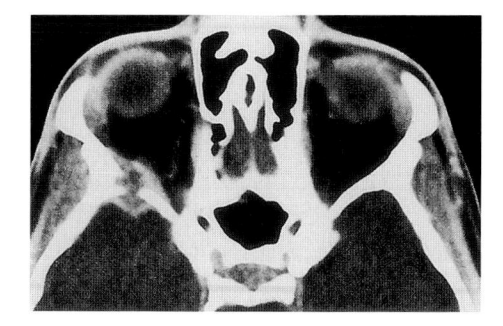

is generally good. Children with this condition usually present between ages 2 and 5 years.

Letterer-Siwe disease is the most severe and malignant variety, usually affecting infants younger than 2 years. It is characterized by soft tissue lesions of multiple viscera (liver, spleen) but rarely involves the eye.

Huang F, Arceci R. The histiocytoses of infancy. *Semin Perinatol.* 1999;23:319–331.

Benign Tumors

Capillary hemangioma

Capillary hemangioma is one of the most common benign orbital tumors in childhood, with a female-to-male predominance of at least 2:1. Pathological examination shows proliferated endothelial cells and small vascular channels, contrasting with the large blood-filled spaces found in adult-onset cavernous hemangioma of the orbit. Most periocular capillary hemangiomas involve primarily the upper eyelid, with variable extension into the orbit and surrounding tissues. Usually, the skin has a characteristic raised, red, dimpled appearance *(strawberry nevus)*, but some lesions are entirely subcutaneous, appearing as a smooth, firm swelling or fullness with dark red to bluish discoloration of the overlying skin (Fig 26-5). Axial proptosis or other displacement of the globe indicates a significant intraorbital component. The mass may swell when the baby cries as a result of venous congestion from increased intrathoracic pressure. Many affected children show similar lesions elsewhere on the skin.

About 30% of capillary hemangiomas are evident at birth, and 95% are recognized by age 6 months. Typically, they appear quite small and insignificant at first but then undergo a period of alarmingly rapid growth during the first few months of life. Maximum size is usually reached between ages 6 and 12 months. Spontaneous involution begins during the second year of life, initially manifested as lightening or graying of color in the central portion of the lesion. This process leads to complete regression in about 40% of cases by age 4 years and 80% by age 8 years.

Approximately half of children with eyelid or orbital hemangiomas develop some degree of amblyopia, usually resulting from anisometropic astigmatism oriented toward the lesion (ie, a superonasal lesion of the right eye would require plus-cylinder correction with an axis of about 45°). Ptosis is common and can cause deprivation amblyopia. Strabismus develops in approximately one third of cases. Optic atrophy, exposure kera-

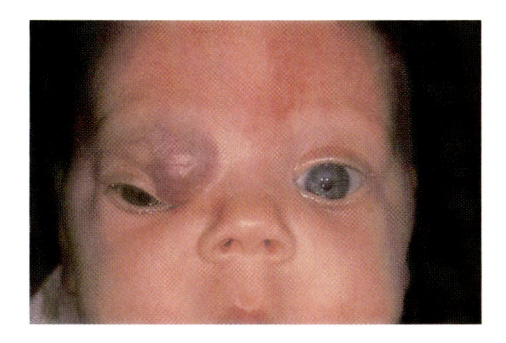

Figure 26-5 Capillary hemangioma in a 2-month-old girl involving the right upper eyelid and orbit with displacement of the globe and induction of 8 D of astigmatic refractive error.

titis, and ulceration of the skin with bleeding and secondary infection are relatively rare complications in severe cases. Massive capillary hemangiomas may be associated with thrombocytopenia as a result of platelet sequestration within the lesion *(Kasabach-Merritt syndrome)*. *PHACES syndrome* (*p*osterior fossa malformations, *h*emangiomas, *a*rterial anomalies, *c*oarctation of the aorta and other cardiac defects, *e*ye abnormalities, and *s*ternum abnormalities) can be associated with increased intraocular pressure.

Early treatment is indicated for capillary hemangioma when amblyopia is a serious concern and conventional measures (refractive correction, patching) are judged inadequate. Treatment should be performed in conjunction with the child's pediatrician, who is familiar with the proper dosages and possible side effects of the medications employed.

The therapeutic approach currently preferred by many pediatric ophthalmologists is intralesional injection of corticosteroids. A total volume of about 1–2 mL of short- and longer-acting agents (usually 40 mg triamcinolone acetate and 6 mg of a preparation consisting of betamethasone acetate and betamethasone phosphate) combined in 1:1 mixture is injected percutaneously with a fine needle deep into the lesion. After corticosteroid injection, shrinkage of the tumor proceeds most rapidly during the first 2 weeks but it can continue at a slower rate for several months. Sometimes the response is dramatic, leading to almost complete disappearance of the lesion, but more often the size reduction is moderate; occasionally, little or no improvement occurs. Injection may be repeated up to three or four times at intervals of 6 weeks or longer if initial treatment produces a partial but inadequate effect. No definite correlation between responsiveness to treatment and any characteristic of the lesion or patient has been recognized.

Infrequent but potentially serious reported complications of intralesional corticosteroid injection include depigmentation of the overlying skin and subcutaneous fat atrophy (both of which may be temporary), eyelid necrosis, and central retinal artery occlusion by particles of the drug. Subcutaneous whitish crystalline deposits often persist for months at the injection site. The possibility of pituitary-adrenal suppression that may retard growth must be kept in mind, especially with small infants.

Oral corticosteroid administration (recommended dosages of prednisone range from 1 to 3 mg/kg/day or equivalent) is an alternative to injection that deserves consideration, particularly if the lesion is extensive; however, withdrawal of medication may cause rebound enlargement. In some cases, treatment of periocular hemangiomas with recombinant interferon-α2b or topical clobetasol propionate has been effective. When systemic or intralesional corticosteroids are to be used, the child's pediatrician should be notified.

In selected patients, the tumor has been completely or partially excised as a primary treatment. Hemangiomas that are small, well circumscribed, and not superficial are the best candidates for surgical removal. Because of the highly vascular nature of these tumors, excision is often difficult and meticulous dissection is necessary. Excision of residual tumor tissue with reconstructive surgery after steroid treatment may be necessary if significant disfigurement persists. This cosmetic intervention should be delayed until school age to take advantage of the natural regression that occurs with these tumors.

Haik BG, Karcioglu ZA, Gordon RA, Pechous BP. Capillary hemangioma (infantile periocular hemangioma). *Surv Ophthalmol.* 1994;38:399–426.

Kushner BJ. Hemangiomas. *Arch Ophthalmol.* 2000;118:835–836.

Lymphangioma

The second most common orbital tumor of vascular origin in childhood is lymphangioma. This lesion consists largely of lymph-filled channels lined by endothelium and separated by thin delicate walls containing small blood vessels that are easily disrupted and tend to hemorrhage spontaneously or after minor trauma. Lymphangiomas tend to infiltrate orbital tissues extensively, but occasionally these tumors are localized to the eyelids or conjunctiva (Fig 26-6). In most cases, orbital lymphangioma initially manifests with gradual development of mild proptosis during the first few years of life. Episodes of rapid enlargement with markedly increased proptosis can result from either hyperplasia of lymphoid tissue within the mass (typically induced by upper respiratory infection) or intralesional bleeding. Such a development occurring between ages 5 and 15 years may in fact be the first indication of a problem.

Complete excision of an orbital lymphangioma is difficult. No treatment is indicated when the only symptom is mild proptosis, and biopsy should be avoided if possible because of the risk of inducing hemorrhage. Surgical evacuation of the hematoma should be considered when CT or MRI shows large blood-filled cavities, indicating acute hemorrhagic deterioration, if it is accompanied by intractable pain, nausea, and vomiting or if development of an afferent pupillary defect indicates that the optic nerve is threatened. Otherwise, conservative management, such as activity restriction, cold compresses, or lubricating ointment for corneal exposure, is recommended.

   Muallem MS, Garzozi HJ. Conservative management of orbital lymphangioma. *J Pediatr Ophthalmol Strabismus.* 2000;37:41–43.
   Wright JE, Sullivan TJ, Garner A, et al. Orbital venous anomalies. *Ophthalmology.* 1997; 104:905–913.

Other vascular tumors

Other orbital tumors composed of vascular elements are rare in childhood. *Hemangiopericytoma* is a generally benign lesion with a tendency to become locally invasive, which makes the long-term prognosis guarded. *Orbital varix* is a venous malformation that usually does not become clinically evident until early adulthood, although this tumor may cause intermittent proptosis in childhood, typically associated with the prone position or Valsalva maneuver.

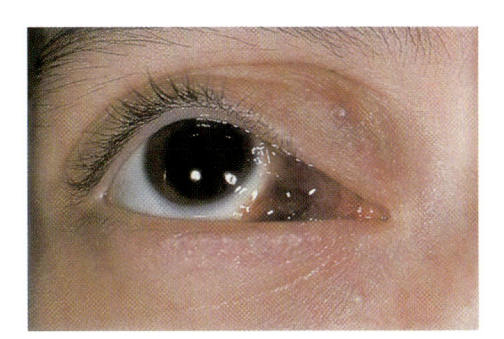

Figure 26-6 Lymphangioma with hemorrhage involving the right orbit, upper eyelid, and conjunctiva in a 15-year-old girl.

Tumors of bony origin

A variety of uncommon benign orbital tumors of bony origin may present during the early years of life with gradually increasing proptosis. *Fibrous dysplasia* and *ossifying fibroma* are similar disorders characterized by destruction of normal bone and its replacement by fibroosseous tissue. In both conditions, orbital radiography and CT show varying degrees of lucency and sclerosis.

Fibrous dysplasia has a slow progression that ceases when skeletal maturation is complete. The most serious complication is visual loss caused by optic nerve compression, which may occur acutely. Periodic assessment of vision, pupil function, and optic disc appearance is indicated. Surgical treatment is indicated for functional deterioration or significant disfigurement.

Histopathologically, ossifying fibroma is distinguished by the presence of osteoblasts. Ossifying fibroma tends to be a more locally invasive lesion than fibrous dysplasia; some authorities recommend early excision.

Brown tumor of bone is an osteoclastic giant cell reaction resulting from hyperparathyroidism. *Aneurysmal bone cyst* is a degenerative process in which normal bone is replaced by cystic cavities containing fibrous tissue, inflammatory cells, and blood, producing a characteristic radiographic appearance.

Tumors of connective tissue origin

Benign orbital tumors originating from connective tissue are rare in childhood. *Juvenile fibromatosis* may present as a mass in the inferior anterior portion of the orbit. These tumors, sometimes called *myofibromas* or *desmoid tumors,* are composed of relatively mature fibroblasts. They tend to recur locally after excision and can be difficult to control, but they do not metastasize.

Tumors of neural origin

Optic nerve glioma is the most important orbital tumor of neural origin in childhood. About 50% of these cases are associated with type 1 neurofibromatosis. *Plexiform neurofibroma* nearly always occurs in the context of neurofibromatosis and not infrequently involves the eyelid and orbit. (These tumors are discussed fully in Chapter 27.) Orbital *meningioma* and *schwannoma* (neurilemoma, neurinoma) are rare prior to adulthood and also usually appear in patients with neurofibromatosis. Meningioma typically presents with progressive visual loss, mild proptosis, and restriction of ocular motility; a large majority of patients are female. Childhood meningiomas tend to be locally aggressive and should be totally excised if possible, unless the involved eye retains good vision.

Dutton JJ. Gliomas of the anterior visual pathway. *Surv Ophthalmol.* 1994;38:427–452.

Ectopic Tissue Masses

The term *choristoma* is applied to growths consisting of normal cells and tissues appearing at an abnormal location. They may result from abnormal sequestration of germ layer tissue during embryonic development or from faulty differentiation of pluripotential cells. Masses composed of such ectopic tissue growing in the orbit can also be a consequence of herniation or outpouching of tissue from adjacent structures.

Cystic lesions

Dermoid cysts are benign developmental choristomas thought to be the most common space-occupying orbital lesions of childhood. These cysts are congenital, arising from rests of primitive dermal elements that have been sequestered in fetal suture lines at the time of closure. The tissue forms a cyst lined with keratinized epithelium and dermal appendages, including hair follicles, sweat glands, and sebaceous glands. Cysts containing squamous epithelium without dermal appendages are called *epidermoid cysts.*

Orbital dermoid cysts have been classified into juxtasutural, sutural, and soft tissue types. The juxtasutural type is adjacent but not demonstrably attached to the bony suture line. This is the most common type in children and is the most common type to arise in the superonasal and superotemporal quadrants (Fig 26-7). A sutural dermoid cyst extends into the bony suture line. Soft tissue or complicated dermoids usually present in adulthood.

Clinically, the juxtasutural dermoid cyst in children presents as a painless mass that is unattached to overlying skin and is mobile, smooth, and nontender. Episodes of inflammation may occur with small ruptures of the cyst wall and consequent extrusion of cyst contents into the surrounding tissue. Most patients have no visual symptoms. Sutural and soft tissue dermoids present differently. The soft tissue dermoid grows slowly over many years and often presents with proptosis. Sutural dermoids may present as a mass or as proptosis with chewing from pressure of the masseter on the extraocular portion of the tumor. CT confirms the diagnosis, revealing a well-circumscribed lesion with a low-density lumen and often bony remodeling. Deeper orbital lesions may show complete bony defects.

Management of dermoid cysts is surgical. Surgery is delayed until the risk of general anesthesia is outweighed by the possibility of accidental rupture from trauma, usually around age 1 year. For the juxtasutural dermoid cyst, an infrabrow or eyelid crease incision is used and the cyst is carefully dissected. If possible, rupture of the cyst at the time of surgery is avoided to limit lipogranulomatous inflammation and scarring. If the cyst is entered, the site should be irrigated. Sutural cysts often cannot be removed intact because of their communication into or through bone. Care is taken to remove all

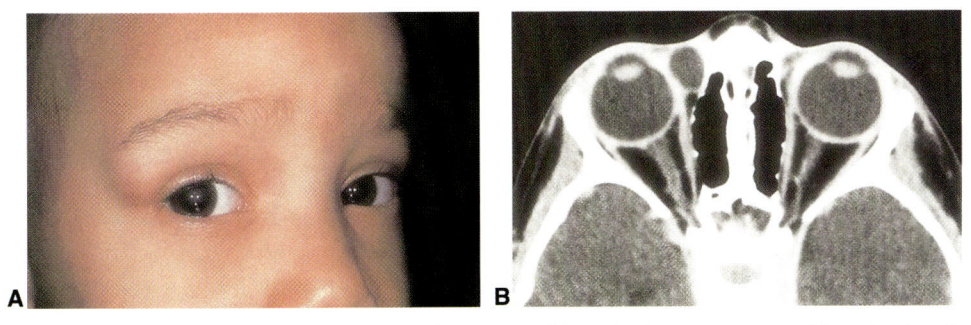

Figure 26-7 A, Periorbital dermoid cyst, right eye, with typical superotemporal location in a 3-year-old girl. **B,** Axial CT image showing a dermoid cyst of the superonasal anterior orbit, right eye, in a 6-year-old boy.

remaining cyst lining to limit the possibility of recurrence. Soft tissue cysts are removed by way of a transconjunctival or lateral orbitotomy.

> Shields JA, Kaden IH, Eagle RC Jr, et al. Orbital dermoid cysts: clinicopathologic correlations, classification, and management. The 1997 Josephine E. Schueler Lecture. *Ophthal Plast Reconstr Surg.* 1997;13:265–276.

Teratomas

Choristomatous tumors that contain multiple tissues derived from all three germinal layers (ectoderm, mesoderm, and endoderm) are known as *teratomas*. Skin and dermal appendages, neural tissue, muscle, and bone are typically present; endodermal elements such as respiratory and intestinal tract epithelium are less consistently found. Most teratomas are partially cystic with varying fluid content. Orbital teratomas account for a very small fraction of both orbital tumors and teratomas in general, which usually arise in the gonads or sacrococcygeal region. The clinical presentation of orbital teratomas is particularly dramatic, however, with massive proptosis evident at birth (Fig 26-8). In contrast with teratomas in other locations, which tend to show malignant growth, most orbital lesions are benign. Surgical excision, facilitated by prior aspiration of fluid, can often be accomplished without sacrificing the globe. Permanent optic nerve damage from stretching and compression usually results in poor vision in the involved eye.

Ectopic lacrimal gland

A rare choristomatous lesion, ectopic lacrimal gland may present with proptosis in childhood. Cystic enlargement and chronic inflammation sometimes aggravate the problem.

Sudoriferous cyst

Originating from ectopic apocrine gland tissue resembling that found in the eyelid glands of Moll, the sudoriferous cyst is a rare lesion of the eyelid or anterior orbit in childhood.

Colobomatous cyst

Also known as *microphthalmos with cyst,* the colobomatous cyst is composed of tissues that originate from the eye wall of a malformed globe with posterior segment coloboma. Most fundus colobomas show some degree of scleral ectasia, resulting from a deficiency of tissue in the region where apposing edges of the embryonic neuroectodermal fissure have failed to fuse properly. In extreme cases, a bulging globular appendage grows to

Figure 26-8 Congenital cystic teratoma originating in the left orbit of a 1-day-old girl.

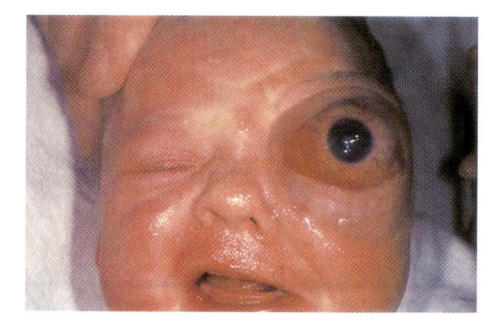

become as large as or larger than the globe itself, which is invariably microphthalmic, sometimes to a marked degree.

Like other colobomatous malformations, microphthalmos with cyst may occur either as an isolated congenital defect or in association with a variety of intracranial or systemic anomalies. Frequently, the other eye shows evidence of coloboma as well. The wall of a colobomatous cyst consists of thin sclera lined by rudimentary tissue of neuroectodermal origin, occasionally incorporating hyperplastic glial tissue accumulations; the cyst contains aqueous fluid with a few suspended cells. The usual location is inferior or posterior to the globe, with which the cyst is always in contact. The cyst interior communicates with the vitreous cavity, sometimes through a channel so small it is undetectable even with high-resolution imaging.

Posteriorly located colobomatous cysts may or may not cause proptosis, depending on the size of the globe and the cyst. Inferiorly located cysts present as a bulging of the lower eyelid or a bluish subconjunctival mass (Fig 26-9). Occasionally, the globe is pushed so far superiorly that it disappears behind the upper eyelid. If fundus examination does not make the diagnosis obvious, other possibilities can be excluded by using CT, MRI, or ultrasonography to demonstrate a cystic lesion with the uniform internal density of vitreous attached to the globe. No treatment is necessary unless disfigurement is a problem. Aspiration of cyst fluid provides relief of varying duration; reaccumulation may be retarded or prevented by placement of a cosmetic shell behind the eyelids. For more definitive treatment, surgical excision is indicated. The globe can sometimes be preserved; in other cases, the globe must be removed with the cyst.

Weiss A, Martinez C, Greenwald M. Microphthalmos with cyst: clinical presentations and computed tomographic findings. *J Pediatr Ophthalmol Strabismus*. 1985;22:6–12.

Mucocele

Mucoceles are cystic lesions that originate from the paranasal sinuses and may expand over time, potentially causing destruction of bone and possibly eroding into the orbit or intracranial space. These lesions most commonly arise from the frontal or anterior eth-

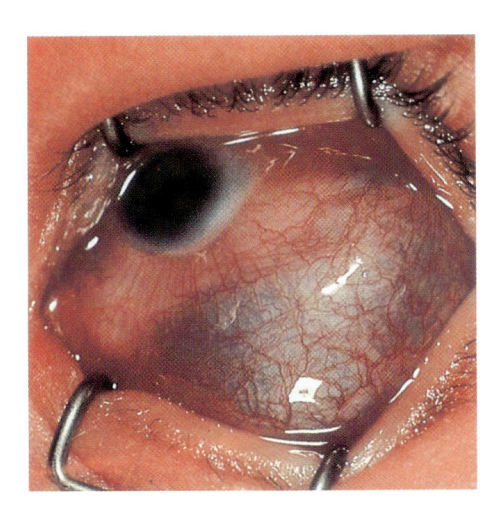

Figure 26-9 Colobomatous cyst (microphthalmos), left eye.

moidal sinuses with inferior or medial displacement of the globe. The differential diagnosis includes encephalocele with skull base deformity. Treatment involves reestablishing normal sinus drainage and removing the cyst wall.

Encephalocele or meningocele

Encephaloceles or meningoceles in the orbital region may result from a congenital bony defect that permits herniation of intracranial tissue or may develop after trauma that disrupts the bone and dura mater of the anterior cranial fossa. Intraorbital location leads to proptosis or downward displacement of the globe. Anterior presentation takes the form of a subcutaneous mass, typically located above the medial canthal ligament. Pulsation of the globe or the mass from the transmission of intracranial pulse pressure is characteristic. Neuroimaging readily confirms the diagnosis of this rare condition.

Childhood Orbital Inflammations

Several noninfectious, nontraumatic disorders that may simulate an orbital mass lesion deserve brief mention. *Graves disease*, the most common cause of proptosis in adults, rarely occurs in prepubescent children but occasionally affects adolescents (Fig 26-10). (See also Chapter 11.)

Idiopathic orbital inflammatory disease (orbital pseudotumor)

Idiopathic orbital inflammatory disease is an inflammatory cause of proptosis in childhood that differs significantly from the adult form. The typical pediatric presentation is acute and painful, resembling orbital cellulitis more than tumor or Graves ophthalmopathy (Fig 26-11). Bilaterality and episodic recurrence are common, as are associated systemic manifestations such as headache, fever, nausea and vomiting, and lethargy. Uveitis is common and occasionally constitutes the dominant manifestation. Imaging studies

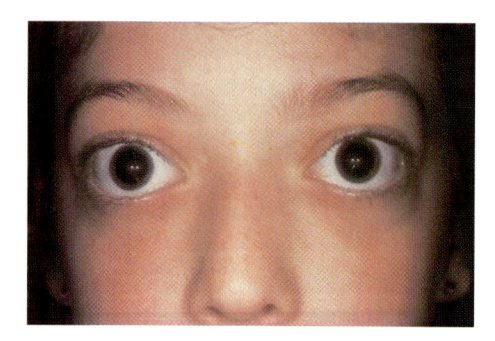

Figure 26-10 Graves disease with bilateral exophthalmos in a 15-year-old girl.

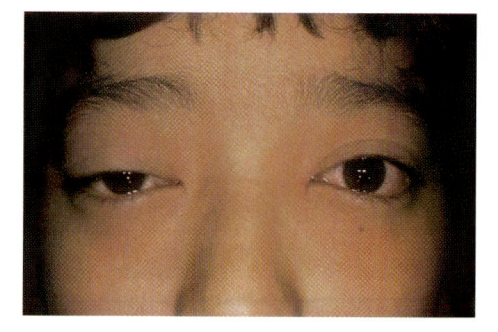

Figure 26-11 Bilateral idiopathic orbital inflammatory disease (orbital pseudotumor) in an 11-year-old boy with a 1-week history of eye pain. Ocular rotation was markedly limited in all directions. CT confirmed proptosis and showed enlargement of all extraocular muscles. Laboratory workup was negative for thyroid disease and rheumatologic disorders. Complete resolution occurred after 1 month of corticosteroid treatment.

may show increased density of orbital fat, thickening of posterior sclera and Tenon's layer, or enlargement of extraocular muscles. Treatment with a systemic corticosteroid usually provides prompt and dramatic relief.

Orbital myositis

Orbital myositis describes idiopathic orbital inflammatory disease that is confined to one or more extraocular muscles. The clinical presentation depends on the amount of inflammation. Diplopia, conjunctival chemosis, and orbital pain are common. Symptoms can be subacute for weeks or can progress quite rapidly. Visual function is rarely involved unless massive muscle enlargement is present. CT or MRI findings consist of diffusely enlarged muscles with the enlargement extending all the way to the insertion (unlike thyroid myopathy, which mainly involves the muscle belly). Corticosteroid treatment usually results in prompt resolution of symptoms, but prolonged treatment (4–6 weeks) is often necessary to avoid recurrence.

Eyelid and Epibulbar Tumors

Malignant tumors arising from eyelid skin or conjunctiva *(basal cell carcinoma, squamous cell carcinoma, melanoma)* are relatively common in adults, but they are extremely rare in childhood. These tumors are discussed elsewhere in the BCSC (see Section 4, *Ophthalmic Pathology and Intraocular Tumors*; Section 7, *Orbit, Eyelids, and Lacrimal System*; and Section 8, *External Disease and Cornea*). Pediatric cases are likely to be associated with underlying systemic disorders that predispose to malignancy, such as basal cell nevus syndrome or xeroderma pigmentosum. In addition, rhabdomyosarcoma may present atypically as an eyelid or conjunctival mass.

Benign lesions of the ocular surface and surrounding skin are frequent, and these may be classified as originating from epithelium, melanocytes, or vascular tissue.

Papillomas

Papillomas are benign epithelial proliferations that usually appear as sessile masses at the limbus or as pedunculated lesions of the caruncle, fornix, or palpebral conjunctiva. Papillomas may be transparent, pale yellow, or salmon-colored, sometimes speckled with red dots. Papillomas in children usually result from viral infection, similar to verrucae, and are likely to disappear spontaneously. Surgical excision is indicated if there is persistent associated conjunctivitis or keratitis or if new lesions continue to appear. Recurrence following surgical excision is common.

Conjunctival epithelial inclusion cysts

Usually resulting from surgery or trauma, conjunctival epithelial inclusion cysts are filled with clear fluid. Excision is indicated only if they are a source of bothersome symptoms.

Epibulbar dermoid tumors

Although both are classified as choristomas, dermoid tumors are completely distinct from dermoid cysts. Limbal dermoids are evident at birth as whitish dome-shaped masses, straddling the limbus in the inferotemporal quadrant in about three quarters of cases, with a diameter of about 2–10 mm and a thickness of 1–3 mm. They are composed of keratinizing surface epithelium with an underlying dermislike layer that frequently contains a few hair follicles and a small amount of fatty tissue. Little if any postnatal growth occurs. Apart from their undesirable appearance, limbal dermoids may cause ocular irritation and interfere with vision by inducing astigmatism or haziness of adjacent clear cornea.

There is no urgency in removing epibulbar dermoids unless irritating symptoms persist. Epibulbar limbal dermoids are removed by shelling out the lesion from the corneal side along its readily identifiable cleavage plane and excising the episcleral portion flush with the plane of surrounding tissue. In general, the surgeon need not remove underlying clear corneal tissue, mobilize surrounding tissue, or apply a patch graft over the resulting surface defect. Cornea and conjunctiva heal within a few days to several weeks, generally with some scarring and imperfect corneal transparency; nevertheless, the appearance is improved considerably.

Lipodermoid (dermolipoma)

A conjunctival lesion, the lipodermoid is usually located near the temporal fornix and is composed of adipose tissue and dense connective tissue. The overlying conjunctival epithelium is normal, and hair follicles are absent. Lipodermoids may be extensive, sometimes involving orbital tissue, lacrimal gland, and extraocular muscle. Both limbal dermoids and conjunctival lipodermoids are frequently associated with Goldenhar syndrome (Fig 26-12). In patients with Goldenhar syndrome, the lesions are accompanied by a variety of other anomalies, including ear deformities (preauricular appendages, aural fistulas), maxillary or mandibular hypoplasia (hemifacial microsomia), vertebral deformities, notching of the upper eyelid, and Duane syndrome.

Lipodermoids rarely require excision. If surgery is undertaken, the surgeon should attempt to remove only the portion of the lesion visible within the palpebral fissure, disturbing fornical conjunctiva and Tenon's layer as little as possible to minimize scarring. Even with a conservative operative approach, cicatrization may be a problem that requires surgical revision.

Conjunctival nevi

Conjunctival nevi are relatively common in childhood, occurring mainly in light-skinned persons. The lesions may be flat or elevated. Histopathologically, most of these nevi are

Figure 26-12 Small inferior limbal dermoid and larger lipodermoid involving the temporal conjunctival fornix, right eye, in a child with Goldenhar syndrome.

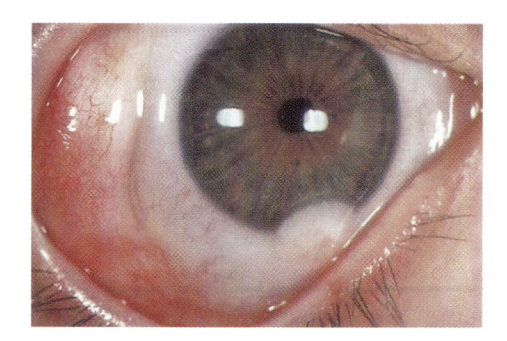

compound (nevus cells are found in both epithelium and substantia propria); others are junctional (nevus cells confined to the interface between epithelium and substantia propria). The color is typically brown, but approximately one third are nonpigmented, having a pinkish appearance. The lesions are occasionally noted at birth but more commonly develop during later childhood or adolescence (Fig 26-13).

No well-documented cases of malignant transformation of a conjunctival nevus have occurred in a patient younger than 20 years. Malignant melanoma of the conjunctiva and primary acquired melanosis, a premalignant nevoid lesion of adulthood, are extremely rare in childhood.

Congenital nevocellular nevi of the skin (giant hairy nevus)

Congenital nevocellular nevi can occur on the eyelids and may cause amblyopia or undergo malignant transformation (Fig 26-14). The risk of malignant transformation increases with the size of the lesion, with large lesions (>20 cm) having a 5%–20% risk of malignant transformation. Observation is often recommended for small (<1.5 cm) and medium-sized (1.5–20 cm) lesions, although complete excision removes the possibility of malignant transformation.

Ocular melanocytosis (melanosis oculi)

A congenital pigmentary lesion, ocular melanocytosis is characterized by unilateral patchy but extensive slate-gray or bluish discoloration of the sclera (not conjunctiva). Intraocular pigmentation is also increased, which contributes to a higher incidence of glaucoma and possibly increases the risk of malignant melanoma. Some patients, particularly persons of Asian ancestry, may have associated involvement of eyelid and adjacent skin with dermal hyperpigmentation that produces brown, bluish, or black discoloration without thickening or other abnormality *(oculodermal melanocytosis, nevus of Ota)*. Small patches of slate-gray scleral pigmentation, typically bilateral and without clinical significance, are common in black and Asian children. Melanosis of skin and sclera is occasionally associated with Sturge-Weber syndrome and Klippel-Trénaunay-Weber syndrome.

Port-wine stain (nevus flammeus)

A congenital vascular nevus, the port-wine stain typically involves the eyelid skin and episclera in Sturge-Weber syndrome (see the discussion of this condition in Chapter 27) but is seen more often as an isolated cutaneous anomaly on the eyelids or elsewhere.

Elsas FJ, Green WR. Epibulbar tumors in childhood. *Am J Ophthalmol.* 1975;79:1001–1007.
McDonnell JM, Carpenter JD, Jacobs P, et al. Conjunctival melanocytic lesions in children. *Ophthalmology.* 1989;96:986–993.
Panton RW, Sugar J. Excision of limbal dermoids. *Ophthalmic Surg.* 1991;22:85–89.

Inflammatory Conditions

Inflammatory masses of the eyelids and ocular surface are much more common than tumors. Although *chalazia* occur less frequently in children than in adults, the pediatric ophthalmologist must be prepared to encounter these masses. Because surgical treatment

366 • Pediatric Ophthalmology and Strabismus

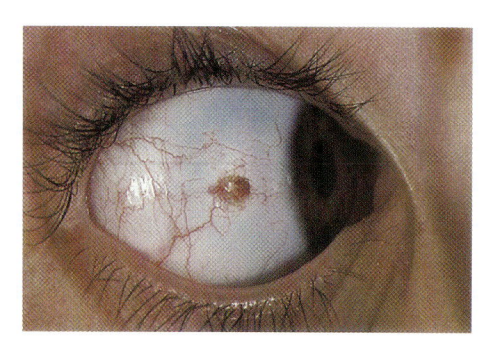

Figure 26-13 Pigmented nevus of the bulbar conjunctiva, right eye, recently developed in a 4-year-old girl.

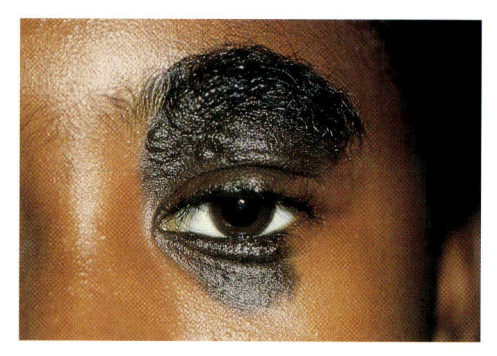

Figure 26-14 Congenital nevocellular nevus (giant hairy nevus) of the eyelid.

usually requires general anesthesia, conservative management is worth an extended trial. Most lesions resolve spontaneously over a period of weeks to months with frequent application of warm compresses. Doxycycline can be used safely in children who are at least 8 years old but should be avoided in younger children. *Pyogenic granuloma* is a pedunculated fleshy pink growth of granulation tissue that develops, sometimes rapidly and exuberantly, from the conjunctiva overlying a chalazion.

Phlyctenular keratoconjunctivitis and *ligneous conjunctivitis* are two uncommon inflammatory disorders of the conjunctiva that typically occur in young patients and may result in formation of ocular surface masses. *Nodular episcleritis* occasionally is seen in childhood. Eyelid and epibulbar lesions can develop in juvenile xanthogranuloma, which is discussed below. See also BCSC Section 8, *External Disease and Cornea*.

Intraocular Tumors

Iris and Ciliary Body Lesions

Both primary and secondary malignant tumors of the iris are very rare in children. Approximately 1% of *malignant uveal melanomas* occur in patients younger than 20 years. *Leukemic infiltration* of iris tissue may create a mass lesion, which is one of the less common ocular manifestations of pediatric leukemia. Solid tumors almost never metastasize to the uveal tract in childhood.

A number of relatively common and entirely benign iris lesions may generate concern about the possibility of malignancy in childhood. Pigmented *iris nevi* and *freckles* large enough to be noticed by family members or primary care physicians sometimes require repeated observation to provide reassurance concerning their harmless nature. Children with type 1 neurofibromatosis occasionally develop melanocytic lesions similar to the common Lisch nodule that are large enough to be considered benign tumors. *Nodules of iris pigmented epithelium* at the pupillary margin may be present as an insignificant congenital anomaly or may develop after prolonged use of miotic drops (eg, echothiophate for treatment of strabismus).

Juvenile xanthogranuloma

Juvenile xanthogranuloma is a nonneoplastic histiocytic proliferation that develops in infants younger than 2 years. It is characterized by the presence of Touton giant cells. Skin involvement is typically but not invariably present in the form of one or more small round papules, orange or tan in color. Iris lesions are relatively rare and virtually always unilateral. The fleshy yellow-brown mass may be small and localized or diffusely infiltrative of the entire iris, with resulting heterochromia. Spontaneous bleeding with hyphema is a characteristic clinical presentation. Secondary glaucoma may cause acute pain and photophobia and ultimately significant visual loss (Fig 26-15).

Juvenile xanthogranuloma is a self-limited condition that usually regresses spontaneously by age 5 years, but treatment is indicated for ocular involvement to avoid complications. Topical corticosteroids and agents that lower intraocular pressure, given as necessary, are generally sufficient to control the problem; surgical excision or radiation should be considered if intractable glaucoma is present.

Medulloepithelioma (diktyoma)

The medulloepithelioma originates from the nonpigmented epithelium of the ciliary body and most often presents as an iris mass during the first decade of life. Secondary glaucoma, hyphema, and ectopia lentis are less frequent initial manifestations. This rare lesion shows a spectrum of clinical and pathological characteristics, ranging from benign to malignant. Although metastasis is rare, local invasiveness can lead to death. Teratoid elements are often present. Enucleation is usually required and is curative in a large majority of cases.

> Broughton WL, Zimmerman LE. A clinicopathologic study of 56 cases of intraocular medulloepitheliomas. *Am J Ophthalmol.* 1978;85:407–418.
>
> Shields CL, Shields JA, Milite J, et al. Uveal melanoma in teenagers and children. A report of 40 cases. *Ophthalmology.* 1991;98:1662–1666.

Choroidal and Retinal Pigment Epithelial Lesions

A pigmented fundus lesion in a child is usually benign. Flat *choroidal nevi* are common as an incidental fundus finding in children and need not be viewed as a particular cause for concern. Patients with type 1 neurofibromatosis often have flat tan-colored spots in the choroid.

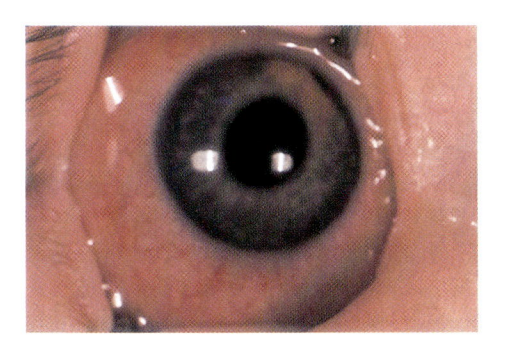

Figure 26-15 Juvenile xanthogranuloma of iris, right eye, in a 1-year-old boy with a 3-day history of redness and light sensitivity. Note small hyphema layered superonasally adjacent to the tan-colored iris lesion. Intraocular pressure was 30 mm Hg. The lesion regressed without further complications over 6 months with topical corticosteroid treatment.

Congenital hypertrophy of the retinal pigment epithelium (CHRPE) is a sharply demarcated, flat hyperpigmented lesion that may be isolated or multifocal. Such lesions are sometimes grouped, in which case they are also known as *bear tracks*. A specific subgroup of these lesions has been associated with familial adenomatous polyposis (Gardner syndrome). Patients with Gardner syndrome are at very high risk for adenocarcinoma of the colon by age 50 years. The CHRPE lesions associated with Gardner syndrome have a halo of surrounding depigmentation with a tail of depigmentation that is oriented radially and directed toward the optic nerve. Patients with Gardner syndrome may also have skeletal hamartomas and various other soft tissue tumors. The presence of four or more CHRPE lesions not restricted to one sector of the fundus or bilateral involvement should raise suspicion of familial polyposis syndrome.

Combined hamartoma of the retina and retinal pigment epithelium is an ill-defined, elevated, variably pigmented tumor that may be either juxtapapillary or located in the retinal periphery. In the peripheral location, dragging of the retinal vessels is a prominent feature. Tumors have a variable composition of glial tissue and retinal pigment epithelium. This condition can be associated with neurofibromatosis, incontinentia pigmenti, X-linked retinoschisis, and facial hemangiomas.

Melanocytoma is a darkly pigmented tumor with little or no growth potential that usually involves the optic disc and adjacent retina. Malignant melanoma of the choroid is extremely rare in children.

Choroidal osteoma is a benign bony tumor of the uveal tract that may occur in childhood, usually presenting with decreased visual acuity. Isolated localized *choroidal hemangioma* is extremely rare in childhood. Diffuse hemangioma of the choroid associated with Sturge-Weber syndrome is discussed in Chapter 27.

Retinoblastoma

Retinoblastoma is the most common malignant ocular tumor of childhood and one of the most common of all pediatric solid tumors, with an incidence of about 1 in 15,000. Retinoblastoma is typically diagnosed during the first year of life in familial and bilateral cases and between 1 and 3 years of age in sporadic unilateral cases. Onset later than age 5 is rare, but primary retinoblastoma can present in adulthood. The most common initial sign is leukocoria (white pupil), which is usually first noticed by the family and described as a glow, glint, or cat's-eye appearance (Fig 26-16A). In approximately 25% of cases, strabismus (esotropia or exotropia) is the first sign. Less common presentations include vitreous hemorrhage, hyphema, ocular or periocular inflammation, glaucoma, proptosis, and hypopyon. BCSC Section 4, *Ophthalmic Pathology and Intraocular Tumors*, also discusses retinoblastoma in depth.

Retinoblastoma is a neuroblastic tumor, biologically similar to neuroblastoma and medulloblastoma. Diagnosis of retinoblastoma can usually be based on its ophthalmoscopic appearance. Intraocular retinoblastoma can exhibit a variety of growth patterns. With *endophytic* growth, it appears as a white to cream-colored mass that breaks through the internal limiting membrane and has either no surface vessels or small, irregular tumor vessels (Fig 26-16B). Endophytic retinoblastoma is sometimes associated with *vitreous seeding*, in which individual cells or fragments of tumor tissue become separated from

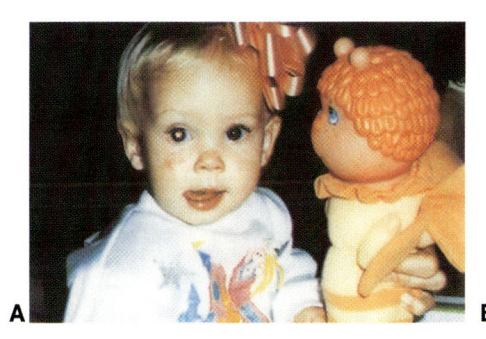

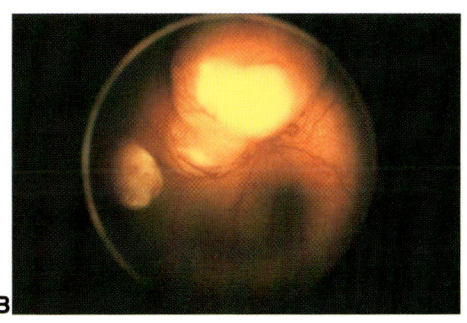

Figure 26-16 A, Leukocoria of the right eye shown in family photograph of a 1-year-old girl with retinoblastoma. **B,** Wide-angle fundus photograph showing multiple retinoblastoma lesions, left eye. *(Photograph courtesy of A. Linn Murphree, MD.)*

the main mass, as shown in Figure 26-17A. Vitreous seeds may be few and localized or so extensive that the clinical picture resembles endophthalmitis. Occasionally, malignant cells find their way into the anterior chamber and form a pseudohypopyon.

Exophytic tumors are usually yellow-white and occur in the subretinal space so that the overlying retinal vessels are commonly increased in caliber and tortuosity (Fig 26-17B). Exophytic retinoblastoma growth is often associated with subretinal fluid accumulation that can obscure the tumor and closely mimic the appearance of an exudative retinal detachment suggestive of advanced Coats disease. Retinoblastoma cells have the potential to implant on previously uninvolved retinal tissue and grow, thereby creating an impression of multicentricity in an eye with only a single primary lesion.

Large tumors often show signs of both endophytic and exophytic growth. Small retinoblastoma lesions appear as a grayish mass and are frequently confined between the internal and external limiting membranes. In rare cases, extensive tumor spread may occur within the retina to produce a diffuse infiltrating growth pattern.

Pretreatment evaluation of a patient with presumed retinoblastoma requires CT of the head and orbits. A bone marrow aspirate and lumbar puncture are also sometimes performed. The demonstration of typical intraocular calcification by CT usually confirms the diagnosis and can assist in evaluating possible extraocular extension and potential intracranial disease (Fig 26-18). Aspiration of ocular fluids for diagnostic testing should be performed only under the most unusual circumstances because such procedures can disseminate malignant cells.

Both of the patient's parents and all siblings should also be examined (Table 26-2). In about 1% of cases, a parent may be found to have an unsuspected fundus lesion that represents either spontaneously regressed retinoblastoma or a benign growth known as *retinoma* or *retinocytoma* that can be an expression of the retinoblastoma gene.

The retinoblastoma gene maps to a locus within the q14 band of chromosome 13 and codes for a protein that functions as a dominant suppressor of tumor formation. Approximately 60% of retinoblastoma cases arise from somatic nonhereditary mutations in retinal cells. These mutations generally result in unifocal and unilateral tumors. The remaining 40% occur in persons who possess an inheritable form of retinoblastoma.

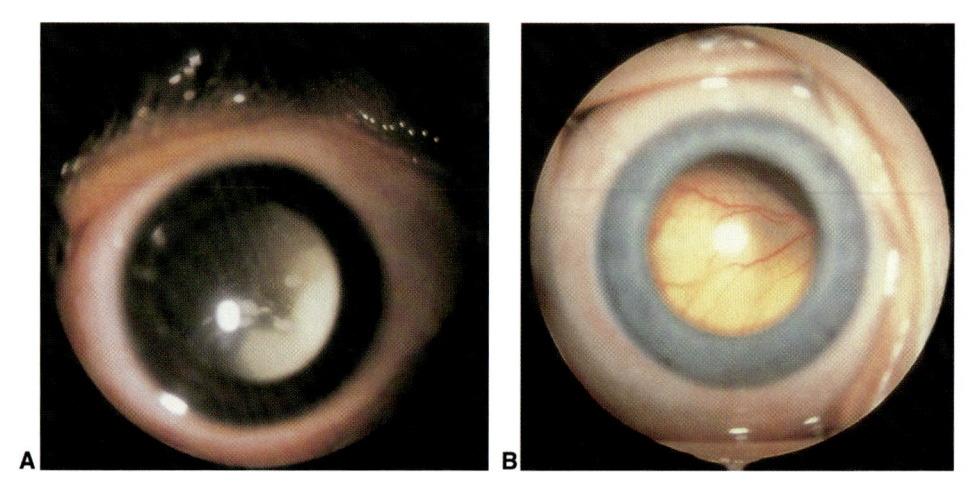

Figure 26-17 **A,** Endophytic retinoblastoma with vitreous seeding. **B,** Exophytic retinoblastoma with overlying detached retina.

Figure 26-18 Axial CT image showing retinoblastoma filling most of the posterior segment of left eye, with localized calcification.

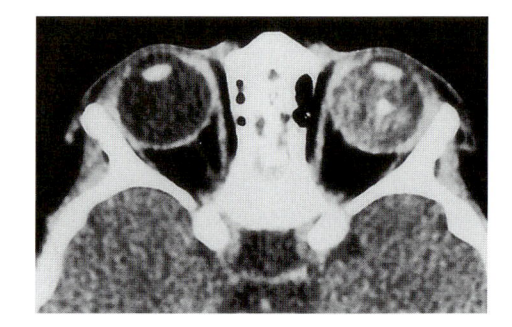

Mutations may occur during embryonic development and therefore may not be associated with a family history of retinoblastoma. Although not yet widely available, genetic testing for individuals and families suspected of carrying the heritable mutation has the potential to improve treatment plans and genetic counseling.

> Smith BJ, O'Brien JM. The genetics of retinoblastoma and current diagnostic testing. *J Pediatr Ophthalmol Strabismus.* 1996;33:120–123.

The differential diagnoses of leukocoria are given in Table 26-3. The most common retinal lesion simulating retinoblastoma is Coats disease. The presence of crystalline material, extensive subretinal fluid, and peripheral vascular abnormalities combined with lack of calcium on CT suggests Coats disease. *Astrocytic hamartoma* and *hemangioblastoma* are benign retinal tumors that may simulate the appearance of small retinoblastomas. Both are usually associated with the neurocutaneous syndromes discussed in Chapter 27.

The characteristic histopathologic features of retinoblastoma include *Flexner-Wintersteiner rosettes*, which are usually present, and *fleurettes*, which are less common. Both represent limited degrees of retinal differentiation. *Homer-Wright rosettes* are also fre-

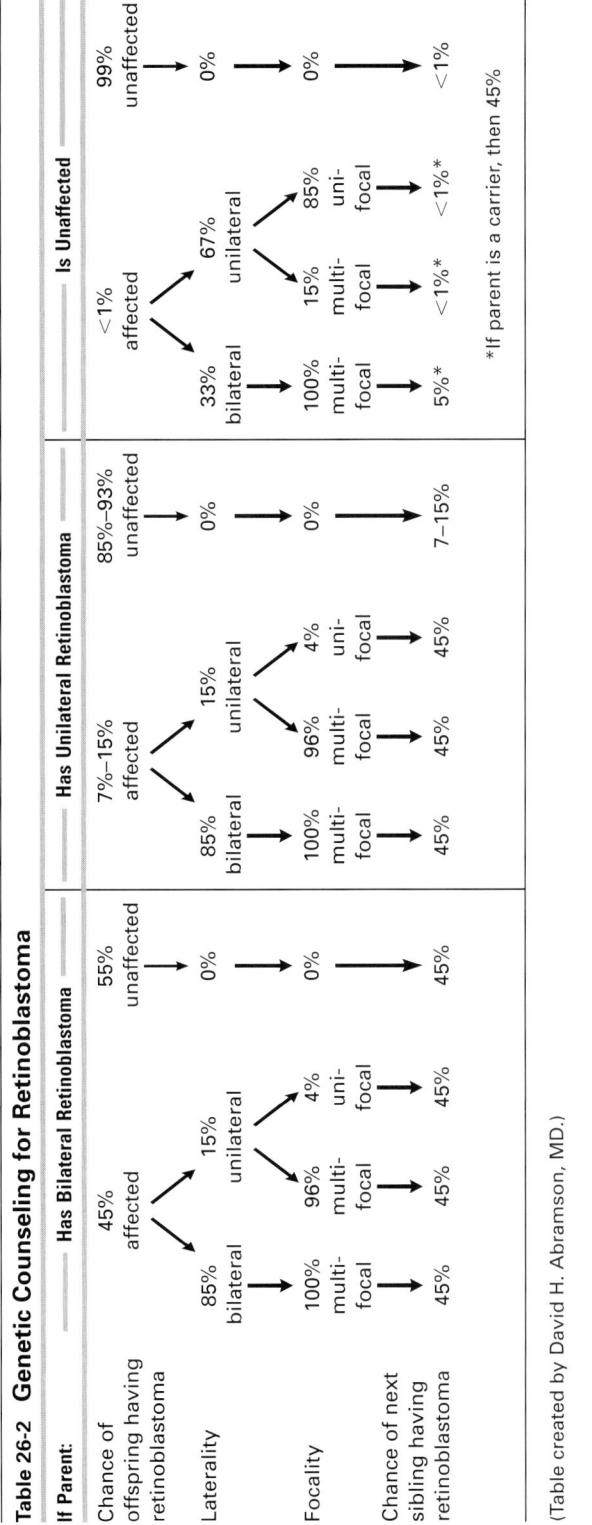

Table 26-2 Genetic Counseling for Retinoblastoma

If Parent:	Has Bilateral Retinoblastoma	Has Unilateral Retinoblastoma	Is Unaffected
Chance of offspring having retinoblastoma	45% affected → / 55% unaffected → 0%	7%–15% affected → / 85%–93% unaffected → 0%	<1% affected → / 99% unaffected → 0%
Laterality	85% bilateral / 15% unilateral	85% bilateral / 15% unilateral	33% bilateral / 67% unilateral
Focality	100% multifocal → 0% ; 96% multifocal / 4% unifocal	100% multifocal → 0% ; 96% multifocal / 4% unifocal	100% multifocal → 0% ; 15% multifocal / 85% unifocal
Chance of next sibling having retinoblastoma	45% ; 45% ; 45% ; 45%	45% ; 45% ; 45% ; 7–15%	5%* ; <1%* ; <1%* ; <1%

*If parent is a carrier, then 45%

(Table created by David H. Abramson, MD.)

Table 26-3 Differential Diagnosis of Leukocoria

Clinical Diagnosis in Suspected Retinoblastoma
Retinoblastoma
Persistent hyperplastic primary vitreous
Retinopathy of prematurity
Cataract
Coloboma of choroid or optic disc
Uveitis
Larval granulomatosis (toxocariasis)
Congenital retinal fold
Coats disease
Organizing vitreous hemorrhage
Retinal dysplasia
Corneal opacity
Familial exudative vitreoretinopathy (FEVR)
High myopia/anisometropia
Myelinated nerve fibers
Norrie disease
Retinal detachment

quently present but are less specific for retinoblastoma because they are common in other neuroblastic tumors. Calcification of varying extent is usually present. In some patients with bilateral retinoblastoma, a third primary tumor, *pineoblastoma*, can be found in the pineal gland. Such cases of trilateral retinoblastoma can be seen at initial presentation or can occur years after successful ocular treatment.

Management of retinoblastoma

The treatment of retinoblastoma has changed significantly in recent years. The major goals of treatment are primarily to save the patient's life and secondarily to salvage the patient's eye and vision if possible. Although enucleation is still a major form of treatment for retinoblastoma, many other treatment modalities exist today. The choice of treatment depends on the size, location, and extent of the tumor.

> Shields CL, Shields JA. Recent developments in the management of retinoblastoma. *J Pediatr Ophthalmol Strabismus.* 1999;36:8–18.
>
> Usalito M, Wheeler S, O'Brien J. New approaches in the clinical management of retinoblastoma. *Ophthalmol Clin North Am.* 1999;12:255–264.

Enucleation Enucleation is usually employed in patients with large unilateral tumors, especially when the involved eye is judged to have no visual potential. Enucleation has also traditionally been performed in the eye with more advanced disease in patients with bilateral retinoblastoma. Recently, chemotherapy combined with local therapy has been used successfully in some cases. The technique should be gentle, avoiding the use of clamps, snares, or cautery. The surgeon should obtain as long a section of optic nerve as is possible. This is best achieved via a temporal approach with slightly curved enucleation scissors.

The results of enucleation for retinoblastoma are excellent, with a cure rate greater than 95%. Survival decreases if the cut end of the nerve contains tumor cells.

> Shields JA, Shields CL, De Potter P. Enucleation technique for children with retinoblastoma. *J Pediatr Ophthalmol Strabismus*. 1992;29:213–215.

External-beam radiotherapy Retinoblastoma cells are highly radiosensitive. External-beam radiotherapy is a method of delivering whole-eye irradiation to treat advanced retinoblastoma, particularly with diffuse vitreous seeding. The tumor may recur. Side effects include cataract, radiation retinopathy, optic neuropathy, chronic dry eye, and atrophy of muscles and subcutaneous tissue. The risk of secondary tumors is increased in patients who receive external-beam radiotherapy. This risk is most pronounced in children who are younger than 12 months at the time of irradiation.

Plaque radiotherapy A form of brachytherapy, plaque radiotherapy is limited to tumors less than 16 mm in base diameter and 8 mm in thickness. This technique can be used as a primary or secondary treatment. The overall tumor control rate is about 90%, but patients have been carefully selected. Side effects include radiation retinopathy and optic neuropathy and are more prominent in children who have been exposed to chemotherapy.

Cryotherapy and laser photoablation Small tumors may respond to local therapy. Cryotherapy can be used in small anterior tumors that are 3.5 mm or less in diameter and 2.0 mm or less in thickness. Laser photocoagulation is useful in tumors 4.5 mm or less in base diameter and 2.5 mm or less in thickness. Complications include retinal tears and detachments, preretinal fibrosis, and vascular occlusion. Recurrences can be a problem.

Chemotherapy Traditionally, chemotherapy had been reserved for patients with metastatic disease. Chemotherapy has recently been introduced as a primary treatment to reduce tumor bulk in an attempt to avoid external-beam radiation *(chemoreduction)*. Cytotoxic drugs are given initially for 2–3 months to decrease tumor size. This method is effective even in cases of total retinal detachment.

Follow-up treatment with cryotherapy, laser therapy, or scleral plaque may be necessary for resistant tumors. A combination of chemotherapy and diode laser hyperthermia has also been effective in eradicating small and medium-sized endophytic tumors without vitreous seeds *(thermochemotherapy)*. Several different modalities are sometimes necessary for eyes with large or multiple tumors. Decisions on how to treat retinoblastoma are complex and best approached by a team of experienced specialists.

Treated retinoblastoma sometimes disappears altogether, but more often it persists as a calcified mass (*type 1*, or *cottage cheese*, pattern) or a translucent grayish lesion (*type 2*, or *fish flesh*, pattern, which is difficult to distinguish from untreated tumor). The child with treated retinoblastoma must be followed closely, with frequent examinations under anesthesia, for several years to watch for recurrence, which is of particular concern in cases with vitreous seeding.

Intraocular spread or recurrence of retinoblastoma can be associated with optic nerve or transscleral extension or with massive invasion of the choroid. The most common extraocular sites for disseminated retinoblastoma are the orbit, central nervous system, and cranium. The prognosis for survival with recurrent retinoblastoma is poor, but if diagnosed early, the disease can occasionally be cured with chemotherapy, radiation, or both. Periodic repeated imaging of the head and orbits is advisable for several years after successful treatment.

Monitoring

Close monitoring of patients with retinoblastoma and their family members is crucial. Even patients with unilateral unifocal tumors have an almost 20% chance of developing retinoblastoma in their fellow eye. This risk is diminished with age and is quite small after age 24 months. If the retinoblastoma is the hereditary form, the patient and siblings should be examined every 4 months until age 3 or 4 years and every 6 months until age 6 years. General anesthesia is indicated to obtain a thorough peripheral examination. Most children over age 8 years can be examined yearly in the office.

> Murphree AL, Christensen LE. Retinoblastoma and malignant intraocular tumors. In: Wright KW, ed. *Pediatric Ophthalmology and Strabismus.* St Louis: Mosby; 1995:495–509.

Children with the heritable form of retinoblastoma are also at risk for secondary nonocular tumors later in life. Osteosarcomas and various soft tissue sarcomas may develop up to 30 years after treatment of retinoblastoma, particularly in the orbital region after external-beam radiation therapy but also elsewhere in the body with or without a history of radiation exposure. Primary extraocular tumors associated with retinoblastoma carry a very poor prognosis.

CHAPTER 27

Phakomatoses

The phakomatoses, or *neurocutaneous syndromes*, are a group of disorders featuring multiple discrete lesions of one or a few histologic types that are found in two or more organ systems, including the skin and central nervous system. The lesions are usually hamartomas (abnormal proliferations of tissues normally found in the involved organs). Each syndrome is defined not by the characteristics of the individual lesions but by their multiplicity or association with one another. Eye involvement is frequent and may constitute an important source of morbidity or provide information of critical importance to diagnosis. Four major disorders have traditionally been designated phakomatoses, and all have important eye manifestations:

- Neurofibromatosis (von Recklinghausen disease)
- Tuberous sclerosis (Bourneville disease)
- Angiomatosis of the retina and cerebellum (von Hippel-Lindau disease)
- Encephalofacial or encephalotrigeminal angiomatosis (Sturge-Weber syndrome)

Other conditions sometimes classified as phakomatoses include:

- Incontinentia pigmenti (Bloch-Sulzberger syndrome)
- Ataxia-telangiectasia (Louis-Bar syndrome)
- Racemose angioma (Wyburn-Mason syndrome)

Table 27-1 lists the phakomatoses.

Neurofibromatosis

Persons with neurofibromatosis (NF) manifest characteristic lesions composed of melanocytes or neuroglial cells, which are both primarily derivatives of neural crest mesenchyme. Although the melanocytic and glial lesions in NF are often called *hamartomas*, this designation is questionable in that most lesions do not become evident until years after birth and many are histologically indistinguishable from low-grade neoplasms originating in the same tissues.

NF has two distinct forms (NF-1 and NF-2) that are distinguished by differences in genetics, diagnostic criteria, morbidity, and treatment. Both are familial disorders that show autosomal dominant inheritance with very high penetrance (virtually 100% in NF-1). However, a large percentage of cases (nearly half in NF-1) are sporadic, presum-

Table 27-1 The Phakomatoses

Condition	Description	Associated Ocular Condition	Associated Conditions and Risks	Transmission
von Hippel-Lindau disease (retinal angiomatosis)	Retinal angioma supplied by dilated tortuous arteriole and venule; may be multiple	Retinal exudates, hemorrhages, retinal detachment, glaucoma	Cerebellar capillary hemangiomas, malformation of visceral organs	Autosomal dominant, chromosome 3p25
Sturge-Weber syndrome (encephalofacial angiomatosis)	Capillary hamartia (nevus flammeus) of skin, conjunctiva, episclera, and/or uveal tract, and of meninges	Glaucoma (especially with upper eyelid involvement by nevus flammeus)	Diffuse meningeal hemangioma with seizure disorder, hemiplegia or hemianopia, or mental retardation	Sporadic
Neurofibromatosis (von Recklinghausen disease)	Occasionally congenital, widespread hamartomas of peripheral nerves and tissue of neural crest derivation	Neurofibromas of eyelid and orbit, uveal melanocytic nevi, retinal glial hamartomas, congenital glaucoma, optic nerve glioma, absence of greater wing of sphenoid with pulsating exophthalmos	Similar hamartomas of central nervous system, peripheral and cranial nerves, gastrointestinal tract; malignant transformation possible	Autosomal dominant NF-1: chromosome 17q11.2
Tuberous sclerosis (Bourneville disease)	Mental deficiency, seizures, and adenoma sebaceum	Angiofibromas of eyelid skin; glial hamartomas of retina and optic disc	Adenoma sebaceum (angiofibromas), cerebral glial hamartomas	Autosomal dominant, chromosome 9q34
Ataxia-telangiectasia (Louis-Bar syndrome)	Progressive cerebellar ataxia, ocular and cutaneous telangiectasis, pulmonary infections	Conjunctival telangiectasis, anomalous ocular movements, and nystagmus	Dysarthria, coarse hair and skin, immunologic deficiency, and mental and growth retardation	Autosomal recessive, chromosome 11q22
Wyburn-Mason syndrome (racemose angioma)	Retinal and midbrain arteriovenous (AV) communication (aneurysms and angiomas) and facial nevi	AV communication (racemose angioma) of retina, with vision loss depending on location of AV communication	AV aneurysm at midbrain; intracranial calcification	Sporadic
Incontinentia pigmenti (Bloch-Sulzberger syndrome)	Cutaneous; dental, central nervous system, and ocular changes	ROP-like vasculopathy may progress to retinal detachment and retrolental membrane	"Splashed paint" hyperpigmented maculas, microcephaly, seizures, and mental deficiency	X-linked dominant

(Modified from Isselbacher K, Braunwald E, Wilson JD, eds. *Harrison's Principles of Internal Medicine.* 13th ed. New York: McGraw-Hill; 1994:2207–2210).

ably reflecting the high rate of mutation known to be true for the responsible gene. The genetic locus of NF-1 is on the long arm of chromosome 17, and that of NF-2 is on the long arm of chromosome 22. The NF-1 gene has been isolated and cloned. The function of this gene is still poorly understood, but it is thought to code for a protein involved in regulation of cellular proliferation.

Type 1 *(NF-1)*, sometimes called *peripheral neurofibromatosis*, is by far the more common, with a prevalence of 1 in 3000–5000. Details of NF-1's clinical and pathological manifestations follow.

Melanocytic Lesions

Almost all adults with NF-1 have melanocytic lesions involving both the skin and the eye. The most common cutaneous expression, *café-au-lait spots*, appear clinically as flat, sharply demarcated, uniformly hyperpigmented macules of varying size and shape. At least a few are usually present at birth, but their number and size increase during the first decade of life. Clusters of small café-au-lait spots, or *freckling*, in the axillary or inguinal regions are particularly characteristic of NF-1, occurring in a majority of patients over 10 years old.

Many unaffected persons have one to three café-au-lait spots, but greater numbers are rare except in association with NF. In the past, NF was often diagnosed solely on the basis of multiple café-au-lait spots, but it is now recognized that a few persons with this finding never develop other stigmata of the disease and may have offspring with a similarly limited condition, suggesting the existence of a genetic disorder distinct from NF-1. Currently, NF-1 is diagnosed only when two or more criteria from the following group of seven are met:

- Six or more café-au-lait spots >5 mm in diameter in prepubescents or >15 mm in diameter in postpubescents
- Two or more neurofibromas of any type or one plexiform neurofibroma
- Freckling of axillary, inguinal, or other intertriginous areas
- Optic nerve glioma
- Two or more iris Lisch nodules
- A distinctive osseous lesion, such as sphenoid bone dysplasia or thinning of the long-bone cortex, with or without pseudarthrosis
- A first-degree relative with NF-1 according to the above criteria

Neurofibromatosis. Conference Statement. National Institutes of Health Consensus Development Conference. *Arch Neurol.* 1988;45:575–580.

Occasionally, eyelid skin or conjunctiva is hyperpigmented in NF-1, but melanocytic lesions of the uveal tract are far more common ocular manifestations. In the iris, these lesions take the form of small (usually ≤1 mm), sharply demarcated, dome-shaped excrescences known as *Lisch nodules* (Fig 27-1). Clinically, Lisch nodules usually appear to have smooth surfaces and a translucent interior suggesting a gelatinous consistency, but in some persons they look solid and wartlike. Color varies but can be described as tan in most cases. In heavily pigmented brown irides, the nodules tend to stand out against the smooth, dark anterior surface and are often visible to the unaided eye. When overall iris stromal pigmentation is lighter, Lisch nodules can be partly hidden within recesses

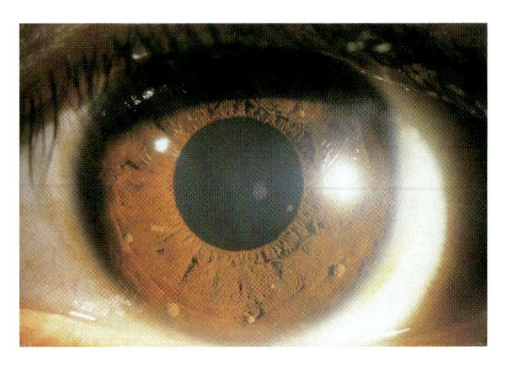

Figure 27-1 Lisch nodules of iris, left eye, in child with type 1 neurofibromatosis.

in the lacy stromal tissue and may be overlooked unless a slit lamp is used to search for them. They may be difficult to differentiate from small clumps of normal pigmented tissue, especially when they are few and the patient is less than fully cooperative. Histopathologically, the lesions consist primarily of uniform spindle-shaped melanin-containing cells, indistinguishable from those found in iris nevi and low-grade spindle-cell melanomas.

Most Lisch nodules develop during childhood or adolescence. They are seen infrequently before age 3 years, appear in a majority of cases of NF-1 between 5 and 10 years of age, and are present in nearly 100% of affected adults. The finding of two or more Lisch nodules is a diagnostic criterion for NF-1, but an affected adult's eye typically has dozens and occasionally 100 or more (see also Chapter 20).

Choroidal lesions have been reported to occur in one third to one half of adults with NF-1. These lesions are described as flat with indistinct borders and hyperpigmented in relation to the surrounding fundus but ranging from yellow-white to dark brown in color. Their number varies from 1 to 20 per eye, with each lesion typically one to two times the size of the optic disc. Direct histopathological correlation for this clinical finding is lacking, but it is presumed to represent localized concentration of melanocytes similar to a choroidal nevus.

Like café-au-lait spots, none of the common ocular melanocytic lesions of NF-1 has any clinical significance beyond establishing the diagnosis. Neither the vision nor the health of the eye is affected by these lesions, regardless of their extent. Persons with NF-1 are thought to be predisposed to uveal melanoma as well as a number of other malignant neoplasms. However, the incidence of iris, and especially choroidal, tumors is still quite low.

Glial Cell Lesions

Nodular neurofibromas

Among lesions of neuroglial origin in NF-1, *nodular cutaneous* and *subcutaneous neurofibromas*, or *fibroma molluscum*, are by far the most common. These are soft papulonodules, often pedunculated, with color ranging from that of normal skin to violescent. They typically begin to appear in late childhood and increase in number throughout adolescence and adulthood; nearly all adults with NF-1 have at least a few. In some cases, hundreds of these lesions are present, causing considerable disfigurement.

Plexiform neurofibromas

Of much greater clinical significance than nodular neurofibromas are the less common *plexiform neurofibromas*, which occur in approximately 30% of patients with NF-1. These neurofibromas are very rarely seen in other contexts. These lesions appear clinically as extensive subcutaneous swellings with indistinct margins. Hyperpigmentation or hypertrichosis of the overlying skin is common, as is hypertrophy of underlying soft tissue and bone *(regional gigantism)*. The consistency of plexiform neurofibromas is typically soft and not easily distinguished from that of normal tissue; the oft-repeated statement that they feel like a bag of worms applies in only a minority of cases.

Plexiform neurofibromas develop earlier than nodular lesions, frequently becoming evident in infancy or childhood. These neurofibromas often show considerable enlargement over time, resulting in severe disfigurement and functional impairment. Rarely, the lesion undergoes malignant degeneration, producing a neurofibrosarcoma capable of widespread metastasis.

Approximately 10% of plexiform neurofibromas involve the face, commonly the upper eyelid and orbit. At onset, the involved upper eyelid is thicker than normal and usually appears mildly ptotic (Fig 27-2). Its inner surface may override the lower eyelid margin and lashes when the eye is closed. Characteristically, the greater involvement of its temporal portion gives the eyelid margin an S-shaped configuration and an overall appearance of an eyelid that is too big for the eye. The lesion undergoes considerable and sometimes massive growth during childhood and adolescence, although extension across the facial midline is rare. Complete ptosis may eventually result from the increasing bulk and weight of the upper eyelid. Irritation of the upper palpebral conjunctiva caused by rubbing against the lower lashes can create significant discomfort. Glaucoma in the ipsilateral eye is found in as many as half of cases.

Complete excision of a plexiform neurofibroma involving the eyelid is generally not possible. Treatment is directed toward the relief of specific symptoms and is likely to be partially successful at best. Topical ointment helps to reduce conjunctival irritation. Distorted and chronically inflamed conjunctiva sometimes requires resection. Surgical

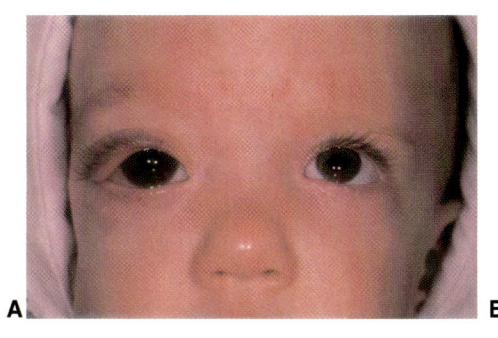

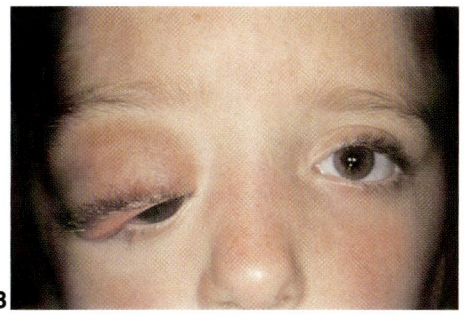

Figure 27-2 Plexiform neurofibroma involving the right upper eyelid, associated with ipsilateral buphthalmos, in girl with NF-1. **A,** Age 8 months. **B,** Age 8 years.

debulking and frontalis suspension procedures can reduce ptosis sufficiently to permit binocular vision, but the resulting benefit is often only temporary.

Optic glioma

Low-grade pilocytic astrocytoma involving the optic nerve, chiasm, or both (optic glioma) is among the most characteristic and potentially serious complications of NF-1. Symptomatic optic gliomas (ie, tumors producing significant visual loss, proptosis, or other complications) occur in 1%–5% of persons with NF-1. When CT or MRI is performed prospectively on unselected NF-1 patients, abnormalities of the optic nerve (often bilateral) or chiasm, indicating the presence of glioma, are found in approximately 15% of cases.

Typically, the entire orbital portion of an involved optic nerve shows cylindrical or fusiform enlargement (Fig 27-3). A relatively narrow central core usually differs from surrounding tissue because of the characteristic growth pattern of optic nerve glioma in NF-1: most cellular proliferation occurs in the perineural intradural space *(arachnoidal gliomatosis)* associated with production of abundant mucinous material that gives this tissue the signal characteristics of water. This core shows higher density in CT; with MRI, the core shows higher density on T1-weighted images and lower density on T2-weighted images.

Increased length of the intraorbital nerve segment results in exaggerated sinuousness or *kinking* that often creates an appearance of discontinuity or localized constriction on axial images. These appearances distinguish optic glioma reliably from the principal differential diagnostic alternative, *optic nerve sheath meningioma*, which also occurs with increased frequency in NF. However, optic nerve sheath meningioma occurs much less commonly than optic glioma and rarely in childhood.

Gliomas involving the intracranial optic nerve or chiasm in NF-1 produce enlargement of these structures on both CT and MRI and, frequently, abnormal signal intensity on MRI, which is now the preferred means of diagnosis. Associated contiguous involvement of the orbital portion of one or both optic nerves usually occurs, and extension into the optic tracts and posterior visual pathways is often evident, especially on MRI.

Optic gliomas that become symptomatic in patients with NF-1 nearly always do so before age 10 years, often apparently following a brief period of rapid enlargement. Even without treatment, many gliomas then appear to enter a phase of stability or much slower growth, and spontaneous improvement has been documented in a few cases.

Figure 27-3 Axial CT image showing bilateral optic glioma with chiasmal involvement, associated with severe bilateral visual loss, in an adolescent boy with NF-1. Note the relatively low density of tissue surrounding the central core of the enlarged optic nerve.

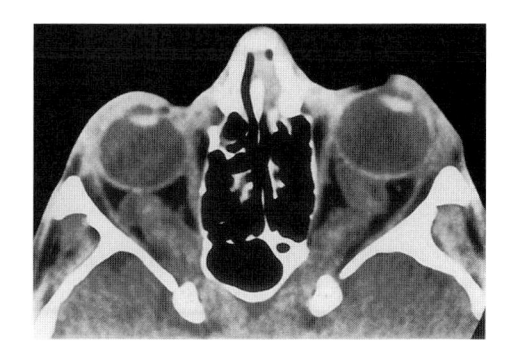

Tumors confined to the optic nerve at the time of clinical presentation infrequently extend into the chiasm subsequently and very rarely develop extradural extension or distant metastasis; mortality is virtually nil. Treatment remains controversial. Many authorities recommend complete excision through a transfrontal approach that preserves the globe but sacrifices any remaining vision on the involved side, but it has not been convincingly demonstrated that this approach improves the prognosis for sight in the other eye. Most patients treated with subtotal orbital excision for relief of proptosis also do well.

In addition to bilateral visual loss, tumors primarily involving the chiasm may produce significant morbidity, including hydrocephalus and hypothalamic dysfunction leading to precocious puberty or hypopituitarism. Glioma of the chiasm carries a reported mortality rate of 50% or higher. In the past, most deaths occurred within months of diagnosis, but recent series show longer survival, reflecting earlier detection and improved management of complications in addition to treatment of the tumor itself that may be more effective. Megavoltage radiation therapy appears to retard or reverse progression in many cases, but it is not firmly established that this therapy can substantially reduce the ultimate rate of tumor-related blindness and death, which may occur as late as 20 years after presentation. In an effort to avoid complications of brain irradiation in early childhood, chemotherapy has been investigated as an alternative treatment modality with encouraging preliminary results.

Other neuroglial abnormalities

Abnormal proliferation of peripheral neuroglial or other neural crest–derived cells may occur in relation to deeper tissues and visceral organs as well as skin (spinal and gastrointestinal neurofibromas, pheochromocytoma). Prominence of corneal nerves, thought to represent glial hypertrophy, may be noted on slit-lamp examination in as many as 20% of cases. A frequent histopathological finding in the choroid is the presence of so-called *ovoid bodies*, onionlike formations that appear to consist of hyperplastic Schwann cells surrounding peripheral nerve axons. Rarely, a localized neurofibroma develops within the orbit in association with NF. Retinal hamartomas indistinguishable from those seen in tuberous sclerosis have also been found in patients with NF-1.

Other Manifestations

NF-1 is associated with an increased, but still generally low, incidence of a number of conditions that cannot be explained by abnormal proliferation of neural crest–derived cells. These conditions include a variety of benign tumors that may involve skin or eye (juvenile xanthogranuloma, capillary hemangioma) and several forms of malignancy (leukemia, rhabdomyosarcoma, pheochromocytoma, Wilms tumor). Also relatively common are bony defects (scoliosis, pseudarthrosis of the tibia, and hypoplasia of the sphenoid bone, which may result in ocular pulsation) and a number of ill-defined abnormalities of the central nervous system (macrocephaly, aqueductal stenosis, seizures, and usually minor intellectual deficits).

The most significant ophthalmic disorder in this category is glaucoma, which is usually unilateral. In most cases, glaucoma is associated with ipsilateral plexiform neurofibroma of the upper eyelid or with the iris abnormality known as *congenital iris ectropion* (see Fig 20-9 and discussion in Chapter 20). *Buphthalmos,* or enlargement of the cornea and the globe as a whole, is seen if IOP is elevated during the first 2 years of life. In some cases, excessive growth of the eyeball may also be a manifestation of regional hypertrophy, at least in part. Corneal edema and high myopia can result from high pressure in early or later childhood.

The pathogenesis of glaucoma in NF-1 is unknown. Abnormal trabecular meshwork development in some patients can lead to early-onset childhood or congenital glaucoma. In other patients, synechial closure of the angle may result from neurofibromatous tissue posterior to the iris or neurofibromatous infiltration of the angle directly. Medical management of the glaucoma can be attempted but frequently fails. A variety of surgical procedures have been employed with moderate success; achievement of adequate pressure control often requires several operations. Useful vision is seldom retained in the involved eye. Contributing to this poor prognosis are frequently associated, significant orbital and optic nerve abnormalities, as well as refractory amblyopia (anisometropic or deprivation).

A child or adult who appears to have any one of the abnormalities typically associated with NF-1 should undergo an eye examination that includes the following:

- Assessment of vision (acuity and color discrimination)
- Pupillary light reaction, including careful scrutiny for relative afferent defect
- Slit-lamp examination with particular attention to the iris
- Ophthalmoscopy to identify disc pallor or edema and choroidal lesions
- Measurement of IOP, when indicated by other findings

The discovery of Lisch nodules has been used to confirm the presence of NF-1 in a patient with café-au-lait spots, and the absence of such nodules in an adult patient has been said to virtually rule out the diagnosis. However, the use of iris changes as a diagnostic marker for NF-1 has been questioned. Iris changes in patients with known NF-1 are more diverse than the classic descriptions of Lisch nodules, and interobserver reliability for the diagnosis of NF-1 based on iris findings is often poor.

Although the role of routine screening with MRI remains controversial, abnormalities of vision, pupil function, or optic disc appearance indicate a need for neuroimaging studies to look for optic glioma. An appropriate interval for periodic ophthalmologic reassessment in childhood is 1–2 years unless a significant abnormality requires closer observation. New onset of significant eye involvement is very unlikely in adults, but blood pressure should be regularly monitored because of the risk of pheochromocytoma.

NF-2 is less common than NF-1 by a factor of at least 10. NF-2 has been termed *central NF* and is diagnosed by presence of bilateral acoustic neuromas (eighth nerve tumors) or a first-degree relative with NF-2 and presence of a unilateral acoustic neuroma, neurofibroma, meningioma, schwannoma, glioma, or early-onset cataract (posterior subcapsular cataract).

Patients with NF-2 typically present in their teens to early adulthood with symptoms related to the eighth nerve tumor(s), including decreased hearing or tinnitus. Ocular findings may predate the onset of symptoms. Therefore, the alert ophthalmologist may be able to help diagnose the potential for central nervous system tumors before they become symptomatic. The most characteristic eye finding in NF-2 is lens opacity, especially posterior subcapsular cataract or wedge cortical cataracts. Other less common findings are retinal hamartoma and combined hamartomas of the retina and RPE. Lisch nodules of the iris can occur in NF-2 but are not expected.

> Beauchamp GR. Neurofibromatosis type 1 in children. *Trans Am Ophthalmol Soc.* 1995; 93:445–472.
>
> Kaiser-Kupfer MI, Freidlin V, Datiles MB, et al. The association of posterior capsular lens opacities with bilateral acoustic neuromas in patients with neurofibromatosis type 2. *Arch Ophthalmol.* 1989;107:541–544.
>
> Lewis RA, Riccardi VM. Von Recklinghausen neurofibromatosis. Incidence of iris hamartomata. *Ophthalmology.* 1981;88:348–354.
>
> Listernick R, Charrow J, Greenwald MJ, et al. Natural history of optic pathway tumors in children with neurofibromatosis type 1: a longitudinal study. *J Pediatr.* 1994;125:63–66.
>
> National Institutes of Health Consensus Development Conferences Statement on Acoustic Neuroma, Dec. 11–13, 1991. Consensus Development Panel. *Arch Neurol.* 1994;51: 201–207.

Tuberous Sclerosis (Bourneville Disease)

Tuberous sclerosis (TS) is a familial disorder associated with a variety of abnormalities involving the skin, eye, central nervous system, and other organs. Estimates of the prevalence of TS range from as high as 1:6000 to 1:100,000 or lower. Two distinct gene mutations giving rise to TS have been identified: 9q34 (TSC-1) and 16p13.3 (TSC-2). Prenatal testing for these mutations is not currently available. Transmission as an autosomal dominant trait has been documented in numerous pedigrees, but new mutations account for as many as 80% of cases.

The three classic findings, known as *Vogt triad,* are mental retardation, seizures, and facial angiofibromas, though all three are present in only about 30% of patients with TS. The disease is characterized by benign tumor growth in multiple organs, predominantly the skin, brain, heart, kidney, and eye. Primary features of this disorder, any one of which is sufficient to diagnose TS, are:

- Facial angiofibroma
- Ungual fibromas (multiple)
- Cortical tuber
- Subependymal nodule (giant cell astrocytoma)
- Multiple subependymal nodules protruding into the ventricle
- Multiple retinal astrocytomas

Several distinct skin lesions are characteristic of TS (Fig 27-4). The earliest cutaneous sign to appear is the *white spot,* or *hypopigmented macule,* which is present in almost all cases at birth or in infancy. These lesions are sharply demarcated with a shape that often resembles an ash leaf. Ultraviolet light from a Wood's lamp increases the visibility of white spots in light-skinned persons. Histopathologically, these spots have decreased melanin but normal numbers of melanocytes.

Facial angiofibromas often called *adenoma sebaceum* begin to appear in childhood and increase progressively in number; they are present in three quarters of adolescents

384 • Pediatric Ophthalmology and Strabismus

and adults with TS. These lesions are often mistaken for common acne. Subungual and periungual fibromas are also common after puberty; gingival fibromas may occur as well. A thickened plaque of skin known as a *shagreen patch*, or *collagenoma*, occurs in approximately one quarter of cases, typically in the lumbosacral area. Plaques involving the forehead that sometimes extend into the eyelids may be present at birth.

Seizures occur in 80% of patients with TS, and they may be difficult to control. Severe mental retardation is present in 50% of patients, but intelligence is often normal. Characteristic findings in neuroimaging studies include nodular periventricular or basal ganglion calcifications (representing benign astrocytomas) and tuberous malformations of the cortex (Fig 27-5). Malignant astrocytomas occur infrequently. Obstruction of the foramen of Monro by tumor may produce hydrocephalus, and cardiac tumors *(rhabdomyomas)* can lead to early death or severe disability. Lesions of bone and kidney are common but usually produce no significant disturbance of function.

Hypopigmented lesions analogous to white spots of the skin are occasionally seen in the iris or choroid, but the most frequent and characteristic ocular manifestation of TS is the *retinal phakoma* (Fig 27-6). Pathologically, this growth arises from the innermost

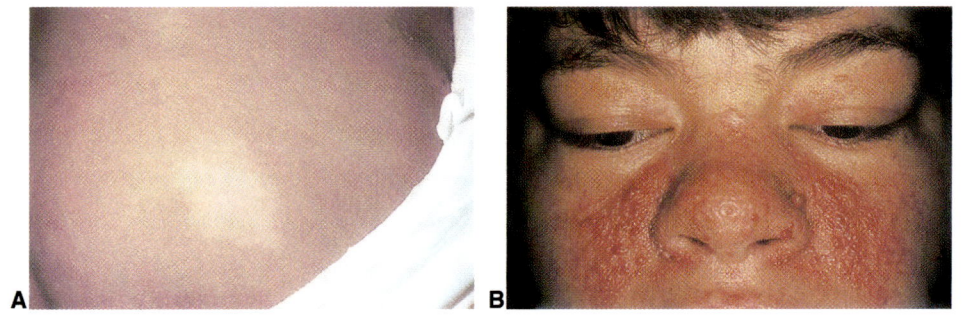

Figure 27-4 Cutaneous lesions of tuberous sclerosis. **A,** Hypopigmented macule. **B,** Adenoma sebaceum of the face.

Figure 27-5 Brain lesions of tuberous sclerosis. **A,** Axial CT image showing small periventricular calcifications in the basal ganglia bilaterally. **B,** Axial T2-weighted MRI showing two tuberous malformations of the right hemisphere cortex.

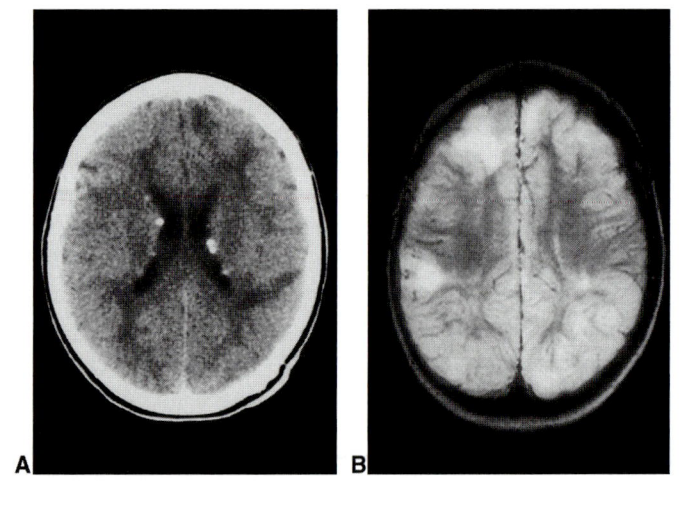

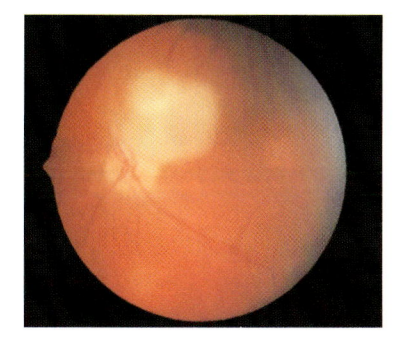

Figure 27-6 Fundus lesions of tuberous sclerosis, left eye. In addition to the large phakoma partially overlying the optic disc, a small hypopigmented lesion appears in the temporal macula and a barely visible second phakoma partially obscures a retinal blood vessel near the edge of the photograph directly below the disc.

layer of the retina and is composed of nerve fibers and relatively undifferentiated cells that appear to be of glial origin; the growth is frequently called an *astrocytic hamartoma.* Phakomas can develop anywhere in the fundus but are usually found near the posterior pole, involving the retina, the optic disc, or both. They vary in size from about half to twice the diameter of the disc. Vision is rarely affected significantly.

Retinal phakomas usually have one of two distinct appearances, although intermediate forms can occur. The first type is typically found in very young children and is relatively flat with a smooth surface, indistinct margins, and gray-white color. These lesions are translucent to a degree that at times makes them difficult to detect ophthalmoscopically. The examiner can most easily locate them by tracing retinal vessels from the disc peripherally and scrutinizing points at which a vessel is partially obscured by overlying tissue. The examiner can then perceive domelike elevations with the binocular indirect ophthalmoscope by carefully observing the surface light reflection while shifting viewing direction slightly. The second type of phakoma is sharply demarcated and more elevated than the first type, with an irregular surface that has been compared to a mulberry or a cluster of tapioca grains or fish eggs. These lesions are opaque, glistening, and yellow-white as a result of calcification. They are found relatively more often in older patients and on or adjacent to the optic disc. The term *giant drusen* has been applied to disc involvement by a mulberry phakoma because of its resemblance to the common but unrelated condition known as *drusen* (or *hyaline bodies*) of the optic nerve head.

The reported frequency of phakomas in persons with TS varies greatly, but data from recent series suggest that they are present in one third to more than one half of cases. One to several may be found in a single eye, and the rate of bilateral involvement is about 40%. There is no evidence that the number of lesions increases with age, although individual tumors have been documented to grow over time. Phakomas are not pathognomonic of TS: they occur occasionally in association with neurofibromatosis and in the eyes of unaffected persons.

Alcorn DM. Ocular oncology. *Ophthalmol Clin North Am.* 1999;12:2.

von Hippel–Lindau Disease (Retinal Angiomatosis)

von Hippel–Lindau (VHL) disease is an autosomal-dominantly inherited disorder manifesting both benign and malignant tumors of many organ systems. The most common abnormalities are vascular tumors *(hemangioblastomas)* of the retina and central nervous system, most often the cerebellum. These tumors have only limited proliferative capacity, but exudation across thin vessel walls in the lesions leads to the formation of fluid accumulations that may attain considerable size and compromise vital structures. Cysts and tumors occur frequently in numerous other organs, including the kidneys *(renal cell carcinoma)*, pancreas, liver, epididymis, and adrenal glands *(pheochromocytoma)*. Despite its well-accepted classification as a neurocutaneous syndrome, VHL disease rarely has significant cutaneous manifestations, although café-au-lait spots and port-wine stains *(nevus flammeus)* are seen occasionally. Mental deficiency is not a feature of the disease. The VHL gene is a tumor suppressor found on chromosome 3. The incidence of VHL is approximately 1 in 36,000 births. Associated malignant tumors make it a potentially fatal disease.

Pedigree studies suggest that ocular involvement occurs in most cases of VHL disease. (Identical eye disease without familial transmission or systemic involvement is three to four times more common than the complete syndrome.) The retinal lesions originally described by von Hippel usually become visible ophthalmoscopically between ages 10 and 35 years, with an average age of onset of 25 years, about a decade before the peak clinical incidence of cerebellar disease. Tumors are multiple in the same eye in about one third of cases and bilateral in as many as half of cases. Tumors typically occur in the peripheral fundus, but lesions adjacent to the optic disc have also been described.

The incipient retinal lesion appears as a minor nonspecific vascular anomaly or a small reddish dot in the fundus that gradually enlarges into a flat or slightly elevated grayish disc. The lesion ultimately acquires the fully developed appearance of a pink globular mass one to three or more disc diameters in size. The hallmark of the mature tumor is a pair of markedly dilated vessels (artery and vein) running between the lesion and the optic disc, indicating significant arteriovenous shunting (Fig 27-7). Recent observations suggest that characteristic paired or twin retinal vessels of normal caliber may be present before the tumor becomes visible.

Histopathologically, retinal angiomas consist of relatively well-formed capillaries; however, fluorescein angiography shows these vessels to be leaky. Transudation of fluid into the subretinal space causes lipid accumulation, retinal detachment, and consequent loss of vision in many involved eyes. Secondary degenerative changes, including cataract and glaucoma, often occur in blind eyes with long-standing retinal detachment; ultimately, enucleation may become necessary.

Retinal angiomas can be effectively treated with cryotherapy or laser photocoagulation in two thirds or more of cases, particularly when the lesions are still small. Multiple treatment sessions may be necessary to achieve complete success. Early diagnosis increases the likelihood of successful treatment, yet the ocular lesions of VHL are asymptomatic prior to retinal detachment. Therefore, children known to be at risk for the disease should undergo periodic ophthalmologic evaluation beginning at about age 5 years.

CHAPTER 27: Phakomatoses • 387

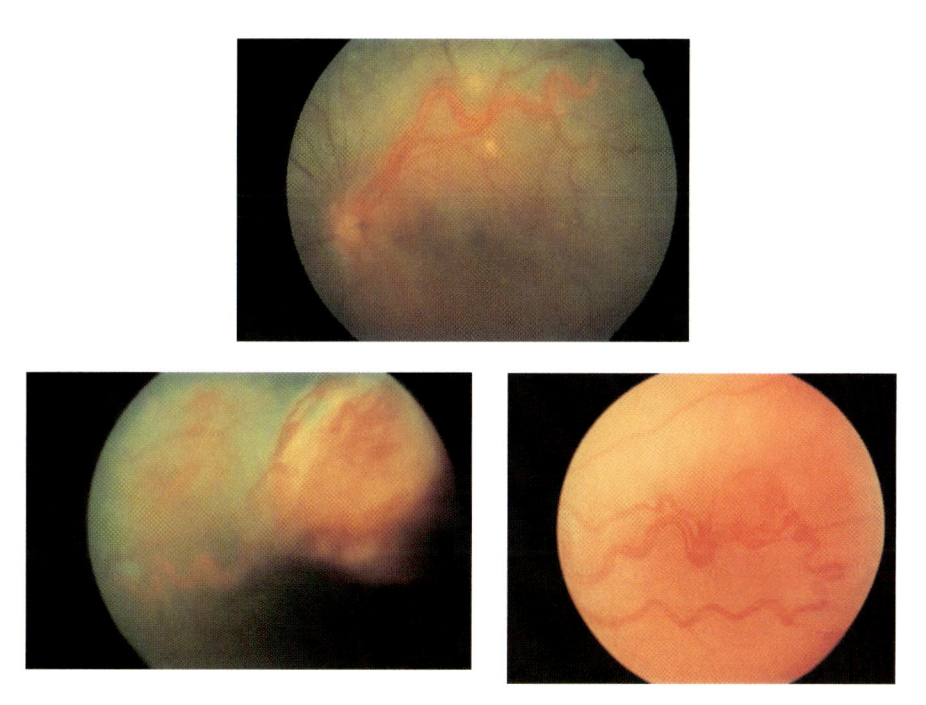

Figure 27-7 von Hippel–Lindau disease (retinal angiomatosis), left eye.

Systemically, early tumor diagnosis can significantly reduce morbidity and mortality. The Cambridge Screening Protocol recommends that patients with VHL undergo annual complete physical examination and dilated eye examinations, renal ultrasonography, and 24-hour urine collection for vanillylmandelic acids. These patients should undergo neuroimaging every 3 years to age 40 and every 5 years thereafter. At-risk relatives should also undergo thorough annual screening for the disorder. Molecular genetic testing has been suggested for patients with early-onset cerebellar hemangioblastoma (<30 years old), early-onset retinal angioma, or familial clear cell renal carcinoma.

Filling-Katz MR, Choyke PL, Oldfield E, et al. Central nervous system involvement in von Hippel–Lindau disease. *Neurology.* 1991;41:41–46.

Maher ER, Yates JR, Harries R, et al. Clinical features and natural history of Von Hippel–Lindau disease. *Q J Med.* 1990;77:1151–1163.

Sturge-Weber Syndrome (Encephalofacial Angiomatosis)

Sturge-Weber syndrome (SWS) consists of a facial cutaneous angioma (port-wine stain) with an ipsilateral leptomeningeal vascular malformation that typically results in the following:
- Cerebral calcification
- Seizures, which may show a jacksonian pattern, progressing from focal to grand mal

- Focal neurologic deficits (hemianopia, hemiparesis)
- A highly variable degree of mental deficiency (with normal intelligence in many affected persons)

SWS is unique among the four major neurocutaneous syndromes in that it is not a genetically transmitted disorder. Lesions are always present at birth, however. The distribution of cutaneous and cerebral involvement suggests a disturbance very early in embryonic development (4–8 weeks' gestation), when primitive facial structures overlie the future occipital lobes of the developing brain. The prevalence of SWS is not reliably known.

Calcium deposits characteristic of SWS form after birth in brain parenchyma, usually involving the occipital lobe and varying portions of the parietal, temporal, and occasionally frontal lobes. Curvilinear densities, paralleling cerebral convolutions to produce the so-called *railroad-track sign*, can be demonstrated by means of CT earlier and more consistently than by conventional radiographs, but these densities are often not detectable before age 2 years. MRI is less sensitive than CT for identifying calcification but may provide better delineation of other abnormalities associated with the angiomatous malformation that can confirm the diagnosis in very young children (Fig 27-8). These abnormalities include cerebral volume reduction, abnormal signal intensity in cortex and white matter, prominent deep venous system, and enlarged choroid plexus.

The Sturge-Weber skin lesion, which can be quite disfiguring, consists of dilated and excessively numerous but well-formed capillaries in the dermis. The lesion usually involves the forehead and upper eyelid on the same side as the cerebral vascular malformation, with varying extension to the ipsilateral lower eyelid and maxillary and mandibular regions (Fig 27-9). The sharply demarcated area of the port-wine nevus frequently does not conform to the distribution of the trigeminal divisions, and involvement of the contralateral face, the scalp, and the trunk and extremities is common. (The designation *Klippel-Trénaunay-Weber syndrome* is sometimes applied to cases with extensive lesions of the extremities, although this syndrome may not be a true phakomatosis.) Hypertrophy

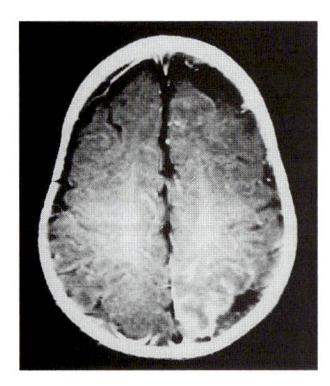

Figure 27-8 Axial gadolinium-enhanced T1-weighted MRI shows vascular malformation with underlying cortical atrophy in the left occipital lobe of a 4-month-old girl with Sturge-Weber syndrome.

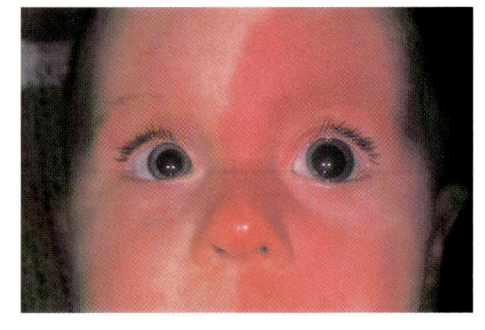

Figure 27-9 Facial port-wine nevus involving the left eyelids, associated with ipsilateral buphthalmos in an infant girl with Sturge-Weber syndrome.

of soft tissue and bone underlying the angioma is common in childhood, and thickening of the involved skin (sometimes with a nodular pattern) may develop later in life. Treatment of affected skin with the pulsed dye laser has been shown to markedly reduce vascularity, considerably improving appearance without causing significant damage to dermal tissue.

Many children have a port-wine stain but do not have SWS.

Ocular Involvement

Any portion of the ocular circulation may be anomalous in SWS when the skin lesion involves the eyelids. Increased conjunctival vascularity commonly produces a pinkish discoloration. Frequently, an abnormal plexus of episcleral vessels appears, although it may be hidden by the overlying tissue of Tenon's layer. The retina sometimes shows tortuous vessels and arteriovenous communications.

The choroid is the site of the most significant purely vascular anomaly of the eye associated with SWS. In a majority of cases of SWS with ocular involvement, increased numbers of well-formed choroidal vessels give the fundus a uniform bright red or red-orange color that has been compared to tomato catsup (Fig 27-10). Typically, the region of the posterior pole is involved; in some cases there is gradual transition to a normal vascular pattern in the periphery, whereas in others the entire fundus seems to be affected. Choroidal angiomatosis usually remains asymptomatic in childhood. During adolescence or adulthood, however, the choroid sometimes becomes markedly thickened. Degeneration or detachment of the overlying retina with severe visual loss may follow, but the frequency of this progression is not established. No treatment is known to effectively prevent or reverse such deterioration, although scattered application of laser photocoagulation, which has proved useful in the management of circumscribed choroidal angiomas not associated with SWS, may help.

Glaucoma is the most common and serious ocular complication, occurring in approximately half of cases. The cause of elevated IOP is uncertain but is likely secondary to elevated episcleral venous pressure, hyperemia of the ciliary body with hypersecretion of aqueous, or developmental anomaly of the anterior chamber angle. Involvement of the upper-lid skin seems to raise the likelihood of glaucoma. Onset of glaucoma can be

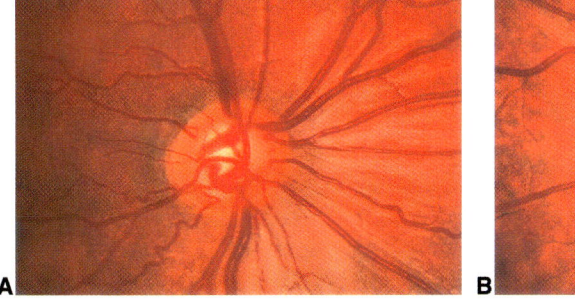

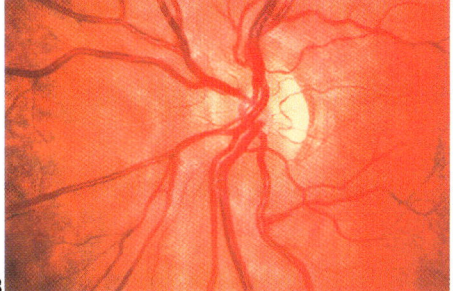

Figure 27-10 Fundus appearance in an adolescent boy with Sturge-Weber syndrome. **A,** Right eye. Note glaucomatous disc cupping and deeper red color of surrounding choroid, compared with normal fellow eye. **B,** Left eye.

at birth or later in childhood. If IOP is elevated during early infancy, enlargement of the cornea can occur, although presentation with corneal clouding is rare.

Management

When SWS is first documented or suspected, a complete ophthalmologic evaluation is essential, including measurement of IOP. Sedation or general anesthesia may be necessary for uncooperative children. Examination should be repeated periodically throughout childhood even if no ocular abnormality is initially detected. SWS glaucoma is difficult to treat, and there is no universally accepted treatment scheme. Initial therapy with topical drops can be effective, especially when onset occurs later. Surgery is indicated in early-onset cases and when medical treatment is inadequate. Adequate long-term pressure control can frequently be achieved, although multiple operations are typically necessary. Aqueous shunting devices, or setons, have shown promise in the management of otherwise intractable glaucoma in patients with SWS (see BCSC Section 10, *Glaucoma*). A particular hazard of glaucoma surgery in SWS is the risk of massive intraoperative or postoperative exudation or hemorrhage from anomalous choroidal vessels due to rapid ocular decompression. Special care must be taken with implanted drainage devices to prevent excessive early postoperative hypotony. Choroidal or subretinal fluid accumulation after surgery may be dramatic, but spontaneous resorption usually occurs within 1–2 weeks. Angle surgery in the form of goniotomy and trabeculotomy has been used successfully in some patients, presumably those whose glaucoma has some etiologic similarity to typical congenital glaucoma.

> Iwach AG, Hoskins HD Jr, Hetherington J Jr, et al. Analysis of surgical and medical management of glaucoma in Sturge-Weber syndrome. *Ophthalmology.* 1990;97:904–909.
> Sullivan TJ, Clarke MP, Morin JD. The ocular manifestations of the Sturge-Weber syndrome. *J Pediatr Ophthalmol Strabismus.* 1992;29:349–356.

Ataxia-Telangiectasia (Louis-Bar Syndrome)

Ataxia-telangiectasia (AT) is an autosomal recessive disorder that primarily involves the central nervous system (particularly the cerebellum), the ocular surface, the skin, and the immune system. Although rare (prevalence is about 1:40,000), AT is thought to be the most common cause of progressive ataxia in early childhood. Truncal ataxia is usually noted during the second year of life, with subsequent development of dysarthria, dystonia, and choreoathetosis. Progressive deterioration of motor function leads to serious disability by age 10 years. Intellectual impairment, if present, is usually mild.

Recognition of ocular features is often the key to diagnosis of AT. Ocular motor abnormalities are found in nearly all patients with AT and are frequently among the earliest manifestations. Characteristically, the ability to initiate saccades with preservation of vestibulo-ocular movements is poor, very similar to the case with congenital ocular motor apraxia. Strabismus and nystagmus may also be present.

Telangiectasia of the conjunctiva develops in all cases between the ages of 3 and 5 years. Involvement is initially interpalpebral but away from the limbus, eventually becoming generalized (Fig 27-11). Similar, though less obvious, vessel changes can appear

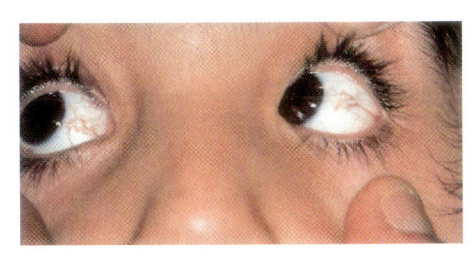

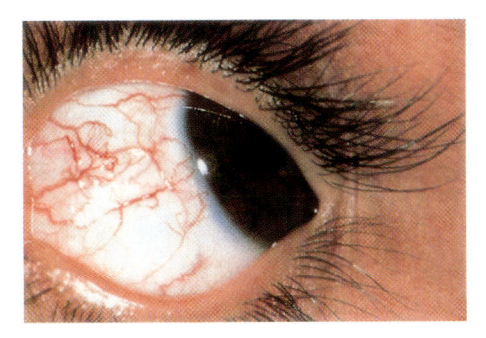

Figure 27-11 Abnormally dilated and tortuous conjunctival vessels, left eye, in a child with ataxia-telangiectasia.

in the skin of the eyelids and other sun-exposed areas. A variety of skin changes that suggest accelerated aging are common in older children and adults with AT.

Persons with AT show greatly increased sensitivity to the tissue-damaging side effects of therapeutic radiation and many chemotherapeutic agents. Defective T cell function in patients with AT is usually associated with hypoplasia of the thymus and decreased levels of circulating immunoglobulin. Recurrent respiratory tract infections are a serious problem, frequently causing death in adolescence or young adulthood even with optimal antimicrobial and supportive treatment. The increased susceptibility to various malignancies, particularly lymphomas and leukemias, contributes to early mortality in one third to one half of cases.

The function of the AT gene or genes, now localized to the long arm of chromosome 11, is unknown but probably relates to DNA repair. AT heterozygosity is present in an estimated 1%–3% of the population. Although gene carriers are generally healthy and cannot be identified except in the context of a known AT pedigree, they are at significantly increased risk for common forms of malignancy and show greater-than-normal sensitivity to radiation. In women heterozygous for the AT gene, breast cancer is about seven times more frequent than in noncarriers and accounts for nearly 10% of all cases in the United States.

Gatti RA, Boder E, Vinters HV, et al. Ataxia-telangiectasia: an interdisciplinary approach to pathogenesis. *Medicine*. 1991;70:99–117.

Harley RD, Baird HW, Craven EM. Ataxia telangiectasia. Report of seven cases. *Arch Ophthalmol*. 1967;77:582–592.

Incontinentia Pigmenti (Bloch-Sulzberger Syndrome)

Incontinentia pigmenti (IP) is a syndrome involving the skin, brain, and eye that shows the unusual inheritance pattern of X-linked dominance with a presumed lethal effect on the hemizygous male fetus. Nearly all affected persons are female, with mother-to-daughter transmission in familial cases. BCSC Section 2, *Fundamentals and Principles of Ophthalmology*, details this inheritance pattern in the chapters on genetics.

392 • Pediatric Ophthalmology and Strabismus

The cutaneous manifestations of IP are distinctive. The skin usually appears normal at birth, but erythema and bullae develop during the first few days of life, usually on the extremities, and persist for weeks to months. A second distinct phase characterized by verrucous changes begins at about 2 months of age, subsiding after a few more months. Finally, clusters of small hyperpigmented macules in a characteristic splashed-paint distribution make their appearance, most prominently on the trunk (Fig 27-12).

Histopathologically, the early vesicular lesions show local accumulation of unusually large macrophages and eosinophils accompanied by peripheral blood eosinophilia. In the lesions of the pigmentary stage, which persist for years before gradually fading, free melanin granules are found abnormally scattered in the dermis. Although present in all cases, skin involvement varies considerably in extent, occasionally being so limited that it is completely overlooked at one or more of its stages.

About one third of patients with IP have central nervous system problems that may include microcephaly, hydrocephalus, seizures, and varying degrees of mental deficiency. Dental abnormalities (missing and malformed teeth) are found in roughly two thirds of cases. Other, less common findings include scoliosis, skull deformities, cleft palate, and dwarfism.

Ocular involvement occurs in at least one quarter to one third of cases, typically in the form of a proliferative retinal vasculopathy that closely resembles retinopathy of prematurity. At birth, the only detectable abnormality may be incomplete peripheral retinal vascularization. Abnormal arteriovenous connections, microvascular abnormalities, and neovascular membranes develop at or near the junction of vascular and avascular retina (Fig 27-13). Rapid progression sometimes leads to total retinal detachment and retrolental membrane formation *(pseudoglioma)* within the first few months of life. Other affected eyes show gradual deterioration over a period of several years; still others have proliferative lesions of limited extent that may persist for decades. Microphthalmos, cat-

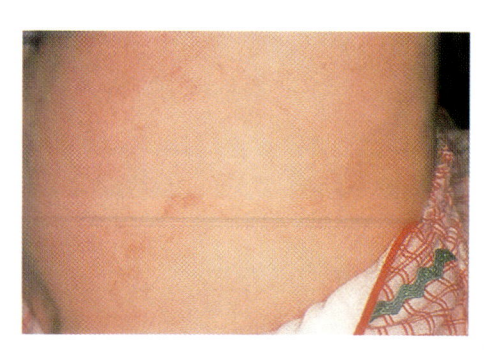

Figure 27-12 Pigmented skin lesions of incontinentia pigmenti.

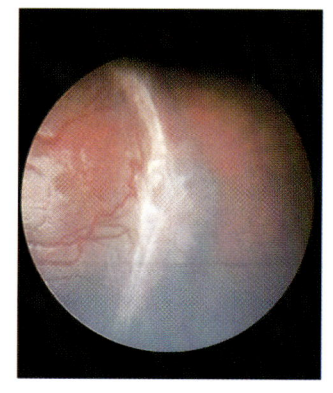

Figure 27-13 Vascular abnormalities of the temporal retina, right eye, in a 2-year-old child with incontinentia pigmenti. Note avascularity peripheral to the circumferential white vasoproliferative lesion, which showed profuse leakage on fluorescein angioscopy.

aract, glaucoma, optic atrophy, strabismus, and nystagmus occur occasionally, representing secondary consequences of endstage retinopathy in most if not all cases.

The retinopathy of IP has been managed by photocoagulation or cryotherapy in a small number of cases with varying degrees of reported success. No consensus exists as to whether treatment should be applied primarily to the avascular peripheral retina, as in the currently preferred approach to management of retinopathy of prematurity, or to the proliferative lesions themselves.

Catalano RA. Incontinentia pigmenti. *Am J Ophthalmol.* 1990;110:696–702.

Wyburn-Mason Syndrome (Racemose Angioma)

Wyburn-Mason syndrome is a nonhereditary arteriovenous malformation of the eye and brain, typically involving the optic disc or retina and the midbrain. Skin lesions are present in a minority of cases. The complete syndrome is considerably less common than an isolated occurrence of similar ocular or intracranial disease.

Seizures, mental changes, hemiparesis, and papilledema may result from the central nervous system lesions, which are frequently a source of hemorrhage, unlike the hemangioma of SWS.

Ocular manifestations are unilateral and congenital but may progress somewhat during childhood. The typical lesion consists of markedly dilated and tortuous vessels that shunt blood flow directly from arteries to veins; these vessels do not leak fluid (Fig 27-14). Vision ranges from normal to markedly reduced in the involved eye, and intraocular hemorrhage and secondary neovascular glaucoma are possible complications. No treatment is indicated for primary lesions.

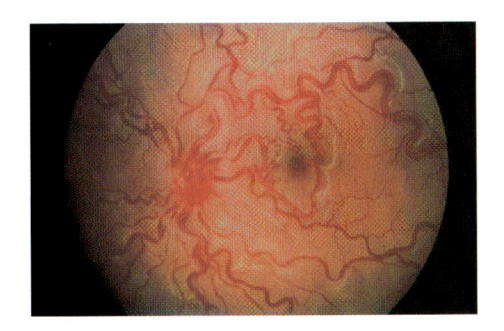

Figure 27-14 Racemose angioma of the retina, left eye.

CHAPTER 28

Craniofacial Malformations

Approach to the Child With Craniofacial and Ocular Malformations

Children with congenital malformations and syndromes involving craniofacial structures are at a significant risk for ocular anomalies. The number of syndromes and isolated malformations is enormous, and the spectrum of eye problems is vast. Therefore, the reader may find it helpful to develop an approach to the dysmorphic child rather than to attempt to memorize all the ocular pathological changes reported in the literature. It is useful to consider these findings in two large categories: *intrinsic ocular pathology* and *secondary ocular complications*.

Intrinsic Ocular Pathology

With intrinsic ocular pathology, the ocular findings are primary, not secondary, and they are related to the basic defect. The underlying insult, genetic or environmental, results in damage to the developing ocular tissues or their failure to form. Examples include:

- Myopia and retinal pathological changes in Stickler syndrome
- Anterior segment developmental anomalies associated with systemic anomalies, fetal alcohol syndrome, chromosomal anomalies
- Ocular colobomas in many syndromes and ocular muscle anomalies of position or size in craniosynostosis syndrome
- Cranial nerve/ocular motility involvement in Möbius syndrome, thalidomide embryopathy, Duane syndrome with systemic abnormalities

Secondary Ocular Complications

Complications secondary to changes in size, shape, or position of bony and soft tissue orbital structures may occur as disruption or deformation during development, or they may be acquired after birth. These complications are derived changes that can be anticipated from the malformations present in the surrounding tissues. Complications are not necessarily specific to a syndrome but the result of a type of deformity or mechanical factors. Thus, the same anomaly may occur in various types of syndromes. Complications include:

- Corneal exposure resulting from extreme proptosis or eyelid defects
- Refractive errors associated with soft tissue anomalies of the eyelid and adnexa
- Ocular motility deviations associated with abnormal position or shape of the orbits
- Papilledema or optic atrophy secondary to increased intracranial pressure or local factors *(craniosynostosis)*
- Ocular anomalies that are caused by environmental factors during embryogenesis (corneal opacities and eyelid colobomas in some patients with amniotic band syndrome)

Cohen MM Jr. *The Child with Multiple Birth Defects.* 2nd ed. New York: Oxford; 1997.

Selected Craniofacial Syndromes

Craniosynostosis

Craniosynostosis is the premature closure of one or more cranial sutures in the embryonic period or early childhood. The involved synostosed suture or sutures determine the shape of the skull because growth is inhibited perpendicular to the closed suture. Compensatory growth occurs not only at the open sutures but also in weakened areas of the cranial vault. Varying patterns of suture closure may result in a wide spectrum of skull shapes. Mental retardation may occur, but many patients show normal intellectual capacity.

A few important terms associated with premature suture closure are:

- *Plagiocephaly*—unilateral closure of a coronal suture results in skull asymmetry
- *Brachycephaly*—bilateral closure of coronal sutures results in a short, wide skull
- *Scaphocephaly*—premature closure of the sagittal suture results in a long, narrow skull

Other important terms describing craniofacial structural anomalies are:

- *Hypertelorism*—increased separation of the bony orbits. This is an anatomical description that can be a part of many craniofacial syndromes or other midline defects, not a diagnostic entity. *Hypotelorism* refers to a decreased distance between the orbits.
- *Telecanthus*—increased distance between the medial canthi. This may be secondary to hypertelorism but can be a primary soft tissue abnormality.

Craniosynostosis can occur as a primary isolated anomaly, or it can be associated with systemic malformations resulting from a variety of etiologic conditions (eg, metabolic diseases, chromosomal anomalies, nutritional factors, or mendelian genetic syndromes). The most frequently encountered group, the *craniosynostosis syndromes,* usually show an autosomal dominant transmission (eg, Apert, Crouzon, Pfeiffer, Saethre-Chotzen syndromes), although a few show autosomal recessive inheritance (eg, Marshall syndrome). Mutations in the fibroblast growth factor receptors (FGFR 1–3) have been found in several of the syndromes.

CHAPTER 28: Craniofacial Malformations • 397

Common systemic features of this syndrome group include abnormally shaped skull, midfacial hypoplasia, hypertelorism, oral and dental problems, and respiratory difficulties (Fig 28-1). Syndactyly is a feature of a number of the syndromes, including Apert, Saethre-Chotzen, and Pfeiffer.

Ocular complications

Poor vision in one or both eyes is common in patients with craniosynostosis. The poor vision may be present at birth, develop slowly or rapidly (usually in childhood), or occur as a complication of reconstructive orbital surgery. Several low-frequency anomalies (eg, cataracts, retinal pigmentary changes, keratoconus, ptosis) have also been reported.

Proptosis in craniosynostosis results from a reduced volume of the bony orbital space secondary to a variety of anatomical factors and differs from proptosis secondary to orbital masses. Although the ophthalmic complaints and complications are similar in both causes, the definitive treatment may be different. The severity of the proptosis in patients with craniosynostosis is not uniform and frequently increases with age because of the impaired growth of the bony orbit.

Because the eyelids may not afford adequate protection for the globe, the most serious complication of severe proptosis is corneal exposure. Exposure keratitis results; if this is inadequately managed, perforation of the globe and irreversible damage to the eye sometimes occurs. The progression of proptosis caused by craniosynostosis syndromes may be slow, permitting conservative treatment such as use of lubricating ointment. However, if the exorbitism is severe or rapidly progressive, emergency tarsorrhaphy may

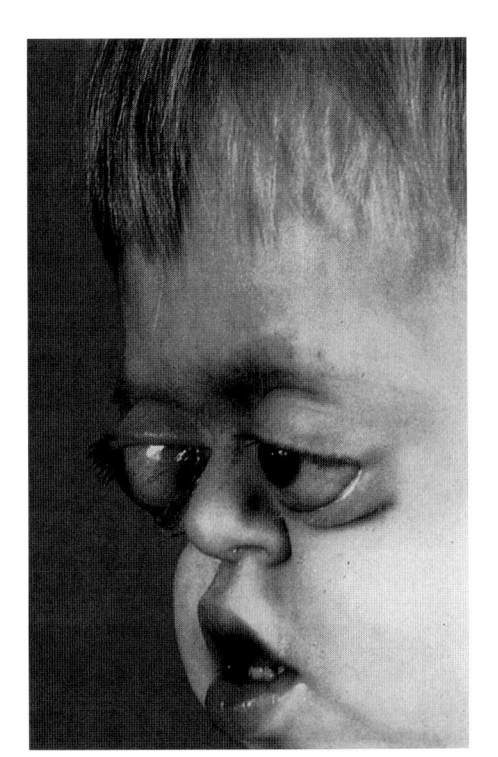

Figure 28-1 Side view of patient with Crouzon syndrome showing midfacial hypoplasia, very prominent eyes that developed severe corneal exposure and ulceration, and so-called *parrot beak*. *(Reproduced by permission from Miller MT. Ocular malformations in craniofacial malformations.* Int Ophthalmol Clin. *1984;24:148.)*

be indicated. This procedure is still not a definitive treatment because the underlying cause of shallow orbit has not been eliminated.

Rarely, the eye is completely dislocated because of the extremely shallow orbit, constituting a medical emergency because of the problems of corneal exposure and possible compromise of the blood supply to the eye, conjunctiva, or both. The clinician can sometimes retroplace the eye by gently bringing the upper eyelid over the globe with a finger. If conjunctival prolapse occurs, treatment must be aimed at keeping the exposed conjunctiva moist.

Closure of certain crucial cranial sutures, especially the coronal, frequently results in increased intracranial pressure and papilledema. If this is not reversed, optic atrophy occurs. Some authors suggest that optic atrophy is always secondary to high intracranial pressure; others think that local changes in the optic canal can also cause damage to the optic nerve in some cases. Optic atrophy is infrequent if the sagittal suture is the only one involved or if suture closure is unilateral.

A mild, chronic type of papilledema without retinal hemorrhages has also been described. This form of papilledema is difficult to differentiate from pseudopapilledema. Papilledema may also disappear without residual signs. The apparent increased frequency of tortuous vasculature reported in craniosynostosis has been suggested as evidence of previous papilledema. Chapter 25 also discusses papilledema and pseudopapilledema.

Strabismus and amblyopia

Patients with craniosynostosis show a variety of horizontal deviations in primary position; exotropia is the most frequent. The most consistent finding, however, is a marked V pattern, most commonly with a large exotropia on upgaze and a small exotropia, orthophoria, or esotropia on downgaze. This V pattern is often accompanied by a marked apparent overaction or pseudooveraction of the inferior oblique muscles, frequently caused by abnormal insertions of the rectus muscles. In some patients, testing of ocular movements reveals definite limitation in various fields of action, especially in connection with the superior rectus muscle. In a number of patients, CT or MRI has shown abnormally inserted or unusually small ocular muscles. This is frequently secondary to excyclorotation of the orbits. Amblyopia is common secondary to strabismus or refractive differences between the two eyes. Recognition of the risk factors aids in prevention or reversal with treatment.

Management

Reconstructive surgery for severe craniofacial malformation has seen major advances in recent decades. This surgery is frequently extensive and involves en bloc movement of the facial structures. The status of the visual system should be documented preoperatively, and certain relationships, such as intercanthal and interpupillary distance as well as palpebral fissure, should be measured. Postoperatively, the function of the visual system should be reevaluated and appropriate treatment instituted.

In many centers, a specialized craniofacial team—including facial plastic surgeons, neurosurgeons, ophthalmologists, and oral surgeons—collaborates to determine the timing of the reconstructive surgery by prioritizing the child's multiple problems. However, the team may choose to intervene earlier than they would have normally chosen in cases of vision-threatening corneal exposure and ulceration. Postoperative corneal damage, which may go unnoticed because of transient or permanent decrease in corneal sensation, may be caused by bandage abrasion of the cornea or exposure from incomplete protection by the eyelids due to postoperative edema. The position of the eye or the canthi may also change, and ptosis and new symptoms of lacrimal system obstruction may ensue.

Additionally, reconstructive surgery that involves moving the orbits may significantly change the degree or type of strabismus, thereby modifying the indicated form of strabismus surgery. Another consideration is that improved binocular function may not be attainable in these patients because of their unusual and incomitant form of ocular muscle imbalance. Thus, early strabismus surgery is of no particular advantage, and deferring treatment until craniofacial surgery is completed may be appropriate.

Cohen MM. *The Child with Multiple Birth Defects*. 2nd ed. New York: Oxford; 1997:178–196.
Posnick JC, Ruiz R. The craniofacial dysostosis syndromes: current surgical thinking and future directions [review]. *Cleft Palate Craniofac J*. 2000;37:434.

The ophthalmologist should be familiar with several craniofacial syndromes. These include Crouzon, Apert, and Pfeiffer syndromes. All are inherited in an autosomal dominant fashion and involve various mutations of the fibroblast growth factor receptor (FGFR) genes.

Crouzon syndrome

Crouzon syndrome involves premature closure of one or more of the metopic, sagittal, or lambdoidal sutures, but the characteristic appearance of a brachycephalic skull results from bilateral coronal suture closure. Patients also have shallow orbits, resulting in varying degrees of proptosis and midface hypoplasia, which in turn results in significant malocclusion.

Apert syndrome

The characteristic facial appearance results from cartilage dysplasia at the cranial base, which causes premature closure of midline structures from the anterior to the posterior extent of the skull. In addition, patients with Apert syndrome have complex syndactyly of the hands and feet as well as frequent joint abnormalities of elbows and shoulders.

Pfeiffer syndrome

Pfeiffer syndrome is less common than Crouzon and Apert syndromes and yields greater variation in craniofacial expressivity. Pfeiffer syndrome is usually associated with broad thumbs and great toes and occasionally with syndactyly of one or both hands.

Other Craniofacial Anomalies

Waardenburg syndrome

Patients with Waardenburg syndrome, an autosomal dominant disorder, may have any of the following:
- Lateral displacement of the inner canthi and lacrimal puncta
- Confluent eyebrows
- Heterochromia iridis (complete or partial)

- Congenital bilateral sensorineural deafness (complete or partial)
- White forelocks
- Fundus hypopigmentation

Hemifacial microsomia

Other terms for hemifacial microsomia are *hemifacial hypoplasia, oculoauriculovertebral dysplasia, first and second arch syndrome,* and *Goldenhar syndrome.* Findings include microtia, macrostomia, and mandibular anomalies (Fig 28-2). Ear tags are common; inner-ear anomalies occur in some cases. Vertebral anomalies are common; the central nervous system occasionally is affected. Involvement is unilateral in 70%–80% of cases. Ocular manifestations may range from clinical anophthalmos to minor fissure asymmetry.

Goldenhar syndrome

Also known as *oculoauriculovertebral dysplasia,* Goldenhar syndrome is proposed to represent a variant of the hemifacial microsomia group, with characteristic epibulbar dermoids or lipodermoids, usually in the inferotemporal quadrant. Limbal dermoids are reported more frequently than lipodermoids, and they can be bilateral (approximately 25% of cases). They occasionally impinge on the visual axis but more commonly interfere with visual acuity by causing astigmatism and predisposing to secondary strabismus from

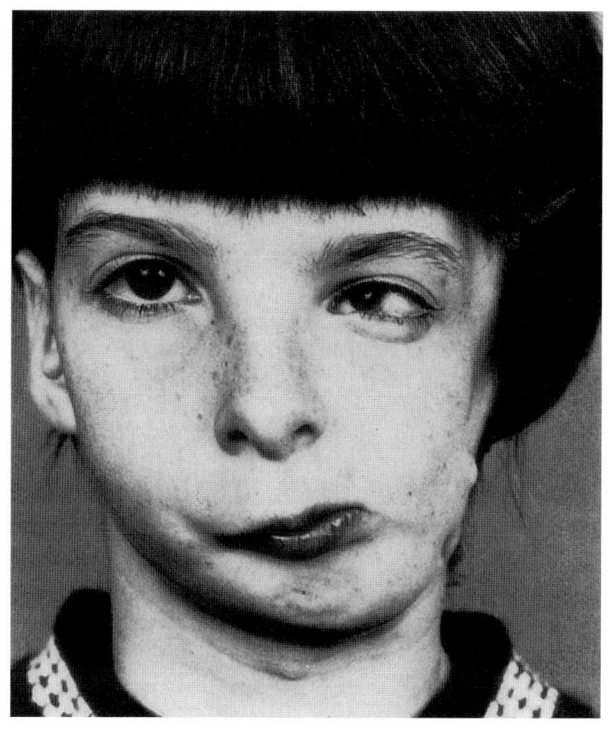

Figure 28-2 Hemifacial microsomia, Goldenhar variant. Patient has facial asymmetry, a hypoplastic left ear, an ear tag near the right ear, conjunctival lipodermoid in the left eye, and esotropia. Patient also has a left Duane syndrome.

anisometropic amblyopia. Another common finding is an upper eyelid coloboma, almost always on the more affected side. Duane syndrome has been reported in some patients with Goldenhar syndrome. Low-incidence anomalies include decreased corneal sensitivity, cataract, and iris abnormalities.

Hallermann-Streiff syndrome

Also known as *oculomandibulofacial dyscephaly*, Hallermann-Streiff syndrome is characterized by mandibular hypoplasia, a beaked nose, and bilateral cataracts often associated with microphthalmos, microcornea, or both. Spontaneous resorption of the lens has been reported frequently; occasionally, patients present with apparent congenital aphakia. Glaucoma may complicate the ocular findings. Additional anomalies may include atrophy of the facial skin, hypotrichosis, and marked dwarfism with dental and nasal abnormalities. All cases have been sporadic, and the cause is unknown.

Pierre Robin sequence (anomaly, deformity)

The Pierre Robin sequence is characterized by micrognathia, glossoptosis, and cleft palate. These abnormalities occur in a variety of syndromes, and associated ocular anomalies include retinal detachment, microphthalmos, congenital glaucoma, cataracts, and high myopia. The Pierre Robin sequence is a frequent finding in *Stickler syndrome.*

Mandibulofacial dysostosis (Treacher Collins–Franceschetti syndrome)

Mandibulofacial dysostosis is characterized by bilateral involvement of facial structures, including malar and mandibular hypoplasia, microstomia, coloboma in the outer third of the lower lid, and external- and middle-ear anomalies (Fig 28-3).

In the severe form, the zygomatic bone is underdeveloped and may be absent. A fissure in the maxilla and a defect in the lower margin of the orbit are often present. Hypoplasia of the supraorbital rim has also been observed.

In about 50% of patients, the lateral canthus is displaced downward, producing the characteristic antimongoloid slant. At times, the lower eyelid coloboma produces the illusion of a slant. Deficiency in the cilia medial to the eyelid coloboma may also occur, as may a number of low-incidence anomalies such as iris coloboma and absence of lower lacrimal puncta and meibomian glands. The syndrome is inherited as an autosomal dominant trait with incomplete penetrance and varying expressivity.

> Dixon MJ. Treacher Collins syndrome. *J Med Genet.* 1995;32:806–808.
> Gorlin RJ, Cohen MM, Levin LS. *Syndromes of the Head and Neck.* 3rd ed. New York: Oxford; 1990.

Fetal Alcohol Syndrome

A pattern of malformations has been observed in children born to women with a history of heavy alcohol use during pregnancy. Alcohol and other teratogens can produce a wide range of effects on the developing fetus, depending on consumption or dose, timing of intake, genetic background, and other factors. The presence of certain dysmorphic features along with other symptoms and signs has been designated fetal alcohol syndrome (Fig 28-4). The more consistent characteristics of fetal alcohol syndrome include:

402 • Pediatric Ophthalmology and Strabismus

Figure 28-3 Mandibulofacial dysostosis (Treacher Collins–Franceschetti syndrome). Note downward slant of palpebral fissure, low-set abnormal ears, notch or curving of the inferotemporal eyelid margin, and maxillary and mandibular hypoplasia. *(Reproduced by permission from Peyman GA, Sanders DR, Goldberg MF.* Principles and Practice of Ophthalmology. *Philadelphia: Saunders; 1980:2411.)*

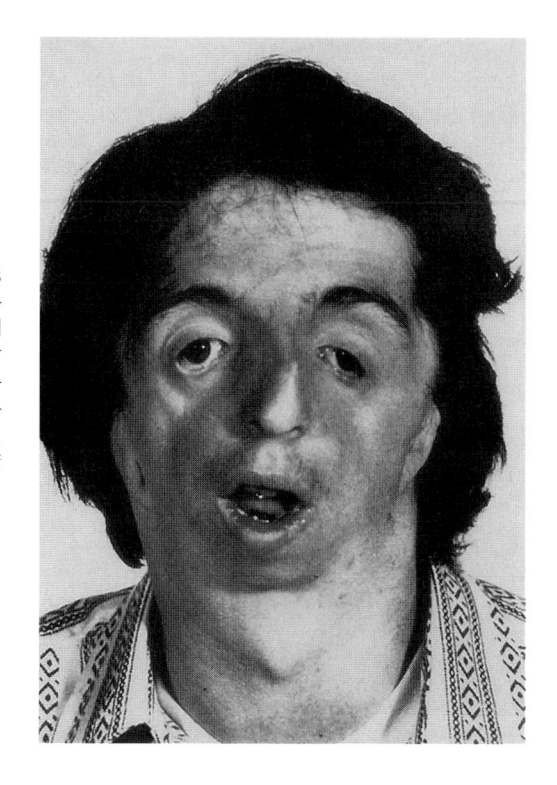

Figure 28-4 Fetal alcohol syndrome. Asymmetrical ptosis; telecanthus; strabismus; long, flat philtrum; anteverted nostrils. This child also had Peters anomaly of the left cornea and myopia of the right eye. *(Reproduced by permission from Miller MT. Fetal alcohol syndrome.* J Pediatr Ophthalmol Strabismus. *1981;18:6–5.)*

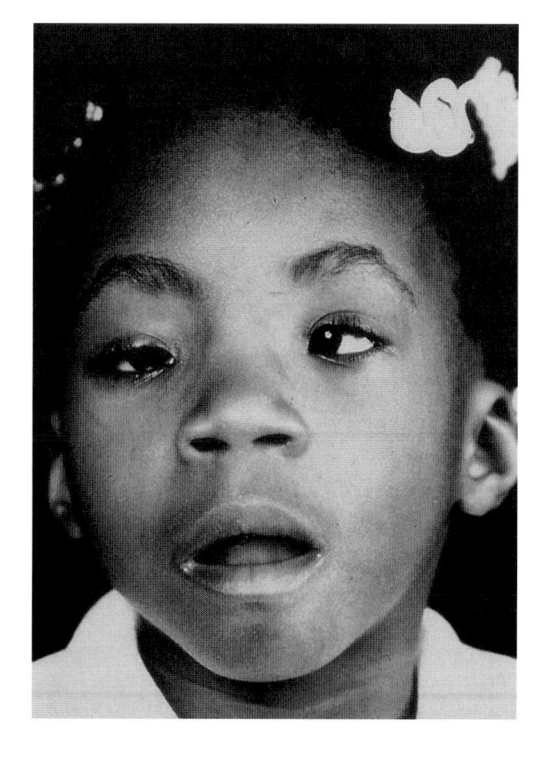

- Facial abnormalities with short palpebral fissures, thin vermilion border of upper lip, and epicanthal folds
- Mental retardation (mild to severe)
- Small weight and height at birth that persist in the postnatal period
- Abnormalities of cardiovascular and skeletal systems

Ocular involvement can include hypoplasia of the optic nerve head and increased tortuosity of retinal vasculature. Optic disc anomalies are the most common malformations of the fundus (up to 48%). Frequently, the disc is small with sharp and often irregular margins; the condition may be unilateral or bilateral. A combination of anomalies of the optic disc and the retinal vessels is a typical finding in the fundus of a child with fetal alcohol syndrome.

Stromland K, Hellstrom A. Fetal alcohol syndrome—an ophthalmological and socioeducational prospective study. *Pediatrics.* 1996;97:845–850.

Fetal Hydantoin Syndrome

Offspring of women treated with hydantoins for convulsive disorders show a varying pattern of altered growth, decreased mental performance, unusual facies, and systemic malformations. Although severe ocular abnormalities are rare, strabismus, ptosis, hypertelorism, optic nerve hypoplasia, and epicanthal folds have been reported. These children also frequently have microcephaly and a nasal bridge that is broad, depressed, or both. Although congenital anomalies occur in 4%–5% of children born to epileptic mothers not taking anticonvulsants (compared with a normal incidence of 2%–3%), the rate increases to 6%–11% if the mother is taking anticonvulsants.

Davies SM. Epilepsy and pregnancy. *Am Fam Physician.* 1986;34:179–183.
Jones KL. Fetal hydantoin effects. In: Jones KL, ed. *Smith's Recognizable Patterns of Human Malformation.* 5th ed. Philadelphia: Saunders; 1997:559.

CHAPTER 29

Ocular Findings in Inborn Errors of Metabolism

With advances in ophthalmology and medicine over the past 50 years, and the elimination of infectious diseases and cataract as major causes of blindness in the United States and other industrialized countries, genetic and metabolic disorders affecting the eye have assumed a much larger role in visual impairment and blindness. Ophthalmologists must therefore learn more about the ophthalmic manifestations of genetic and metabolic disorders. Genetic disorders are also discussed in detail in BCSC Section 2.

Inborn errors of metabolism are a group of disorders characterized by the genetic absence, either physical or functional, of one or more enzymes. This enzyme deficiency creates a block in one of the many metabolic or biochemical pathways critical to the normal growth, development, or functioning of the organism. Clinically, the enzyme deficiency may produce the observed ocular changes in one of three ways, as shown in Figure 29-1.

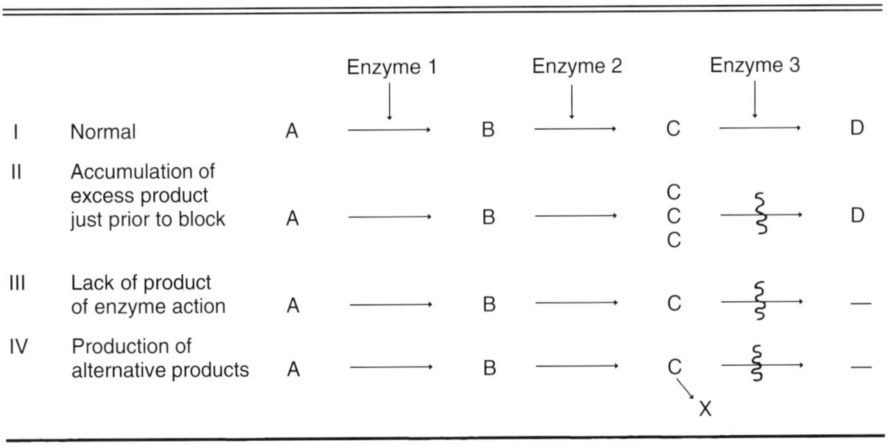

		Enzyme 1	Enzyme 2	Enzyme 3	
I	Normal	A →	B →	C →	D
II	Accumulation of excess product just prior to block	A →	B →	C C C ⟿	D
III	Lack of product of enzyme action	A →	B →	C ⟿	—
IV	Production of alternative products	A →	B →	C ⟿ ↘ X	—

Figure 29-1 In the normal state, substance A is converted by enzyme 1 to substance B, which is converted by enzyme 2 to substance C, etc. The absence of functional enzyme 3 may result in an accumulation of excess product C just prior to the block, as is clinically observed in alkaptonuria. Alternatively, deficiency of enzyme 3 may result in a lack of the product of this enzyme's action, as in albinism. Finally, a deficiency of enzyme 3 may block the normal conversion of product C to product D and result in the up-regulation of alternative pathways, which produce abnormal products or products normally present in very low quantity. These abnormal products may be toxic and produce disease manifestations as in phenylketonuria.

Table 29-1 Ocular Findings in Mucopolysaccharidoses, Mucolipidoses, Lipidoses, Gangliosidoses, and Miscellaneous Disorders

Disease	Enzyme Deficiency	Corneal Clouding	Motility Disorders	Cherry-Red Spot	RPE Degeneration	Optic Atrophy	Other	Inheritance
Mucopolysaccharidoses								
MPH IH, IS Hurler (2528)* Scheie	α-iduronidase	+++	–	–	+++	+	glaucoma papilledema	AR
MPS II Hunter (30990)	iduronate sulfatase	–	–	–	++	+	–	XR
MPS III Sanfilippo (25290)	A: heparan N-sulfatase B: N-acetyl-α-D-glucosaminidase	+	–	–	++	rare	late blindness	AR
MPS IV	A: N-acetyl-galactosamine-6-sulfatase B: β-galactosidase	++	–	–	rare	rare	–	AR
Morquio (25300)								
MPS VI Maroteaux-Lamy (25320)	arylsulfatase B	++	–	–	–	+	papilledema glaucoma	AR
MPS VII Sly (25322)	β-glucuronidase	+	–	–	–	–	–	AR
Mucolipidoses								
Type I (25240) sialidosis (type 2) cherry-red-spot myoclonus syndrome	neuraminidase	–	+	+	+	–	hearing loss	AR
Type II I-cell disease (25250)	multiple lysosomal enzymes	++	–	–	–	–	Hurler-like	AR
Type III pseudo-Hurler polydystrophy (25260)	multiple lysosomal enzymes	+++	–	–	–	–	Hurler-like puffy eyelids (25260)	AR
Type IV (25265)	partial ganglioside sialidase	+++	–	–	++	+	photophobia	AR
Lipidoses								
Niemann-Pick disease (25720)	sphingomyelinase	+	nystagmus	+	–	+	eventual vision loss	AR
Fabry disease (30150)	α-galactosidase A	whorl-like	–	–	–	–	angiokeratoma, spokelike cataract, aneurysmal conjunctival vessels	XR
Gaucher disease (Type 1 23080) (Type II 23090) (Type III 23100)	glucocerebrosidase	–	paralytic strabismus, looped saccades	–	+	–	pinguecula, conjunctival pigmentation	AR
Metachromatic leukodystrophy (25010)	arylsulfatase A	–	nystagmus	+	–	+	blindness, decreased pupil reaction	AR
Krabbe disease (24520)	galactocerebrosidase	–	nystagmus	rare	–	+	cortical blindness	AR
Fucosidosis (23000)	α-L-fucosidase	–	–	–	+	–	Hurler-like features, angiokeratoma tortuous conjunctival vessels	AR

Disease	Enzyme Deficiency	Conjunct. Tortuosity	Corneal Clouding	Motility Disorders	Cherry-Red Spot	RPE Degeneration	Optic Atrophy	High Myopia	Blindness	Inheritance
Gangliosidoses										
Generalized (GM₁) gangliosidosis										
(1) Type I (23050)	β-galactosidase A, B, and C	+	±	ET, nystagmus	50% of patients	−	+	+	+	AR
(2) Type II (23060) Derry disease juvenile GM₁	β-galactosidase B and C	−	−	ET, nystagmus	−	+	±	−	late	AR
(3) Type III (23065) adult GM₁	β-galactosidase (partial)	±	rare	−	−	−	−	−	−	AR
GM₂ gangliosidosis										
(1) Type I (27280) Tay-Sachs disease	hexosaminidase A	−	−	nystagmus, ophthalmoplegia	+	−	+	−	+	AR
(2) Type II (26880) Sandhoff disease	hexosaminidase A and B	−	rare	ET	+	−	±	−	+	AR
(3) Type III (23065) juvenile GM₂ Bernheimer-Seitelberger disease	hexosaminidase A (partial)	−	−	−	−	+	+	−	late	AR

Disease	Enzyme Deficiency	Corneal Clouding	Motility Disorders	Cherry-Red Spot	RPE Degeneration	Optic Atrophy	Other	Inheritance
Miscellaneous Disorders								
Galactosialidosis	β-galactosidase neuraminidase	+	−	+	−	+	dwarfism, seizures, coarse facies	AR
Ceroid lipofuscinosis (20420)								
Hagberg-Santavuori disease	PPT-1	−	+	Macular bull's eye	+	+	blindness	AR
Jansky-Bielschowsky disease	PPT-1	−	+		+	+	blindness	AR
Spielmeyer-Vogt disease	unknown	−	+		+	+	blindness	AR
Kufs disease	unknown	−	−	−	−	−		AR
Cystinosis (21980)	unknown	crystals	−	−	++	−	conjuctival crystals, renal problems	AR
Galactosemia (23040)	gal-1-PO₄ uridyl transferase	−	−	−	−	−	cataracts if not treated	AR
Mannosidosis (24850)	α-mannosidase	++	−	−	−	pallor, blurred margin	Hurler-like, spokelike cataract	AR
Homocystinuria (23620)	cystathionine β-synthase	−	−	−	+	−	dislocated lens, cataract	AR
Refsum disease (26650)	phytanic acid α-hydrolase	−	−	−	++	−	cataract, night blindness	AR

*These code numbers refer to the system developed by Victor MuKusick (McKusick VA, Francomano CA, Antonarakis SE. *Mendelian Inheritance in Man: Catalogs of Autosomal Dominant, Autosomal Recessive, and X-linked Phenotypes.* 10th ed. Baltimore: The Johns Hopkins University Press; 1992).
Plus (+) and minus (−) signs indicate the relative likelihood of occurrence of ocular findings in these systemic disorders.

Inborn errors of metabolism are generally inherited as recessive disorders. The presence of half the normal quantity of an enzyme, as is expected in patients with one normal gene and one defective one, results in adequate metabolic function. Enzyme activity can be measured in suspected carriers: documentation of enzyme levels that are half of normal is frequently diagnostic of the carrier state. Furthermore, measurement of enzyme levels in fetal cells obtained through amniocentesis has allowed prenatal detection of many of these metabolic conditions. Different clinical pictures can be caused by different but allelic mutations or compound mutations wherein each of the pair of chromosomes has a different mutation in the same gene. In some disorders, the control of an enzyme is defective, rather than the enzyme itself.

Ophthalmologists must be aware of the ophthalmic manifestations of inborn errors of metabolism, both in carriers and in affected persons. Eye findings may be the earliest signs in a number of systemic disorders such as the phakomatoses, connective tissue disorders, metabolic disorders, and albinism. Early diagnosis of these conditions permits genetic counseling regarding the risk of recurrence of a particular disorder in the family, as well as aids in determining prognosis and clinical expectations. In addition, through genetic counseling, services such as prenatal testing using amniocentesis can be made available to an affected family.

Table 29-1 summarizes the common ophthalmic manifestations of the major inborn errors of metabolism that affect the eye. Evaluation of suspected patients should include:

- Complete ocular and family history
- Examination of other family members for additional evidence or findings that confirm the carrier state
- Complete ocular examination focusing on the expected findings
- Appropriate directed laboratory testing

Treatment

Recently, bone marrow transplantation and enzyme replacement therapy have been found to be helpful in some of the mucopolysaccharidoses, making accurate diagnosis even more imperative. Consultation with a geneticist is warranted for any patient with ocular findings suggestive of an inborn error of metabolism.

In vitro studies of cells from albino mice have been successful in repairing the tyrosinase gene, allowing previously amelanotic cells to produce melanin. Early in vivo animal studies look promising. With the rapid pace of genetic research, many metabolic disorders may be treatable.

Alexeev V, Yoon K. Stable and inheritable changes in genotype and phenotype of albino melanocytes induced by an RNA-DNA oligonucleotide. *Nat Biotechnol.* 1998;16:1343–1346.

Cowan MJ. Bone marrow transplantation for the treatment of genetic diseases. *Clin Biochem.* 1991;24:375–381.

Scriver CR, Beaudet AL, Sly WS, et al, eds. *The Metabolic and Molecular Bases of Inherited Disease.* 7th ed. New York: McGraw-Hill; 1995.

CHAPTER 30

Ocular Trauma in Childhood

Trauma is one of the most important causes of ocular morbidity in childhood. Only strabismus ranks higher in frequency among reasons for pediatric eye surgery, and only amblyopia is responsible for more early monocular vision loss. Children 11–15 years old have a particularly high incidence of severe eye injury compared with other age groups. Injured boys outnumber girls by a factor of 3 or 4 to 1.

Most ocular trauma in younger children occurs during casual play with other children. Older children and adolescents are most likely to be injured while participating in sports. A majority of serious childhood eye injuries could thus in principle be prevented by appropriate adult supervision and by regular use of protective eyewear for sports. Fireworks and BB guns are among the less frequent causes of pediatric ocular trauma, but they are likely to cause severe injuries.

> O'Neill JF. Eye safety in the pediatric population. *Ophthalmol Clin North Am.* 1999;12:413–419.
>
> Vinger PF. Athletic eye injuries and appropriate protection. In: *Focal Points: Clinical Modules for Ophthalmologists.* San Francisco: American Academy of Ophthalmology; 1997: vol 15, no 8.
>
> Woods T: Protective eyewear. *Ophthalmol Clin North Am.* 1999;12:381–406.

The management of eye trauma in very young patients requires several special considerations. First, the difficulty of evaluation and treatment is often considerably increased by inadequate cooperation. Even school-age children, stressed by the recent injury, may strenuously resist any approach to the eye. Overcoming the child's opposition by force risks exacerbating the damage caused by penetrating wounds or blunt impact. In a child older than 3 years, a forceful approach may make it exceedingly difficult to establish the rapport needed for subsequent treatment. Examination in cases likely to involve minor injury can be facilitated by instilling topical anesthesia and by giving the child a chance to calm down in quiet surroundings. When preliminary assessment indicates that prompt surgical treatment may be necessary, it is appropriate to defer detailed physical examination of the eye until the patient is in the operating room under general anesthesia.

A second issue in the care of children with eye trauma is the potential for the injury or its treatment to lead to visual loss from amblyopia. In children younger than 5 years, visual-deprivation amblyopia associated with traumatic cataract or other media opacity may be more likely to cause severe long-term reduction of acuity than the original physical damage. Minimizing the interval between the injury and restoration of optimal media clarity and optics, including adequate aphakic refractive correction, must be a high priority. Monocular occlusion following injury should be kept to a minimum as well; the expected benefit from an occlusive dressing must be weighed against the risk of disturbing binocular function or inducing amblyopia.

Child Abuse

Although most eye injuries in childhood are accidental or innocently caused by other children, a significant portion result from physical abuse by adults. Child abuse is a pervasive problem in our society, with an estimated 2 million victims per year in the United States. Abusive behavior in a parent or other caregiver usually reflects temporary loss of control during a period of anger or stress rather than premeditated cruelty. Lack of knowledge of the proper way to care for or discipline a child is also a frequent contributing factor. In the relatively rare *Munchausen syndrome by proxy,* the child is physically harmed by a psychopathic parent to create signs of illness in an effort to manipulate medical care providers.

A reliable history is often difficult to obtain when child abuse has occurred. Suspicion should be aroused when repeated accounts of the circumstances of injury or histories obtained from different individuals are inconsistent or when the events described seem to conflict with the extent of injuries (eg, bruises on multiple aspects of the head after a fall) or with the child's developmental level (eg, a 2-month-old rolling off a bed or a 6-month-old climbing out of a high chair).

Any physician who suspects that child abuse might have occurred is required by law in every U.S. state and Canadian province to report the incident to a designated governmental agency. Once this obligation has been discharged, the ophthalmologist is probably best advised to leave full investigation of the situation to appropriate specialists or authorities.

The presenting sign of child abuse involves the eye in approximately 5% of cases, and ocular manifestations are detected in the course of evaluating many others. Blunt trauma inflicted with fingers, fists, or implements such as belts or straps is the usual mechanism of nonaccidental injury to the ocular adnexa or anterior segment. Periorbital ecchymosis, subconjunctival hemorrhage, and hyphema should raise suspicion of recent abuse if the explanation provided is less than completely plausible. Cataract and lens dislocation may be signs of repeated injury or trauma inflicted more remotely in the past. A majority of rhegmatogenous retinal detachments that occur in childhood have a traumatic origin; abuse should be suspected when such a finding is encountered in a child without a history of injury or an apparent predisposing factor such as high myopia.

> Levin AV. The ocular findings in child abuse. In: *Focal Points: Clinical Modules for Ophthalmologists.* San Francisco: American Academy of Ophthalmology; 1998: vol 16, no 7.

Shaking Injury

A unique complex of ocular, intracranial, and sometimes other injuries occurs in infants who have been abused by violent shaking. Since the essential features of what is now generally known as shaken baby syndrome were identified in the early 1970s, it has become widely recognized as one of the most important manifestations of child abuse.

Victims of shaking injury are always under 3 years old and usually under 12 months. When a reliable history is available, it typically involves a parent or other caregiver who shook an inconsolably crying baby in anger and frustration. Often, however, the only information provided is that the child's mental status deteriorated or that seizures or respiratory difficulty developed. It may be related that an episode of relatively minor trauma occurred, such as a fall from a bed. Even without a supporting history, the diagnosis of shaken baby syndrome can still be made with confidence on the basis of characteristic clinical findings. It must be kept in mind, however, that answers to important questions concerning the timing and circumstances of injury and the identity of the perpetrator frequently cannot be inferred from medical evidence alone.

Intracranial injury in shaken infants almost always includes subdural hematoma, typically bilateral over the cerebral convexities or in the interhemispheric fissure. Evidence of subarachnoid bleeding is also often apparent. In many cases, cerebral parenchymal damage is manifest on neuroimaging, acutely as edema, ischemia, or contusion and in later stages as atrophy. These findings are thought to result from repetitive abrupt deceleration of the child's head as it whiplashes back and forth during the shaking episode. Some authorities, citing the frequency with which shaken baby syndrome victims also show evidence of having received blows to the head, think that impact is an essential component. Displacement of the brain in relation to the skull and dura mater ruptures bridging vessels, and compression against the cranial bones produces further damage. The infant's head is particularly vulnerable to such effects because of its relatively large mass in relation to the body and poor stabilization by neck muscles.

Ocular involvement

The most common ocular manifestation of shaking injury, present in a large majority of cases, is retinal hemorrhage. Preretinal, nerve fiber layer, deep retinal, or subretinal localization may be seen. Hemorrhages tend to be concentrated in or near the macular region but not uncommonly are so extensive that they occupy nearly the entire fundus (Fig 30-1). Vitreous hemorrhage may also develop, usually as a secondary phenomenon resulting from migration of blood that was initially intraretinal. Occasionally, the vitreous becomes almost completely opacified by dispersed hemorrhage within a few days of injury. Retinal hemorrhages in shaken infants resolve over a period ranging from 1 or 2

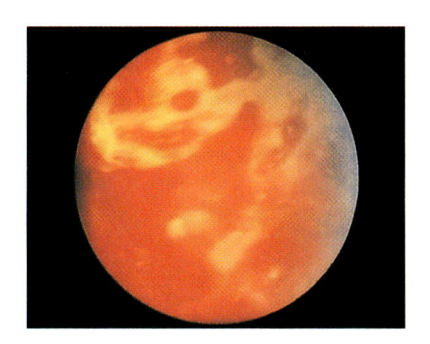

Figure 30-1 Extensive retinal hemorrhages, left eye, in a 2-month-old infant thought to have been violently shaken. Temporal portion of the disc is visible near the left edge of the photograph.

weeks to several months but may persist for many months or even years. Vitrectomy should be considered if amblyopia is possible.

Some eyes of shaken infants show evidence of retinal tissue disruption in addition to hemorrhage. Full-thickness folds in the neurosensory retina, typically with circumferential orientation around the macula that creates a craterlike appearance, are highly characteristic. Splitting of the retina *(traumatic retinoschisis)*, either deep to the nerve fiber layer or superficial (involving only the internal limiting membrane), may create partially blood-filled cavities of considerable extent, also usually in the macular region (Fig 30-2). Full-thickness retinal breaks and detachment are rare. Retinal folds usually flatten out within a few weeks of injury, but schisis cavities can persist indefinitely.

A striking feature of shaken baby syndrome is the typical lack of external evidence of trauma. The ocular adnexa and anterior segments appear entirely normal. Occasionally, the trunk or extremities show bruises representing the imprint of the perpetrator's hands. In a minority of cases, broken ribs or characteristic metaphyseal fractures of the long bones result from forces generated during shaking. It must be kept in mind, however, that many shaken babies are also victims of other forms of abuse. In particular, signs of impact to the head must be carefully sought.

When extensive retinal hemorrhage accompanied by perimacular folds and schisis cavities is found in association with intracranial hemorrhage or other evidence of trauma to the brain in an infant, shaking injury can be diagnosed with confidence regardless of other circumstances. Extensive retinal hemorrhage without other ocular findings strongly suggests that intracranial injury has been caused by shaking, but alternative possibilities such as a coagulation disorder must be considered as well. Severe accidental head trauma (eg, sustained in a fall from second-story level or a motor vehicle collision) is infrequently accompanied by retinal hemorrhage, which is virtually never extensive. Retinal hemorrhage is rare and has never been documented to be extensive following cardiopulmonary resuscitation by trained personnel. Spontaneous subarachnoid hemorrhage occurs rarely

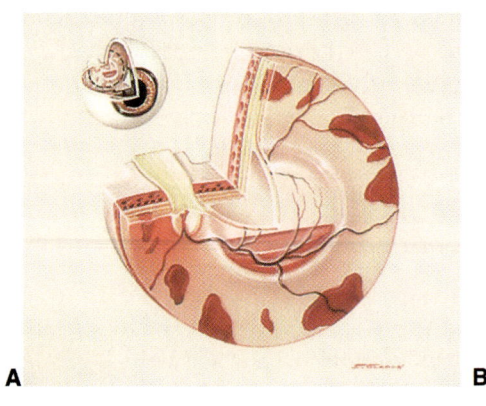

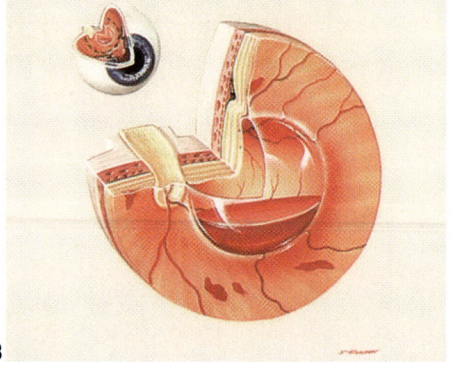

Figure 30-2 Traumatic retinoschisis. **A,** Deep splitting of the retina, typically associated with severe permanent visual impairment and loss of ERG b-wave. **B,** Superficial splitting, with separation of the internal limiting membrane and a full-thickness perimacular fold. Recovery of good vision is common. *(Reproduced by permission from Greenwald MJ. The shaken baby syndrome.* Semin Ophthalmol. *1990;5:202–213. Illustrations by S. Gordon.)*

in young children and may be associated with some degree of intraocular bleeding. Retinal hemorrhages resulting from birth trauma are common in newborns but seldom persist beyond age 1 month.

> Emerson MV, Pieramici DJ, Stoessel KM, et al. Incidence and rate of disappearance of retinal hemorrhage in newborns. *Ophthalmology.* 2001;108:36–39.

Prognosis

In one large study, 29% of children with shaken baby syndrome died from their injuries. Poor visual and pupillary response were correlated with a higher risk of mortality. Survivors often suffered permanent impairment ranging from severe retardation and quadriparesis to mild learning disability and motor disturbances. Visual loss from traumatic retinoschisis, optic nerve damage, or cortical injury occurred in 20% of patients, but nearly complete recovery of vision was common. Dense vitreous hemorrhage, usually associated with deep traumatic retinoschisis, carried a poor visual prognosis. Vitrectomy should be deferred if bright flash electroretinography shows loss of the b-wave.

> Caffey J. The whiplash shaken infant syndrome: manual shaking by the extremities with whiplash-induced intracranial and intraocular bleeding, linked with residual permanent brain damage and mental retardation. *Pediatrics.* 1974;53:396–403.
>
> Kivlin JD, Simons KB, Lazoritz S, et al. Shaken baby syndrome. *Ophthalmology.* 2000; 107:1246–1254.

Superficial Injury

Corneal abrasion is one of the most common ocular injuries among children, as it is among older persons. Use of a pressure patch to keep the eyelids closed so that an abrasion will heal faster is of questionable value for the preschool child. Obtaining and maintaining the desired effect is difficult in this age group, and if the patch loosens, contact between the cotton eye pad and the ocular surface may actually aggravate the problem. Even moderately large traumatic corneal epithelial defects usually heal within 1–2 days in young children without patching. Use of topical cycloplegic drops and antibiotic ointment may help reduce discomfort and risk of infection.

Cigarette burns of the cornea are the most common thermal injuries to the ocular surface in childhood. Usually, these occur in the age range of 2–4 years and are accidental, not manifestations of abuse. These burns result from the toddler's running into a cigarette held at eye level by an adult. Despite the alarming initial white appearance of coagulated corneal epithelium, cigarette burns typically heal rapidly and without scarring. Treatment is the same as for mechanical abrasions.

Chemical burns in childhood are generally caused by organic solvents or soaps found in household cleaning agents. Even those involving almost total loss of corneal epithelium are likely to heal in a week or less with or without patching. Acid and alkali burns in children, as in adults, can be much more serious. The initial and most important step in management of all chemical injuries is copious irrigation and meticulous removal of any particulate matter from the conjunctival fornices. See also BCSC Section 8, *External Disease and Cornea.*

Corneal foreign bodies in children can sometimes be dislodged with a forceful stream of irrigating solution from a small bottle; sharp instruments can thus be avoided. When mechanical removal proves necessary, it is important that the patient not move during the procedure.

Penetrating Injury

Unless an adult has witnessed a traumatic incident, the history cannot be relied on to exclude the possibility of penetrating injury to the globe. The anterior segment and fundus must be thoroughly inspected in suspicious circumstances, using general anesthesia if necessary. An area of subconjunctival hemorrhage or chemosis or a small break in the skin of the eyelid may be the only surface manifestation of scleral perforation by a sharp-pointed object, such as a dart or scissors blade (Fig 30-3). Distortion of the pupil may be the most evident sign of a small corneal or limbal perforation. CT of the orbits should be considered if there is any reason to suspect a deeply situated foreign body.

Corneoscleral lacerations in children are repaired according to the same principles as for adults. Corneal wounds heal relatively rapidly in very young patients, however, and sutures should be removed correspondingly early.

Fibrin clots often form quickly in the anterior chamber of a child's eye after a penetrating injury to the cornea, and these can simulate the appearance of fluffy cataractous lens cortex to a remarkable degree. To avoid unnecessarily rendering the eye aphakic (and thereby compromising visual rehabilitation), lens removal should not be performed in the course of primary wound repair unless the clinician is absolutely certain that the anterior capsule has been ruptured. Even if lens cortex is exposed, postponing cataract surgery for 1–2 weeks until severe posttraumatic inflammation has quieted down may result in a smoother recovery and reduced risk of complications, without significantly worsening the visual prognosis. See also BCSC Section 11, *Lens and Cataract.*

Full-thickness eyelid lacerations should be repaired meticulously, and general anesthesia may be required, even in older children. Otherwise, working near the eyes with sharp instruments and draping the face to create a sterile field are likely to frighten the patient and add to the difficulty of the repair. Clearly superficial wounds can be repaired in the emergency room. Use of 6–0 plain gut or synthetic absorbable sutures is an acceptable alternative if the physician wishes to avoid the need for removal of nonabsorbable sutures.

Blunt Injury

Hyphema

The management of hyphema in infants and children requires special considerations. As with all forms of pediatric trauma, the precise occurrence that led to intraocular bleeding may be difficult to determine. The possibility of abuse must be considered, as must the possibility of nontraumatic etiology: retinoblastoma, juvenile xanthogranuloma of the iris, and bleeding diathesis resulting from leukemia or other blood dyscrasia are relatively

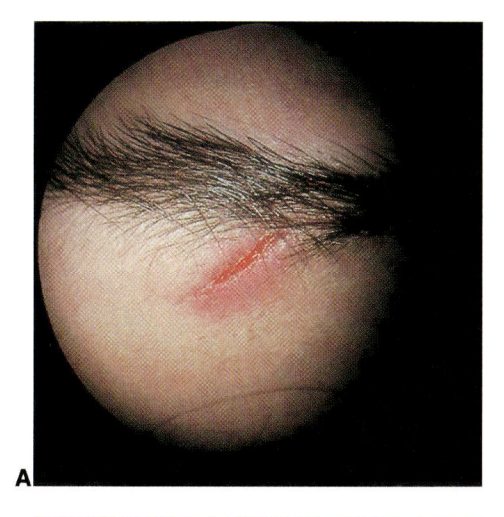

Figure 30-3 A, Small skin entry wound created by a thrown dart, right brow region in a 7-year-old boy. **B,** Conjunctival exit wound indicates complete perforation of the eyelid. **C,** Extensive injury to the anterior segment of the same eye.

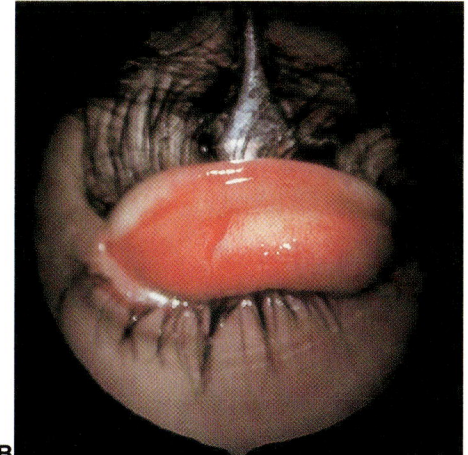

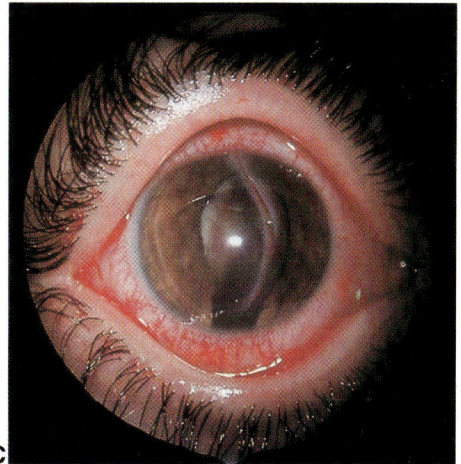

rare but important causes of spontaneous hyphema during the early years of life. Ultrasonography or CT should be performed to rule out intraocular tumor in suspicious cases wherein the iris and fundus cannot be adequately seen, and a complete blood count should be performed routinely, with coagulation studies, if a bleeding disorder is suspected.

Intraocular pressure (IOP), an important parameter for therapeutic decision making with traumatic hyphema, is often difficult to monitor in the pediatric patient. The risks of inaccurate measurements and of further traumatizing the injured eye may outweigh the potential value of obtaining results in uncooperative children. With small blood collections, concern about pressure tends to be greatest in patients with sickle cell trait or disease (Fig 30-4). Such patients may develop sickling in the anterior chamber, elevating IOP and retarding resorption of blood, or in the retinal circulation, causing vascular occlusion.

Figure 30-4 Small hyphema, right eye, in an adolescent girl with sickle trait. Note corneal edema resulting from high intraocular pressure.

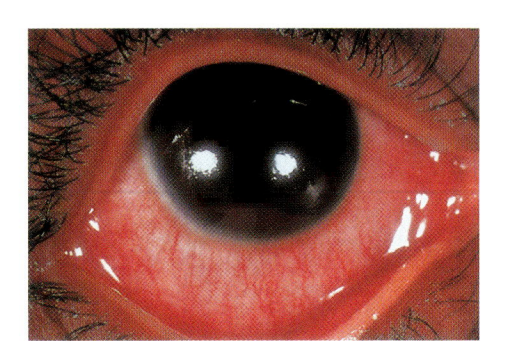

It was once common practice to hospitalize all patients with hyphema and place them on bed rest with bilateral patching of the eyes. Such extreme restriction has never been shown to improve prognosis, however, and is likely to be unproductive in children. On the other hand, some decrease in normal childhood running, jumping, and rough play is both reasonable and appropriate. Hospitalization during the first 5 days after injury, when risk of rebleeding is greatest, remains justifiable and is one way to ensure the opportunity for daily follow-up evaluation. Outpatient management with daily follow-up is an acceptable alternative.

Medical management of hyphema remains controversial in children as in adults. Many ophthalmologists routinely use cycloplegic and corticosteroid drops to facilitate fundus examination, improve comfort, and reduce the risk of inflammatory complications and possibly of rebleeding as well. The value of these topical agents is unproved, however, and some clinicians prefer to use them selectively for control of pain or obvious inflammation or avoid them altogether to minimize manipulation of the eye. Pressure-lowering medication is appropriate for eyes known or strongly suspected to be hypertensive. Aspirin-containing compounds should be scrupulously avoided because of their antiplatelet action.

Oral administration of an antifibrinolytic agent (ε-aminocaproic acid, 50 mg/kg every 4 hours to a maximum of 30 g daily; or tranexamic acid, 25 mg/kg every 8 hours to a maximum of 4.5 g daily, for 5 days) has been shown to reduce the incidence of rebleeding in traumatic hyphema. On the other hand, one study found an insignificant decrease in the incidence of rebleeding among patients treated with tranexamic acid. Gastric upset and hypotension may be significant side effects of oral ε-aminocaproic acid. Recently, topical aminocaproic acid has been demonstrated to be an effective alternative. Oral prednisolone has also been advocated in a dosage of 0.75 mg/kg/day in two divided doses (to a maximum of 40 mg/day in children).

Surgical evacuation of hyphema is usually performed in adults when early corneal blood staining is detected or when significant IOP elevation has persisted for 5–7 days. The difficulty of detecting early blood staining in a child and the risk that corneal staining may cause severe deprivation amblyopia coupled with the problems of accurately measuring IOP justify earlier surgical intervention whenever a total hyphema persists for 4–5 days. Various operative techniques have been employed; none has been shown to offer particular advantages in childhood.

Late glaucoma is a potential complication of traumatic hyphema in children, as in adults, and may present no symptoms. Gonioscopy should be performed after the eye has healed and the child can cooperate. Routine annual follow-up should be continued in children who are found to have an angle recession. It is important to remember that children with hyphemas may also have other significant injuries, including damage to the retina and optic nerve.

> Crouch ER Jr, Crouch ER. Management of traumatic hyphema: therapeutic options. *J Pediatr Ophthalmol Strabismus.* 1999;36:238–250.
> Farber MD, Fiscella R, Goldberg MF. Aminocaproic acid versus prednisone for the treatment of traumatic hyphema. A randomized clinical trial. *Ophthalmology.* 1991;98:279–286.
> Rahmani B, Jahadi HR. Comparison of tranexamic acid and prednisolone in the treatment of traumatic hyphema: a randomized clinical trial. *Ophthalmology.* 1999;106:375–379.
> Shiuey Y, Lucarelli MJ. Traumatic hyphema. *Ophthalmology.* 1998;105:851–855.

Orbital Fractures

Children, like adults, may sustain isolated fractures of orbital bone after blunt impact in the region of the eye. Careful examination of the eye is important to rule out associated ocular damage. CT should be performed to evaluate the fracture and possible associated injuries. The involvement of other specialties, including otolaryngology and neurosurgery, may be helpful in some cases. If there is severe enophthalmos or if the eye movements are extremely compromised, consideration should be given to primary repair of orbital fractures during the first 2 weeks following injury. In many cases, however, the motility will recover or strabismus surgery can be considered after several months if it proves necessary.

The most common orbital fracture in early childhood involves the orbital roof, which is rarely fractured in older patients. Isolated roof fractures typically result from impact to the brow region in a fall, often from a height of only a few feet. The principal external manifestation is hematoma in the upper eyelid (Fig 30-5). For further discussion of diagnosis and management of orbital trauma, see Chapter 9 of this book and BCSC Section 7, *Orbit, Eyelids, and Lacrimal System.*

> Bansagi ZC, Meyer DR. Internal orbital fractures in the pediatric age group: characterization and management. *Ophthalmology.* 2000;107:829–836.
> Jordan DR, Allen LH, White J, et al. Intervention within days for some orbital floor fractures: the white-eyed blowout. *Ophthal Plast Reconstr Surg.* 1998;14:379–390.

418 • Pediatric Ophthalmology and Strabismus

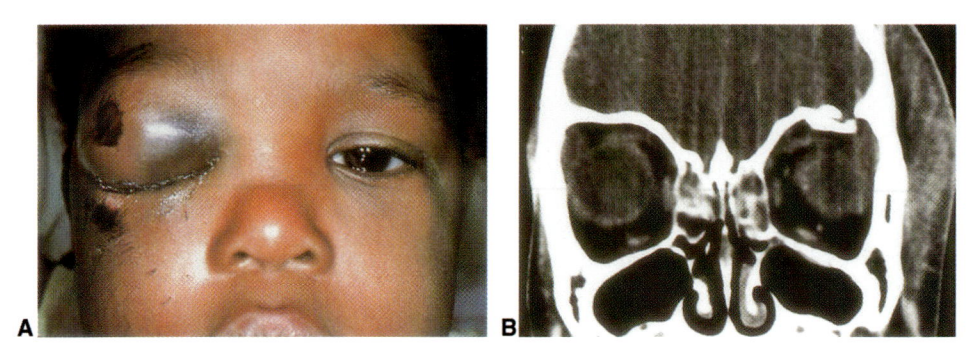

Figure 30-5 Orbital roof fracture in infants who fell with frontal impact. **A,** Marked right upper eyelid swelling from hematoma originating in the superior orbit adjacent to a linear fracture. **B,** Coronal CT image of a different patient, showing a bone fragment displaced into left orbit.

CHAPTER 31

Decreased Vision in Infants and Children

Several causes must be considered when an infant has not developed good visual attention or ability to fixate and follow objects by age 3–4 months. Many of these causes are covered elsewhere in this volume in the Chapters on cataracts, glaucoma, retinal disorders, and malformations. Some of these conditions are relatively easily diagnosed by standard ophthalmic examinations. However, other ocular abnormalities are subtle and difficult to detect.

Normal Visual Development

Visual development is a highly complex maturation process. Structural changes occur in both the eye and the central nervous system. Laboratory and clinical research has shown that normal vision develops as a result of both genetic coding and experience in a normal visual environment.

Vision in the infant usually is assessed qualitatively by clinical appraisal and additionally by psychophysical tests such as optokinetic nystagmus (or *OKN*) responses, visually evoked cortical potentials (*VEP* or *VER*), and preferential looking techniques. A blink reflex to bright light should be present several days after birth. The pupillary light reflex is usually present after 31 weeks' gestation, but it can be difficult to evaluate because of miosis in the newborn.

At about 6 weeks of age, the normal baby should be able to make and maintain eye contact with other humans and react with facial expressions. Infants 2–3 months old should be interested in bright objects. Premature infants can be expected to reach these landmarks later, depending on their degree of prematurity.

Disconjugate eye movements may be noted initially, but they should not persist after age 4 months. Skew deviation and *sunsetting* (tonic downward deviation of both eyes) have been observed as transient deviations in the newborn period. Signs of actual poor visual development include wandering eye movements, lack of response to familiar faces and objects, and nystagmus. Staring at bright lights and forceful rubbing of the eyes in an otherwise visually disinterested infant *(oculodigital reflex)* are other signs of poor visual development and suggest an ocular cause for the deficiency.

Weinacht S, Kind C, Monting JS, et al. Visual development in pre-term and full-term infants: a prospective masked study. *Invest Ophthalmol Vis Sci.* 1999;40:346–353.

Approach to the Infant With Decreased Vision

A careful history, beginning with a review of vision problems in the family, is essential. If the patient is male, the possibility of an X-linked disorder should be explored. If a sibling has a similar condition not present in previous generations, this suggests an autosomal recessive disease.

Details of the pregnancy should be reviewed: important factors include maternal infection, radiation, drugs, or trauma. Perinatal problems including prematurity, intrauterine growth retardation, fetal distress, bradycardia, meconium staining, and oxygen deprivation are important. The clinician also should inquire about the presence of systemic abnormalities or delayed developmental milestones.

Examination of the infant directs special attention to visual fixation, crispness and equality of pupillary light responses, ocular alignment and motility, and the presence of nystagmus or roving eye movements. A detailed fundus examination also is necessary.

An infant with a normal but immature visual system may be unresponsive to even a very bright light, a state indistinguishable from blindness. By moving a red light horizontally or vertically in front of the infant, the clinician can sometimes elicit a fixation-and-following response in an otherwise unresponsive baby.

Pupillary responses are sluggish with anterior visual pathway disease such as optic nerve hypoplasia or atrophy, optic nerve coloboma, and morning glory disc anomaly . *Paradoxical pupillary phenomenon* (constriction to darkness) implies diffuse retinal disease such as cone dystrophy. Pupillary responses are normal in infants with cortical visual impairment.

Nystagmus (a rhythmic pendular or jerk movement pattern) as an indicator of decreased vision usually begins at age 2–3 months, not at birth. Nystagmus implies the presence of at least some visual function (nystagmus does not occur in total blindness). In contrast, roving eye movements suggest total or near-total blindness. Both of these conditions are different from congenital motor nystagmus (no organic eye abnormality), which is associated with only a mild to moderate reduction in visual acuity, although it can appear as early as the first month of life. Chapter 12 discusses nystagmus in detail.

Visual deficits in one or both eyes can cause abnormal binocular alignment. In the infant younger than 1 year, the most common misalignment is exotropia. Beyond the age of 1 year, esotropia is most common.

When an infant presents with poor vision and ocular structures that appear normal, a number of retinal disorders should be considered, including Leber congenital amaurosis, achromatopsia, blue-cone monochromatism, and X-linked or autosomal recessive congenital stationary night blindness. Electroretinography can aid in the diagnosis of these disorders, and some investigators advocate ERG testing for all infants with visual inattentiveness and normal eye structures. Other researchers think that, in infancy, ERGs should be reserved only for patients thought to have Leber congenital amaurosis. Obtaining quality ERGs in infants is difficult, and the examiner must be aware of the normal developmental variations that occur in these electrophysiologic tests in the first year of life. Serial testing may be important before definitive diagnostic and prognostic information is provided.

For infants with low vision, additional testing might include visually evoked cortical potentials, ultrasonography, CT, or MRI. In some cases, specialized laboratory studies are indicated, which should be obtained in consultation with a pediatric neurologist, an endocrinologist, a neurosurgeon, and a geneticist.

The most common causes of reduced vision in infants are listed here, and several are discussed individually below:

- Anterior segment anomalies
- Glaucoma
- Cataract
- Optic nerve hypoplasia
- Optic atrophy
- Leber congenital amaurosis
- Achromatopsia (rod monochromatism)
- Congenital infection syndrome/TORCH syndrome
- Cortical visual impairment
- Delay in visual maturation
- Retinopathy of prematurity (see Chapter 24)
- X-linked retinoschisis (see Chapter 24)
- Congenital motor nystagmus (see Chapter 12)
- Albinism (see Chapter 24)
- Coloboma (see Chapters 20 and 25)

Anterior Segment Anomalies, Glaucoma, Cataract

The common feature of childhood anterior segment anomalies, glaucoma, and cataract is stimulus deprivation severe enough to result in permanently reduced vision. Complete ptosis and lens or corneal opacification (eg, Peters anomaly, sclerocornea, glaucoma) are prominent among the causes. Even with only partial loss of clarity, image degradation can be significant and result in amblyopia.

If the condition is unilateral or not of comparable severity in both eyes, an additional component of inhibition of the more disadvantaged eye is present. Although some of these abnormalities often are beyond correction, prompt attention to the remediable ones is required during the critical window (within several weeks of birth). See also Chapters 6, 19, 21, and 22.

Optic Nerve Hypoplasia

Disturbed optic nerve development can range from a minimal decrease in size to complete absence of the nerve *(aplasia)*, causing varying degrees of reduced visual function in infants. In hypoplasia, the optic disc appears somewhat pale and small and may be circumscribed by a yellow-white ring, surrounded by pigmentation. This encircling ring has been described clinically as the *double ring sign*. It is not apparent in every case.

The condition can be unilateral or bilateral, and there is no sex predilection. When hypoplasia is unilateral, strabismus is often present, and one element of partial loss may be secondary to a superimposed amblyopia. Nystagmus frequently accompanies severe bilateral involvement.

A relative afferent pupillary defect usually is present with asymmetrical involvement, and the ERG usually appears normal. The visually evoked cortical potential is subnormal, reflecting the disturbed conduction of visual impulses via the optic nerve. Imaging studies may demonstrate a small optic foramen or optic nerve but are not required when the ophthalmologic findings are definite.

Optic nerve hypoplasia is associated with other developmental abnormalities, including hydrocephalus, hydranencephaly, anencephaly, and congenital tumors of the anterior visual pathways. The brain may be affected by midline defects, including agenesis of the septum pellucidum, malformations of the corpus callosum, and enlargement of the chiasmal cistern.

The *de Morsier syndrome (septo-optic dysplasia)* includes optic nerve hypoplasia, absence of the septum pellucidum, agenesis of the corpus callosum, and pituitary dwarfism. Endocrine abnormalities may occur when the midline defect extends into the hypothalamus, with resulting panhypopituitarism, growth hormone deficiency, diabetes insipidus, and hypoglycemia. Recent studies have identified ectopia of the posterior pituitary gland, revealed on MRI, as a predictor of endocrine abnormalities in patients with optic nerve hypoplasia.

Neuroimaging is recommended for children with bilateral optic nerve hypoplasia. When the condition is unilateral, the incidence of midline brain abnormalities is much smaller, but many neurologists would obtain such studies in this instance also.

The cause of optic nerve hypoplasia remains unknown. Maternal ingestion of phenytoin, quinine, and LSD has been implicated. Optic nerve hypoplasia is common in infants with fetal alcohol syndrome and has been reported in the offspring of mothers with diabetes. Another postulated cause of optic nerve hypoplasia is degeneration of ganglion cell axons due to an insult occurring prior to the 13th week of gestation. See also Chapter 25.

> Hellstrom A, Wiklund LM, Svennson E. The clinical and morphologic spectrum of optic nerve hypoplasia. *J AAPOS*. 1999;3:212–220.

Optic Atrophy

Various inherited and noninherited conditions can cause optic atrophy. Congenital and acquired forms occur and can be an isolated defect or a facet of systemic disease.

Secondary optic atrophy has been attributed to hydrocephalus, brain tumors, perinatal hypoxia, central nervous system malformations such as porencephaly, and toxins (eg, lead, quinine, and methyl alcohol) and has been associated with metabolic storage diseases and with trauma, including child abuse. See Chapter 25.

Leber Congenital Amaurosis

Leber congenital amaurosis is responsible for an estimated 10% of cases of congenital blindness. Infants with Leber congenital amaurosis may have severe visual impairment at birth, although the visual deficit is noted more typically at age 2–3 months with the onset of a coarse, searching sensory nystagmus. The pupillary reactions to direct light are poor, and the pupils may paradoxically constrict in the dark. The oculodigital habit is common, with gouging of the eyes by a finger or fist in an effort to induce entoptic stimulation of the retina. The inheritance pattern is autosomal recessive.

Initially, the fundus can appear completely normal, although a diffuse pigmentary change, optic nerve pallor, or both may be noted. A blond fundus and an atrophic appearance of the macula are additional characteristics. With time, optic atrophy, narrowing of the retinal vessels, and diffuse retinal pigmentary changes indistinguishable from retinitis pigmentosa develop. Other findings include cataracts, hyperopia, and glaucoma.

The ERG appears abnormal, showing either completely flat or low voltage, and the base value of the electro-oculogram is low, with no rise after light adaptation. Such a result may not be clearly distinguishable from normal in an infant younger than 12–15 months. Histologic examination reveals severe disorganization or absence of the rods and cones.

Associated neurologic conditions include abnormal electroencephalogram results, microcephaly, hydrocephaly, seizures, and other cerebral abnormalities. Possible associated skeletal changes are acrocephaly, hemifacial hypoplasia, polydactyly, kyphoscoliosis, arachnodactyly, and osteoporosis. Muscular hypotony and kidney abnormalities with oligophrenia also may occur. See also Chapter 24.

> Heher KL, Traboulsi EI, Maumenee IH. The natural history of Leber congenital amaurosis: age-related findings in 35 patients. *Ophthalmology*. 1992;99:241–245.

Achromatopsia (Rod Monochromatism)

Achromatopsia is a retinal disorder characterized by total color blindness, with all colors perceived as varying brightnesses of gray. The condition is inherited as an autosomal recessive trait. Photophobia of varying degree, nystagmus, and visual acuity in the 20/200 range are common. The degree of nystagmus may decrease at near fixation, giving better visual acuity than at distance.

Fundus examination usually is normal when the child is young, although an abnormal foveal reflex may develop later. A central scotoma can be demonstrated. The ERG usually shows a normal scotopic recording and an abnormal photopic response. The electro-oculogram typically appears normal.

Histopathologic examination reveals a markedly reduced population of cones. Those that are present are often abnormally structured. The rods are normal. The condition is nonprogressive and has no associated neurologic abnormalities. See also Chapter 24.

Congenital Infection Syndrome/TORCH Syndrome

Marked reduction in visual acuity often is associated with congenital infections (primarily toxoplasmosis, rubella, cytomegalovirus, herpes simplex, and syphilis) and with severe disruption of the visual pathways from encephalitis, meningitis, arachnoiditis, optic neuritis, and sometimes chorioretinitis. Chapter 17 discusses these conditions in detail.

Cortical Visual Impairment

Infants with cortical visual impairment demonstrate varying degrees of visual attentiveness. Both the family and the ophthalmologist may be uncertain as to whether the baby can see. Examination reveals normal ocular structures, normal pupillary responses, and searching eye movements.

The ERG appears normal; the visually evoked cortical potential may be normal or subnormal. Neuroimaging may reveal changes such as atrophy and porencephaly in the occipital (striate or parastriate) cortex, damage to the optic radiations, or periventricular leukomalacia. This last condition is a prominent cause of visual impairment in children born prematurely. In some cases, no such findings are present and the prognosis may be more favorable.

Cortical visual impairment may be congenital or acquired. Prenatal and perinatal causes include intrauterine infection (see Chapter 17), cerebral dysgenesis, asphyxia, intracranial hemorrhage, hydrocephalus, and infection. Acquired causes include trauma and child abuse (see Chapter 30), shunt malfunction, meningitis, and encephalitis.

Cortical visual impairment may be transient or permanent and can be an isolated finding or associated with multiple neurologic handicaps. Descending optic atrophy (transsynaptic degeneration) may coexist.

> Good WV, Jan JE, DeSa L, et al. Cortical visual impairment in children. *Surv Ophthalmol.* 1994;38:351–364.
>
> Jacobson LK, Dutton GN. Periventricular leukomalacia: an important cause of visual and ocular motility dysfunction in children. *Surv Ophthalmol.* 2000;45:1–13.

Delay in Visual Maturation

Sometimes, when eye examination results are totally normal but fixation is poor, the problem is merely delayed maturation of the visual system. In such children, neurologic examination results may be normal except for poor visual attention, but some patients have evidence of other neurologic impairment.

If the infant's visual behavior does not begin to progress toward normal within a few months, further investigation is warranted. Visually evoked cortical potentials recorded very early in life may initially be abnormal; this determination is more valid as the child approaches 12 months of age, and such testing can be omitted when the infant's visual behavior is clearly progressing toward normal.

Acquired Vision Loss Later in Childhood

When a child with normal visual development in infancy subsequently loses vision, the search for a treatable disorder is of paramount concern. Table 31-1 lists many of the conditions that can lead to acquired amaurosis. Amblyopia, the most prevalent cause of treatable vision loss in children, is discussed in Chapter 5 and elsewhere in this volume. Childhood cataract acquired as a developmental, familial, traumatic, or metabolic disorder is discussed in Chapter 22.

Vision screening programs in schools, primary care medical offices, and community outreach programs should be supported and monitored. Visual recovery often is directly related to early, accurate detection of the visual loss. Table 31-2 lists resources for further information.

> Hutcheson KA, Drack AV. Diagnosis and management of the infant who does not see. In: *Focal Points: Clinical Modules for Ophthalmologists.* San Francisco: American Academy of Ophthalmology; 1998: vol 16, no 12.

Table 31-1 Acquired Childhood Amaurosis

Congenital Malformations
  Congenital hydrocephalus
  Encephalocele, particularly occipital type

Tumors
  Retinoblastoma
  Optic glioma
  Perioptic meningioma
  Craniopharyngioma
  Chiasmal glioma
  Posterior and intraventricular tumors when complicated by hydrocephalus

Neurodegenerative Diseases: Abiotrophies
  Cerebral storage disease
  Gangliosidoses, particularly Tay-Sachs disease (infantile amaurotic familial idiocy), Sandhoff disease, generalized gangliosidosis
  Other lipidoses and ceroid lipofuscinoses, particularly the late-onset amaurotic familial idiocies such as those of Jansky-Bielschowsky and of Spielmeyer-Vogt
  Mucopolysaccharidoses, particulary Hurler syndrome and Hunter syndrome
  Leukodystrophies (dysmyelination disorders), particularly metachromatic leukodystrophy and Canavan disease
  Demyelinating scleroses (myelinoclastic diseases), especially Schilder disease and Devic neuromyelitis optica
  Special types: Dawson disease, Leigh disease, Bassen-Kornzweig syndrome, Refsum disease
  Retinal degenerations of obscure pathogenesis: retinitis pigmentosa and its variants, and Leber congenital type
  Optic atrophies of obscure pathogenesis: congenital autosomal recessive type, infantile and congenital autosomal dominant types, Leber disease, and atrophies associated with hereditary ataxias—the types of Behr, of Marie, and of Sager-Brown

Infectious or Inflammatory Processes
  Encephalitis, especially in the prenatal infection syndromes due to *Toxoplasma gondii,* cytomegalovirus, rubella virus, *Treponema pallidum*
  Meningitis; arachnoiditis
  Optic neuritis
  Chorioretinitis

Hematologic Disorders
  Leukemia with CNS involvement

Vascular and Circulatory Disorders
  Collagen vascular diseases
  Arteriovenous malformations: intracerebral hemorrhage, subarachnoid hemorrhage

Trauma
  Contusion or avulsion of optic nerves or chiasm
  Cerebral contusion or laceration
  Intracerebral, subarachnoid, or subdural hemorrhage

Drugs and Toxins
  Lead
  Quinine
  Methyl alcohol

(Adapted from Nelson LB, Calhoun JH, Harley RD, eds. *Pediatric Ophthalmology.* 3rd ed. Philadelphia: Saunders; 1991.)

Table 31-2 Sources of Information on Low Vision

NAPVI (National Association of Parents of the Visually Impaired)
(800) 562-6265
(Some areas have a state organization as well: NAPVI can direct the parent.)

Prevent Blindness America
160 East 56th Street
New York, NY 10022 (212) 980-2020 or (800) 331-2020

National Information Center for Children and Youth With Handicaps (NICCYH)
PO Box 1492
Washington, DC 20013 (800) 999-5599

National Association for the Visually Handicapped, Inc. (Western Office)
3201 Balboa Street
San Francisco, CA 94121 (415) 221-3201
(Large-print textbooks, library material on request. Sources of information and guidance on resources for the visually handicapped.)

National Association for the Visually Handicapped (NAVH)
22 West 21st St.
New York, NY 10010 (212) 889-3141

National Organization for Albinism and Hypopigmentation (NOAH)
1530 Locust St., #29
Philadelphia, PA 19102 (215) 545-2322
http://www.albinism.org

Recording for the Blind, Inc.
20 Roszel Road
Princeton, NJ 08540 (609) 452-0606

American Foundation for the Blind, Inc.
11 Pennsylvania Plaza, Suite 300
New York, NY 10001
(212) 502-7600 or (800) 232-5463
(For the publication *Reach Out and Teach,* call (800) 232-3044.)

Library of Congress National Library Service for the Blind and Physically Handicapped
1291 Taylor St. NW
Washington, DC 20542
(202) 707-5100 or (800) 424-8567
(Recorded poetry and literature talking books.)

American Printing House for the Blind
1839 Frankfort Avenue
PO Box 6085
Louisville, KY 40206 (502) 895-2405 or (800) 223-1839
Fax: (502) 899-2274
(Large-print textbooks, tapes, braille books, and tangible aids.)

Lighthouse for the Blind
(Independent organizations in every state; check local directories for listings.)

The Family Resource Coalition of America
200 S. Michigan Avenue
16th floor
Chicago, IL 60604 (312) 341-0900
(Provides identification of parent support groups all over the country.)

(Continued)

Table 31-2 Sources of Information on Low Vision (Continued)

Retinoblastoma Support News (newsletter for families of children with retinoblastoma) and *Parent To Parent* (newsletter for families of blind and visually impaired children) published by:
The Institute for Families of Blind Children
Children's Hospital of Los Angeles
Division of Ophthalmology, Box 111
P.O. Box 54700
Los Angeles, CA 90054-0700 (213) 669-4649

National Toll-Free Numbers

American Council of the Blind (800) 424-8666

Better Hearing Institute (800) 327-9355 (EAR-WELL)

Epilepsy Information Line (800) EFA-1000

Cystic Fibrosis Foundation (800) 344-4823

National Down Syndrome Society (800) 221-4602

Down Syndrome Information Center (888) 999-3759

National Easter Seal Society (800) 221-6827

National Health Information Clearinghouse (800) 336-4797

Spina Bifida (800) 621-3141

United Cerebral Palsy Association (800) 872-5827

National Fragile X Foundation (800) 688-8765

American Kidney Fund (800) 638-8299

The Arc (formerly Association for Retarded Citizens) (800) 433-5255

Sickle Cell Association (800) 421-8453

Retinitis Pigmentosa (RP) Association International (800) 344-4877

Sources of Large-Print Books
New York Times Large Print Weekly
229 West 43rd Street
New York, NY 10036 (800) 631-2580

Library for the Blind
919 Walnut Street
Philadelphia, PA 19107 (215) 925-3213

Reader's Digest Large Print Edition
(800) 678-9746

Basic Texts

Pediatric Ophthalmology and Strabismus

Brodsky MC, Baker RS, Hamed LM. *Pediatric Neuro-Ophthalmology.* New York: Springer-Verlag; 1996.

Buckley EG, Freedman S, Shields MB. *Atlas of Ophthalmic Surgery.* Vol III: *Strabismus and Glaucoma.* St Louis: Mosby; 1995.

Calhoun JH, Nelson LB, Harley RD. *Atlas of Pediatric Ophthalmic Surgery.* Philadelphia: Saunders; 1987.

Cibis GW, Tongue AC, Stass-Isern ML. *Decision Making in Pediatric Ophthalmology.* St Louis: Decker; 1993.

Del Monte MA, Archer SM. *Atlas of Pediatric Ophthalmology and Strabismus Surgery.* New York: Churchill Livingstone; 1993.

Helveston EM. *Surgical Management of Strabismus: An Atlas of Strabismus Surgery.* 4th ed. St Louis: Mosby; 1993.

Helveston EM, Ellis FD. *Pediatric Ophthalmology Practice.* 2nd ed. St Louis: Mosby; 1984.

Isenberg SJ, ed. *The Eye in Infancy.* 2nd ed. St Louis: Mosby-Year Book; 1994.

Jones KL. *Smith's Recognizable Patterns of Human Malformation.* 5th ed. Philadelphia: Saunders; 1997.

Leigh RJ, Zee DS. *The Neurology of Eye Movements.* 3rd ed. New York: Oxford; 1999.

Miller NR, Newman NJ. *Walsh and Hoyt's Clinical Neuro-Ophthalmology.* 5th ed. Baltimore: Williams & Wilkins; 1999.

Nelson LB, ed. *Harley's Pediatric Ophthalmology.* 4th ed. Philadelphia: Saunders; 1998.

Pratt-Johnson JA, Tillson G. *Management of Strabismus and Amblyopia: A Practical Guide,* 2nd ed. New York: Thieme; 2001.

Renie WA, eds. *Goldberg's Genetic and Metabolic Eye Disease.* 2nd ed. Boston: Little, Brown & Co; 1986.

Spencer WH, ed. *Ophthalmic Pathology: An Atlas and Textbook.* 4th ed. Philadelphia: Saunders; 1996.

Tasman W, Jaeger EA, eds. *Duane's Clinical Ophthalmology* [CD-ROM set]. Lippincott Williams & Wilkins; 2002.

Taylor D. *Pediatric Ophthalmology.* 2nd ed. Cambridge, MA: Blackwell Science; 1997.

von Haam E, Helveston EM. *Strabismus: A Decision Making Approach.* St Louis: Mosby; 1994.

von Noorden GK. *Binocular Vision and Ocular Motility: Theory and Management of Strabismus.* 6th ed. St Louis: Mosby; 2002.

von Noorden GK. *von Noorden–Maumenee's Atlas of Strabismus.* 4th ed. St Louis: Mosby; 1983.

Wright KW, ed. *Color Atlas of Stabismus Surgery: Strategies and Techniques,* 2nd ed. *Strabismus.* Torrance, CA: Wright; 2000.

Wright KW, Spiegel PH, eds. *Pediatric Ophthalmology and Strabismus,* 2nd ed. New York: Springer; 2002.

Related Academy Materials

Focal Points: Clinical Modules for Ophthalmologists

Archer S. Esotropia (Module 12, 1994).
Bartley GB. Periorbital animal bites (Module 3, 1992).
Beck AD, Lynch MG. Pediatric glaucoma (Module 5, 1997).
Borchert MS. Nystagmus in childhood (Module 8, 1991).
Brooks SE. Transposition procedures (Module 10, 2001).
Dinning WJ. Uveitis and juvenile chronic arthritis (Module 5, 1990).
Dunn JP. Uveitis in children (Module 4, 1995).
Haldi BA, Mets MB. Nonsurgical treatments of strabismus (Module 4, 1997).
Hutcheson KA, Drack AV. Diagnosis and management of the infant who does not see (Module 12, 1998).
Isenberg SJ. How to examine the eye of the neonate (Module 1, 1989).
Keech RV. Practical management of amblyopia (Module 2, 2000).
Lambert SR, Boothe RG. Amblyopia: basic and clinical science perspectives (Module 8, 1994).
Levin AV. The ocular findings in child abuse (Module 7, 1998).
Mets MB, Noffke AS. Ocular infections of the external eye and cornea in children (Module 2, 2002).
Meyer DR. Congenital ptosis (Module 2, 2001).
Palmer EA. Current management of retinopathy of prematurity (Module 3, 1993).
Quinn GE, Young TL. Retinopathy of prematurity (Module 11, 2001).
Rapoza PA, Chandler JW. Neonatal conjunctivitis: diagnosis and treatment (Module 1, 1988).
Ruttum MS. Childhood cataracts (Module 1, 1996).
Silkiss RZ. Craniofacial anomalies (Module 11, 1992).
Spencer JB. A practical approach to refraction in children (Module 4, 1993).
Stefanyszyn MA. Orbital tumors in children (Module 8, 1990).
Steinkuller PG. Orbital cellulitis (Module 11, 1991).
Stevens JCL. Retinoblastoma (Module 1, 1990).
Sutula FC. Management of tearing in children (Module 11, 1989).
Walton DS. Childhood glaucoma (Module 10, 1990).
Wilson ME. Exotropia (Module 11, 1995).
Wilson ME. Management of aphakia in childhood (Module 1, 1999).

Publications

Lane SS, Skuta GL, eds. *ProVision: Preferred Responses in Ophthalmology*, Series 3 (Self-Assessment Program, 1999).

Skuta GL, ed. *ProVision: Preferred Responses in Ophthalmology,* Series 2 (Self-Assessment Program, 1996).

Wilson FM II, ed. *Practical Ophthalmology: A Manual for Beginning Residents.* 4th ed. (1996).

Multimedia

Eye Care Skills on CD-ROM (all seven titles from the Eye Care Skills for the Primary Care Physician Series) (1999).

Wright KW, Drack AV, McKeown CA, Repka MX. *Leo Clinical Update Course on Pediatric Ophthalmology and Strabismus* (CD-ROM, 1998).

Slide-Scripts

Day SH. *Understanding and Preventing Amblyopia* (Eye Care Skills for the Primary Care Physician Series, 1987).

Young SE. *Managing the Red Eye* (Eye Care Skills for the Primary Care Physician Series, 1994).

Continuing Ophthalmic Video Education

Bergin DJ. *Management and Surgery of Congenital and Acquired Ptosis* (1990).
Price RL, Beauchamp GR. *Strabismus Surgery: Oblique Procedures* (1989).
Price RL, Beauchamp GR. *Strabismus Surgery: Rectus Recession and Resection* (1989).
Reinecke RD. *Nystagmus: Fundamentals of Clinical Evaluation* (2000).
Wilson ME. *Ocular Motility Evaluation of Strabismus and Myasthenia Gravis* (1993).

Preferred Practice Patterns

Preferred Practice Patterns Committee, Pediatric Ophthalmology Panel. *Amblyopia* (2002).

Preferred Practice Patterns Committee, Pediatric Ophthalmology Panel. *Esotropia and Exotropia* (2002).

Preferred Practice Patterns Committee, Pediatric Ophthalmology Panel. *Pediatric Eye Evaluations* (2002).

LEO Specialty Clinical Updates Online

Repka MX, West CE, Alcorn DM, et al. *Pediatric Ophthalmology and Strabismus* (2002).

To order any of these materials, please call the Academy's Customer Service number at (415) 561-8540, or order online at www.aao.org.

Credit Reporting Form

Basic and Clinical Science Course, 2004–2005 Section 6

The American Academy of Ophthalmology is accredited by the Accreditation Council for Continuing Medical Education to provide continuing medical education for physicians.

The American Academy of Ophthalmology designates this educational activity for a maximum of 40 category 1 credits toward the AMA Physician's Recognition Award. Each physician should claim only those hours of credit that he/she actually spent in the activity.

The American Medical Association has determined that non-US licensed physicians who participate in this CME activity are eligible for AMA PRA category 1 credit.

If you wish to claim continuing medical education credit for your study of this section, you may claim your credit online or fill in the required forms and mail or fax them to the Academy.

To use the forms:

1. Complete the study questions and mark your answers on the Section Completion Form.
2. Complete the Section Evaluation.
3. Fill in and sign the statement below.
4. Return this page and the required forms by mail or fax to the CME Registrar (see below).

To claim credit online:

1. Log on to the Academy website (www.aao.org).
2. Go to Education Resource Center; click on CME Central.
3. Follow the instructions.

Important: These completed forms or the online claim must be received at the Academy within 3 years of purchase.

I hereby certify that I have spent _____ (up to 40) hours of study on the curriculum of this section and that I have completed the Study Questions.

Signature: _____
Date
Name: _____

Address: _____

City and State: _____ Zip: _____

Telephone: (_____) _____ Academy Member ID# _____
area code

Please return completed forms to: **Or you may fax them to:** 415-561-8557
American Academy of Ophthalmology
P.O. Box 7424
San Francisco, CA 94120-7424
Attn: CME Registrar, Clinical Education

2004–2005
Section Completion Form

Basic and Clinical Science Course

Answer Sheet for Section 6

Question	Answer	Question	Answer	Question	Answer
1	a b c d	18	a b c d	35	a b c d
2	a b c d	19	a b c d	36	a b c d
3	a b c d	20	a b c d	37	a b c d
4	a b c d	21	a b c d	38	a b c d e
5	a b c d	22	a b c d	39	a b c d
6	a b c d	23	a b c d	40	a b c d
7	a b c d	24	a b c d e	41	a b c d
8	a b c d	25	a b c d e	42	a b c d
9	a b c d	26	a b c d	43	a b c d
10	a b c d	27	a b c d	44	a b c d
11	a b c d	28	a b c d	45	a b c d
12	a b c d e	29	a b c d	46	a b c d
13	a b c d e	30	a b c d	47	a b c d
14	a b c d e	31	a b c d	48	a b c d
15	a b c d e	32	a b c d	49	a b c d
16	a b c d e	33	a b c d	50	a b c d
17	a b c d e	34	a b c d		

Section Evaluation

Please complete this CME questionnaire.

1. To what degree will you use knowledge from BCSC Section 6 in your practice?
   - ☐ Regularly
   - ☐ Sometimes
   - ☐ Rarely
2. Please review the stated objectives for BCSC Section 6. How effective was the material at meeting those objectives?
   - ☐ All objectives were met.
   - ☐ Most objectives were met.
   - ☐ Some objectives were met.
   - ☐ Few or no objectives were met.
3. To what degree is BCSC Section 6 likely to have a positive impact on health outcomes of your patients?
   - ☐ Extremely likely
   - ☐ Highly likely
   - ☐ Somewhat likely
   - ☐ Not at all likely
4. After you review the stated objectives for BCSC Section 6, please let us know of any additional knowledge, skills, or information useful to your practice that were acquired but were not included in the objectives. [Optional]

5. Was BCSC Section 6 free of commercial bias?
   - ☐ Yes
   - ☐ No
6. If you selected "No" in the previous question, please comment. [Optional]

7. Please tell us what might improve the applicability of BCSC to your practice. [Optional]

Study Questions

Although a concerted effort has been made to avoid ambiguity and redundancy in these questions, the authors recognize that differences of opinion may occur regarding the "best" answer. The discussions are provided to demonstrate the rationale used to derive the answer. They may also be helpful in confirming that your approach to the problem was correct or, if necessary, in fixing the principle in your memory. Where relevant, additional references are given.

1. A 7-year-old girl is brought in for evaluation of a left "lazy eye." The parents describe intermittent outward drifting of the eye since the girl was 4 years old. Recently, the frequency and duration of the deviation have increased. Visual acuity is 20/50 OU, which corrects to 20/20 OU with −1.5 sphere OU. The exotropia measures 30 X′ and 35 X(T). Stereopsis is 40 arc seconds. The best initial treatment of this patient is

    a. single-vision glasses of −1.5 sphere OU
    b. single-vision glasses of −3.5 sphere OU
    c. alternate patching, 4 hours per day
    d. patching of the right eye only, 4 hours per day

2. A 4-year-old girl is brought in for evaluation of new-onset right esotropia. There was no antecedent viral illness or head injury. Her pediatrician has already performed CT, the results of which were normal. The parents show you several photographs of how the child looked before with straight eyes. In each photograph, she has a consistent face turn 15° left. The right eye abducts fully. The most likely diagnosis is

    a. congenital palsy, right cranial nerve VI
    b. acute idiopathic palsy, right cranial nerve VI, resolved
    c. Duane syndrome type 1 OS
    d. Duane syndrome type 2 OD

3. A 5-month-old healthy full-term infant is brought in for evaluation of esotropia. The deviation measures 50 ET′ by Krimsky testing and is constant in the office. The child cross-fixates equally well with each eye. The cycloplegic refraction is +1.0 sphere OU. Surgery should be performed

    a. immediately
    b. around 1 year of age, in order to allow time for spontaneous resolution
    c. between 1 and 2 years of age, so that if inferior oblique overaction or dissociated vertical deviations develop they can be treated at the same time (ie, during one surgery)
    d. as soon as the child is old enough to permit a reliable alternate-cover test

4. A 9-month-old healthy full-term infant is brought in for evaluation of esotropia. The crossing started variably around 6–7 months of age and now is nearly constant. Vision is central, steady, and maintained in each eye. The deviation measures 30 ET′ by alternate cover testing. The ocular rotations show −1 limitation of voluntary abduction OU. The cycloplegic refraction is +4.0 sphere OU. The first step in treatment is

   a. neuroimaging
   b. full-time alternate occlusion
   c. glasses containing +4.0 sphere OU
   d. glasses containing +2.0 sphere OU

5. A 2-year-old girl is brought in for examination because her mother and brother have neurofibromatosis type 1 and the family wishes to determine whether this child is also affected. Her ocular examination results are normal. Which of the following statements is true?

   a. The absence of Brushfield spots means that the child is unaffected.
   b. Optic nerve gliomas in neurofibromatosis usually develop in infancy, so this child is unlikely to be affected by this complication.
   c. The absence of Lisch nodules does not mean that the child is unaffected.
   d. The child should undergo examination under sedation to check intraocular pressure.

6. Vision loss in Riley-Day syndrome is most often due to

   a. cataracts
   b. optic nerve hypoplasia
   c. amblyopia
   d. corneal scarring

7. A 5-year-old child presents with a 5-day complaint of progressive right upper- and lower-lid redness and swelling. Currently, the lids are swollen shut, tender, and warm. He was placed on ampicillin and Benadryl by his pediatrician 3 days earlier, without noticeable improvement. His past medical history is significant for lots of allergies and congestion. The examination is limited because of poor cooperation, and a lid speculum is required to open the right eyelids. There is moderate conjunctival injection; the cornea is clear and iris details are visible; the pupil is round and reactive; the optic disc is normal. By observation, the ocular rotations are grossly full. There is no area of broken skin on the eyelids. The left eye is normal. The next step in treatment is to

   a. ask the pediatrician to change to a stronger oral antibiotic such as amoxicillin/clavulanate potassium (Augmentin)
   b. order MRI
   c. order CT
   d. order a dermatologic consultation

8. All of the following conditions have a characteristic anterior-segment finding *except*

   a. sickle cell disease
   b. Marfan syndrome
   c. galactosemia
   d. Wilson disease

9. The parents of a 7-month-old child complain of intermittent tearing OD only, beginning 3 months ago. Their pediatrician prescribed lacrimal sac massage but noticed a decreased red reflex OD on a follow-up visit. The most likely diagnosis is

   a. congenital glaucoma
   b. infantile cataract
   c. chlamydial conjunctivitis with corneal scarring
   d. retinoblastoma

10. A 5-month-old infant has a capillary hemangioma of the right upper lid involving the temporal third of the lid. The lid margin is deformed in an S-shape and covers about one third of the superior pupil. The child appears amblyopic by fixation preference testing. The most likely cause is

    a. intermittent occlusion during periods of fatigue
    b. intermittent occlusion when the child looks to the right
    c. anisometropic amblyopia due to unequal hyperopia
    d. anisometropic amblyopia due to unequal astigmatism

11. A 2-year-old child with a history of prematurity and cerebral palsy is brought in for evaluation of possible ocular torticollis. The child maintains a frequent head posture of tilting to the left. He can sit unaided but is not crawling or walking. On examination, his vision is central, steady, maintained OD and central, steady, not maintained OS. There is a constant 45 left esotropia, and bilateral inferior oblique muscle overaction is greater OS than OD. Which of the following best explains the torticollis?

    a. It is nonocular.
    b. It is due to congenital bilateral superior oblique palsies.
    c. It is an effort to avoid the left inferior oblique overaction.
    d. It is due to a V pattern.

12. Dissociated vertical deviation (DVD) is characterized by which of the following features?

    a. extorsion or horizontal component as the eye moves vertically
    b. upward movement to fixate of the adducting eye in lateral gaze
    c. essentially identical movements of the eyes in the alternate-cover test in all positions of gaze
    d. (a) and (b)
    e. (a) and (c)

13. Tucking the superior oblique tendon

    a. is appropriate to correct superior oblique muscle palsy
    b. can result in Brown syndrome
    c. is the procedure of choice when the symptoms and measurements indicate principally a torsional misalignment
    d. (a) and (b)
    e. (b) and (c)

14. Which feature(s) below are not typically found in Brown syndrome?
    a. hyperdeviation in the lower field of gaze
    b. exotropia in straight upgaze
    c. incomplete elevation in straight upgaze
    d. esotropia in downgaze
    e. (a) and (d)

15. Which of the following statements about strabismus secondary to thyroid ophthalmopathy is false?
    a. It can be restrictive.
    b. It can be caused by extraocular muscle weakness.
    c. It usually is surgically corrected early after onset.
    d. It is unrelated to the degree of thyroid function.
    e. Both (b) and (c) are correct.

16. Congenital dacryocele
    a. presents with a mass above the medial canthal ligament
    b. usually responds to systemic antibiotics alone
    c. can be associated with an intranasal mucocele
    d. is best treated with incision and drainage through the skin
    e. usually indicates stenosis of the bony nasolacrimal canal

17. The electroretinogram (ERG) usually appears normal in the following conditions *except*
    a. optic nerve hypoplasia
    b. cortical visual impairment
    c. achromatopsia
    d. delayed visual maturation
    e. (a) and (c)

18. Which of the following statements is false?
    a. Epiblepharon is well-tolerated and only occasionally requires surgical correction.
    b. Telecanthus indicates increased separation between the bony orbits.
    c. Amblyopia resulting from ptosis is usually a result of induced astigmatism rather than occlusion.
    d. The blepharophimosis syndrome is often inherited in an autosomal dominant fashion.

19. Which of the following choroidal lesions may be associated with adenocarcinoma of the colon?
    a. choroidal osteoma
    b. combined hamartoma of the retina and retinal pigment epithelium
    c. melanocytoma
    d. congenital hypertrophy of the retinal pigment epithelium

20. Which of the following diagnostic tests should be performed on all patients with retinoblastoma?
    a. CT of the head and orbits
    b. total-body CT
    c. aspiration of intraocular fluid
    d. bone marrow biopsy

21. Regarding the treatment of retinoblastoma, which of the following statements is true?
    a. Enucleation is no longer an appropriate treatment for retinoblastoma.
    b. External beam irradiation results in a much higher incidence of secondary tumor formation.
    c. Cryotherapy and laser therapy can be used for tumors that are 5 mm in thickness.
    d. Plaque radiotherapy should not be used for retinoblastomas that fail to respond to other methods of treatment.

22. Which of the following statements is false?
    a. Juvenile rheumatoid arthritis is the most commonly identified cause of childhood uveitis.
    b. Steroid administration in children is less likely to result in cataracts or glaucoma than in adults.
    c. Toxoplasmosis is the most commonly identified infectious cause of childhood uveitis.
    d. Toxocariasis is usually caused by *Toxocara canis.*

23. Which of the following is *not* a complication of steroid administration in children?
    a. angle-closure glaucoma
    b. bone fractures
    c. death
    d. altered mental status

24. Which of the following statements regarding the pathophysiology of amblyopia is true?
    a. Changes in the nerve fiber layer of the retina are characteristic of strabismic amblyopia.
    b. The cells in the medial geniculate body corresponding to the amblyopic eye may be smaller and less intensely staining than those corresponding to the sound eye.
    c. The visual acuity of an amblyopic eye may be better when measured in the presence of contour interaction than if measured with isolated optotypes.
    d. The most significant change in the visual cortex of an amblyopic patient is loss of binocular cells, cells that are responsive to stimulation from either eye.
    e. The sensitive period for the development of deprivation amblyopia begins earlier and lasts longer than that for strabismic or anisometropic amblyopia.

442 • Study Questions

25. Which one of the following statements regarding accommodative esotropia is false?
    a. In the gradient method of determining the AC/A ratio, plus or minus lenses can be used to evaluate the effect of accommodation on the deviation at a given distance.
    b. In the heterophoria method for determining the AC/A ratio, measurements of the deviation at distance and near are compared.
    c. It is generally acceptable to perform surgery for fully accommodative esotropia as long as the patient has good fusion.
    d. Executive or flat-top bifocals are preferred over progressive bifocals in young children with nonrefractive accommodative esotropia.
    e. Miotic agents can be used diagnostically in accommodative esotropia or as a short-term substitute for glasses.

26. Regarding patients with congenital nasolacrimal duct obstruction, which of the following statements is false?
    a. Obstruction of the nasolacrimal duct occurs in 2%–4% of full-term infants during the first 2 weeks of life.
    b. Topical antibiotics, lacrimal massage, and nasal decongestants are therapies in the initial treatment of these children.
    c. In-office probing, without general anesthesia, can be done anytime during the first year of life.
    d. The success rate of probe and irrigation alone drops to 33% if not done by 2 years of age.

27. Which of the following conditions is not characteristically associated with childhood glaucoma?
    a. Sturge-Weber syndrome
    b. aniridia
    c. galactosemia
    d. Lowe syndrome

28. A 2-month-old boy presents with epiphora, photophobia, and a band of cloudiness of the right cornea that does not obscure the pupil. Appropriate evaluation should include
    a. corneal biopsy with Oil Red O stain
    b. examination under anesthesia with IOP measurement at the end of the case
    c. refraction
    d. conjunctival scraping for chlamydia

29. You examine a 1-year-old boy with bilateral cataracts. Appropriate evaluation includes
    a. chromosomal analysis and examination of female relatives
    b. serum copper level
    c. urine protein level
    d. red blood cell galactose-1-phosphate uridyl transferase level

30. Which of the following is least likely to cause a subluxation of the lens?
    a. Marfan syndrome
    b. homocystinuria
    c. hyperlysinemia
    d. Weill-Marchesani syndrome

31. A 1-year-old child has a 3-month history of intermittent, rapid, asymmetrical, fine nystagmus. Ophthalmologic and neurologic examination results are otherwise normal. Further evaluation should include MRI of the
    a. cerebellum
    b. chiasmal area
    c. brain stem
    d. foramen magnum

32. Which of the following is *not* a major criterion for the diagnosis of neurofibromatosis type 1?
    a. sphenoid wing dysplasia
    b. posterior subcapsular cataract
    c. single plexiform neurofibroma
    d. optic nerve glioma

33. Which of the following phakomatoses is *not* inherited?
    a. incontinentia pigmenti (Bloch-Sulzberger syndrome)
    b. ataxia-telangiectasia (Louis-Bar syndrome)
    c. racemose angiomatosis (Wyburn-Mason syndrome)
    d. tuberous sclerosis (Bourneville disease)

34. Which of the following is true concerning retinal angiomas associated with von Hippel–Lindau disease?
    a. Their peak clinical incidence coincides with the peak incidence of cerebellar hemangioblastomas.
    b. The tumors are rarely bilateral.
    c. Vision loss is usually secondary to lipid accumulation and serous retinal detachment.
    d. Cryotherapy, laser photocoagulation, or both are ineffective in the treatment of these lesions.

35. The most common horizontal deviation associated with craniosynostosis syndromes is
    a. A-pattern esotropia
    b. A-pattern exotropia
    c. V-pattern esotropia
    d. V-pattern exotropia

36. Crouzon syndrome is most often associated with
    a. plagiocephaly
    b. brachycephaly
    c. scaphocephaly
    d. syndactyly

37. Findings associated with Goldenhar syndrome include all of the following *except*
    a. cleft palate
    b. epibulbar dermoid
    c. eyelid coloboma
    d. Duane syndrome

38. Which antibiotic should be given for suspected neonatal *Neisseria* conjunctivitis?
    a. intravenous ceftriaxone
    b. intravenous penicillin
    c. oral amoxicillin
    d. topical gentamicin
    e. topical ciprofloxacin

39. Which of the following is *not* a major cause of Parinaud oculoglandular syndrome?
    a. *Bartonella henselae*
    b. *Borrelia burgdorferi*
    c. *Francisella tularensis*
    d. *Mycobacterium tuberculosis*

40. Which is a feature of orbital, not preseptal, cellulitis?
    a. eyelid edema
    b. tenderness to palpation
    c. proptosis
    d. conjunctivitis

41. Which of the following is *not* a characteristic of Sturge-Weber syndrome?
    a. glaucoma
    b. choroidal hemangioma
    c. cerebral calcification
    d. posterior subcapsular cataract

42. Overcorrections following strabismus surgery
    a. can be avoided with adjustable sutures
    b. can occur when the resected muscle slips or is lost after surgery
    c. are less common than undercorrections
    d. frequently cause diplopia in young children

43. Scleral perforations during strabismus surgery in children
    a. are frequently followed by retinal detachment
    b. are frequently treated with laser therapy or cryopexy
    c. occur in about 10% of strabismus surgeries
    d. frequently cause postoperative endophthalmitis

44. Localized conjunctival injection and chemosis noted several days postoperatively at the site of eye muscle surgery may be caused by
    a. suture allergy
    b. poor closure of the conjunctival wound
    c. conjunctival inclusion cyst
    d. all of the above

45. Anterior segment ischemia following eye muscle surgery
    a. is especially common following muscle transposition procedures
    b. can occur following surgery on two rectus muscles
    c. typically presents with iritis and an irregular pupil
    d. all of the above

46. Botulinum toxin is particularly useful for
    a. large-angle exotropia
    b. mechanical restrictions
    c. small residual angles following strabismus surgery
    d. dissociated vertical deviations

47. A 3-year-old boy was brought to the emergency room following an injury to the right eye. The history states that he wandered too close when his father was practicing his golf swing. The lids are ecchymotic and cannot be opened. The child is inconsolably terrified. You should
    a. call Child Protective Service
    b. get a papoose board to restrain the child and open the lids with a speculum to investigate for ocular injury
    c. prepare the child for an examination under anesthesia
    d. send the child home for reexamination in several days, when the swelling has subsided

48. All of the following are characteristic of the shaken baby syndrome *except*
    a. the child is younger than 12 months
    b. parenchymal brain damage and intracranial hemorrhage are common
    c. ocular adnexae and anterior segments are typically involved
    d. retinal hemorrhage is typical, especially in the posterior pole

49. All of the following suggest an occult perforating injury *except*
    a. an eyelid laceration with intact conjunctiva
    b. an irregular pupil
    c. loss of ocular rotations
    d. all of the above suggest perforation

50. Hyphema following blunt trauma in a child
    a. should be treated on an inpatient basis, with bilateral patching and bedrest
    b. should be treated with long-acting cycloplegics and topical steroids on an outpatient basis
    c. is more common in children with sickle cell hemoglobin
    d. should be evacuated if a total hyphema in a young child persists more than 4 or 5 days

Answers

1. Answer—a. Uncorrected myopia often worsens control of exotropia by blurring distance vision and by decreasing the accommodative requirement for intermediate and near fixation. In response b, overminused glasses were prescribed to promote increased accommodative demand at all fixation distances. Although overminused glasses may be helpful and necessary, they are not indicated as the initial treatment. Antisuppression patching (either of the dominant eye or alternating) can also improve control of exotropia but is unlikely to have much effect in the face of uncorrected myopia. Therefore, the best initial treatment of this child is to correct her myopia.

2. Answer—c. Because the child can currently abduct the right eye fully, she does not have a congenital palsy of right cranial nerve VI. An acute right CN VI palsy should provoke a head turn right, not left, to obtain fusion and avoid diplopia. Duane syndrome type 2 involves limited adduction of the affected eye, not limited abduction; given the complaint of right esotropia, it is unlikely that the child has right a Duane syndrome type 2 OD. A surprising number of children with Duane syndrome type 1 are brought in for evaluation of crossing of the normal eye. The parents and pediatrician fail to recognize that there is an abduction deficit when the child gazes toward the affected eye (in this case, left gaze), and they assign the problem to the eye with normal motility. This child has a long-standing ocular torticollis consistent with Duane syndrome type 1 OS (turn left to keep the left eye somewhat adducted). Girls are more commonly affected than boys, and the left eye is more commonly affected than the right eye. Palpebral fissure widening on attempted abduction and narrowing on adduction confirm the diagnosis. Despite the history of a new problem, if the clinical examination is consistent with Duane syndrome, neuroimaging is not indicated.

3. Answer—a. A neurologically normal child nearing 6 months of age with a large-angle esotropia, who has established cross-fixation, is very unlikely to experience spontaneous improvement. Depending on the personality of the child, it may be several more months before alternate-cover testing of any accuracy can be performed, and the measurements are unlikely to be more than 5 different from the results of a good Krimsky test. In order to maximize the likelihood of some level of binocular function, the child's eye should be surgically straightened as soon as possible. There is no reason for delay. Subsequent eye misalignments can be dealt with by subsequent surgeries, and the parents should be informed that more than one operation may be needed during childhood.

4. Answer—c. The time of onset is not consistent with a diagnosis of "true" congenital esotropia. Although the limited voluntary abduction might raise the issue of a central nervous system process causing bilateral cranial nerve VI palsies, abduction should be tested using a doll's head maneuver before neuroimaging is obtained. Many infants with esotropia cross-fixate rather than abduct and get out of the habit of abduction. Full-time alternate occlusion will not restore the child to orthotropia and thus is not indicated. A small subset of children with accommodative esotropia present in infancy rather than the more typical range of 18–36 months. If the condition is caught early enough, these patients respond well to spectacles containing the full cycloplegic refraction. Prescribing less than the full cycloplegic refraction may work if the child is highly hyperopic (eg, >+6 sphere OU), but in this case to eliminate a near angle of 30, success is most likely with full refractive correction.

Answers • 447

5. **Answer—c.** Brushfield spots are seen in Down syndrome, not neurofibromatosis. Optic nerve gliomas associated with neurofibromatosis generally develop in the first 1–2 decades of life, rarely in toddlerhood. Glaucoma with neurofibromatosis is seen in association with plexiform neurofibromas of the eyelids (a secondary form of glaucoma); in the absence of a lid lesion, there is no reason to suspect that this child has elevated IOP and no reason to sedate her to measure IOP. Answer c is correct: Lisch nodules eventually develop in over 90% of patients with neurofibromatosis type 1, but they are rarely present in early childhood. Lisch nodules are therefore a sensitive, but not a specific, finding for neurofibromatosis at this age.

6. **Answer—d.** Riley-Day syndrome is a congenital disorder of the autonomic nervous system. Cataracts and optic nerve hypoplasia are not primary manifestations of the disease. Vision loss is principally due to complications from the cornea anesthesia and anhidrosis. Affected children suffer from neutrotrophic keratitis, which is complicated by dryness. Repeated slow-healing corneal erosions occur, which lead to corneal scarring. Amblyopia may be superimposed in cases of asymmetrical corneal clarity but is rarely the most important element of vision loss in these children.

7. **Answer—c.** The pediatrician's initial diagnosis was probably preseptal cellulitis, which can often be treated orally if caught early and monitored carefully. Ampicillin is not the most potent first-line agent for this condition. However, answer a is still incorrect because in this case the child most likely does not have simple preseptal cellulitis, and continued outpatient treatment is inappropriate. There are clear infectious signs, and a dermatologic consultation will be of little benefit in management. The most likely correct diagnosis is a subperiosteal abscess from ethmoid sinusitis. The external signs can be indistinguishable from those of preseptal cellulitis. Although limitation of eye movement is considered a hallmark of this condition, it is difficult to elicit a history of pain on eye movement or double vision from young children, and it is often impossible to perform a detailed assessment of ocular rotations given the clinical circumstances. These patients can have a history of chronic nasal congestion or sinus infections. A CT scan with coronal views, rather than MRI, is the best way to image a subperiosteal abscess. This is fortunate because a 5-year-old child usually requires deep sedation or general anesthesia for MRI but not for CT.

8. **Answer—a.** Marfan syndrome is associated with lens subluxation. Galactosemia causes infantile cataracts, often beginning as oil droplet cataracts. Wilson disease causes a sunflower cataract due to copper deposition on the lens capsules, in addition to the Kayser-Fleischer ring. Sickle cell disease is a thromboembolic disorder that primarily affects the retinal circulation, not the anterior segment, although neovascularization of the iris can develop in severe cases secondary to widespread retinal ischemia.

9. **Answer—a.** Nasolacrimal duct obstructions present within 2–4 weeks of life. A history of epiphora onset at 4 months old is atypical for this condition, and other diagnoses must be considered. Congenital or infantile cataracts do not cause epiphora. Chlamydial conjunctivitis acquired by passage through the birth canal can start slowly in newborns but is usually overtly symptomatic within a few weeks of life. Retinoblastoma does not cause epiphora unless it is associated with very high IOP and corneal edema, in which case other signs of ocular inflammation are usually present. The most likely diagnosis is congenital glaucoma. This can be mistaken by pediatricians for nasolacrimal duct obstruction, particularly if obvious corneal edema or buphthalmos are absent when the parents first complain of tearing.

10. Answer—d. Upper lid lesions can cause amblyopia due to pupil occlusion. Usually, the lid must cover half or more of the pupil at all times to be significantly amblyopic. Even infants adopt head turns or chin-up postures to avoid pupil occlusion, if possible. Although intermittent occlusive ptosis may be a contributing factor, a far more likely cause in this case is induced astigmatism from the mass pressing on the soft pediatric eye wall. This complication should not be overlooked: children with nonocclusive lid hemangiomas require careful follow-up and repeated refractions to permit detection and treatment of aniso-astigmatic amblyopia.

11. Answer—a. This child has esotropia associated with significant cerebral palsy and motor delays. Although it is often not possible to perform cover testing in various positions of gaze, simple observation usually establishes that there is no fusional position (no head posture where the eyes are sufficiently aligned to allow for a degree of binocular function). Primary inferior oblique overaction is common in childhood esotropia and is not due to superior oblique palsies. Because the child is right eye dominant and nonfusing, he suppresses the left eye and has no reason to try to avoid the left inferior oblique overaction. Children with V-pattern esotropia who have binocular function use a chin-down posture, not a head tilt. In this case, the torticollis is nonocular and is likely another muscular manifestation of the cerebral palsy.

12. Answer—e. Choice a describes the complex motion that characterizes this entity. Choice c is likewise a part of the description of DVD. Choice b describes an important difference that distinguishes DVD from other vertical misalignments.

13. Answer—d. Tucking is a tightening procedure intended to improve superior oblique muscle action. Because all of the tendon fibers are included in the procedure, tucking cannot be employed selectively only for the torsional component of the deviation. Tucking too much or too close to the trochlea can hinder the movement of the tendon through that structure; hence, tucking generally is performed in the portion of the tendon adjacent to the nasal border of the superior rectus muscle or more distally.

14. Answer—e. Absence of hyperdeviation in the lower field, where there is no occasion for the short or otherwise restricted superior oblique tendon to generate a limited rotation, is characteristic of all but the most severe cases of Brown syndrome. Divergence in straight upgaze is an important sign helping to distinguish Brown syndrome from inferior oblique muscle palsy; it was considered by Brown to be a defining feature of this condition and is not associated with the opposite horizontal deviation in downgaze.

15. Answer—c. The restrictive changes that occur in the extraocular muscles in this condition are preceded and accompanied by an inflammatory phase that adds a variable weakening effect to their action. Neither phase is closely related to the patient's overall thyroid status.

16. Answer—c. Masses presenting above the medial canthal ligament in infancy are usually dermoid cysts or encephaloceles. It is important to rule out this last condition by imaging, as it would be a serious error to attempt excision of a mass in this area without knowing that it does not communicate intracranially. Systemic antibiotics without drainage do not affect lacrimal system blockage definitively. Percutaneous incision and drainage too often results in fistula formation and should be avoided unless the skin is already seriously compromised. Bony stenosis of the nasolacrimal canal typically gives signs of a chronic partial obstruction rather than of an acute total closed-end obstruction.

17. Answer—c. This is the only disorder that involves the retinal photoreceptors directly. Low vision from disorders of the central portions of the visual pathway, as well as those which primarily implicate the inner retinal layers, typically are not reflected in abnormalities of the ERG.

18. Answer—b. Telecanthus is a wide intercanthal distance. Hypertelorism indicates increased separation between the bony orbits.

19. Answer—d.

20. Answer—a. CT of the head and orbit is necessary to confirm the presence of intraocular calcification and to detect any extraocular or intracranial disease. Aspiration of intraocular fluid can spread tumor and should be avoided.

21. Answer—b. Enucleation is still frequently used to treat large tumors in eyes with poor visual potential or when other methods of treatment have failed. Cryotherapy and laser therapy are usually reserved for small tumors, less than 2.0–2.5 mm in thickness. Plaque radiotherapy can be used as a secondary treatment for retinoblastoma but may be associated with a higher incidence of radiation retinopathy and optic neuropathy when used in children who have already undergone chemotherapy.

22. Answer—b. Steroid administration is more likely to result in cataracts or glaucoma in children than in adults.

23. Answer—a. Although open-angle glaucoma can occur following steroid administration in children, angle-closure glaucoma is uncommon.

24. Answer—e. The critical period for the development of deprivation begins earlier and lasts longer than that for strabismic or anisometropic amblyopia. Furthermore, a shorter period of time is necessary for visual deprivation to cause amblyopia than is the case for strabismic or anisometropic amblyopia. Evidence that the retina is involved in amblyopia is inconclusive. The lateral geniculate body, not the medial geniculate body, is involved in amblyopia. The visual acuity of an amblyopic patient worsens with contour interaction (crowding). The most significant cortical change in amblyopia is loss of cells responsive to stimulation from the amblyopic eye.

25. Answer—c. It would be controversial to substitute surgery for glasses in a patient with fully accommodative esotropia. Surgery for the accommodative excess portion of the deviation at near to enable an older child to wear single-vision glasses or contact lenses is less controversial. Surgery for any nonaccommodative portion of an esodeviation, as long as it has been confirmed that the patient is wearing the full hyperopic correction, is commonly performed.

26. Answer—c. Nasal lacrimal duct obstruction is a very common abnormality in the newborn infant and presents as apparent conjunctivitis. Nasolacrimal duct obstruction usually responds to treatment with topical antibiotics and massage of the lacrimal sac. Early probing is often curative but its effectiveness decreases markedly after age 1 year. In-office probing can be performed in children younger than 6 months but becomes increasingly difficult as the child gets older. By 9–12 months of age, the child is usually too big to hold down and forcibly probe.

27. Answer—c. Hereditary ocular conditions that affect the anterior segment anatomy are often associated with childhood glaucoma. Aniridia and Lowe syndrome have marked structural abnormalities of the anterior segment involving the lens, iris, and aqueous outflow system. Over time, glaucoma often develops. Sturge-Weber syndrome can cause glaucoma by two mechanisms. First, the episcleral venous pressure is elevated because of ocular vascular abnormalities; second, the trabecular meshwork is often abnormal in these patients. Galactosemia can cause cataracts by interfering with normal lens metabolism, but the anatomy otherwise is normal and glaucoma is not an issue except as a complication of cataract surgery.

28. Answer—c. The classic presentation for congenital glaucoma is epiphora, light sensitivity, and a hazy cornea. Chlamydial infections are normally transmitted from the mother and are present soon after birth. IOP should be measured at the beginning of the examination under anesthesia because anesthesia has a rapid lowering effect on IOP. Refraction might show a myopic anisometropia, which helps confirm the diagnosis and may require treatment to prevent amblyopia.

29. Answer—d. Bilateral congenital cataracts are either inherited (due to a metabolic or infectious cause) or developmental. The genetics of cataracts are not well-known, and although cataracts can be associated with a chromosomal defect, this is rare and analysis is usually not indicated. The one treatable metabolic disorder is galactosemia, which can be detected by looking at the red blood cell enzymes.

30. Answer—c. The most common cause of subluxed lenses is simple ectopia lentis, which can be familial. Marfan syndrome, Weill-Marchesani syndrome, and homocystinuria are rare but always are included in the differential diagnosis. The association with hyperlysinemia is very weak and probably not real.

31. Answer—b. Spasmus nutans is a bilateral, often very asymmetrical, fine horizontal nystagmus. The nystagmus can be intermittent and difficult to see. It normally is idiopathic starting about age 3–4 months and resolves by age 3–4 years. The nystagmus can be seen in patients who have gliomas of the chiasm. These cases are always associated with decreased vision and optic atrophy. However, because these findings can be subtle in a very young baby, neuroimaging is often recommended when the diagnosis is uncertain.

32. Answer—b. Posterior subcapsular or wedge cortical lens opacities are associated with neurofibromatosis type 2 and are not a feature of type 1. Other major diagnostic criteria for neurofibromatosis type 1 include the presence of two or more Lisch nodules, six or more café-au-lait spots, axillary or inguinal freckling, and a family history of a first-degree relative with neurofibromatosis type 1.

33. Answer—c. Wyburn-Mason and Sturge-Weber syndromes are the only two phakomatoses that have no genetic inheritance pattern. Tuberous sclerosis, von Hippel–Lindau disease, and neurofibromatosis are typically autosomal dominant. Ataxia-telangiectasia has autosomal recessive transmission, and incontinentia pigmenti is X-linked dominant.

34. Answer—c. Retinal angiomas are often located in the peripheral fundus and may be asymptomatic when small. As the lesion grows, its capillaries may become more incompetent and allow for transudation of fluid. If the retinal edema and exudates are extensive enough to involve the macula, vision becomes compromised. The peak incidence of retinal angioma occurs a decade before its cerebellar counterpart. The tumors are bilateral in up to 50% of cases. Treatment with cryotherapy or laser photocoagulation may be especially efficacious with smaller lesions.

35. Answer—d. The craniosynostoses are often associated with excyclorotation of the orbits and abnormal insertions of the horizontal rectus muscles. This may result in a V-pattern exotropia, in which the exotropia increases in upgaze and is minimized in downgaze.

36. Answer—b. Premature bilateral coronal suture closure results in brachycephaly, a characteristic feature of Crouzon syndrome. Plagiocephaly denotes the asymmetry caused by premature closure of a unilateral coronal suture, whereas scaphocephaly is the abnormal skull shape caused by premature sagittal suture closure. Syndactyly is associated with numerous other syndromes, including Apert, Pfeiffer, and Saethre-Chotzen syndromes.

37. Answer—a. Goldenhar syndrome (oculoauriculovertebral dysplasia) is a variant of hemifacial microsomia and is characterized by epibulbar dermoids or lipodermoids, usually in the inferotemporal quadrant. Other findings include upper-eyelid coloboma and Duane syndrome. Cleft palate is not a feature of Goldenhar syndrome but is a part of the Pierre Robin sequence (micrognathia, glossoptosis, and cleft palate) that is common in Stickler syndrome.

38. Answer—a. If untreated, children affected with *Neisseria gonorrhoeae* conjunctivitis can develop life-threatening complications, such as sepsis and meningitis. Antibiotic therapy should therefore be systemic. Topical medications may be used as an adjunct but should certainly not be considered primary therapy. Although intravenous penicillin was once considered the treatment of choice of *Neisseria* infections, resistant strains have made ceftriaxone a better choice. Fluoroquinolones should be avoided in this age group because of potential bone toxicity.

39. Answer—b. The major causes of Parinaud oculoglandular syndrome include cat-scratch fever, tularemia, and tuberculosis. Other causes include syphilis, chlamydia, leprosy, Epstein-Barr virus, and rarely fungi.

40. Answer—c. Preseptal cellulitis is an inflammatory process of the tissues anterior to the orbital septum that can occur secondary to trauma, severe conjunctivitis, or upper-respiratory or sinus infection. Orbital cellulitis is an infection of the orbit involving the tissues posterior to the orbital septum. Both may present with eyelid edema and tenderness to palpation, but proptosis is not a feature of preseptal cellulitis. Full ocular motility and absence of pain on eye movement help distinguish preseptal from orbital cellulitis.

41. Answer—d. Sturge-Weber syndrome (SWS, or encephalofacial angiomatosis) is a sporadic disorder characterized by a port-wine stain with an ipsilateral leptomeningeal vascular malformation. Children with SWS typically have cerebral calcification (railroad-track sign), seizures, hemiparesis or hemianopia, and variable mental deficiency. A majority also have choroidal angiomatosis that has been likened to tomato catsup. Glaucoma is the most common and serious ocular complication and occurs in approximately half of cases. Posterior subcapsular cataract occurs in neurofibromatosis type 2, not SWS.

42. Answer—c. Undercorrections are much more common than overcorrections. Overcorrections can occur after suture adjustment. Slippage of a resected muscle causes an undercorrection. Though definitely an issue in adults, diplopia is not a problem in young children.

43. Answer—b. Retinal detachments (especially in children) and endophthalmitis are rare even in cases with known scleral perforation. Although the incidence was as high as 10% in the 1970s, spatulated needles have made the complication much less common recently. Most surgeons recommend cryopexy or laser therapy, although some do not.

44. Answer—d. They all can present in this fashion.

45. Answer—d. Transposition procedures and other surgeries involving three or more rectus muscles pose a special risk of anterior segment ischemia. Such ischemia can occur even following two-muscle surgery, although typically in elderly patients with poor circulation or blood dyscrasias. Iritis and sector iris atrophy are characteristic of anterior segment ischemia.

46. Answer—c. Botulinum has been shown to be relatively ineffective in the other conditions listed but can often resolve a small residual angle strabismus in the first few months following surgery.

47. Answer—c. The presentation does not suggest child abuse. Forcing an examination in a terrified child with a possibly ruptured globe risks further injury. Sending the child home is inappropriate because he may have suffered serious ocular damage.

48. Answer—c. Adnexae and anterior segments are typically uninvolved. The other choices are characteristic of the syndrome.

49. Answer—d. A sharp object can perforate the sclera posterior to the conjunctival cul de sac through a lid laceration. Other choices are typical of perforating injuries.

50. Answer—d. Hospitalization, patching, bedrest, cycloplegia, and steroids are all controversial in the treatment of hyphemas, which should be individualized according to the risk of complications. Hyphemas are not more common in sickle cell disease or trait, but they are more dangerous because of impeded resorption and risk of retinal vascular occlusion. Because of the risk of corneal blood staining and the difficulty obtaining accurate pressure measurements, total hyphemas in young children should be evacuated in this time frame.

Index

(i = image; t = table)

A pattern, 80, 125, 131–136, 133i, 134i
  definition of, 131
  esotropia, 134i
    treatment of, 136
  exotropia, 133i
    treatment of, 136
  superior oblique overaction causing, 131, 133i
  surgical treatment of, 132–135, 136, 173, 174
Abducens nerve palsy. *See* Sixth nerve (abducens) palsy, 92
Abduction, 33
  extraocular muscles in
    inferior oblique, 17, 19i, 20t
    lateral rectus, 13, 14i, 20t
    superior oblique, 16, 18i, 20t
  gaze position and, 31–32, 32i
Abetalipoproteinemia, Leber congenital amaurosis and, 317
Abrasions, corneal, 413
Abuse, child, ocular trauma and, 410–413, 411i, 412i
AC. *See* Accommodative convergence
AC/A. *See* Accommodative convergence/accommodation ratio
Accommodative convergence, 35
Accommodative convergence/accommodation ratio, 35, 81
  in intermittent exotropia, 107, 108, 110
  management of abnormalities of, 82
  measurement of, 81–82
  in nonrefractive accommodative esotropia, 96–97
Accommodative esotropia, 92t, 95–98
  nonrefractive, 92t, 96–98
  partially accommodative, 92t, 98–99
  refractive, 92t, 96
Acetazolamide, for glaucoma, 268
Achromatopsia (rod monochromatism), 317–318, 423
Acquired immunodeficiency syndrome. *See* HIV infection/AIDS
Active force generation, 84
Acular. *See* Ketorolac tromethamine
Acyclovir, for herpes simplex virus infections, 207, 215
Adduction, 33
  extraocular muscles in
    inferior rectus, 14, 16i, 20t, 30
    medial rectus, 13, 14i, 20t
    superior rectus, 14, 15i, 20t, 30
  gaze position and, 30–32, 32i
Adenoma sebaceum, in tuberous sclerosis, 383, 384i
Adenomatous polyposis, familial (Gardner syndrome), retinal manifestations of, 368
Adenoviruses
  epidemic keratoconjunctivitis caused by, 212–213
  pharyngoconjunctival fever caused by, 213
Adherence syndrome, after strabismus surgery, 180
Adipose tissue, in orbit, 23i, 25
Adjustable suture techniques, 167
Adnexa. *See* Ocular adnexa
Adrenergic agents, for glaucoma, 268
Afterimage test, retinal correspondence evaluated with, 57–59, 60i

Agenesis, definition of, 195
Aging, Lisch nodule prevalence and, 251, 252i
Agonist muscles, 33
Ahmed implant, for glaucoma, 267
Aicardi syndrome, 319
AIDS. *See* HIV infection/AIDS
Alagille syndrome, posterior embryotoxon in, 239
Albinism, 327–330, 330i, 328–329t
  brown, 328t
  in Chédiak-Higashi syndrome, 329t
  Cross syndrome (oculocerebral hypopigmentation), 328t
  with deafness, 329t
  in Hermansky-Pudlak syndrome, 328t
  iris transillumination in, 257–258, 327, 330i
  minimal pigment, 329t
  ocular, 327, 329t
    autosomal recessive, 329t
    X-linked, 327, 329t
  oculocutaneous, 327, 329t
  with pigment, 328t
  retinal manifestations of, 327, 330i
  temperature-sensitive, 329t
  tyrosinase-negative/positive, 327, 328t
  X-linked, 327
Alcohol (ethanol), malformations associated with maternal use of, 401–403, 402i
Alexander's law, 151
Alignment, ocular
  tests of, 74–80
    confounding factors and, 80
  unsatisfactory, after strabismus surgery, 176
Allen pictures, for visual acuity testing, 72t, 73
Allergic conjunctivitis, 220
Allergic reactions, 220–223, 220i, 221i, 223t
  allergic conjunctivitis, 220
  atopic keratoconjunctivitis, 221
  to suture materials, in strabismus surgery, 178, 178i, 179i
  vernal keratoconjunctivitis, 221–222, 221i
Allergic shiners, 221
Alpha-tocopherol. *See* Vitamin E
Alphagan. *See* Brimonidine
Alport disease/syndrome, 331
  lenticonus in, 272–273, 331
Alternate cover test (prism and cover test), 75–77, 76i
  for intermittent exodeviation evaluation, 107–108
Alternating fixation, 11
Alternating heterotropia, 75
Alternating nystagmus, periodic, 157
Alternating suppression, 51
Alveolar rhabdomyosarcoma, 352
Amaurosis
  acquired, 425, 426t
  Leber congenital, 316–317, 317i, 423
    RPE65 defects causing, 317
Amblyopia, 63–70
  abnormal visual experiences and, 46–48, 63–64
  anisometropic, 65

453

visual development affected by, 48
bilateral high refractive error and, 65
classification of, 64–66
compliance with therapy and, 68, 69–70
in craniosynostosis, 398
deprivation, 65–66
  in eye trauma, 409
  visual development affected by, 47
diagnosis of, 66, 71–90. *See also* Ocular motility, assessment of
ex anopsia. *See* Deprivation amblyopia
hemangiomas and, 355–357
history/presenting complaint in, 71–72
isometropic, 65
meridional, 65
occlusion, 66
  in eye trauma, 410
recurrence of, 70
in retinopathy of prematurity, 307
strabismic, 48, 64–65
treatment of, 67–70
  cataract surgery and, 276–277
  complications of, 69
  unresponsiveness to therapy and, 70
Amblyoscope
  corneal light reflex evaluated with, 77
  retinal correspondence evaluated with, 59–60, 61*i*
Aminocaproic acid/ε-aminocaproic acid, for hyphema, 416
Amniotocele, of lacrimal sac (congenital dacryocystocele), 228, 229*i*
Amplitude, fusional, 41, 41*t*
Anesthesia (anesthetics)
  general, for extraocular muscle surgery, 175
  local (topical/regional)
    in adjustable suture technique, 168
    for extraocular muscle surgery, 175
    for foreign body removal, 5
  malignant hyperthermia caused by, 183–184, 185*t*
  retrobulbar
    for extraocular muscle surgery, 175
    strabismus after, 149
Aneurysmal bone cyst, orbital involvement and, 358
Angiofibromas, facial, in tuberous sclerosis, 383, 384*i*
Angiomas (angiomatosis)
  encephalofacial (Sturge-Weber disease/syndrome), 376*t*, 387–390, 388*i*, 389*i*
  nevus flammeus in, 365, 387–388, 388*i*
  racemose (Wyburn-Mason syndrome), 376*t*, 393, 393*i*
  retinal (von Hippel-Lindau disease), 376*t*, 386–387, 387*i*
  retinoblastoma differentiated from, 368–372
Angle-closure glaucoma, 266
Angle kappa (positive and negative), 80, 81*i*
  in retinopathy of prematurity, 80, 313, 314*i*
Aniridia, 249, 249*i*
  nystagmus and, 150, 249
  Wilms tumor and, 249
Anisometropia, amblyopia caused by (anisometropic amblyopia), 65
  visual development affected by, 46–48
Ankyloblepharon, 197, 198*i*
  filiforme adnatum, 197

Anomalies, congenital. *See specific type and* Congenital anomalies
Anomalous retinal correspondence, 39, 51–53, 52*i*
  harmonious, 55, 60, 61*i*
  testing for, 52–53, 54–60, 61*i*
  unharmonious, 56, 60, 61*i*
Antagonist muscles, 33
  contralateral, 34
Anterior chamber, 191. *See also* Anterior segment
Anterior chamber cleavage syndrome. *See* Anterior segment, dysgenesis of
Anterior ciliary arteries, 17–18
  extraocular muscles supplied by, 18–19
Anterior lenticonus, in Alport syndrome, 273, 324
Anterior megalophthalmos, 238
Anterior segment. *See also* Anterior chamber
  development of, 237
  disorders of, 237–248, 413
  dysgenesis of, 239–242
    central developmental abnormalities and, 241–242, 243*i*
    peripheral developmental abnormalities and, 239–242, 240*i*
  examination of
    in cataract, 283, 283*t*
    in glaucoma, 263
  ischemia of, after strabismus surgery, 180–181, 182*i*
Anterior uveitis, 292–297, 292*t*, 303*t*
  differential diagnosis of, 292*t*
  herpetic disease and, 297
  HLA-B27–related diseases and, 296–297
  juvenile rheumatoid arthritis and, 293–295, 293*t*, 294*i*, 296*i*
  laboratory tests for, 303*t*
  sarcoidosis and, 295–296
  sympathetic ophthalmia and, 297
  syphilis and, 297
  trauma causing, 295
Anteriorization (extraocular muscle), and recession, 167*t*
Anticipation (genetic), evaluation of congenital/juvenile ocular anomalies and, 193–194
Anticonvulsant drugs, anomalies associated with maternal use of, 403
Antifibrinolytic agents, for hyphema, 416
Antifibrotic agents, with trabeculectomy, for glaucoma, 267
Antihistamines, for ocular allergy, 222, 223*t*
Apert syndrome, 396–397
  V pattern associated with, 132
Aphakia
  congenital, 271
  contact lenses for correction of, 285
  spectacle lenses for correction of, 285
Aphakic glaucoma, 266, 288
Aphakic spectacles, 285
Apoptosis, 196
Applanation tonometer/tonometry, in glaucoma, 263
Apraclonidine, for glaucoma, 268
Apraxia, ocular motor, congenital, 148
Arachnoid cysts, nystagmus caused by, 152*t*
Arachnoidal gliomatosis, 380
ARC. *See* Anomalous retinal correspondence
Arc of contact, 30

Arterial system, of extraocular muscles, 17–18
    surgery and, 25–27
Arthritis, juvenile rheumatoid. *See* Juvenile rheumatoid
        arthritis
Association (genetic), 195
Asthenopia, strabismus surgery and, 165–166
Astigmatism
    in glaucoma, 269
    with-the-rule, after strabismus surgery, 176
Astrocytoma (astrocytic hamartoma)
    nystagmus caused by, 152*t*
    retinoblastoma differentiated from, 368–372
    in tuberous sclerosis, 384–385
AT. *See* Ataxia-telangiectasia
AT gene, 391
Ataxia-telangiectasia (Louis-Bar syndrome), 376*t*,
        390–391, 391*i*
Atopic keratoconjunctivitis, 222
Atovaquone, for toxoplasmosis, 205
ATP binding cassette (ABC) transporters, in Stargardt
        disease, 321
Atrophy, optic. *See* Optic atrophy
Atropine
    for amblyopia, 68
    for cycloplegia/cycloplegic refraction, 87, 88, 88*t*
    for refractive accommodative esotropia, 96
Axenfeld anomaly. *See* Axenfeld-Rieger syndrome
Axenfeld-Rieger syndrome, 239–241, 240*i*
    posterior embryotoxon in, 239, 240*i*
Axes
    of Fick, 29, 29*i*
    visual, 39

Bacterial conjunctivitis, 211–212, 212*t*
Baerveldt implant, for glaucoma, 267
Bagolini striated glasses, in suppression/anomalous
        retinal correspondence evaluation, 57, 58*i*
Balloon dacryoplasty (balloon catheter dilation), for
        congenital nasolacrimal duct obstruction, 235
Band keratopathy
    in juvenile rheumatoid arthritis, 293–294, 294*i*
    in uveitis, surgery for, 303–304
Bartonella henselae (*Rochalimea* spp), cat scratch
        disease caused by, 216
Bassen-Kornzweig syndrome, Leber congenital
        amaurosis and, 317
Bear tracks (grouped pigmentation of retina), 368
Behr optic atrophy, 344
Bergmeister's papillae, 341
Bernheimer-Seitelberger disease (GM$_2$ gangliosidosis
        type III), 333, 407*t*
Best vitelliform dystrophy, 321–322, 322*i*
    bestrophin defect causing, 321
    electro-oculogram in, 321
Bestrophin, mutations in, 321
Beta (β)-hemolytic group A streptococci (*Streptococcus
        pyogenes*), orbital cellulitis caused by, 218
Betaxolol, for glaucoma, 268
Betoptic. *See* Betaxolol
Bielschowsky head-tilt test, 86*i*, 87
    in superior oblique muscle palsy, 120
Bifixation, in monofixation syndrome, 53
Bifocal lenses
    for nonrefractive accommodative esotropia, 96–98

    for refractive accommodative esotropia, 96
Binocular eye movements, 33–35, 35*i*, 36*i*. *See also
        specific type*
    conjugate (versions), 33–35, 35*i*, 36*i*
    disjugate (vergences), 34–35
Binocular fixation pattern, for amblyopia detection, 66
Binocular vision
    abnormalities of, 49–50. *See also specific type*
    assessment of, 83–89
    physiology of, 39–42
    single
        Panum's area of, 40, 41*i*
        testing field of, 84, 85*i*
Binocular Visual Acuity Test (BVAT), 84
Biomicroscopy, slit-lamp
    in cataract, 283, 283*t*
    in glaucoma, 263
Birth trauma, nystagmus caused by, 152
Birth weight, retinopathy and, 307–308. *See also*
        Retinopathy, of prematurity
Blepharophimosis syndrome, with epicanthus inversus/
        telecanthus/ptosis (Kohn-Ramono syndrome), 201,
        201*i*
Blepharoptosis. *See* Ptosis
Blepharospasm
    botulinum toxin for, 187
    in glaucoma, 260
Blindness. *See also* Low vision; Visual loss
    cerebral/cortical, 424
    glaucoma causing, 264, 269
    night. *See* Night blindness
    retinopathy of prematurity causing, 314
Blinking (blink reflex), in newborn, 419
Bloch-Sulzberger syndrome (incontinentia pigmenti),
        376*t*, 391–393, 392*i*
Blowout fractures of orbital floor, 127–129, 128*i*
    vertical deviations and, 127–129, 128*i*
Blue-cone monochromatism, 318
Blunt trauma, 414–417, 415*i*, 416*i*
    child abuse and, 410
Bone, brown tumor of, orbital involvement and, 358
Bone cyst, aneurysmal, orbital involvement and, 358
Bone marrow transplantation, for
        mucopolysaccharidoses, 408
Bony tumors, of orbit, 358
Botox. *See* Botulinum toxin
Botryoid rhabdomyosarcoma, 352
Botulinum toxin
    for blepharospasm, 187–188
    for classic congenital (essential infantile) esotropia,
        94
    complications of use of, 188
    for esotropia in sixth nerve palsy, 102
    pharmacology and mechanism of action of, 187
    for strabismus, 187–188
    for undercorrection of intermittent exotropia,
        110–111
Bourneville disease/syndrome (tuberous sclerosis),
        376*t*, 383–385, 384*i*, 385*i*
Bowman probe, 232, 232*i*
Brachycephaly, 396
Brachytherapy, for retinoblastoma, 373
Brain lesions
    nystagmus caused by, 152

in tuberous sclerosis, 383, 384*i*
Brimonidine, for glaucoma, 268
Brinzolamide, for glaucoma, 268
Brodmann's area 17 (striate cortex), 42, 45*i*
  development of, 44–46, 46*i*
Brodmann's areas 18 and 19, 42
Brown albinism, 328*t*
Brown (superior oblique tendon sheath) syndrome, 123–125, 123*i*, 125*t*
Brown tumor of bone, orbital involvement and, 350
Brückner test
  for cataract, 283
  for strabismus and amblyopia, 77
Brushfield spots, 254
Bulbar conjunctiva, in vernal keratoconjunctivitis, 221–222
Buphthalmos (megaloglobus)
  in glaucoma, 264–265
  in neurofibromatosis, 381–382
Burkitt lymphoma, of orbit, 354
Burns
  chemical, 413
  of cornea, accidental cigarette burns, 415
Busacca nodules, in sarcoidosis, 258
BVAT (Binocular Visual Acuity Test), 84

Café-au-lait spots, in neurofibromatosis, 377
Canaliculi, lacrimal, 227
  common, 227
Cancer chemotherapy, for retinoblastoma, 373–374
Capillary hemangiomas, of orbit, 355–356, 355*i*
Capsulectomy, for cataract, 284, 286*i*
Capsulorrhexis, 286
Capsulotomy, 286, 287*i*
  Nd:YAG laser, 286
Carbonic anhydrase inhibitors, for glaucoma, 268
Cardinal positions of gaze, 30, 80
  yoke muscles and, 33–34, 34*i*, 80
Cat-scratch disease, Parinaud oculoglandular syndrome and, 216, 216*i*
Cataract, 271–290, 272*i*, 421
  age at onset and, 278
  amblyopia caused by, 67
  congenital and infantile, 277–278, 278*i*, 280*i*, 282–283
  corticosteroid use and, 301, 303
  diabetic, 324–325
  etiology of, 271, 273*t*, 278*t*
  evaluation of, 192–193, 282–283, 283*t*, 284*i*, 285*t*
  hereditary factors in, 277–278, 278*t*
  intraocular lens implantation and, 286–288, 287*i*
  in juvenile rheumatoid arthritis, 293, 294, 294*i*
  lamellar, 280, 281*i*
  location of, 278
  in Lowe syndrome, 330
  morgagnian, 205
  morphologic types of, 279–282
  in neurofibromatosis type 2, 375, 377
  nuclear, 281, 281*i*
  in persistent hyperplastic primary vitreous, 282, 282*i*, 306
  polar, 279, 281*i*
  posterior lenticonus/lentiglobus and, 272–273, 281–282, 282*i*

rubella, 205–206
surgery for, 278–282, 282*i*. See also Cataract surgery
  traumatic, 277
Cataract surgery, 278–282, 283*t*
  for amblyopia, 67
  complications of, 288
  glaucoma after, 266, 288
  intraocular lens implantation and, 286–288, 287*i*
  juvenile rheumatoid arthritis–associated iridocyclitis/uveitis and, 293
  outcome of, 288–289, 289*i*
  in persistent hyperplastic primary vitreous, 306
  postoperative care and, 285
  uveitis and, 301
Cavernous sinus thrombosis, 218–219
Ceftriaxone, for gonococcal conjunctivitis, 210
Cell death, programmed (PCD/apoptosis), 196
Cellulitis
  orbital, 218–220, 218*i*
    fungal (mucormycosis), 220, 220*i*
    after strabismus surgery, 178, 178*i*
  preseptal, 217
    after strabismus surgery, 178
Center of rotation, 29, 29*i*
Central (pupillary) cysts, 253
Central fusional disruption (horror fusionis), 50, 112
Central posterior keratoconus (posterior corneal depression), 241–242
Central suppression, 50
Central vision loss, in leukemia, 326
Cerebral/cortical blindness, 424
Ceroid lipofuscinosis, 407*t*
Chalazion, 365
CHARGE association, 251, 340
CHED. *See* Congenital hereditary endothelial dystrophy
Chédiak-Higashi syndrome, 329*t*
Chelation therapy, for band keratopathy, in juvenile rheumatoid arthritis, 294
Chemical conjunctivitis, in neonates, 211
Chemical injury (burns), 413
Chemodenervation. *See also* Botulinum toxin
  for strabismus and blepharospasm, 187–188
Chemoreduction, for retinoblastoma, 373–374
Chemotherapy, cancer, for retinoblastoma, 373
Cherry-red spot, 331
  in gangliosidoses, 332
Cherry-red spot myoclonus syndrome, 406*t*
Chiasm (optic), glioma of, in neurofibromatosis, 380–381, 380*i*
Chickenpox. *See* Varicella
Children
  abuse of
    cataract and, 277
    gonococcal conjunctivitis and, 211
    ocular trauma and, 409–418, 412*i*
  decreased/low vision in, 419–428
  examination of, 3–5, 192–194
    preparation for, 3
    rapport and, 3–5
  eye development in, 191–192, 192*i*, 193*i*
Chlamydia trachomatis, conjunctivitis caused by, 210
Chloroma (granulocytic sarcoma), 354
Cholinesterase inhibitors, for nonrefractive accommodative esotropia, 97

Chondrosarcoma, of orbit, 352
Chorioretinitis, in syphilis, 208
Choristomas
　dermoid, 359–360, 359i, 363–364
　of orbit, 358, 360. *See also specific type*
Choroid
　hemangiomas of, 368
　in leukemia, 325
　in neurofibromatosis, 367, 378
　osteoma of, 368
　in Sturge-Weber syndrome, 389, 389i
　tumors of, 367–368
Choroidal nevi, 367
Choroiditis, in ocular histoplasmosis, 300
Chromosome abnormalities
　cataract associated with, 277, 278t
　iris coloboma associated with, 250–251
Chronic cyclitis. *See* Intermediate uveitis
Chronic progressive external ophthalmoplegia, 143, 145t
CHRPE. *See* Congenital hypertrophy of retinal pigment epithelium
CHSD. *See* Congenital hereditary stromal dystrophy
Ciancia syndrome, 92t, 94
CID. *See* Cytomegalic inclusion disease
Cigarette burns of cornea, 413
Ciliary arteries, anterior, 17–18
　extraocular muscles supplied by, 17–18
Ciliary body, neoplastic disorders of, 367
Classic congenital esotropia, 91–95, 92t, 93i
Clindamycin, for toxoplasmosis, 204
Clostridium botulinum, toxin derived from, 187. *See also* Botulinum toxin
CMV. *See* Cytomegalovirus
CN. *See* Congenital nystagmus
CNBG3 gene, in achromatopsia, 318
CNGA3 gene, in achromatopsia, 318
Coats disease, 314–315, 315i
　retinoblastoma differentiated from, 370
Cogan's lid twitch, 144
Collagenoma, in tuberous sclerosis, 384
Colobomas
　eyelid, 197, 198i
　　in mandibulofacial dysostosis (Treacher Collins–Francheschetti syndrome), 401
　Fuchs (tilted disc syndrome), 340–341, 340i
　in Goldenhar syndrome, 197, 400–401
　iris, 250–251, 250i
　lens, 272, 272i
　optic nerve/optic disc, 339, 339i
Colobomatous cyst (microphthalmos with cyst), 360–361, 361i
Color blindness
　achromatopsia (rod monochromatism), 318, 423
　blue-cone monochromatism, 318
Combined deviations, 11
Comitant (concomitant) deviation, 10
Common canaliculus, 227
Compliance with therapy, for amblyopia, 68, 69–70
Compromised host, ocular infection in, cytomegalovirus retinitis, 207
Computed tomography (CT scan)
　in orbital evaluation, 349–352
　in retinoblastoma, 369, 370i

Concomitant (comitant) deviation, 10
Confusion, visual, 49, 49i
Congenital anomalies, 195–196, 426t. *See also specific type*
　of cornea, 238–242
　craniofacial malformations, 395–403
　definition of, 196
　evaluation of child with, 192–194
　of eyelid, 197–202
Congenital aphakia, 265
Congenital (infantile) esotropia, 91–95, 92t
　classic (essential), 91–94, 92t, 93i
Congenital exotropia, 111–112, 111i
Congenital fibrosis syndrome, 145–146, 146i
Congenital glaucoma, 245, 259–265, 261i, 262i, 262t. *See also* Glaucoma
Congenital hereditary endothelial dystrophy, 245
Congenital hereditary stromal dystrophy, 245
Congenital hypertrophy of retinal pigment epithelium (CHRPE), 368
Congenital infection syndrome, reduced vision and, 424
Congenital iris ectropion syndrome, 257–258, 257i
　glaucoma and, 381–382
Congenital lacrimal fistula, 228
Congenital miosis (microcoria), 255–256
Congenital mydriasis, 256
Congenital nevocellular nevi of skin (giant hairy nevus), 365, 366i
Congenital nystagmus, 155–160
　motor, 155–156, 156t, 156i
Congenital ocular motor apraxia, 148
Congenital ptosis, 201–202, 201i
Congenital rubella syndrome, 205, 206i
Congenital stationary night blindness, 318–319
Congenital strabismus, 10
Congenital syphilis, 208–209, 247, 247i
　corneal manifestations of, 246, 246i
　uveitis and, 297
Congenital tarsal kink, 198–199, 199i
Conjugate eye movements (versions), 33–34, 35i, 36i. *See also specific type*
Conjunctiva
　cysts of, 363
　　after strabismus surgery, 179, 179i
　incisions in, for extraocular muscle surgery, 175–176
　nevus of, 364–365, 366i
　scarring of after strabismus surgery, 179–180, 179i
　telangiectasia of, in ataxia-telangiectasia, 390–391, 391i
Conjunctival inclusion cysts, 363
　after strabismus surgery, 178, 178i
Conjunctivitis, 211–217, 212t. *See also* Keratoconjunctivitis
　adenoviruses causing, 212
　allergic, seasonal, 220–221
　bacterial
　　in children, 211–212
　　in neonates, 209–211, 209i
　chemical, 211
　chlamydial, 210
　gonococcal
　　in children, 212
　　in neonates, 209, 209i

Haemophilus causing, 211
herpes simplex virus causing
  in children, 207–208, 211, 214*i*
  in neonates, 211
herpes zoster causing, 214–215, 215*i*
in infectious mononucleosis, 215
influenza virus causing, 215
ligneous, 366
mumps causing, 215
neonatal (ophthalmia neonatorum), 209*i*, 211
in Parinaud oculoglandular syndrome, 216, 216*i*
in pharyngoconjunctival fever, 213
in rubeola, 215
after strabismus surgery, 178
streptococcal, 211–212
in trachoma, 217
trachoma-inclusion (TRIC), 210
varicella-zoster virus causing, 215, 216*i*
vernal, 221–222, 221*i*
viral, 212–216
Connective tissue tumors, of orbit, 358
Consecutive esodeviation, 92*t*, 101
Consecutive exotropia, 112
Constant exotropia, 111–113
Contact, arc of, 30
Contact lenses, for aphakia, 285
Contour interaction (crowding phenomenon), 64
Contour interaction (crowding) bars, for amblyopia evaluation, 66, 67*i*, 73
Contour stereopsis tests, 83–84
Contralateral antagonist, 34
Convergence, 34
  assessment of, 80–82
  fusional, 35, 41, 41*t*
  near point of, 81
Convergence insufficiency, exotropia and, 108, 113
Convergence paralysis, exotropia and, 114
Convergence-retraction nystagmus, 159
Convergent strabismus, 9
Copper, deposition of in Wilson disease, 247
Corectopia, 256
  ectopia lentis and, 256, 273–274, 274*i*
Cornea
  abrasions of, 413
  congenital/developmental anomalies of, 238–241
    of size and shape, 238
  curvature of, 191, 192*i*
  development of, 237
  diameter of, 191, 192*i*, 237, 260–261
    abnormalities of, 238–241, 260–261
  disorders of, 237–247
  edema of, in glaucoma, 260, 262*t*
  enlargement of, in glaucoma, 260, 261*i*, 262*t*
  examination of, in glaucoma, 261, 262*t*
  exposure of, in craniosynostosis-induced proptosis, 397
  foreign body in, 414
  in glaucoma, 260, 261*i*, 262*t*
  opacification of, 242–245, 243*t*
  perforating injury of, 414
    management of, 414
  posterior depression of (central posterior keratoconus), 241–242
  systemic diseases affecting, 246–247

Corneal dystrophies, congenital hereditary
  endothelial, 244
  stromal, 245
Corneal light reflex tests, 77
Corneal ulcers, in vernal keratoconjunctivitis, 222
Corneoscleral laceration, repair of, 414
Correspondence, 39–41, 41*i*
Cortical evoked potentials, visual, in infants, 191, 419
Cortical visual impairment (cortical blindness), 424
Corticosteroids (steroids)
  adverse effects of, 301, 303
  for capillary hemangiomas, 356
  after cataract surgery, 288
  for hyphema, 416
  for ocular allergy, 222–223
  for toxocariasis, 300
  for toxoplasmosis, 204–205, 299
  for uveitis, 301, 303
    intermediate, 298
    juvenile rheumatoid arthritis–associated, 294
Cottage cheese pattern, in treated retinoblastoma, 373
Cover tests, 74–77, 75*i*, 76*i*
  for intermittent exotropia evaluation, 107
Cover-uncover test, 74, 75*i*
CPEO. *See* Chronic progressive external ophthalmoplegia
Cranial nerve III, palsy of. *See* Third nerve (oculomotor) palsy
Cranial nerve IV, palsy of. *See* Fourth nerve (trochlear) palsy
Cranial nerve VI, palsy of. *See* Sixth nerve (abducens) palsy
Craniofacial dysostosis (Crouzon syndrome), 397*i*, 399
  V pattern associated with, 132–135
Craniofacial malformations, 395–403. *See also specific type*
  Apert syndrome, 399
  approach to child with, 395–396
  craniosynostosis, 395, 396–399, 397*i*
  Crouzon syndrome, 397*i*, 399
  in fetal alcohol syndrome, 401–403, 402*i*
  in fetal hydantoin syndrome, 403
  Goldenhar syndrome. *See* Goldenhar syndrome
  Hallermann-Streiff syndrome, 401
  hemifacial microsomia, 400, 400*i*
  intrinsic ocular pathology in, 395
  mandibulofacial dysostosis (Treacher Collins–Franceschetti syndrome), 401, 402*i*
  Pfeiffer syndrome, 399
  Pierre Robin sequence (anomaly/deformity), 401
    Stickler syndrome and, 323, 401
  secondary ocular complications in, 395–396
  Waardenburg syndrome, 399
Craniopharyngiomas, nystagmus caused by, 152*t*
Craniosynostosis, 395, 396–399, 397*i*
  syndromes associated with, 396–397, 397*i*, 399
Crede (silver nitrate) prophylaxis, 211
Crolom. *See* Cromolyn
Cromolyn, for ocular allergy, 222, 223*t*
Cross syndrome (oculocerebral hypopigmentation), 328*t*
Crossed diplopia, 54, 55*i*
Crouzon syndrome (craniofacial dysostosis), 397*i*, 399
  V pattern associated with, 132–135

Crowding (contour interaction) bars, for amblyopia evaluation, 66, 67*i*, 73
Crowding phenomenon (contour interaction), 64
CRX gene, in Leber congenital amaurosis, 317
CRYO-ROP study, 307–308
Cryotherapy
 for glaucoma, 267
 for retinoblastoma, 373
 for retinopathy of prematurity, 311*t*, 313–314, 313*t*
Cryptophthalmos, 197, 197*i*
CSM method, for visual acuity assessment, 72
CSNB. *See* Congenital stationary night blindness
Cupping of optic disc
 cup/disc ratio and, 191
  in glaucoma, 262*t*, 263–264, 265*i*
  in megalopapilla, 341
 physiologic, 192
Curvature (corneal), 191, 193*t*
Cyclitis, chronic. *See* Intermediate uveitis
Cycloablation, for glaucoma, 267
Cyclocryotherapy, for glaucoma, 267
Cyclomydril. *See* Cyclopentolate
Cyclopentolate, for cycloplegia/cycloplegic refraction, 87, 87*t*
Cycloplegia/cycloplegics
 for hyphema, 416
 side effects of, 88
Cycloplegic refraction, 87, 88*t*
 in classic congenital (essential infantile) esotropia, 93
Cyclovertical muscle palsies, three-step test in, 85, 86*i*, 87
Cyclovertical strabismus, surgery planning and, 170
Cystathionine β-synthase, abnormality of in homocystinuria, 274
Cysteamine, for cystinosis, 246
Cystinosis, 407*t*
 corneal disorders in, 246, 246*i*
 cysteamine for, 246
Cytomegalovirus/cytomegalic inclusion disease, 206, 206*i*

Dacryocele/dacryocystocele, 228, 229*i*
Dacryoplasty, balloon (balloon catheter dilation), for congenital nasolacrimal duct obstruction, 235
Dantrolene, for malignant hyperthermia, 184, 185*t*
Daraprim. *See* Pyrimethamine
de Morsier syndrome (septo-optic dysplasia), 342, 422
Deafness, albinism and, 329*t*
Deformation, definition of, 196
Degradation, optical, for amblyopia, 68
Dellen, after strabismus surgery, 180, 180*i*
Denervation and extirpation, 167*t*
Deorsumduction/deorsumversion. *See* Depression of eye
Depression of eye (downgaze), 33
 extraocular muscles controlling
  inferior rectus, 14, 16*i*, 20*t*
  superior oblique, 14, 18*i*, 20*t*
Deprivation amblyopia, 65–66
 in eye trauma, 409
 visual development affected by, 47
Depth perception
 stereo acuity testing of, 83–84
 stereopsis differentiated from, 42

Dermoids (dermoid cysts/tumors), 245, 359–360, 359*i*, 363–364
 corneal, 245
  infantile opacities and, 245
 epibulbar, 363–364
 Goldenhar syndrome and, 245, 364, 364*i*
 limbal, 245, 355–356
  Goldenhar syndrome and, 245, 364, 364*i*, 400–401
 of orbit, 359–360, 359*i*
Dermolipomas (lipodermoids), 364, 364*i*
 Goldenhar syndrome and, 245, 364, 364*i*, 400–401
Derry disease (GM$_1$ gangliosidosis type II), 332, 407*t*
Descemet's membrane/layer, injuries to, infantile corneal opacities and, 242–244, 243*t*
Desmoid tumors (myofibromas), of orbit, 358
Developmental field, definition of, 196
Developmental glaucoma, 265–266. *See also* Glaucoma
Deviations. *See also specific type and* Esodeviations; Exodeviations
 combined, 11
 comitant (concomitant), 10
 horizontal, 11
  dissociated, 112–113, 113*i*
 incomitant (noncomitant), 10
  esodeviations, 92*t*, 101–102
  surgery planning and, 170–175
 primary, 34
 secondary, 34
 skew, in infants, 419
 terminology in description of, 9–11
 torsional, 11
 vertical, 11. *See also* Vertical deviations
  dissociated, 113, 113*i*
Dextrocycloversion, 33
Dextroversion (right gaze), 33
DHD. *See* Dissociated horizontal deviation
Diabetes mellitus, 324–325
 cataracts associated with, 325
Diabetic retinopathy, 324–325
Diagnostic positions of gaze, 80–81, 81*i*
Diamox. *See* Acetazolamide
Diktyoma (medulloepithelioma), 367
Diode laser
 cycloablation with, for glaucoma, 267
 hyperthermia with, for retinoblastoma, 373
Dipivefrin (dipivalyl epinephrine), for glaucoma, 268
Diplopia, 40, 41*i*, 49–50
 crossed, 54, 55*i*
 heteronymous, 54, 55*i*
 homonymous, 54, 55*i*
 Panum's area and, 41*i*
 paradoxical, 52, 52*i*
 after strabismus surgery, 52, 176–177
 strabismus surgery for elimination of, 166
 testing for, 54–56, 55*i*. *See also* Red filter (glass/lens) test
 after third nerve (oculomotor) palsy surgery, 140–141
 uncrossed, 54, 55*i*
Disconjugate eye movements (vergences), 34. *See also specific type*
 in infants, 419
Dislocated lens, 273–277, 273*t*. *See also* Ectopia lentis
Disruption, definition of, 196

Dissimilar image tests, 77–78
Dissimilar target tests, 79–80
Dissociated horizontal deviation, 112, 113*i*, 118
Dissociated nystagmus, 160
Dissociated vertical deviation, 113, 113*i*, 118–119, 118*i*
  surgery for, 173–174
Distance visual acuity, testing, 72–74, 72*t*
  nystagmus and, 154
Distichiasis, 199, 200*i*
Disuse anopsia. *See* Deprivation amblyopia
Divergence, 35
  fusional, 35, 41*t*
Divergence excess exotropia, 107
Divergence insufficiency/paralysis, esodeviation and, 92*t*, 100
Divergent strabismus, 9
Dorsal midbrain (Parinaud) syndrome, nystagmus in, 159
Dorzolamide, for glaucoma, 268
Double elevator palsy/paresis (monocular elevation deficiency), 125–127, 127*i*
Double Maddox rod testing, 79
  in superior oblique muscle palsy, 120
Double ring sign, in optic nerve hypoplasia, 341, 342*i*, 422
Double vision. *See* Diplopia
Down syndrome (trisomy 21/trisomy G syndrome), Brushfield spots in, 254
Downbeat nystagmus, 159
Downgaze. *See* Depression of eye
Doxycycline, for chalazia, 365–366
Drusen, 347, 348*i*
  dominant (familial), 322, 339
  giant, in tuberous sclerosis, 385
  pseudopapilledema and, 347, 348*i*
Duane syndrome, 137–140, 138*i*, 139*i*
  esotropic, 92*t*, 138, 138*i*, 139
  exotropic (retraction), 112, 138, 138*i*
  Goldenhar syndrome and, 137, 401
Ductions, 33. *See also specific type*
  forced. *See* Forced ductions
DVD. *See* Dissociated vertical deviation
Dysautonomia, familial (Riley-Day syndrome), 247
Dyscoria, 256
Dysfunctional over- or underaction, vertical deviations caused by, 115
Dysplasia, definition of, 196
Dysraphia, definition of, 195
Dystrophies
  Best vitelliform, 321, 322*i*
    bestrophin defect causing, 321
    electro-oculogram in, 321
  corneal. *See* Corneal dystrophies
  familial renal-retinal, 331
  macular. *See* Macular dystrophy
  stromal, congenital hereditary, 245
  vitreoretinal, Goldmann-Favré, 324

"E game," for visual acuity testing, 72*t*, 73
Eccentric fixation, in strabismic amblyopia, 65
Ecchymoses, periorbital, in neuroblastoma, 353, 353*i*
Echothiophate
  for glaucoma, 268
  for nonrefractive accommodative esotropia, 97
  for refractive accommodative esotropia, 96
Ectopia lentis, 273–274, 274*i*
  et pupillae, 256, 273–274, 274*i*
  in homocystinuria, 274–276, 275*i*
  in hyperlysinemia, 276
  in Marfan syndrome, 274, 275*i*
  simple, 273
  in sulfite oxidase deficiency, 276
  treatment of, 276–277
  in Weill-Marchesani syndrome, 276
Ectopic lacrimal gland, 360
Ectopic tissue masses, orbital, 358–363
Ectropion, congenital, 197
  iris (ectropion uveae), 257, 257*i*
    glaucoma and, 381–382
Edrophonium, in myasthenia gravis diagnosis, 144, 144*i*
Ehlers-Danlos syndrome, keratoglobus in, 238
Electro-oculogram, in Best vitelliform dystrophy, 321–322
Electromyography, 32
  in myasthenia gravis, 143–145
Electroretinogram
  in infant with decreased vision, 420
  in Leber congenital amaurosis, 317, 423
Elevated intraocular pressure, in glaucoma, 263, 267
Elevation of eye (upgaze), 33, 33–34
  extraocular muscles controlling
    inferior oblique, 15–16, 18*i*, 20*t*
    superior rectus, 14, 15*i*, 20*t*
  monocular deficiency of (double elevator palsy), 125–127, 127*i*
Embryonal rhabdomyosarcoma, 352
Embryotoxon, posterior, 239, 240*i*
  in Axenfeld-Rieger syndrome, 239, 240*i*
Empirical horopter, 40, 41*i*
En grappe nerve endings, 19
En plaque nerve endings, 19
Encephaloceles, of orbit, 362
Encephalofacial angiomatosis (Sturge-Weber syndrome), 376*t*, 387–390, 388*i*
  nevus flammeus in, 365, 387, 388, 388*i*
Endophthalmitis, after strabismus surgery, 177
  scleral perforation and, 177, 177*i*
Endothelial dystrophies, congenital hereditary, 244
Entropion, congenital, 198
Enucleation, for retinoblastoma, 372
Eosinophilic granuloma, of orbit, 354, 354*i*
Ependymoma, nystagmus caused by, 152*t*
Epiblepharon, 198
Epibulbar tumors, 363–366
  dermoids, 363–364
Epicanthus, 199, 200*i*
  inversus, 199
    with blepharophimosis/telecanthus/ptosis (Kohn-Ramono syndrome), 201, 201*i*
  palpebralis, 199, 200*i*
  supraciliaris, 199
  tarsalis, 199, 200*i*
Epidemic keratoconjunctivitis, 212–213
Epidermoid cysts, of orbit, 359
Epinephrine, for glaucoma, 268
Epiphora. *See* Tearing
Episcleritis, nodular, 366

Epithelial inclusion cysts, conjunctival, 363
 after strabismus surgery, 179, 179*i*
ERG. *See* Electroretinogram
Erythema, multiforme major (Stevens-Johnson syndrome), 223–224, 225*i*
Erythromycin, for neonatal conjunctivitis, 211
 prophylaxis and, 211
Eso (prefix), definition of, 9
Esodeviations, 91–103, 92*t. See also specific type and* Esotropia
 divergence insufficiency/paralysis, 92*t*, 100–101
 incomitant, 92*t*, 101–103
 medial rectus muscle restriction causing, 92*t*, 103
 negative angle kappa and, 80, 81*i*
 sensory deprivation, 92*t*, 100
 sixth nerve (abducens) palsy causing, 92*t*, 101–102
 surgery for, 170–171, 171*t*
Esophoria, 89
Esotropia, 89, 92*t. See also* Esodeviations
 A-pattern, 134*i*
  treatment of, 136
 accommodative, 92*t*, 95–99
 acute, 92*t*, 99
 basic (acquired), 92*t*, 99
 cyclic, 92*t*, 100
 divergence insufficiency/paralysis, 92*t*, 100–101
 in Duane syndrome, 92*t*, 138*i*, 138–139
 incomitant, 92*t*, 101–103
 infantile (congenital), 91–95, 92*t*, 420–421
  essential (classic), 91–94, 92*t*, 93*i*
 intermittent, 91
 medial rectus muscle restriction causing, 92*t*, 103
 in Möbius syndrome, 92*t*, 147
 nonaccommodative, 92*t*, 99–101
 with nystagmus, 92*t*, 94–95, 156
 sensory deprivation, 92*t*, 100
 sixth nerve (abducens) palsy causing, 92*t*, 101–102
 spasm of near synkinetic reflex and, 92*t*, 101
 surgical (consecutive), 92*t*
 V-pattern, 133*i*
  treatment of, 135–136
Essential infantile esotropia, 91–94, 92*t*, 93*i*
Euryblepharon, 199
Ewing sarcoma, of orbit, 353
Ex anopsia. *See* Deprivation amblyopia
Examination
 under anesthesia
  for eye trauma, 409
  for retinoblastoma, 373
  for Sturge-Weber syndrome, 390
 ophthalmic, 3–5. *See also specific type of test*
  for glaucoma, 261, 263–264, 264*i*
  for nystagmus, 152–155, 153*t*, 154*t*
  for retinoblastoma, 373
Excyclo (prefix), definition of, 10
Excycloduction. *See* Extorsion
Excyclovergence, 34
Exo (prefix), definition of, 9
Exodeviations, 105–114. *See also specific type and* Exotropia
 esodeviation following surgery for (surgical/consecutive esodeviation), 92*t*, 101
 overcorrection in, value of, 110, 172
 positive angle kappa and, 80, 81*i*

sensory deprivation, 92*t*, 100
surgery for, 171–172, 171*t*, 172*t*
in third nerve (oculomotor) palsy, 140
Exophoria, 105
Exorbitism, 351. *See also* Proptosis
Exotropia
 A-pattern, 132*i*, 133*i*
  treatment of, 136
 congenital, 111–112, 111*i*
 consecutive, 112
 constant, 111–113
 convergence insufficiency and, 108, 113
 convergence paralysis and, 114
 in craniosynostosis, 398
 dissociated horizontal deviation and, 112–113, 113*i*
 in Duane syndrome, 112, 138–139, 139*i*
 in infants, 420
 intermittent, 105–111, 106*i*
 neuromuscular abnormalities causing, 112
 sensory, 112
 V-pattern, 133*i*
  treatment of, 136
Exposure keratitis, in craniosynostosis-induced proptosis, 397–398
External beam radiation, for retinoblastoma, 373
Extirpation and denervation, 167*t*
Extorsion (excycloduction), 33
 extraocular muscles in
  inferior oblique, 15, 19*i*, 20*t*
  inferior rectus, 14, 16*i*, 20*t*
Extorsional strabismus, 10
Extraocular muscle surgery, 165–185, 185*t. See also* Strabismus surgery
 for A pattern, 132–135
 adjustable suture techniques for, 167–168
 anatomical implications and, 25–28, 26*i*, 27*i*
 anesthesia for, 175
 for classic congenital (essential infantile) esotropia, 93–94
 conjunctival incisions for, 175–176
 for constant exotropia, 111
 esodeviation after, 92*t*, 101
 for esotropia in sixth nerve palsy, 102
 exotropia after, 112
 in Graves/thyroid ophthalmopathy, 142–143
 indications for, 165–166
 for inferior oblique muscle palsy, 125
 for intermittent exotropia, 109
 for monocular elevation deficiency (double elevator palsy), 126–127
 for nonrefractive accommodative esotropia, 97
 for nystagmus, 162–163, 162*t*
 for partially accommodative esotropia, 98
 prior surgery and, 169–170
 for refractive accommodative esotropia, 96
 strengthening procedures in, 166–167
 for superior oblique muscle palsy, 121–122
 techniques for, 166–168
 for third nerve (oculomotor) palsy, 140–141
 transposition procedures in, 168, 174
 for V pattern, 132–135
 weakening procedures in, 166, 167*t*
Extraocular muscles, 13–28, 21*i. See also specific type and* Eye movements; Ocular motility

actions of, 13–17, 20t
  gaze position and, 31–33, 32i
  primary/secondary/tertiary, 30, 31t
anatomy of, 13–28, 21i
  fine structure, 18–22
arterial system of, 17–18
blood supply of, 17–18
  surgery and, 27
dysfunctional over- or underactions of, vertical deviations caused by, 115
fascial relationships of, 22–25
fiber types in, 19, 22
innervation of, 13–17, 20t
  surgery and, 25, 26i, 27
insertions of, 13–17, 20t
  advancing, as strengthening procedure, 166–167
lost, during surgery, 182
orbital relationships of, 22–25, 22i
origins of, 13–17, 20t
paralysis/paresis of, three-step test in evaluation of, 85, 86i
physiology of, 32–33
slipped, after surgery, 182–183, 183i
surgery of. *See* Extraocular muscle surgery; Strabismus surgery
venous system of, 18
Eye
  axial length of, 191, 192i
  color of, age affecting, 191
  development of, 191–194, 192i, 193i, 193t
  dimensions of, 191, 192i, 193t
  injury to. *See* Trauma
Eye drops, 5
Eye movements, 33–36. *See also specific type and* Ocular motility
  assessment of, 74–89, 419
  binocular, 33–36, 35i, 36i. *See also specific type*
    conjugate (versions), 33–34, 35i, 36i
    disconjugate (vergences), 34–35
  monocular (ductions), 33
  recruitment after, 32
  supranuclear control of, 36–37
Eye muscles. *See* Extraocular muscles
Eye patches. *See* Patching
Eyelashes, accessory. *See* Distichiasis
Eyelids
  coloboma of, 197, 198i
  disorders of, congenital, 197–202
  drooping. *See* Ptosis
  fusion of (ankyloblepharon), 197, 198i
  inflammatory conditions affecting, 365–366
  lacerations of, 414
  lower
    ectropion of, 197
    entropion of, 198
  plexiform neurofibroma involving, 379–380, 379i
  strabismus surgery affecting position of, 181, 182i
  tumors of, 363–366
  upper
    coloboma of, 197, 198i
    entropion of, 198

Fabry disease, 406t
Facial angiofibromas, in tuberous sclerosis, 383, 384i
Facial angioma (port-wine stain), in Sturge-Weber syndrome, 365, 387, 388i, 389
Facial defects. *See* Craniofacial malformations
Facultative suppression, 51
Fadenoperation (posterior fixation suture), 167t
False passage, probing of nasolacrimal duct obstruction and, 234
Familial adenomatous polyposis (Gardner syndrome), retinal manifestations of, 368
Familial (dominant) drusen, 322, 347
Familial dysautonomia (Riley-Day syndrome), 247
Familial exudative vitreoretinopathy, 323–324
Familial iridoplegia, 256
Familial oculorenal syndromes, 330–331
Familial renal–retinal dysplasia/dystrophy, 331
Family history
  in congenital/juvenile ocular anomalies, 192–193
  in nystagmus, 152, 153t
Fanconi syndrome, 246
FAS. *See* Fetal alcohol syndrome
Fascia bulbi. *See* Tenon's capsule
Fat, orbital, 22i, 25
Felderstruktur muscle fibers, 19
Fetal alcohol syndrome, 401–403, 402i
Fetal hydantoin syndrome, 403
Fetal vasculature, persistent (persistent hyperplastic primary vitreous), 282–283, 282i, 306–307, 307i. *See also* Persistent hyaloid artery/system
FEVR. *See* Familial exudative vitreoretinopathy
FGFR 1–3 receptors, mutations in, in craniosynostosis syndromes, 396
FHS. *See* Fetal hydantoin syndrome
Fibrillenstruktur muscle fibers, 19
Fibrin clots, after penetrating trauma, 414
Fibroblast growth factor receptors, mutations in, in craniosynostosis syndromes, 396
Fibroma
  molluscum, 378
  ossifying, of orbit, 358
  in tuberous sclerosis, 383–385
Fibromatosis, juvenile, of orbit, 358
Fibroplasia, retrolental. *See* Retinopathy, of prematurity
Fibrosarcoma, of orbit, 352
Fibrosis, congenital, 145–146, 146i
Fibrous dysplasia, of orbit, 358
Fick, axes of, 29, 29i
Field of action/field of activation, 30–31
First and second arch syndrome (hemifacial microsomia), 400, 400i. *See also* Goldenhar syndrome
Fish flesh pattern, in treated retinoblastoma, 373
Fissures, palpebral, 191
  congenital widening of (euryblepharon), 199
  slanting of, 200–201
  surgery affecting, 27, 27i
Fistulas, lacrimal, congenital, 228
Fixation (visual)
  alternating, 11
  eccentric, 65
  monocular, 11
  recruitment during, 32
FKHL7 gene, in Axenfeld-Rieger syndrome, 241
Flame hemorrhages, in leukemia, 325–326, 326i
Fleurettes, in retinoblastoma, 370

Flexner-Wintersteiner rosettes, in retinoblastoma, 370
Fluorescein, in congenital nasolacrimal duct obstruction evaluation, 229
Foldable intraocular lens, 288
Forced ductions, 84
Foreign body
  anesthesia for removal of, 5
  corneal, 414
  uveitis differentiated from, 303*t*
Foreign body granuloma, after strabismus surgery, 178, 178*i*
Fornix incision, for extraocular muscle surgery, 175–176
Fourth nerve (trochlear) palsy, superior oblique muscle palsy and, 119
Fovea, 191
  hypoplasia of, 319
    in albinism, 327
Foveal retinoschisis, 322
Fractures. *See specific type or structure affected*
Freckle
  iris, 366
  in neurofibromatosis, 377
Fresnel prisms
  for esotropia in sixth nerve palsy, 102
  for nystagmus, 160
  for overcorrection of intermittent exotropia, 110
Fuchs coloboma (tilted disc syndrome), 340–341, 341*i*
Fucosidosis, 406*t*
Fundus
  evaluation of
    in cataract, 284
    in nystagmus, 155, 155*t*
    in premature infants, 308, 310*i*, 311*t*
  flavimaculatus, 320–321, 321*i*
  salt-and-pepper
    in rubella, 205, 206*i*
    in syphilis, 208, 297
Fungi, orbital cellulitis (mucormycosis) caused by, 220, 220*i*
Fusion, 40, 41*t*, 42
  peripheral, in monofixation syndrome, 53–54
  tenacious proximal, in intermittent exotropia, 107
Fusional amplitudes, 41, 41*t*
Fusional convergence, 35, 41, 41*t*
Fusional convergence training, for intermittent exotropia, 109
Fusional divergence, 35, 41*t*, 82
Fusional vergence, 41, 41*t*, 82

Galactosemia, 407*t*
  cataracts in, 284, 284*i*
Galactosialidoses, 407*t*
β-Galactosidase enzymes, deficiency of, in gangliosidoses, 332
Ganciclovir, for cytomegalovirus retinitis, 207
Gangliosidoses, 332, 407*t*
Gardner syndrome (familial adenomatous polyposis), retinal manifestations of, 368
Gaucher disease, 406*t*
Gaze, positions of, 30
  assessment of, 80, 81*i*
  cardinal, 30, 80
    yoke muscles and, 34, 35*i*, 80
  diagnostic, 80, 82*i*
  extraocular muscle action affected by, 31, 32*i*
  midline, 80
  primary, 13, 30, 80, 82*i*
  secondary, 30
  tertiary, 30
  variation of deviation with, 10
General anesthesia, for extraocular muscle surgery, 175. *See also* Anesthesia
Generalized gangliosidosis (GM$_1$ gangliosidosis type I), 332, 407*t*
Genetic counseling
  in albinism, 327
  in retinoblastoma, 370, 371*t*
Genetics, clinical
  cataract and, 277–284, 277*i*
  evaluation of congenital/juvenile ocular anomalies and, 192–194
  primary congenital glaucoma and, 259–265
Geniculate body/nucleus/ganglion, lateral, 42–44, 43*i*, 45*i*
  development of, 44, 46*i*
German measles. *See* Rubella
Germinomas, nystagmus caused by, 152*t*
Gestational age, retinopathy and, 307–308. *See also* Retinopathy, of prematurity
Giant cells, Touton, in juvenile xanthogranuloma, 367
Giant drusen, in tuberous sclerosis, 385
Giant hairy nevus (congenital nevocellular nevi of skin), 365, 366*i*
Gigantism, regional, 379
Glasses. *See* Spectacle lenses (spectacles)
Glaucoma, 259–269, 413
  aphakic, 266, 288
  clinical features of, 260–264, 261*i*, 262*i*, 262*t*, 264*i*, 265*i*
  congenital, 245, 259–265, 261*i*, 262*i*, 262*t*
  developmental, 265–266
  corticosteroid use and, 301–302
  diagnosis of, 260–264, 261*i*, 262*i*, 262*t*, 264*i*, 265*i*
  evaluation of, 192–193
  genetic basis of, 259–260
  infantile, 245
  in leukemia, 326
  in Lowe syndrome, 330
  medical therapy of, 267–268
  natural history of, 264–265
  in neurofibromatosis, 381–382
  pathophysiology of, 260
  primary, 259–265, 261*i*, 262*i*, 262*t*
    developmental, 265–266
  prognosis and follow-up for, 269
  retinopathy of prematurity and, 314
  secondary, 259, 266
  in Sturge-Weber syndrome, 389–390
  surgery for, 267
    uveitis and, 304
  treatment of, 266–268
GLC3 gene, primary congenital glaucoma and, 259
Glial cells, retinal, lesions of in neurofibromatosis, 378–383, 380*i*
Gliomas
  chiasmal, in neurofibromatosis, 380–381, 380*i*
  nystagmus caused by, 152*t*

optic nerve, 358, 380–381, 380*i*
  in neurofibromatosis, 358, 380–381
  orbital involvement in, 358, 380
Gliomatosis, arachnoidal, 380
GM$_1$ gangliosidosis type I (generalized), 332, 407*t*
GM$_1$ gangliosidosis type II (Derry disease), 332, 407*t*
GM$_2$ gangliosidosis type I (Tay-Sachs disease), 332, 407*t*
GM$_2$ gangliosidosis type II (Sandhoff disease), 332, 407*t*
GM$_2$ gangliosidosis type III (Bernheimer-Seitelberger disease), 332, 407*t*
Goldenhar syndrome (oculoauricular/oculoauriculovertebral dysplasia), 400–401. *See also* Hemifacial microsomia
  colobomas and, 197, 392
  dermoids/dermolipomas in, 245, 364, 364*i*, 400–401
  Duane syndrome and, 137
Goldmann applanation tonometry, 263
Goldmann-Favré disease/syndrome (vitreoretinal dystrophy), 324
Gonioscopy, in glaucoma, 263, 264*i*
Goniotomy, for glaucoma, 267
Gonococcal conjunctivitis
  in children, 212
  in neonates, 209, 209*i*
Gradient method, for accommodative convergence/accommodation ratio measurement, 81
Granulocytic sarcoma (chloroma), 354
Granulomas
  eosinophilic, of orbit, 354, 354*i*
  foreign body, after strabismus surgery, 178–179, 178*i*
  pyogenic, 366
  in toxocariasis, 300, 302*i*
Grating acuity, in strabismic amblyopia, 64
Graves disease, 141–143, 142*i*, 145*t*, 362, 362*i*
  proptosis and, 142, 362–363, 362*i*
  after muscle recessions, 143
  strabismus and, 141–143, 142*i*, 145*t*
Group A beta-hemolytic streptococci (*Streptococcus pyogenes*), orbital cellulitis caused by, 217
Grouped pigmentation of retina (bear tracks), 368
Guanylate cyclase gene, photoreceptor-specific (*RETGC1* gene) in Leber congenital amaurosis, 317

H$_1$-receptor blockers, for ocular allergy, 222, 223*t*
Haab striae, 260–261, 261*i*
Haemophilus influenzae, 217
  conjunctivitis caused by, 211
  orbital cellulitis caused by, 218
  preseptal cellulitis caused by, 217
Hagberg-Santavouri disease, 407*t*
Hallermann-Streiff syndrome (oculomandibulofacial dyscephaly), 401
Hamartomas
  astrocytic (astrocytomas)
    nystagmus caused by, 152*t*
    retinoblastoma differentiated from, 370
    in tuberous sclerosis, 385
  combined, of retina and retinal pigment epithelium, 368
Hand-Schüller-Christian disease, orbital involvement in, 354
Harada-Ito procedure, 167

Harmonious anomalous retinal correspondence, 55, 55*i*, 60
Hasner, valve of, 227
Head-tilt test, Bielschowsky, 86*i*, 87
  in superior oblique muscle palsy, 120
Hearing loss, albinism and, 329*t*
Hemangioblastomas, with retinal angiomatosis (von Hippel–Lindau disease), 376*t*, 386–387, 387*i*
  retinoblastoma differentiated from, 370
Hemangiomas (hemangiomatosis)
  of choroid, 368
  of orbit, capillary, 355–356, 355*i*
Hemangiopericytoma, of orbit, 357
Hemifacial microsomia/hypoplasia, 400, 400*i*. *See also* Goldenhar syndrome
Hemorrhages
  intracranial, in shaking injury, 411
  retinal
    in leukemia, 325–327, 326*i*
    in shaking injury, 411–412, 411*i*
    salmon patch, syphilitic keratitis and, 247
  vitreous, in shaking injury, 411–412
Hepatolenticular degeneration (Wilson disease), 247
Hereditary cataract, 277, 277*i*
Hereditary dystrophies
  endothelial, 244
  stromal, 245
Hereditary optic atrophy, 344–345
Hereditary progressive arthro-ophthalmopathy (Stickler syndrome), 317–318
  Pierre Robin sequence (anomaly/deformity) and, 318, 401
Hering's law of motor correspondence, 34, 36*i*
Hermansky-Pudlak syndrome, 328*t*
Herpes simplex virus, 207–208
  conjunctivitis caused by
    in children, 207, 213–214, 214*i*
    in neonates, 213–214, 214*i*
  iridocyclitis caused by, 297
  perinatal infection caused by, 207
  type 1, 207
  type 2, 207
  uveitis caused by, 297
Herpes zoster. *See also* Varicella-zoster virus
  conjunctivitis and, 214–215, 215*i*
  uveitis and, 297
Hess screen test, 79
  in superior oblique muscle palsy, 120
Heterochromia iridis, 254–255, 254*i*, 254*t*
  in leukemia, 326
Heteronymous diplopia, 54, 55*i*
Heterophoria method, for accommodative convergence/accommodation ratio measurement, 81–82
Heterophorias/phorias, 9
  cover-uncover test in assessment of, 74, 75*i*
  definition of, 9
Heterotropia, 9
  alternating, 75
  simultaneous prism-cover test in assessment of, 76
Hexosaminidase, deficiency of, in gangliosidoses, 332
Hirschberg test, 77, 77*i*
Histiocytosis, Langerhans cell (histiocytosis X/diffuse soft tissue histiocytosis), orbital involvement in, 354–355, 355*i*

Histo spots, 300
Histocompatibility antigens (HLA antigens)
  in anterior uveitis, 296
  in juvenile rheumatoid arthritis, 293–294
Histoplasma capsulatum (histoplasmosis), ocular, 300
  histo spots in, 300
  uveitis and, 300
History
  in amblyopia, 71–72
  in cataract, 283
  in child abuse, 410
  in congenital/juvenile ocular anomalies, 192–194
  in nystagmus, 152, 153*t*
  in strabismus, 71–72
HIV infection/AIDS, cytomegalovirus retinitis in, 207
HLA antigens. *See* Human leukocyte (HLA) antigens
Holes, optic (optic pits), 343, 343*i*
Homatropine, for cycloplegia/cycloplegic refraction, 87, 88*t*
Homer-Wright rosettes, in retinoblastoma, 370–371
Homocystinuria, 274–276, 275*i*, 407*t*
  enzyme defect in, 274, 407*t*
  ocular findings in, 274–275, 275*i*, 407*t*
Homonymous diplopia, 54, 55*i*
Horizontal deviations, 11
  A pattern and V pattern, 131–136
  dissociated, 112–113, 113*i*
Horizontal incomitance, strabismus surgery planning and, 169
Horizontal rectus muscles, 13, 13*i*, 14*i*, 20*t*
  A pattern associated with dysfunction of, 131
  action of, 13, 14*i*, 20*t*, 30, 31*t*
    gaze position and, 31, 32*i*
  anatomy of, 13, 13*i*, 14*i*, 20*t*
  surgery of
    for A- and V-pattern deviations, 132, 133*i*, 134–135, 174
    for nystagmus, 162–163
  V pattern associated with dysfunction of, 131
Horizontal strabismus. *See* Horizontal deviations
Horner syndrome, in neuroblastoma, 353, 353*i*
Horner-Trantas dot, in vernal keratoconjunctivitis, 222
Horopter, empirical, 40, 41*i*
Horror fusionis (central fusional disruption), 50, 112
HOTV test, 72*t*, 73
HSV. *See* Herpes simplex virus
Human immunodeficiency virus infection. *See* HIV infection/AIDS
Human leukocyte (HLA) antigens
  in anterior uveitis, 296
  in juvenile rheumatoid arthritis, 293–294
Hunter syndrome, 406*t*
Hurler syndrome, 406*t*
  corneal opacities in, 244, 244*i*
Hutchinson's triad, 208
Hyaloid artery/system, 341
  persistence/remnants of. *See also* Persistent hyperplastic primary vitreous
Hyaloid corpuscle (Mittendorf's dot), 341
Hydantoin, anomalies associated with maternal use of, 403
Hyper (prefix), definition of, 9
Hyperlysinemia, 276

Hyperopia
  intermittent exotropia and, 108
  nonrefractive accommodative esotropia and, 96
  refractive accommodative esotropia and, 96
Hyperplasia, definition of, 195
Hypertelorism (telorbitism), 396
  telecanthus differentiated from, 200
Hypertensive retinopathy, in renal disease, 331
Hyperthermia
  diode laser, for retinoblastoma, 373
  malignant, 183–185, 185*t*
Hypertropia, 115
  vertical rectus muscle surgery for, 173
Hyphema, 414–417, 416*i*
Hypo (prefix), definition of, 9
Hypopigmented macule, in tuberous sclerosis, 383–385, 384*i*
Hypoplasia, definition of, 195
Hypotropia, 115
  in superior oblique muscle overaction, 116–117, 117*i*
  vertical rectus muscle surgery for, 173

I-cell disease, 406*t*
Idiopathic intracranial hypertension (pseudotumor cerebri), 346
Idiopathic orbital inflammation. *See* Orbital inflammatory syndrome
Illiterate E chart ("E game"), for visual acuity testing, 72*t*, 73
Illumination test, for cataract, 283
Immunotherapy/immunosuppression, for uveitis, 299
  intermediate, 298–299
  juvenile rheumatoid arthritis–associated, 294–295
Implant surgery, for glaucoma, 267
Inborn errors of metabolism, 405, 405*t*, 406*t*, 408
  enzyme defect in, 405, 405*t*, 406*t*
  ocular findings in, 405–408, 405*t*, 406*t*
Incisions, for extraocular muscle surgery, 175–176
Inclusion conjunctivitis, trachoma (TRIC), 210–211
Inclusion cysts, epithelial, conjunctival, 363
  after strabismus surgery, 179, 179*i*
Incomitant (noncomitant) deviations, 10
  esodeviations, 92*t*, 101–102
  strabismus surgery planning and, 169
  vertical, 115
    strabismus surgery planning and, 169
Incontinentia pigmenti (Bloch-Sulzberger syndrome), 376*t*, 391–393, 392*i*
Incyclo (prefix), definition of, 9
Incycloduction. *See* Intorsion
Incyclovergence, 34
Induced tropia test, 73
Infantile (congenital) esotropia, 91–95, 92*t*
  essential (classic), 91–95, 92*t*, 93*i*
Infantile glaucoma, 245, 259–265, 261*i*, 262*t*. *See also* Glaucoma
Infantile phytanic acid storage disease (Refsum disease), 407*t*
  Leber congenital amaurosis and, 317
Infants
  decreased/low vision in, 419–429
  ocular trauma in shaken baby syndrome and, 410–411, 411*i*
  visual acuity in, 191–192
  visually evoked cortical potentials in, 191–192, 419

Infection (ocular), 203–225, 424, 426t. *See also specific type*
  conjunctivitis, 211–217, 212t
  intrauterine and perinatal, 203–209
  ophthalmia neonatorum, 209–211, 209i
  orbital and adnexal, 217–220, 219i
  after strabismus surgery, 178
Infectious mononucleosis, conjunctivitis in, 215
Inferior oblique muscles, 15–16, 19i, 20t
  action of, 16, 19i, 20t
  anatomy of, 15–16, 19i, 20t
  surgery and, 25, 26i
  field of action/activation of, 30–31
  overaction of, 115–116
    V pattern associated with, 131, 132i, 133i
    vertical deviations caused by, 115–116, 116i
  palsy of, 125, 125t
  surgery of, 172–173
    for dissociated vertical deviation, 173–174
    for V-pattern esotropia, 135–136
    for vertical deviations, 116
Inferior orbital vein, 18
Inferior rectus muscles, 14, 16i, 20t
  A pattern associated with dysfunction of, 131
  action of, 14, 16i, 20t
  anatomy of, 14, 16i, 20t
  surgery and, 26i, 27i
  paresis of, in orbital floor fractures, 128–129
  resection of, for dissociated vertical deviation, 173–174
  restriction of, in monocular elevation deficiency (double elevator palsy), 126
Inflammation. *See specific type or structure affected*
Influenza virus, conjunctivitis caused by, 215
Infracture, of turbinate, for congenital nasolacrimal duct obstruction, 234–235
Infraduction. *See Depression of eye*
Infraorbital artery, extraocular muscles supplied by, 17
INO. *See Internuclear ophthalmoplegia*
Instrument (proximal) convergence, 35
Insulin-dependent diabetes mellitus. *See Diabetes mellitus, type 1*
Intermediate uveitis (pars planitis), 292t, 297–299, 298i, 302t
  diagnosis of, 298
  laboratory tests for, 303t
  treatment of, 298
Intermittent tropias, 10
  esotropia, 91
  exotropia, 105–111, 106i
Intermuscular septum, 22i, 25
  surgery and, 26–27
Internuclear ophthalmoplegia, 147–148
  nystagmus in, 147
Interstitial keratitis, in congenital syphilis, 247, 247i
Intorsion (incycloduction), 33
  extraocular muscles in
    superior oblique, 14, 17i, 20t
    superior rectus, 14, 16i, 20t
Intorsional strabismus, 9
Intracranial hemorrhages, in shaking injury, 411–413
Intracranial hypertension (increased intracranial pressure), 346. *See also Papilledema*
  idiopathic (pseudotumor cerebri), 346

Intracranial tumors, nystagmus caused by, 152t
Intraocular foreign body, uveitis differentiated from, 302t
Intraocular lenses, 286–289, 287i
  foldable, 288
  power of, 287
Intraocular pressure
  in glaucoma, 263–264
  normal range for, 263
  traumatic hyphema and, 415–416
Intraocular tumors, 366–374
  choroidal and retinal pigment epithelial lesions, 367–368
  iris and ciliary body lesions, 366
  lymphoma, uveitis differentiated from, 302t
  retinoblastoma, 368–374, 369i, 370i, 371t
Intrauterine ocular infection, 203–209. *See also specific type*
Intubation, silicone, for congenital lacrimal duct obstruction/tearing, 235–236
IO. *See Inferior oblique muscles*
IOLs. *See Intraocular lenses*
Iopidine. *See Apraclonidine*
IP. *See Incontinentia pigmenti*
IR. *See Inferior rectus muscles*
Iridocyclitis. *See also Anterior uveitis*
  in herpetic disease, 297
  in juvenile rheumatoid arthritis, 293
Iridoplegia, familial, 256
Iris
  abnormalities of, 249–258
  absence of (aniridia), 249, 249i
    nystagmus and, 150, 249
  coloboma of, 250–251, 250i
  color of, in infants, 191
  cysts of, 252–253, 253i
  ectropion of, congenital, 257, 257i
    glaucoma and, 381–382
  flocculi, 253
  juvenile xanthogranuloma affecting, 252, 367, 367i
  leukemic involvement differentiated from, 326
  in leukemia, 325–326, 366
  melanoma of, 366
  neoplastic disorders of, 366–367
  nodules of. *See Iris nodules*
  pigment epithelium of. *See Iris pigment epithelium*
  stroma of, cysts of, 253
  transillumination of, 257
    in albinism, 257, 327, 330, 330i
Iris freckle, 366
Iris nevus, 366
Iris nodules, 251–252, 252i. *See also Lisch nodules*
  in neurofibromatosis, 377, 378i
  with posterior synechiae, 258
Iris pigment epithelium
  cysts of, 252, 253i
  nodules of, 366
Iritis. *See Anterior uveitis; Iridocyclitis*
Isoflurophate, for refractive accommodative esotropia, 96
Isometropia, amblyopia caused by, 65

Jansky-Bielschowsky disease/syndrome, 399t
Jaw winking, Marcus Gunn, 202

Jerk nystagmus, 151, 153*i*. *See also* Nystagmus
JRA. *See* Juvenile rheumatoid arthritis
Juvenile fibroma/fibromatosis, of orbit, 358
Juvenile glaucoma, primary, 259. *See also* Glaucoma
Juvenile macular degeneration (Stargardt disease/fundus flavimaculatus), 320–321, 320*i*, 321*i*
Juvenile-onset diabetes mellitus. *See* Diabetes mellitus, type 1
Juvenile retinoschisis, 322, 323*i*
Juvenile rheumatoid arthritis, 293–295, 293*t*, 294*i*, 296*t*
  diagnosis of, 293, 294*i*
  iridocyclitis in, 293
  management of, 294–295, 296*t*
  pauciarticular, 293, 293*t*, 296*t*
  polyarticular, 293, 293*t*, 296*t*
  prevalence of, 293
  systemic (Still disease), 293, 293*t*, 296*t*
  uveitis in, 293, 294–295, 293*t*, 294*i*, 296*t*
Juvenile xanthogranuloma (nevoxanthoendothelioma), 367, 367*i*
  of iris, 252, 367, 367*i*
    leukemic involvement differentiated from, 326
  uveitis differentiated from, 302*t*
JXG. *See* Juvenile xanthogranuloma

Kasabach-Merritt syndrome, 356
Kawasaki syndrome (mucocutaneous lymph node syndrome), 224–225
Kayser-Fleischer ring, 247
Kearns-Sayre syndrome, 143
Keratitis
  in congenital syphilis, 247, 247*i*
  exposure, in craniosynostosis-induced proptosis, 397–398
  herpes simplex, 207
Keratoconjunctivitis
  atopic, 222–223
  epidemic, 212–213
  phlyctenular, 366
  vernal, 221–222, 221*i*
Keratoconus, 238
  central posterior (posterior corneal depression), 241–242
Keratoglobus, 238
Keratometry values, 191, 192*i*
Keratopathy, band, in juvenile rheumatoid arthritis, 294–295, 294*i*
Kestenbaum (Kestenbaum-Anderson) procedure, 162–163, 162*t*
Ketorolac tromethamine, for ocular allergy, 222
Keyhole pupil (iris coloboma), 250–251, 250*i*
Klippel-Trénaunay-Weber syndrome, 388–389
Knapp procedure
  inverse, for inferior rectus muscle paresis, 129
  for monocular elevation deficiency (double elevator palsy), 127
Koeppe lens, for gonioscopy, 263
Koeppe nodules, in sarcoidosis, 258
Kohn-Ramono syndrome, 201, 201*i*
Krabbe disease/leukodystrophy, 406*t*
Krimsky test, 77, 78*i*
Kufs disease, 407*t*

Lacerations
  corneoscleral, repair of, 414
  eyelid, 414
Lacrimal artery, extraocular muscles supplied by, 17
Lacrimal–cutaneous fistula, congenital, 228
Lacrimal drainage system/lacrimal ducts, 227–236. *See also* Nasolacrimal duct
  developmental abnormalities of, 227–228
  disorders of, 227–236, 229*i*, 238*i*
Lacrimal glands, ectopic, 360
Lacrimal probing
  for congenital dacryocele, 229
  for congenital nasolacrimal duct obstruction, 231–234, 233*i*
Lacrimal puncta. *See* Puncta
Lacrimal sac (tear sac), 227
Lacrimal sac massage
  for congenital dacryocystocele, 229
  for congenital nasolacrimal duct obstruction, 230
Lacrimal system, silicone intubation of, for congenital lacrimal duct obstruction/tearing, 235–236
Lamellar cataracts, 280, 281*i*
Lancaster red-green test, 79
  in superior oblique muscle palsy, 120
Lang stereopsis tests, 84
Langerhans cell histiocytosis (histiocytosis X), orbital involvement in, 354–355
Laser capsulotomy (Nd:YAG), 286
Laser photoablation, for retinoblastoma, 373
Laser therapy (laser surgery). *See also specific procedure*
  for glaucoma, 267
  for retinopathy of prematurity, 311*t*, 313
Latanoprost, for glaucoma, 268
Latent dissociated vertical deviation, 118
Latent/manifest latent nystagmus, 92*t*, 95, 157–158
Latent strabismus, 9
Lateral geniculate body/nucleus, 42, 43–44, 43*i*, 45*i*, 47
  development of, 44, 46*i*
Lateral incomitance, strabismus surgery planning and, 169
Lateral muscular branch, of ophthalmic artery, extraocular muscles supplied by, 17
Lateral rectus muscles, 13, 14*i*, 20*t*
  A pattern associated with dysfunction of, 131
  action of, 13, 14*i*, 20*t*
  anatomy of, 13, 14*i*, 20*t*
  field of action/activation of, 30–31
  paralysis of
    esodeviation caused by, 101–102
    treatment of, 174
  surgery of
    for A- and V-pattern deviations, 132, 132*i*, 133*i*, 134–136, 174
    for incomitant esodeviation, 102
    for intermittent exotropia, 109–111
  V pattern associated with dysfunction of, 131
Law of motor correspondence, Hering's, 34, 36*i*
Law of reciprocal innervation, Sherrington's, 33
Lea symbols, for visual acuity testing, 73
Leash phenomenon, 137
Leber congenital amaurosis, 316–317, 317*i*, 423
  RPE65 defects causing, 317
Leber hereditary optic neuropathy, 344–345
Leber idiopathic stellate neuroretinitis, 345, 345*i*
Left gaze (levoversion), 33
Lens (crystalline), 191, 192*i*, 193*i*

absence of, 271. *See also* Aphakia
colobomas of, 272, 272*i*
congenital anomalies and abnormalities of, 271–273, 271*t*
dislocated, 273–277, 273*t*. *See also* Ectopia lentis
disorders of, 271–289. *See also specific type*
  in homocystinuria, 274–276, 275*i*
  in hyperlysinemia, 276
  in Marfan syndrome, 274, 275*i*
  opacification of. *See* Cataract
  removal of. *See* Cataract surgery; Lensectomy
  in sulfite oxidase deficiency, 276
  in Weill-Marchesani syndrome, 276
Lensectomy
  for cataracts, 284–285, 286*i*. *See also* Cataract surgery
  for rubella, 205
  for subluxed lenses, 277
Lenticonus
  anterior, in Alport syndrome, 273, 331
  posterior (lentiglobus), 272, 272*i*, 281–282, 282*i*
Lentiglobus, 272, 272*i*, 281–282, 282*i*
Letterer-Siwe disease/syndrome, orbital involvement in, 355
Leukemia, 325–327, 326*i*, 354
  ocular involvement in, 325–327, 326*i*, 354
    choroid, 329
    iris, 326, 366
    optic disc/optic nerve, 326, 327*i*, 354
    orbit, 326, 354
    retina, 325–326
  uveitis differentiated from, 302*t*
Leukocoria, 305–315. *See also specific cause*
  differential diagnosis of, 305, 370, 372, 372*t*
  in retinoblastoma, 368, 369*i*, 372*t*
Leukodystrophy
  Krabbe, 406*t*
  metachromatic, 406*t*
Levator muscle (levator palpebrae superioris), 16
Levocycloversion, 34
Levoversion (left gaze), 33
LGB. *See* Lateral geniculate body
LHON. *See* Leber hereditary optic neuropathy
Lid twitch, Cogan's, 144
Ligaments, Lockwood's suspensory, 25
Light
  corneal reflex to, in ocular alignment testing, 77
  pupillary response to
    in newborn, 419
    in nystagmus evaluation, 154
    paradoxical, 154, 154*t*
Ligneous conjunctivitis, 366
Limbal dermoids, 245, 363–364
  Goldenhar syndrome and, 245, 364, 364*i*, 400–401
Limbal incision, for extraocular muscle surgery, 176
Limbus, vernal conjunctivitis/keratoconjunctivitis affecting, 221–222
Lipidoses, 406*t*
Lipodermoids (dermolipomas), 364, 364*i*
  Goldenhar syndrome and, 245, 364, 364*i*, 400–401
Lipofuscinosis, neuronal ceroid, 407*t*
Lisch nodules, 251, 252*i*
  in neurofibromatosis, 251, 252*i*, 366, 377, 378*i*, 382–383
Listing's plane, 29, 29*i*

LN. *See* Latent nystagmus
Local infiltration anesthesia, for extraocular muscle surgery, 175. *See also* Anesthesia
Lockwood, suspensory ligament of, 25
Longitudinal fasciculus, medial, 147
Lost muscle, surgery and, 182
Louis-Bar syndrome (ataxia-telangiectasia), 376*t*, 390–391, 391*i*
Low birth weight, retinopathy and, 307, 308. *See also* Retinopathy, of prematurity
Low vision, 419–425. *See also* Blindness; Visual loss
  achromatopsia (rod monochromatism) and, 423
  acquired, 425, 426*t*
  albinism and, 327–328
  in anterior segment anomalies, 421
  approach to infant with, 420–421
  cataracts and, 421
  congenital infection syndrome and, 424
  cortical visual impairment and, 424
  craniosynostosis syndromes and, 397
  delayed visual maturation and, 424
  in glaucoma, 421
  Leber congenital amaurosis and, 316–317, 423
  optic atrophy and, 344, 422
  optic nerve hypoplasia and, 341–343, 421–422
  sources of information on, 427*t*, 428*t*
  TORCH syndrome and, 424
Lowe syndrome (oculocerebrorenal syndrome), 330
LPS. *See* Levator muscle
LR. *See* Lateral rectus muscles
Luxed/luxated lens, 273, 273*t*. *See also* Ectopia lentis
Lymphangiomas, orbital, 357, 357*i*
Lymphomas
  orbital, 354
  uveitis differentiated from, 302*t*

M cells (magnocellular cells/neurons), 42–44, 43*i*, 45*i*
  development of, 44
Macula
  diseases of. *See also specific type*
    nystagmus and, 155
  in retinopathy of prematurity, 313, 314*i*
Macular degeneration
  juvenile (Stargardt disease/fundus flavimaculatus), 320, 320*i*, 321*i*
  vitelliform (Best vitelliform dystrophy), 321–322, 322*i*
    bestrophin defect causing, 321
    electro-oculogram in, 321–322
Macular dystrophy, hereditary, 320–322. *See also specific type*
Macular translocation surgery, strabismus and, 149
Macule, hypopigmented, in tuberous sclerosis, 383, 384*i*
Maddox rod testing, 78–79
  double, 79
  in superior oblique muscle palsy, 120
Magnetic resonance imaging (MRI)
  in optic nerve hypoplasia, 342–343
  in orbital evaluation, 350–351
Magnocellular (M) system, 42–44, 43*i*, 45*i*
  development of, 44
Major amblyoscope testing, 78, 79
Malformation, definition of, 195. *See also* Congenital anomalies

Malignant hyperthermia, 183–184, 185t
Malignant melanomas. *See* Melanomas
Mandibulofacial dysostosis (Treacher Collins–Franceschetti syndrome), 401, 402i
Manifest dissociated vertical deviation, 118
Manifest latent nystagmus, 92t, 95, 157–158
Manifest strabismus, 9
  cover-uncover test in assessment of, 74–75, 75i
Mannosidosis, 407t
Marcus Gunn jaw-winking ptosis/syndrome, 202
Marfan syndrome, 274, 275i
  ectopia lentis in, 274i
Marginal myotomy, 167t
Maroteau-Lamy syndrome, 406t
Masked bilateral superior oblique muscle palsy, 119
Masquerade conditions, uveitis and, 301, 302t
Mast cell stabilizers, for ocular allergy, 222, 223t
Maternal drug/alcohol use, malformations associated with, 401, 403, 402i
Maxillary osteomyelitis, 220
Measles (rubeola) virus, conjunctivitis caused by, 215
Medial longitudinal fasciculus, 147
Medial muscular branch, of ophthalmic artery, extraocular muscles supplied by, 19
Medial rectus muscles, 13, 14i, 20t
  A pattern associated with dysfunction of, 131
  action of, 13, 14i, 20t
  anatomy of, 13, 14i, 20t
  field of action/activation of, 13, 14i, 20t
  laceration of during sinus surgery, 149
  restriction of, incomitant esodeviation and, 90t, 103
  surgery of
    for A- and V-pattern deviations, 132, 132i, 133i, 134–136
    for classic congenital (essential infantile) esotropia, 93
    for Duane syndrome, 139
  V pattern associated with dysfunction of, 131
Median plane, 29i, 30
Medullated (myelinated) nerve fibers, 340, 340i
Medulloblastoma, nystagmus caused by, 152t
Medulloepithelioma (diktyoma), 367
Megalocornea, 238
  simple, 238
Megaloglobus (buphthalmos)
  in glaucoma, 264–265
  in neurofibromatosis, 382
Megalopapilla, 341
Megalophthalmos, anterior, 238
Melanocytic tumors, in neurofibromatosis, 377–378, 378i
Melanocytoma, 368
Melanocytosis
  ocular (melanosis oculi), 365
  oculodermal (nevus of Ota/congenital oculomelanocytosis), 365
Melanomas
  conjunctival, 365
  uveal, 366
  uveitis differentiated from, 302t
Meningiomas
  optic nerve, optic glioma differentiated from, 380
  orbital, 358
Meningoceles, orbital, 362

Meridional amblyopia, 65
Mesectodermal dysgenesis. *See* Anterior segment, dysgenesis of
Mesenchymal dysgenesis. *See* Anterior segment, dysgenesis of
Metabolic disorders. *See specific type and* Inborn errors of metabolism
Metachromatic leukodystrophy, 406t
Metastatic eye disease, of orbit, 352–355
MH. *See* Malignant hyperthermia
Microcoria (congenital miosis), 255
Microcornea, 238, 239i
Microphthalmos (microphthalmia)
  in congenital rubella, 205
  with cyst (colobomatous cyst), 360–361, 361i
Microsomia, hemifacial, 400, 400i. *See also* Goldenhar syndrome
Microspherophakia, in Weill-Marchesani syndrome, 276
Microtropias, 53
Midline positions of gaze, 80
Minimal pigment albinism, 329t
Miosis/miotic agents
  congenital (microcoria), 255
  for glaucoma, 268
  for refractive accommodative esotropia, 96
Mitomycin-C, with trabeculectomy, for glaucoma, 267
Mittendorf's dot, 341
MLF. *See* Medial longitudinal fasciculus
MLN. *See* Manifest latent nystagmus
Möbius syndrome, 147
  esotropia in, 92t, 147
Modified Snellen technique, in amblyopia evaluation, 66
Molteno implant, for glaucoma, 267
Monochromatism
  blue-cone, 318
  rod (achromatopsia), 317–318, 423
Monocular cover-uncover test, 74, 75i
Monocular elevation deficiency (double elevator palsy), 125–127, 125t
Monocular eye movements (ductions), 33. *See also specific type*
Monocular fixation, 11
Monocular nystagmus, 160
Monocular recess-resect procedures
  for esodeviation, 171, 171t
  for exodeviation, 171t, 172
Monocular suppression, 51
Monofixation syndrome, 53
  4Δ base-out prism test in evaluation of, 57, 59i
  Worth four-dot test in evaluation of, 56–57
Mononucleosis, infectious, conjunctivitis in, 215
Moraxella, conjunctivitis caused by, 211
Morgagnian cataract, 205
Morning glory disc, 339, 339i
Morquio syndrome, 406t
de Morsier syndrome (septo-optic dysplasia), 342, 422
Motility examination. *See* Ocular motility, assessment of
Motor correspondence, Hering's law of, 34, 36i
Motor fusion, 40, 41t
Motor nystagmus, congenital, 155–156, 156t, 156i
Motor physiology, 29–37

basic principles and terms related to, 29–33
eye movements and, 33–35, 36*i*
strabismus and, 29–37
supranuclear control systems and, 36–37
Motor units, 32
MPS. *See* Mucopolysaccharidoses
MPS IH. *See* Hurler syndrome
MPS IS. *See* Scheie syndrome
MPS II. *See* Hunter syndrome
MPS III. *See* Sanfilippo syndrome
MPS IV. *See* Morquio syndrome
MPS VI. *See* Maroteau-Lamy syndrome
MPS VII. *See* Sly syndrome
MR. *See* Medial rectus muscles
MS. *See* Multiple sclerosis
Mucoceles, lacrimal
  congenital, 228, 229*i*
  orbital invasion by, 361–362
Mucocutaneous lymph node syndrome (Kawasaki syndrome), 224–225
Mucolipidoses, 406*t*
  corneal opacities in, 243*t*, 244
Mucopolysaccharidoses, 406*t*
  corneal opacities in, 243*t*, 244, 244*i*
Mucormycosis, orbit involved in, 220, 220*i*
Multiple sclerosis
  optic nerve involvement and, 345
  uveitis differentiated from, 302*t*
Mumps virus, conjunctivitis caused by, 215
Munchausen syndrome by proxy, ocular trauma and, 410
Muscle capsule, of rectus muscles, 24
  surgery and, 25
Muscle cone, 24, 22*i*
Muscle physiology, 32
Muscle-weakening procedures. *See* Weakening procedures
Myasthenia gravis, 143–144, 144*i*, 145*t*
  diagnosis of, edrophonium in, 144, 144*i*
  strabismus in, 143–144, 144*i*, 145*t*
Mydriasis/mydriatics
  after cataract surgery, 288
  congenital, 256
  for juvenile rheumatoid arthritis–associated uveitis, 294
Myectomy, 167*t*
Myelinated (medullated) nerve fibers, 340, 340*i*
Myoclonus, cherry-red spot in, 406*t*
Myofibromas (desmoid tumors), of orbit, 358
Myopia
  ectopia lentis and, 270
  in glaucoma, 269
  intermittent exotropia and, 108–109
  in Stickler syndrome, 322–323
Myositis, orbital, 363
Myotomy, 167*t*
  marginal, 167*t*

Nasolacrimal canal, balloon catheter dilation of, for congenital nasolacrimal duct obstruction, 234
Nasolacrimal duct, 227
  obstruction of
    balloon catheter dilation (balloon dacryoplasty) for, 235

congenital, 229–236, 230*i*
  nonsurgical management of, 230–231
  surgical management of, 231–236, 233*i*
  turbinate infracture for, 234–235
Nausea and vomiting, postoperative, after strabismus surgery, 183
Nd:YAG laser therapy
  capsulotomy, 286
  cycloablation, 267
Near point of convergence, 81
Near reflex
  assessment of, 81
  spasm of, esotropia and, 92*t*, 101
Near visual acuity, testing, 74
  nystagmus and, 154
Negative angle kappa, 80, 81*i*
Neisseria gonorrhoeae (gonococcus), conjunctivitis caused by
  in children, 212
  in neonates, 209, 209*i*
Neonatal ophthalmia. *See* Ophthalmia, neonatorum
Neostigmine, for myasthenia gravis diagnosis, 144
Nephroblastoma. *See* Wilms tumor
Nerve fibers, medullated (myelinated), 340, 340*i*
Neural tumors
  nystagmus caused by, 152*t*
  orbital, 358
Neurilemoma (neurinoma/schwannoma), of orbit, 358
Neuritis, optic. *See* Optic neuritis
Neuroblastoma, 352–353, 353*i*
  nystagmus caused by, 152*t*
  of orbit, 352–353, 353*i*
Neurocristopathy, definition of, 196
Neurocutaneous syndromes. *See* Phakoma/phakomatoses
Neurofibromas
  nodular cutaneous and subcutaneous, 378
  plexiform, 379–380, 379*i*
    glaucoma and, 379
  of orbit, 358
Neurofibromatosis
  bilateral acoustic (type 2), 375, 382
  von Recklinghausen (type 1), 375–393, 376*t*
    choroidal lesions in, 367, 378
    glaucoma and, 379
    glial cell lesions in, 378–381, 379*i*
    Lisch nodules associated with, 251, 252*i*, 366
    melanocytic lesions in, 377–378, 378*i*
    miscellaneous manifestations of, 381–382
    nodular neurofibromas in, 378–379
    optic nerve gliomas and, 358, 380–381, 380*i*
    orbital involvement in, 358, 379
    plexiform neurofibromas in, 358, 379–380, 379*i*
Neuromuscular abnormalities. *See also specific type*
  constant exotropia and, 112
Neuronal ceroid lipofuscinosis, 407*t*
Neuropathy, Leber hereditary optic, 344–345
Neuroretinitis, Leber idiopathic stellate, 345, 345*i*
Neutral-density filter effect, in strabismic amblyopia, 65
Neutral zone, in congenital motor nystagmus, 156
Nevoxanthoendothelioma. *See* Juvenile xanthogranuloma

Nevus
  choroidal, 367
  conjunctival, 364–365, 366i
  flammeus (port-wine stain), 365
    in Sturge-Weber syndrome, 365, 387–389, 388i
  iris, 366
  nevocellular, congenital (giant hairy nevus), 365, 366i
  of Ota (oculodermal melanocytosis/congenital oculomelanocytosis), 365
  strawberry, 355
NF. See Neurofibromatosis
NF-1 gene, 375, 377
NF-2 gene, 375, 377
Niemann-Pick disease, 406t
Night blindness, congenital stationary, 318
NLD. See Nasolacrimal duct
Nodular episcleritis, 366
Nodular neurofibromas, cutaneous and subcutaneous, in neurofibromatosis, 378–379
Nonaccommodative esotropia, 92t, 96–98
Noncomitant deviations. See Incomitant (noncomitant) deviations
Nonoptic reflex systems, 37
Nonrefractive accommodative esotropia, 92t, 96–98
Nonsteroidal antiinflammatory drugs (NSAIDs), for juvenile rheumatoid arthritis–associated uveitis, 294
Normal retinal correspondence, 39–41, 41i
Norrie disease, 324
NRC. See Normal retinal correspondence
NSAIDs. See Nonsteroidal antiinflammatory drugs
Nuclear cataracts, 281, 281i
Null point, 156
  in congenital motor nystagmus, 156–157
Nystagmus, 151–163
  acquired, 158–160
  in albinism, 327, 330
  in aniridia, 154, 249
  in cataract, 283
  congenital, 155–160
    motor, 155–160, 155t, 156i
  convergence-retraction, 159
  in decreased vision, 412
  definition of, 151
  differential diagnosis of, 160, 161i
  dissociated, 160
  downbeat, 159
  with esotropia, 92t, 94–95, 155–156
  evaluation of, 152, 153t, 154–155
  funduscopic evaluation in, 155
  in hereditary retinal disorders, 315–322
  history in, 152, 153t
  in infants, 316, 316t
  in internuclear ophthalmoplegia, 147–148
  intracranial tumors causing, 152t
  jerk, 151, 153i
  latent/manifest latent, 92t, 95, 157–158
  monocular, 160
  nomenclature associated with, 151–152
  ocular examination in, 152, 154–155, 154t
  ocular motility testing in, 155
  opsoclonus and, 159
  optokinetic, 154, 419
    in congenital motor nystagmus, 155–157
  pendular, 151
  periodic alternating, 157
  prisms for, 160, 162
  pupil assessment in, 154, 154t
  retractorius (dorsal midbrain syndrome), 159
  see-saw, 158–159
  sensory defect, 157
  spasmus nutans, 158
  with strabismus, 155. See also Nystagmus blockage syndrome
  surgery for, 162–163, 162t
  types of, 155–160, 156t
  visual acuity testing in, 154–155
Nystagmus blockage syndrome, 92t, 94–95, 156
  surgery for, 162–163

Objective angle, in amblyoscope testing, 60
Objective visual space, 39
Obligatory suppression, 51
Oblique muscles, 14–16, 17i, 18i, 19i, 20t. See also Inferior oblique muscles; Superior oblique muscles
  action of, 15–17, 17i, 19i, 20t, 30, 31t
    gaze position and, 30–31, 32i
  anatomy of, 15–17, 17i, 18i, 19i, 20t, 30, 31t
    surgery and, 25, 26i
  field of action/activation of, 30–31
  overaction of, 115–117
    A pattern associated with, 131, 133i
    V pattern associated with, 131, 132i, 133i
    vertical deviations caused by, 115–117, 116i
  palsy of, 119–122, 121i, 125t
  weakening procedures for, 172–173
Oblique tenotomy
  for Brown syndrome, 124
  for third nerve (oculomotor) palsy, 141
OCA1A (tyrosinase-negative) albinism, 327, 328t
OCA1B albinism, 328t
OCA1MP (minimal pigment) albinism, 329t
OCA1TS (temperature-sensitive) albinism, 329t
OCA2 (tyrosinase-positive) albinism, 327, 328t
OCA3 (brown) albinism, 328t
Occlusion amblyopia, 66
  in eye trauma, 409
Occlusion therapy, for amblyopia, 67–69
Ocular adnexa, infections of, 217–220
Ocular albinism, 327, 329t
  autosomal recessive, 329t
  X-linked, 327, 329t
Ocular alignment
  tests of, 74–80
    confounding factors and, 80
  unsatisfactory, after strabismus surgery, 176
Ocular allergy, 220–223, 220i, 221i. See also Allergic reactions
Ocular dominance columns, 43–44, 45i
Ocular examination. See Examination, ophthalmic
Ocular histoplasmosis syndrome, 300
Ocular melanocytosis (melanosis oculi), 365
Ocular motility. See also Eye movements
  assessment of, 71–89
    distance acuity measurement and, 72–74, 72t
    eye movement assessment and, 74–89
    history/presenting complaint and, 71–72
    near acuity measurement and, 74
    visual acuity measurement and, 72–74, 72t

disorders of, nystagmus and, 155–160
Ocular motor apraxia, congenital, 148
Ocular toxoplasmosis. See *Toxoplasma* (toxoplasmosis)
Ocular trauma. See Trauma
Ocular tumors. See Tumors
Oculinum. See Botulinum toxin
Oculoauriculovertebral dysplasia. See Goldenhar syndrome; Hemifacial microsomia
Oculocardiac reflex, 183
Oculocerebral hypopigmentation (Cross syndrome), 328*t*
Oculocerebrorenal syndrome (Lowe syndrome), 330
Oculocutaneous albinism, 327, 329*t*, 330
Oculodermal melanocytosis (nevus of Ota), 365
Oculodigital reflex, 419
Oculoglandular syndrome, Parinaud, 216–217, 216*i*
Oculomandibulofacial dycephaly (Hallermann-Streiff syndrome), 401
Oculomotor nerve palsy. See Third nerve (oculomotor) palsy
Oculorenal syndromes, familial, 330–331
Ocusert. See Pilocarpine
OKN. See Optokinetic nystagmus
One toy, one look rule, for pediatric examination, 3
Open-angle glaucoma, 259–265, 261*i*, 262*i*, 262*t*
 after cataract surgery, 269
 clinical manifestations and diagnosis of, 260–265, 261*i*, 262*i*, 262*t*, 264*i*, 265*i*
 genetics of, 259–260
 natural history of, 264–265
 pathophysiology of, 260
 treatment of, 266–268
Operation/reoperation techniques, 168
Ophthalmia
 neonatorum, 209–211, 209*i*
  chlamydial, 210
  gonococcal, 209–210, 209*i*
  herpes simplex causing, 211
 sympathetic, 297
Ophthalmic artery, extraocular muscles supplied by, 17–18
Ophthalmopathy, thyroid (Graves). See Thyroid ophthalmopathy
Ophthalmoplegia
 chronic progressive external, 143, 145*t*
 internuclear, 147–148
  nystagmus in, 147–148
Opsoclonus ("saccadomania"), 159
 in neuroblastoma, 353
Optic atrophy, 343–345, 344*t*, 421
 Behr, 344
 in craniosynostosis, 398
 hereditary, 344
 Leber, 344–345
Optic chiasm. See Chiasm
Optic disc (optic nerve head). See also Optic nerve
 atrophy of. See Optic atrophy
 coloboma of, 339–340
 congenital abnormalities of, 339–345
  in fetal alcohol syndrome, 401, 403
 cupping of, 191, 262*t*, 263–264
  in glaucoma, 26*t*, 263, 265*i*
  in megalopapilla, 341
 disorders of, 339–348, 348*i*

edema of, 346–347, 347*t*
 in leukemia, 326
 in glaucoma, 262*t*, 263–264, 265*i*
 hypoplasia of, 341–343, 342*i*, 421–422
 in leukemia, 326
 in megalopapilla, 341
 morning glory, 339
 tilted (Fuchs coloboma), 340–341, 341*i*
Optic gliomas. See also Optic nerve glioma
 in neurofibromatosis, 358, 380–381, 380*i*
Optic nerve (cranial nerve II). See also Optic disc
 aplasia of, 343
 atrophy of. See Optic atrophy
 coloboma of, 339–340, 340*i*
 congenital abnormalities of, 339–343
 disorders of, 339–348, 348*i*
 evaluation of, in nystagmus, 155
 in glaucoma, 263–264
 glioma of. See Optic nerve glioma
 hypoplasia of, 341–343, 342*i*, 421–422
 in leukemia, 326, 326*i*, 354
 myelination of
  normal, 191
  pathologic, 340, 340*i*
Optic nerve glioma, 358, 380–381
 in neurofibromatosis, 358, 380–381
 orbital involvement in, 358, 380
Optic nerve sheath meningioma, optic glioma differentiated from, 380
Optic neuritis, 345, 345*i*
Optic neuropathy, Leber hereditary, 344–345
Optic pits (optic holes), 343, 343*i*
Optical degradation, for amblyopia, 68
Opticrom. See Cromolyn
Optokinetic nystagmus, 154, 419
 in congenital motor nystagmus, 156
Optotypes, evaluation of visual acuity and, 73
Orbit
 cellulitis affecting. See Orbital cellulitis
 cysts of, 359–360
  dermoid, 359, 359*i*
  epidermoid, 359
  with microphthalmos (colobomatous cyst), 360–361, 361*i*
  sudoriferous, 360
 fascial system of, 22–25, 22*i*
 floor of, fractures of, 127–129, 128*i*
  vertical deviations and, 127–129, 128*i*
 fractures of, 127–129, 128*i*, 417, 418*i*
 infection/inflammation of, 217–220, 362–363, 362*i*
  idiopathic. See Orbital inflammatory syndrome
 leukemic infiltration of, 326, 354
 myositis affecting, 363
 roof of, fractures of, 417, 418*i*
 tumors of, 351–363
  benign, 355–363
  bony, 358
  connective tissue, 358
  differential diagnosis of, 348–351, 350*t*
  ectopic tissue masses, 358–362
  inflammatory disorders simulating, 362–363, 362*i*
  malignant
   metastatic, 352–355
   primary, 351–352

Index • 473

neural, 358
vascular, 355–357
Orbital cellulitis, 218–220, 218i
fungal (mucormycosis), 220, 220i
after strabismus surgery, 178
Orbital inflammatory syndrome (idiopathic orbital inflammation/orbital pseudotumor), 362–363, 362i
Orbital varices, 357
Orbital vein, 18
Orbitopathy, thyroid/thyroid-related immune/Graves. *See* Thyroid ophthalmopathy
Orthophoria, 9
Orthoptics
fusional vergences and, 82–83
for intermittent exotropia, 109
for suppression, 51
for undercorrection of intermittent exotropia, 110–111
Ossifying fibroma, of orbit, 358
Osteoma, choroidal, 368
Osteomyelitis, maxillary, 220
Osteosarcoma, of orbit, 352
Overactions, dysfunctional, vertical deviations caused by, 115
Ovoid bodies, in neurofibromatosis, 381
Oxygen therapy
in malignant hyperthermia, 184, 185t
in retinopathy of prematurity, 307

P cells (parvocellular cells/neurons), 42–44, 43i
development of, 44–46
P gene, defects of in albinism, 327–328
Palpebral fissures, 191
congenital widening of (euryblepharon), 199
slanting of, 200–201
surgery affecting, 25, 26i
Palpebral vernal conjunctivitis/keratoconjunctivitis, 221–222, 221i
Palsy. *See specific type or structure affected and* Paralysis
Panum's area of single binocular vision, 40, 41i
Panuveitis, 291, 292t. *See also* Posterior uveitis; Uveitis
sympathetic ophthalmia and, 297
Papillae, Bergmeister's, 341
Papilledema, 346–348, 347t. *See also* Optic disc (optic nerve head), edema of
in craniosynostosis, 398
drusen differentiated from, 347, 348i
in leukemia, 326, 354
in pseudopapilledema, 346, 347t
in pseudotumor cerebri, 346
Papillomas, eyelid, 363
Paradoxical diplopia, 52, 52i
Paradoxical pupillary constriction to darkness, 420
in nystagmus evaluation, 154, 154t
Paralysis (paresis/paretic syndromes). *See also specific type or structure affected*
Paralytic strabismus, Hering's law and, 34, 36i
Paranasal sinusitis, orbital cellulitis caused by, 218–219, 218i
Paresis. *See specific type and* Paralysis
Parinaud (dorsal midbrain) syndrome, nystagmus in, 159
Parinaud oculoglandular syndrome, 216, 216i
Pars planitis (intermediate uveitis), 291, 292t, 287–299, 303t

diagnosis of, 298
laboratory tests for, 303t
treatment of, 298–299
Partially accommodative esotropia, 92t, 98
Parvocellular (P) system, 42–44, 43i
development of, 44
Patching
for amblyopia, 67–68
after cataract surgery, 288
for esotropia in sixth nerve palsy, 102
for intermittent exotropia, 109
occlusion amblyopia and, 66
in eye trauma, 410
for overcorrection of intermittent exotropia, 111
for undercorrection of intermittent exotropia, 111
PAX6 gene, in aniridia, 249
Pediatric cataract. *See* Cataract
Pediatric glaucoma. *See* Glaucoma
Penalization, for amblyopia, 68
Pendular nystagmus, 151
Penetrating injuries, 414, 415i
Penicillin, for syphilis, 208–209
Perennial allergic conjunctivitis, 221
Perinatal ocular infection. *See also specific type*
Periodic alternating nystagmus, 157
Periorbita (periorbital structures), ecchymosis of, in neuroblastoma, 352–353, 353i
Peripapillary staphyloma, 343
Peripheral fusion, in monofixation syndrome, 53
Peripheral neurofibromatosis, 377. *See also* Neurofibromatosis
Peripheral suppression, 50
Peripheral uveitis. *See* Intermediate uveitis
Peritomy incision, for extraocular muscle surgery, 176
Perkins tonometer, 263
Persistent hyaloid artery/system, 341. *See also* Persistent hyperplastic primary vitreous
Persistent hyperplastic primary vitreous (persistent fetal vasculature), 282–284, 282i, 306, 307i. *See also* Persistent hyaloid artery/system
Persistent pupillary membranes, 255, 255i
Peters anomaly, 242, 243i
Pfeiffer syndrome, 391
PHACES syndrome, 356
Phakoma/phakomatoses, 375–393, 376t. *See also specific type*
retinal, in tuberous sclerosis, 385, 385i
Pharyngoconjunctival fever, 213
Phlyctenular keratoconjunctivitis, 365
Phoria (suffix), definition of, 10
Phorias, 10
cover-uncover test in assessment of, 74, 75i
Phospholine. *See* Echothiophate
Photocoagulation
for retinoblastoma, 373
for retinopathy of prematurity, 311t, 313
Photophobia, in glaucoma, 260
Photoreceptor-specific guanylate cyclase *(RETGC1)* gene, in Leber congenital amaurosis, 317
PHPV. *See* Persistent hyperplastic primary vitreous
Phytanic acid storage disease, infantile (Refsum disease), 407t
Leber congenital amaurosis in, 317
Pierre Robin sequence (anomaly/deformity), 401

Stickler syndrome and, 322, 401
Pigment epithelium. *See* Iris pigment epithelium; Retinal pigment epithelium
Pigmentations, 191
Pilocarpine, for glaucoma, 268
Pineoblastoma, 372
Pits, optic (optic holes), 343, 343*i*
PITX2 gene, in Axenfeld-Rieger syndrome, 241
Plagiocephaly, 396
Plaque radiotherapy, for retinoblastoma, 373
Pleomorphic rhabdomyosarcoma, 352
Plexiform neurofibromas,
　glaucoma and, 379
　in neurofibromatosis, 379–380, 379*i*
　of orbit, 358, 379
Plica semilunaris, incorporation of during strabismus surgery, 180, 181*i*
Plus disease, 308, 309*t*, 309*i*, 310*i*
Pneumococcus. *See Streptococcus, pneumoniae*
Poland syndrome, Möbius syndrome and, 147
Polar cataracts, 279, 281*i*
Polycoria, 256
Polydystrophy, pseudo–Hurler, 406*t*
Polymethylmethacrylate (PMMA), intraocular lenses made from, 288
Polyposis, familial adenomatous (Gardner syndrome), retinal manifestations of, 368
Port-wine stain (nevus flammeus), 365
　in Sturge-Weber syndrome, 367, 387–389, 388*i*
Position maintenance system, 37
Position of rest, 32
Positions of gaze. *See* Gaze, positions of
Positive angle kappa, 80, 81*i*
　in retinopathy of prematurity, 80, 313, 314*i*
Posterior corneal depression (central posterior keratoconus), 241–242
Posterior embryotoxon, 239, 240*i*
　in Axenfeld-Rieger syndrome, 239, 240*i*, 241
Posterior fixation suture (fadenoperation), 167*t*
Posterior keratoconus. *See* Keratoconus, posterior
Posterior lenticonus/lentiglobus, 272–273, 272*i*, 281, 281*i*
Posterior synechiae, 258
　in juvenile rheumatoid arthritis, 293
Posterior uveitis, 291, 291*t*, 299–301, 303*t*
　differential diagnosis of, 302*t*
　histoplasmosis and, 300
　laboratory tests for, 303*t*
　toxocariasis and, 300–301, 302*i*
　toxoplasmosis and, 299
Postoperative (two-stage) adjustment, after strabismus surgery, 168
Power, intraocular lens, 287
PPM. *See* Persistent pupillary membranes
Prednisolone, for hyphema, 416
Prednisone, for toxoplasmosis, 205
Preferential looking, for visual acuity testing, 72*t*, 73, 419
Pregnancy
　cytomegalovirus infection during, 206
　herpes simplex virus infection during, 211
　rubella during, 205
　syphilis during, 208
　toxoplasmosis during, 204

Prematurity, retinopathy of. *See* Retinopathy, of prematurity
Presenting complaint, in strabismus and amblyopia, 71–72
Preseptal cellulitis, 217
　after strabismus surgery, 178
Press-On Prism
　for esotropia in sixth nerve palsy, 102
　for nystagmus, 160
　for overcorrection of intermittent exotropia, 110
Pretectal (Parinaud/dorsal midbrain) syndrome, nystagmus in, 159
Primary glaucoma. *See* Glaucoma; Open-angle glaucoma
Primary position of gaze, 13, 29, 80, 81*i*
Primary visual cortex (striate cortex), 42, 43*i*
　development of, 44, 46*i*
　　abnormal visual experience affecting, 46–48
Prism adaptation test, 88–89
Prism and cover test (alternate cover test), 75–76, 76*i*
　for intermittent exotropia evaluation, 107
　simultaneous, 76
Prisms
　for dissociated vertical deviation evaluation, 118
　for esotropia in sixth nerve palsy, 102
　Fresnel. *See* Fresnel prisms
　for induced tropia test, 73
　for intermittent exotropia, 109
　for monofixation syndrome evaluation, 57, 59*i*
　for nystagmus, 160, 162
　for overcorrection of intermittent exotropia, 110
　for undercorrection of intermittent exotropia, 110
Probing of lacrimal system
　for congenital dacryocele, 229
　for congenital nasolacrimal duct obstruction, 231–234, 233*i*
Programmed cell death (PCD/apoptosis), 196
Progressive external ophthalmoplegia, chronic, 143, 145*t*
Project-O-Chart slide, 84
Propine. *See* Dipivefrin
Proptosis (exophthalmos/exorbitism)
　in craniosynostosis, 397–398
　differential diagnosis of, 350
　in Graves ophthalmopathy (thyrotoxic), 142, 362, 362*i*
　after muscle recessions, 143
　in orbital tumors
　　lymphangioma, 357
　　neuroblastoma, 352–353
　　rhabdomyosarcoma, 351, 352*i*
　　teratoma, 360, 360*i*
Prostaglandins, for glaucoma, 268
Prostigmin. *See* Neostigmine
Proximal (instrument) convergence, 35
Proximal fusion, tenacious, in intermittent exotropia, 107
Pseudoesotropia, 80, 91, 92*t*
Pseudoexotropia, 105
　in retinopathy of prematurity, 313, 314*i*
Pseudogliomas, in incontinentia pigmenti, 392
Pseudo–Hurler polydystrophy, 406*t*
Pseudopapilledema, 346, 347*t*
　in craniosynostosis, 398

drusen and, 347, 348*i*
Pseudopolycoria, 256, 257*i*
Pseudoproptosis, 351
Pseudoretinitis pigmentosa, in congenital syphilis, 208
Pseudostrabismus, 80
  in retinopathy of prematurity, 313
Pseudotumor
  cerebri (idiopathic intracranial hypertension), 346
  orbital (orbital inflammatory syndrome), 362–363, 362*i*
Ptosis (blepharoptosis), 145*t*, 201–202, 201*t*
  with blepharophimosis/epicanthus inversus/telecanthus (Kohn-Ramono syndrome), 201, 201*i*
  botulinum toxin injections causing, 188
  classification of, 201*t*
  congenital, 201–202, 201*t*
  in Graves eye disease (thyroid ophthalmology), 145*t*
  hemangiomas and, 356
  in myasthenia gravis, 144, 144*i*, 145*i*
  in orbital rhabdomyosarcoma, 352
Pull-over (stay) sutures, 168
Puncta, 227
  atresia of, 227–228
  congenital disorders of, 227–228
  supernumerary, 228
Pupillary (central) cysts, 253
Pupillary light reflex (pupillary response to light)
  in newborn, 419
  in nystagmus evaluation, 154
  paradoxical, 154, 154*t*, 420
Pupillary membrane (anterior vascular capsule), persistent, 255, 255*i*
Pupils, 191
  abnormal, size/shape/location and, 255–256, 257*i*
  deformed (corectopia), 256
    ectopia lentis and, 256, 273–274, 275*i*
  examination of, in nystagmus, 154, 154*t*
  keyhole (iris coloboma), 250–251, 250*i*
  response of to light. *See* Pupillary light reflex
Pursuit eye movements/pursuit pathways/system, 37
Pyogenic granuloma, 366
Pyrimethamine, for toxoplasmosis, 204, 299

Racemose angioma/hemangioma (Wyburn-Mason syndrome), 376*t*, 393, 393*i*
Radiation therapy, for retinoblastoma, 373
Railroad-track sign, in Sturge-Weber syndrome, 388
Random Dot "E" test, 84
Random dot stereopsis tests, 84
Randot test, 84
RB. *See* Retinoblastoma
Recess-resect procedures
  monocular
    for esodeviation, 170, 171*t*
    for exodeviation, 171, 171*t*
    for nystagmus, 162, 162*t*
Recession (extraocular muscle), 25, 167*t*
  and anteriorization, 167*t*
Reciprocal innervation, Sherrington's law of, 33
Recruitment, 32
Rectus muscles, 13, 14, 14*i*, 15*i*, 16*i*. *See also specific muscle*
  action of, 13–14, 14*i*, 15*i*, 16*i*, 30–31, 31*t*
    gaze position and, 30, 32*i*

anatomy of, 13–14, 14*i*, 15*i*, 16*i*
surgery and, 27–28, 27*i*
fascial capsules of, 24
field of action/activation of, 31–32
horizontal, 13, 13*i*, 14*i*, 20*t*
  A pattern associated with dysfunction of, 131
  action of, 13, 14*i*, 20*t*, 30, 31*t*
    gaze position and, 30, 32*i*
  anatomy of, 13, 14*i*, 20*t*
  surgery of
    for A- and V-pattern deviations, 132, 134–136, 135*i*, 174
    for nystagmus, 162–163
  V pattern associated with dysfunction of, 131
insertion relationships of, 17, 21*i*
intermuscular septum of, 25, 22*i*
surgery of, 173–174
  for A- and V-pattern deviations, 132, 134–136, 135*i*, 174
  anatomy and, 25, 27*i*, 28
  for classic congenital (essential infantile) esotropia, 93–94
  for Duane syndrome, 139–140
  eyelid position changes after, 181, 182*i*
  for hypotropia and hypertropia, 173–174
  for intermittent exotropia, 110–111
  for nystagmus, 162–163
  for third nerve (oculomotor) palsy, 140–141
vertical, 14, 15*i*, 16*i*, 20*t*
  A pattern associated with dysfunction of, 131
  action of, 14, 15*i*, 16*i*, 20*t*, 30–31, 31*t*
    gaze position and, 30–31, 32*i*
  anatomy of, 14, 15*i*, 16*i*, 20*t*
  surgery of
    for A- and V-pattern deviations, 132
    eyelid position changes after, 181, 182*i*
    for hypotropia and hypertropia, 173–174
  V pattern associated with dysfunction of, 131
Red eye. *See* Conjunctivitis
Red filter (glass/lens) test
  in eye movement assessment, 79
  in suppression/anomalous retinal correspondence evaluation, 54–56, 55*i*
Red-green test, Lancaster, 79
  in superior oblique muscle palsy, 120
Red reflex, in cataract, 283
Refraction, clinical
  in congenital glaucoma, 261
  cycloplegic, 87, 88*t*
Refractive accommodative esotropia, 92*t*, 96
Refractive errors
  changes in after strabismus surgery, 176
  correction of. *See also* Spectacle lenses (spectacles)
    in amblyopia treatment, 67
  high, amblyopia caused by, 65
Refractive surgery, strabismus after, 148–149
Refsum disease/syndrome (infantile phytanic acid storage disease), 407*t*
  Leber congenital amaurosis in, 317
Regional gigantism, 379–380
Renal disease, ocular findings in, 330–331
Renal–retinal dysplasia/dystrophy, familial, 331
Renal transplantation, ocular disorders following, 331
Resection (extraocular muscle), 25

Response accommodative convergence/accommodation ratio, 81–82
Rest, position of, 32
RETGC1 gene, in Leber congenital amaurosis, 317
Reticulum cell sarcoma, uveitis differentiated from, 302*t*
Retina
　disorders of. *See* Retinal disease
　hamartomas of, 368
　in HIV infection/AIDS, 207
　phakoma of, in tuberous sclerosis, 384–385, 385*i*
　splitting of, in shaking injury, 412, 412*i*
　systemic diseases affecting, 324–333
　vascular abnormalities of
　　in incontinentia pigmenti, 392–393, 393*i*
　　in Wyburn-Mason syndrome, 393, 393*i*
　　in von Hippel–Lindau disease, 386–387, 387*i*
Retinal angiomatosis (von Hippel–Lindau disease), 376*t*, 386–387, 387*i*
　retinoblastoma differentiated from, 370
Retinal correspondence
　anomalous, 39, 51–53, 52*i*
　　harmonious, 55, 60, 61*i*
　　testing for, 52–53, 54–60, 61*i*
　　unharmonious, 55–56
　normal, 39–41, 40*i*
Retinal detachment
　in child abuse, 410
　in retinopathy of prematurity, 311*t*, 313–314
　surgery for
　　in retinopathy of prematurity, 311*t*, 313–314
　　strabismus and, 149
　uveitis differentiated from, 302*t*
Retinal disease, 305–337. *See also specific type*
　hereditary, 315–319
　vascular
　　in incontinentia pigmenti, 391–393
　　phakomatoses, 375–393, 376*t*
　　in Wyburn-Mason syndrome, 393
Retinal hemorrhages
　in leukemia, 325–327, 326*i*
　in shaking injury, 411–413, 413*i*
Retinal nerve fibers, myelinated (medullated), 340, 340*i*
Retinal pigment epithelium (RPE)
　hamartoma of, 368
　hypertrophy of, congenital, 368
　tumors of, 367–368
Retinal rivalry, 49, 49*i*
Retinitis
　cytomegalovirus (cytomegalic inclusion disease), 206, 206*i*
　pigmentosa, uveitis differentiated from, 302*t*
　in toxoplasmosis, 203–204, 205*i*, 299
Retinoblastoma, 368–374, 369*i*, 370*i*, 371*t*, 372*t*
　clinical evaluation/diagnosis of, 368
　　computed tomography in, 369, 370*i*
　　differential diagnosis and, 370, 372*t*
　endophytic, 368–369*i*
　exophytic, 369, 369*i*
　genetics of, 368, 371*t*
　leukocoria in, 368, 372*t*
　monitoring patient with, 374
　treatment of, 372–374
　　secondary tumors and, 374

　uveitis differentiated from, 302*t*
　vitreous seeding and, 368–369, 369*i*
Retinoblastoma gene, 369, 371*i*
Retinochoroiditis, cytomegalovirus causing, 206, 206*i*
Retino-geniculo-cortical pathway, 42–44, 43*i*
　development of, 44–46, 46*i*
　　abnormal visual experience affecting, 46–48
Retinoma (retinocytoma), 369
Retinopathy
　in congenital rubella syndrome, 205, 206*i*
　in congenital syphilis, 208
　cytomegalovirus, 206–207
　diabetic, 324–325
　hypertensive, in renal disease, 331
　of incontinentia pigmenti, 392*i*, 393
　in leukemia, 325–327
　of prematurity, 307–314, 309*i*, 309*t*, 310*i*, 312*i*, 314*i*
　　angle kappa and, 80, 313, 314*i*
　　classification of, 308, 309*t*, 311*t*
　　management of, 308–314, 311*t*, 312*i*, 313*i*, 314*i*
　　screening examinations for, 308, 310, 311*t*, 312*i*, 333–337
Retinoschisis
　foveal, 322
　juvenile (X-linked), 322
　traumatic, in shaking injury, 412, 412*i*
Retrobulbar anesthesia. *See also* Anesthesia
　for extraocular muscle surgery, 175
　strabismus after, 149
Retrolental fibroplasia. *See* Retinopathy, of prematurity
Rhabdomyomas, in tuberous sclerosis, 384
Rhabdomyosarcoma, of orbit, 351–352, 352*i*
Rheumatoid arthritis, juvenile. *See* Juvenile rheumatoid arthritis
RIEG1/PITX2 gene, in Axenfeld-Rieger syndrome, 241
Rieger anomaly. *See* Axenfeld-Rieger syndrome
Rieger syndrome. *See* Axenfeld-Rieger syndrome
Right gaze (dextroversion), 33–34
Riley-Day syndrome (familial dysautonomia), 247
Rivalry pattern, 49, 49*i*
RLF (retrolental fibroplasia). *See* Retinopathy, of prematurity
Rod monochromatism (achromatopsia), 317–318, 423
ROP. *See* Retinopathy, of prematurity
Rosenmüller, valve of, 227
Rosettes, in retinoblastoma, 370, 372
Rotation, center of, 29, 29*i*
RPE. *See* Retinal pigment epithelium
RPE65 gene, in Leber congenital amaurosis, 317
Rubella, 205, 206*i*
　congenital, 205, 206*i*
Rubeola (measles) virus, conjunctivitis caused by, 215

SAC. *See* Seasonal allergic conjunctivitis
Saccades/saccadic system, 32, 36
　inability to initiate (ocular motor apraxia), 148
　velocity of, 32
　testing, 84
Salmon patches, in syphilitic keratitis, 247
Salt-and-pepper fundus/retinopathy
　rubella and, 205, 206*i*
　syphilis and, 208
Sandhoff disease (GM$_2$ gangliosidosis type II), 332–333, 407*t*

Sanfilippo syndrome, 406t
Sarcoidosis, 295–296
    iris nodules and posterior synechiae associated with, 258
    uveitis in, 295–296
Sarcoma
    Ewing, 353
    granulocytic (chloroma), 354
    orbital, 351–352
    reticulum cell, uveitis differentiated from, 302t
Satellite lesions, in toxoplasmosis, 204, 299
Scaphocephaly, 388
Scheie syndrome, 406
    corneal opacities in, 244
Schwalbe's line/ring, in posterior embryotoxon, 239, 241
Schwannoma (neurilemoma/neurinoma), of orbit, 358
Sclera, 191
    perforation of, extraocular muscle/strabismus surgery and, 28, 177–178, 177i
Scleral buckle, for retinopathy of prematurity, 307t, 313–314
Sclerocornea, 242, 243t
Scopolamine, for cycloplegia/cycloplegic refraction, 87, 88t
Scotomata, of monofixation syndrome, 53
    4Δ base-out prism test in evaluation of, 57, 59i
Screening tests, examination for retinopathy of prematurity and, 308, 309t, 309i, 310, 333–337
Seasonal allergic conjunctivitis, 220–221
Sebaceous adenomas, in tuberous sclerosis, 383–384, 384i
Secondary glaucoma. See Angle-closure glaucoma; Glaucoma
Secondary positions of gaze, 30
See-saw nystagmus, 158–159
Sensory defects/deprivation
    esodeviation and, 92t, 100
    exotropia and, 112
    nystagmus and, 157
    retino-geniculo-cortical pathway affected by, 46–48
Sensory fusion, 40
Sensory visual system, 39–61, 61i
    abnormalities of binocular vision and, 49–50
        testing, 83–84
    adaptations in strabismus and, 50–60, 61i
    neurophysiological aspects of, 42–49
    physiology of normal binocular vision and, 39–42
Septo-optic dysplasia (de Morsier syndrome), 342, 422
Sequence (congenital anomalies), 195
Sexual abuse, gonococcal conjunctivitis and, 212
Shagreen patch, in tuberous sclerosis, 384
Shaking injury (shaken baby syndrome), 410–413
    ocular involvement in, 411–413, 411i
Sherrington's law of reciprocal innervation, 33
Shield ulcer, in vernal keratoconjunctivitis, 222
Sialidoses, 406t
Sickle cell disease, hyphema in, 415, 416i
Silicone intubation, for congenital lacrimal duct obstruction/tearing, 235–236
Silver nitrate, for ophthalmia neonatorum prophylaxis, 211
    chemical conjunctivitis caused by, 211
Simple megalocornea, 238

Simulated divergence excess exotropia, 108
Simultaneous prism and cover test, 75
Single binocular vision
    Panum's area of, 41i, 40
    testing field of, 84–85, 85i
Sinusitis, orbital cellulitis caused by, 218, 218i
Sixth nerve (abducens) palsy, incomitant esodeviation caused by, 92t, 101–102
Skew deviation, in infants, 419
Sleep test, for myasthenia gravis, 144
Slipped muscle, in strabismus surgery, 182–183, 183i
Sly syndrome, 406t
Smooth pursuit system, 37
Snellen acuity, 72t, 73
Snellen charts, modified, for amblyopia evaluation, 66
Snowbank formation, in intermediate uveitis (pars planitis), 297–299, 298i
SO. See Superior oblique muscles
Sorbitol, in cataract formation, 325
Spasmus nutans, 158
Spectacle lenses (spectacles)
    aphakic, 285
    for intermittent exotropia, 108
    for nonrefractive accommodative esotropia, 96–98
    for overcorrection of intermittent exotropia, 110
    for partially accommodative esotropia, 98
    for refractive accommodative esotropia, 96
Spherophakia, 272, 272i
Spielmeyer-Vogt disease, 407t
Spiral of Tillaux, 17, 21i
SR. See Superior rectus muscles
Staphylococcus aureus
    orbital cellulitis caused by, 218
    preseptal cellulitis caused by, 217
Staphylomas, peripapillary, 343
Stargardt disease (juvenile macular degeneration/fundus flavimaculatus), 320, 320i, 321i
Stay (pull-over) sutures, 168
Stereo acuity testing, 83–84
Stereo Fly test, 84
Stereopsis, 40, 40i, 41, 42
    depth perception differentiated from, 42
    in monofixation syndrome, 54
    testing, 83–84
Steroids. See Corticosteroids
Stevens-Johnson syndrome (erythema multiforme major), 223–224, 225i
Stickler syndrome (hereditary progressive arthro-ophthalmopathy), 322–323
    Pierre Robin sequence (anomaly/deformity) and, 323, 401
Still disease (systemic juvenile rheumatoid arthritis), 293, 293t, 296t
Stimulus accommodative convergence/accommodation ratio, 81–82
Storage diseases. See also specific type
    cherry red spot in, 331–332, 398t
Strabismic amblyopia, 48, 64–65
Strabismus, 9–188. See also Deviations; Diplopia
    A-pattern, 131–136
    abbreviated designations for, 11
    acquired, 11
    amblyopia and, 63–70
    botulinum toxin for, 187–188

in cataract, 283–284
in chronic progressive external ophthalmoplegia, 143, 145t
classification of, 10
congenital, 11
in congenital fibrosis syndrome, 145–146, 145i
in congenital ocular motor apraxia, 148
convergent, 9
in craniosynostosis, 396–397
cyclovertical, surgery planning and, 170
definition of, 9
diagnosis of, 71–89. *See also* Ocular motility, assessment of
dissociated. *See also* Dissociated horizontal deviation; Dissociated vertical deviation
divergent, 9
in Duane syndrome, 137–140, 138i, 139i
esodeviations, 91–103, 92t
exodeviations, 105–114
extorsional, 10
extraocular muscle anatomy and, 13–28, 21i
extraocular muscle field of action/activation and, 30–31
fixus, 146
in Graves eye disease (thyroid ophthalmology), 141–143, 142i, 145t
hemangiomas and, 356
history/presenting complaint in, 71–72
in internuclear ophthalmoplegia, 147–148
intorsional, 9
manifest, 9
cover-uncover test in assessment of, 74–77
in Möbius syndrome, 147
motor physiology and, 29–37
in myasthenia gravis, 143–145, 144i, 145t
nystagmus and, 151–163. *See also* Nystagmus blockage syndrome
in orbital rhabdomyosarcoma, 351–352
paralytic, Hering's law and, 34, 36i
in retinoblastoma, 368–374
secondary, botulinum toxin injections causing, 188
sensory adaptations in, 50–60, 61i
sensory physiology and pathology and, 39–60, 61i
terminology related to, 9–11
in third nerve (oculomotor) palsy, 140–141
treatment of
chemodenervation (botulinum toxin), 187–188
surgical, 165–184, 185t. *See also* Strabismus surgery
V-pattern, 131–136, 132i, 133i
vertical deviations, 9, 115–129
botulinum toxin injections causing, 188
Strabismus surgery, 165–185, 185t. *See also* Extraocular muscle surgery
adjustable suture techniques for, 167–168
anesthesia for, 175
complications of, 176–185, 185t
conjunctival incisions for, 175–176
for esodeviations, 170, 171t
for exodeviations, 171–172, 172t, 173t
extraocular muscle anatomy and, 25–28, 26i, 27i
guidelines for, 170–175
indications for, 165–166
planning, 169–170

prior surgery and, 169–170
rectus muscle procedures, 173–174
strengthening procedures in, 166–167, 167t
techniques for, 166–169
transposition procedures in, 168
weakening procedures in, 166, 167t
oblique muscle, 172–173
Strawberry nevus, 355
Strengthening procedures, 166–168
Streptococcus
pneumoniae (pneumococcus)
conjunctivitis caused by, 211–212
orbital cellulitis caused by, 218
preseptal cellulitis caused by, 217
pyogenes (group A beta-hemolytic)
orbital cellulitis caused by, 218
preseptal cellulitis caused by, 217
Striate cortex, 42, 43i, 45i
development of, 44, 46i
abnormal visual experience affecting, 46–48
Stroma, iris, cysts of, 253
Stromal dystrophies, congenital hereditary, 245
Sturge-Weber disease/syndrome (encephalofacial angiomatosis), 376t, 387–390, 388i
nevus flammeus in, 365, 387, 388i, 389
Subjective visual space, 39
Subluxed/subluxated lens, 271–276, 273t. *See also* Ectopia lentis
Sudoriferous cysts, of orbit, 360
Sulfadiazine, for toxoplasmosis, 204, 299
Sulfite oxidase deficiency, 276
"Sunsetting," in infants, 419
Superior oblique muscles, 14–15, 17i, 18i, 20t
action of, 16, 18i, 20t
anatomy of, 14–15, 17i, 18i, 20t
surgery and, 27, 27i
overaction of, 116–117, 117i
A pattern associated with, 131, 133i
vertical deviations caused by, 116–117, 117i
paresis/palsy of, 119–123, 121i
Hering's law and, 34, 36i
surgery of, 173
for A-pattern deviations, 136, 173
for vertical deviation, 117
Superior oblique tendon sheath syndrome (Brown syndrome), 123–125, 123i, 125t
Superior oblique tenotomy
for Brown syndrome, 124
for third nerve (oculomotor) palsy, 141
Superior orbital vein, 18
Superior rectus muscles, 14, 15i, 20t
action of, 14, 15i, 20t
anatomy of, 14, 15i, 20t
surgery and, 27, 27i
resection of, for dissociated vertical deviation, 173–174
surgery of, eyelid position changes after, 181
V pattern associated with dysfunction of, 131
Supernumerary puncta, 228
Suppression, 50–51
testing for, 51, 54–60, 61i
Supraduction. *See* Elevation of eye
Supranuclear eye movement systems, 36–37
Sursumduction/sursumversion. *See* Elevation of eye

Suspensory ligament of Lockwood, 25
Sutures (surgical)
    adjustable, for strabismus surgery, 167
    allergic reaction to, 178, 178*i*, 179*i*
    pull-over (stay), 168
SWS. *See* Sturge-Weber disease/syndrome
Sympathetic ophthalmia, 297
Syndrome (genetic), definition of, 195
Synechiae, posterior, 258
    in juvenile rheumatoid arthritis, 293
Synergist muscles, 33
Synkinesis, in Marcus Gunn jaw-winking ptosis, 202
Synkinetic reflex. *See* Near reflex
Syphilis, 208–209
    congenital, 208–209
        corneal manifestations of, 247, 247*i*
    intrauterine, 208–209
    uveitis and, 297

Tachyzoites, in toxoplasmosis transmission, 203
Tarsal kink, congenital, 198–199, 199*i*
Tay-Sachs disease (GM$_2$ gangliosidosis type I), 332, 407*t*
Tearing (epiphora)
    congenital, 228, 229, 262*t*
    in glaucoma, 230, 260, 262*t*
    in nasolacrimal duct obstruction, 229, 230
    in punctal atresia, 227–228
Telangiectasias
    conjunctival, in ataxia-telangiectasia, 390–391, 391*i*
    retinal, 314–315
Telecanthus, 200, 396
    with blepharophimosis/epicanthus inversus/ptosis (Kohn-Ramono syndrome), 201, 201*i*
Telorbitism (hypertelorism), 396
    telecanthus differentiated from, 200
Temperature-sensitive albinism, 329*t*
Tenacious proximal fusion, in intermittent exotropia, 107
Tenectomy, 167*t*
Tenon's capsule, 22–23, 23*i*, 24*i*
    extraocular muscle surgery and, 27–28
        excessive advancement and, 179–180
        scarring of (adherence syndrome), 180
Tenotomy, 167
    superior oblique
        for Brown syndrome, 124
        for third nerve (oculomotor) palsy, 131
Tensilon test, for myasthenia gravis diagnosis, 144, 144*i*
Teratogens, definition of, 196
Teratomas, orbital, 360, 360*i*
Tertiary positions of gaze, 30
Tetracyclines, for neonatal conjunctivitis prophylaxis, 211
Thermochemotherapy, for retinoblastoma, 373
Third nerve (oculomotor) palsy, 140–141
    inferior oblique muscle palsy caused by, 125
Three-step test, 85, 86*i*
    in superior oblique muscle palsy, 120
Threshold disease, in retinopathy of prematurity, 311*t*, 312–313, 312*i*, 314*i*
Thyroid ophthalmopathy (Graves disease), 141–143, 142*i*, 145*t*, 362–363, 362*i*
    proptosis and, 141, 362, 362*i*
    after muscle recessions, 142–143
    strabismus and, 141–143, 142*i*, 145*t*
Thyroid orbitopathy. *See* Thyroid ophthalmopathy
Thyroid-related immune orbitopathy. *See* Thyroid ophthalmopathy
Tillaux, spiral of, 17, 21*i*
Tilted optic disc syndrome (Fuchs coloboma), 340–341, 341*i*
Timolol, for glaucoma, 268
Timoptic. *See* Timolol
TNO test, 84
α-Tocopherol. *See* Vitamin E
Tonic convergence, 35
Tono-Pen, 263
Tonometry (tonometer), in glaucoma, 263
    Goldmann, 263
    Perkins, 263
Topical anesthesia. *See also* Anesthesia
    for adjustable suture technique, 168
    for extraocular muscle surgery, 175
TORCHES, 203. *See also specific disorder*
    reduced vision and, 424
Torsion, 30
Torsional deviations, 11
Torsional fusional vergence, 82
Torus, 40, 41*i*
Touton giant cells, in juvenile xanthogranuloma, 367
Toxocara canis/Toxocara cata (toxocariasis), 300–301, 302*i*
    uveitis in, 300–301, 302*i*
Toxoplasma gondii (toxoplasmosis), 203–205, 205*i*, 299
    congenital, 203–205, 205*i*
    treatment of, 204–205, 299
    uveitis in, 291, 299
Toys, for pediatric examination, 3, 4*i*
Trabeculectomy, for glaucoma, 267
    antifibrotic agents used with, 267
Trabeculotomy, for glaucoma, 267
Trachoma, 217
Trachoma-inclusion conjunctivitis (TRIC) agent, 210
Tranexamic acid, for hyphema, 416
Transillumination, iris, 257–258
    in albinism, 257, 327, 330*i*
Transposition procedures, 168, 174
Trantas dot, in vernal keratoconjunctivitis, 222
Trauma, 409–418, 426*t*
    abuse and, 410–413, 411*i*
    blunt injury and, 414–417, 418*i*
    cataract caused by, 277–278
    chemical injuries and, 413
    hyphema and, 414–417, 416*i*
    management of, 409
    orbital fractures and, 127–129, 128*i*, 417
    penetrating injury and, 414, 415*i*
    shaking injury and, 410–411, 411*i*
    superficial injury and, 413–414
    uveitis caused by, 295
Traumatic retinoschisis, in shaking injury, 411*i*, 412
Treacher Collins–Franceschetti syndrome (mandibulofacial dysostosis), 401, 402*i*
Treponema pallidum, 208. *See also* Syphilis
TRIC (trachoma-inclusion conjunctivitis) agent, 210
Trifluridine, for herpes simplex virus infections, 207, 213

Trimethoprim-sulfamethoxazole, for toxoplasmosis, 204
TRIO (thyroid-related immune orbitopathy). *See* Thyroid ophthalmopathy
Trisomy 21 (Down syndrome/trisomy G syndrome), Brushfield spots in, 254
Trochlea, 15, 17*i*, 21*i*
Trochlear nerve palsy. *See* Fourth nerve (trochlear) palsy
Tropia (suffix), definition of, 10
Tropias, 10
 cover-uncover test in assessment of, 74, 75*i*
 induced, testing visual acuity and, 73
 intermittent, 10
  esotropia, 91
  exotropia, 105–111, 106*i*
Tropicamide, for cycloplegia/cycloplegic refraction, 87, 88*t*
True divergence excess exotropia, 107–108
Trusopt. *See* Dorzolamide
TS. *See* Tuberous sclerosis
Tuberous sclerosis (Bourneville disease/syndrome), 376*t*, 383–385, 384*i*, 385*i*
Tucking procedure, 167
Tumors, 349–374, 426*t*
 differential diagnosis of, 324*t*, 349–351
 epibulbar, 363–366
 eyelid, 363–366
 intraocular, 366–370, 372–374
 orbital, 351–363
Turbinates, infracture of, for congenital nasolacrimal duct obstruction, 234–235
Two-stage (postoperative) adjustment, after strabismus surgery, 168
Tyrosinase gene mutations, in albinism, 327
 repair of, 408
Tyrosinase-negative/positive albinism, 327, 328*t*

Uncrossed diplopia, 54, 55*i*
Underactions, dysfunctional, vertical deviations caused by, 115
Unharmonious anomalous retinal correspondence, 55, 55*i*, 60
Upgaze. *See* Elevation
Uvea (uveal tract)
 melanomas of, 366
 in neurofibromatosis, melanocytic tumors and, 377–378, 378*i*
Uveitis, 291–304
 anterior, 291, 292–297, 292*t*, 303*t*
 classification of, 291, 292*t*
 clinical features of, 291, 292*t*
 herpetic, 297
 in histoplasmosis, 300
 intermediate (pars planitis), 292*t*, 297–299, 298*i*, 303*t*
 in juvenile rheumatoid arthritis, 293, 293*t*, 294*i*, 303*t*
 in Kawasaki syndrome, 224–225
 laboratory tests for, 303*t*
 masquerade syndromes and, 301, 302*t*
 posterior, 291, 292*t*, 299–301, 303*t*
 in sarcoidosis, 295–296
 sympathetic ophthalmia and, 297
 syphilitic, 297
 in toxocariasis, 300–301, 302*i*
 in toxoplasmosis, 291, 299
 trauma causing, 295
 treatment of, 301, 303–304

V pattern, 80–81, 131–136, 132*i*, 133*i*
 in craniosynostosis, 398
 definition of, 131
 esotropia, 132*i*
  treatment of, 135–136
 exotropia, 133*i*
  treatment of, 135–136
 surgical treatment of, 132, 134–136, 174
Valacyclovir, for cytomegalovirus retinitis, 207
Valve of Hasner, 227
Valve of Rosenmüller, 227
Varicella (chickenpox), conjunctivitis in, 215–216, 216*i*
Varicella-zoster virus
 conjunctivitis caused by, 215–216, 215*i*, 216*i*
 uveitis caused by, 297
Varices, orbital, 357
Vascular system, of extraocular muscles, 17–18
 surgery and, 27–28
Vascular tumors, of orbit, 355–363
VDRL (Venereal Disease Research Laboratory) test, 208
Vectograph Project-O-Chart slide test, 84
Venereal Disease Research Laboratory (VDRL) test, 208
Venous system, of extraocular muscles, 18
 surgery and, 27–28
VEP/VER. *See* Visually evoked cortical potentials (visual evoked response)
Vergence system, 36–37
 assessment of, 83–84
Vergences, 34–35. *See also specific type*
 in infants, 419
Vernal conjunctivitis/keratoconjunctivitis, 221–222, 221*i*
Versions, 33–34, 35*i*, 36*i*. *See also specific type*
Vertical deviations, 9, 11, 115–129. *See also specific type*
 botulinum toxin causing, 188
 Brown (superior oblique tendon sheath) syndrome and, 123–125, 123*i*, 125*t*
 comitant, 115
 dissociated, 112–113, 113*i*, 118–119, 118*i*
  surgery for, 173–174
 incomitant (noncomitant), 115
  strabismus surgery planning, 169–170
 inferior oblique muscle overaction and, 115–116, 116*i*
 inferior oblique muscle palsy and, 125, 125*t*
 monocular elevation deficiency and, 125–127, 127*i*
 orbital floor (blowout) fractures and, 127–129
 superior oblique muscle overaction and, 115, 116–117, 117*i*
 superior oblique muscle paresis and, 119–122, 121*i*
Vertical fusional vergence, 82
Vertical incomitance, 115
 strabismus surgery planning and, 169
Vertical rectus muscles, 14, 15*i*, 16*i*, 20*t*

A pattern associated with dysfunction of, 131
action of, 14, 15*i*, 16*i*, 20*t*, 30–31, 31*t*
   gaze position and, 30–31, 32*i*
anatomy of, 14, 15*i*, 16*i*, 20*t*
surgery of
   for A- and V-pattern deviations, 132, 134–136
   eyelid position changes after, 181, 182*i*
   for hypotropia and hypertropia, 173
V pattern associated with dysfunction of, 131
Vertical retraction syndrome, 146
Vertical strabismus. *See* Vertical deviations
Vertical vergence movement, 34
VHL. *See* von Hippel–Lindau disease
VHL gene, 386
Vidarabine, for herpes simplex virus infections, 207, 213
Vieth-Müller circle, 39–40, 41*i*
Viruses. *See also specific organism*
   conjunctivitis caused by, 212–216
Vision
   binocular. *See* Binocular vision
   decreased. *See* Low vision
   development of, 44–46, 46*i*
      abnormal visual experience affecting, 46–48
      delayed, 424
      normal, 419
   double. *See* Diplopia
   neurophysiology of, 42–48
Visual acuity
   in albinism, 327–328
   fusional vergences and, 82–83
   in optic nerve hypoplasia, 342
   strabismus surgery planning and, 170
   testing, 72–74, 72*t*
      in amblyopia, 72–74, 72*t*
      in nystagmus, 154
      in strabismus, 72–74, 72*t*
Visual axis, 39
Visual confusion, 49, 49*i*
Visual (calcarine/occipital) cortex, 42, 43*i*
   development of, 44–46, 46*i*
      abnormal visual experience affecting, 46–48
Visual loss/impairment. *See also* Blindness; Low vision
   acquired, 424, 425*t*
   in albinism, 327–328
   in cataract, 277, 283, 288–289
   in craniosynostosis syndromes, 397–398
   in glaucoma, 264–265, 269
   in juvenile rheumatoid arthritis, 293
   in retinopathy of prematurity, 313–314
Visual space, objective and subjective, 39
Visually evoked cortical potentials (visual evoked response), in infants, 191, 419
Vitamin E, retinopathy of prematurity and, 308
Vitelliform dystrophy, Best, 321–322, 322*i*
   bestrophin defect causing, 322
   electro-oculogram in, 321–322
Vitelliform macular dystrophy gene *(VMD2)*, 321
Vitrectomy, for retinal detachment, in retinopathy of prematurity, 311*t*, 313–314
Vitrectorrhexis, for IOL implant, 286
Vitreoretinal dystrophies, Goldmann-Favré, 324

Vitreoretinal traction, in retinopathy of prematurity, 313, 314*i*
Vitreoretinopathies. *See also specific type*
   familial exudative, 323–324
   hereditary, 322–324
Vitreous
   disorders of, 305–337. *See also specific type*
   primary, persistent hyperplasia of (persistent fetal vasculature), 282, 282*i*. *See also* Persistent hyaloid artery/system
Vitreous hemorrhage, in shaking injury, 411
Vitreous seeds, in retinoblastoma, 368, 369*i*
VKC. *See* Vernal conjunctivitis/keratoconjunctivitis
VMD2 (vitelliform macular dystrophy) gene, 321
Vogt triad, in tuberous sclerosis, 383
Voluntary convergence, 35
Vomiting. *See* Nausea and vomiting
von Basedow disease. *See* Graves disease
von Hippel–Lindau disease (retinal angiomatosis), 376*t*, 386–387, 387*i*
   retinoblastoma differentiated from, 370
von Recklinghausen disease. *See* Neurofibromatosis, von Recklinghausen (type 1)
Vortex veins, extraocular muscle surgery and, 28
VZV. *See* Varicella-zoster virus

Waardenburg syndrome, 399–400
WAGR syndrome, 250
Weakening procedures, 166, 167*t*
   inferior oblique muscle, 172–173
      for V-pattern deviations, 135–136
      for vertical deviations, 116
   superior oblique muscle, 173
      for A-pattern deviations, 136, 173
      for vertical deviation, 117
Weill-Marchesani syndrome, 276
"White spot," in tuberous sclerosis, 383, 384*i*
Wildervanck syndrome, Duane syndrome and, 137
Wilms tumor
   aniridia and, 250
   of orbit, 353
Wilson disease (hepatolenticular degeneration), 250
With-the-rule astigmatism, after strabismus surgery, 176
Wofflin nodules, 254
Worth four-dot test, 56–57, 56*i*
   in binocular sensory cooperation evaluation, 83
   in suppression/anomalous retinal correspondence evaluation, 56, 57*i*
Wyburn-Mason syndrome (racemose angioma), 376*t*, 393, 393*i*

x axis, eye movements and, 29, 29*i*
X-linked disorders
   Aicardi syndrome, 319
   albinism, 327, 329*t*
   blue-cone monochromatism, 318
   familial exudative vitreoretinoathy, 323–324
   Norrie disease, 324
   retinoschisis (juvenile retinoschisis), 322, 323*i*
X pattern, 131
   in exotropia, 111

Xalatan. *See* Latanoprost
Xanthogranuloma, juvenile (nevoxantho-
    endothelioma), 367, 367*i*
  of iris, 252, 367, 367*i*
    leukemic involvement differentiated from, 326
  uveitis differentiated from, 302*t*

y axis, eye movements and, 29, 29*i*
Yoke muscles, 33–34, 80
  cardinal positions of gaze and, 34, 35*i*, 80
  Hering's law of motor correspondence and, 34, 36*i*

z axis, eye movements and, 29, 29*i*
Zoster. *See* Herpes zoster